Animal and Translational Models for CNS Drug Discovery

Animal and Translational Models for CNS Drug Discovery

Volume I Psychiatric Disorders (ISBN: 978-0-12-373856-1)
Volume II Neurological Disorders (ISBN: 978-0-12-373855-4)
Volume III Reward Deficit Disorders (ISBN: 978-0-12-373860-8)

(ISBN set: 978-0-12-373861-5)

Animal and Translational Models for CNS Drug Discovery

VOLUME I

Psychiatric Disorders

Edited by

Robert A. McArthur, PhD
Associate Professor of Research
Consultant Behavioral Pharmacologist
McArthur and Associates GmbH, Basel, Switzerland

Franco Borsini, PhD
Head, Central & Peripheral Nervous System and
General Pharmacology Area – R&D Department
sigma-tau S.p.A., Pomezia (Rome), Italy

AMSTERDAM • BOSTON • HEIDELBERG • LONDON • NEW YORK • OXFORD
PARIS • SAN DIEGO • SAN FRANCISCO • SINGAPORE • SYDNEY • TOKYO
Academic Press is an imprint of Elsevier

Academic Press is an imprint of Elsevier
30 Corporate Drive, Suite 400, Burlington, MA 01803, USA
360 Park Avenue South, Newyork, NY 10010-1710, USA
525 B Street, Suite 1900, San Diego, CA 92101-4495, USA
32 Jamestown Road, London NW1 7BY, UK

⊚ This book is printed on acid-free paper.

Library of Congress Cataloging-in-Publication Data
A catalog record for this book is available from the Library of Congress

British Library Cataloguing-in-Publication Data
A catalogue record for this book is available from the British Library.

ISBN: 978-0-12-373861-5 (set)
ISBN: 978-0-12-373856-1 (vol 1)

For information on all Academic Press publications
visit our web site at www.elsevierdirect.com

Typeset by Charon Tec Ltd., A Macmillan Company.
(www.macmillansolutions.com)
Printed and bound in Great Britain by
CPI Antony Rowe, Chippenham and Eastbourne
Transferred to Digital Printing, 2010

Working together to grow
libraries in developing countries

www.elsevier.com | www.bookaid.org | www.sabre.org

ELSEVIER   BOOK AID
            International   Sabre Foundation

This book is dedicated to that happy band of behavioral pharmacologists who over the generations have occasionally seen their compound progress into clinical development, and more rarely still seen it used to treat patients. New skills are being learned and new species creeping into the lab, including the ones "without tails." These offer new opportunities and challenges, but equally so greater satisfaction working at the interface. May all your compounds be winners!

Contents

Volume 1 Animal and Translational Models for CNS Drug Discovery: Psychiatric Disorders

CHAPTER 11 **Preclinical Animal Models of Autistic Spectrum Disorders (ASD)**.......................... **353**

Jennifer A. Bartz, Larry J. Young, Eric Hollander, Joseph D. Buxbaum and Robert H. Ring

What Do *You* Mean by "Translational Research"? An Enquiry Through Animal and Translational Models for CNS Drug Discovery: Psychiatric Disorders

Robert A. McArthur[1] and Franco Borsini[2]

[1]McArthur and Associates GmbH, Basel, Switzerland
[2]sigma-tau S.p.A, Pomezia (Rome), Italy

In the 50-odd years since the introduction of clinically effective medications for the treatment of behavioral disorders such as depression,[1] anxiety[2] or schizophrenia[3] there has recently been growing unease with a seeming lack of substantive progress in the development of truly innovative and effective drugs for behavioral disorders; an unease indicated by escalating research and development expenditure associated with diminishing returns (e.g.,[4] and discussed by Hunter[5] in this book series). There are a number of reasons that may account for this lack of new drugs for CNS disorders (cf.,[6]), but according to the US Food and Drug Administration's (FDA) white paper on prospects for 21st century drug discovery and development,[7] one of the main causes for failure in the clinic is the discrepancy between positive outcomes of candidate drugs in animal models and apparent lack of efficacy in humans, that is, the predictive validity of animal models. Consequently, there have been a number of initiatives from the US National Institutes of Health (NIH) (http://nihroadmap.nih. gov/) and The European Medicines Agency (EMEA),[8] to bring interested parties from Academia and Industry together to discuss, examine and suggest ways of improving animal models of behavioral disorders.[9-14] The value of NIH-supported initiatives, even to the point of participating directly in drug discovery from screening to registration is not to be underestimated, as evidenced by the successful registration of buprenorphine (Subutex®) and buprenorphine/naloxone (Suboxone®) by Reckitt-Benckiser in collaboration with the National Institute on Drug Abuse ([15]see also[16]).[i]

Translational research and experimental medicine are closely related activities that have evolved in answer to the need of improving the attrition rate of novel drugs between the preclinical and clinical stage of development.[5,19-22] In general, translational research defines the *process* through which information and insights flow from clinical observations to refine the development of animal models *as well as* the complementary flow of information and insights gained from animal models to the clinical

---

[i]For a comprehensive discussion of NIH-sponsored initiatives and collaborations and opportunities, please refer to Winsky and colleagues[17] and Jones and colleagues[18] for specifics on NIH-Academic-Industrial collaborations in schizophrenia.

Animal and Translational Models for CNS Drug Discovery,
Vol 1 of 3: Psychiatric Disorders
Robert McArthur and Franco Borsini (eds), Academic Press, 2008

setting, be it through improved diagnosis, disease management or treatment; including pharmacological treatment.[23] Experimental medicine, in terms of drug discovery, refers to studies in human volunteers to (1) obtain mechanistic and pharmacological information of compounds entering into development, (2) explore and define biological markers with which the state and progress of a disorder can be monitored, as well as the effects of pharmacological interventions on its progress and (3) establish models and procedures with which to obtain initial signals of efficacy test.[5,15,22] Though claimed as an innovative paradigm shift, translational research nevertheless, is not a new concept, as pointed out by Millan in this book series.[24] The origins of psychopharmacology abound with numerous examples of how pharmaceutical or medicinal chemists interacted directly with their clinical colleagues to "test their white powder", or clinicians who would knock at the chemists' door for anything new. Kuhn and Domenjoz, for example, describes the initial "Phase II" trials of the novel "sleeping pill" forerunner of imipramine.[25,26] Paul Janssen tells how the observation of the paranoid schizophrenia-like hallucinations experienced by cyclists who were consuming amphetamine to stay alert, led him to search for better amphetamine antagonists, one of which was haloperidol. This compound was subsequently given to a young lad in the midst of a psychotic episode by a local psychiatrist with good results.[27] Though largely overtaken in sales and prescription rates by 2nd generation atypical antipsychotics, Haloperidol (Haldol®) remains one of the standard drugs used in the treatment of schizophrenia.[18,28,29]

Translational research is a two-way process which, nonetheless can lead to differences in emphasis and agenda. We have gathered a number of definitions from different sources listed in Table 1 below to help us determine what one of our authors asked us to do when he was contacted to contribute to this book project, "What do *you* mean by 'translational research'?"

These definitions may emphasize the clinical, or top-down approach to translational research,[20,30] or the bottom-up approach of "bench-to-bedside".[21,31] It is clear though, that translational research has a purpose of integrating basic and clinical research for the benefit of the patient in need. While we welcome this as a general definition of translational research, we acknowledge, as do others (e.g.,[31,32]), that a more pragmatic, working definition is required. Consequently, we define translational research, in the context of drug discovery and research, as the partnership between preclinical and clinical research to align not only "... basic science discoveries into medications",[31] but also the information derived from the clinic during the development of those medications. The purpose of this reciprocal definition is to refine the model systems used to understand the disorder by identifying the right targets, interacting with those targets pharmacologically in both animals and humans and monitoring the responses in each throughout a compound's development (cf.,[5 and 15]). Central to this definition is the acknowledgement that the etiology of behavioral disorders and their description are too diffuse to attempt to model or simulate in their entirety. Consequently, emphasis must be placed on identifying specific symptoms or core features of the disorder to model, and to define biological as well as behavioral responses as indices of state, changes in state and response to pharmacological treatment. This process is made easier if, at the same time, greater effort is made to identify procedures used to measure these biological and behavioral responses that are consistent within and between species.[23,24] Brain imaging is one technique that has cross-species consistency (e.g.,[33,36]), as do various operant conditioning procedures.[37,38]

Table 1 Selected definitions of translational research

Definition	Reference
Translational medicine may also refer to the wider spectrum of patient-oriented research that embraces innovations in technology and biomedical devices as well as the study of new therapies in clinical trials. It also includes epidemiological and health outcomes research and behavioral studies that can be brought to the bedside or ambulatory setting.	30
… connotes an attempt to bring information that has been confined to the laboratory into the realm of clinical medicine.	
To the extent that clinical studies could be designed to answer such questions (generated by information from the laboratory), they would represent types of translational clinical research.	20
… a two-way street where the drive to cure should be complemented by the pursuit to understand human diseases and their complexities.	21,136
1. Basic science studies which define the biological effects of therapeutics in humans	
2. Investigations in humans which define the biology of disease and provide the scientific foundation for development of new or improved therapies for human disease	
3. Non-human or non-clinical studies conducted with the intent to advance therapies to the clinic or to develop principles for application of therapeutics to human disease	
4. Any clinical trial of a therapy that was initiated based on #1–3 with any endpoint including toxicity and/or efficacy.	M. Sznol cited by [21]
… research efforts intended to apply advances in basic science to the clinical research setting. For drug discovery and development, the term refers to research intended to progress basic science discoveries into medications.	31
By bringing together top-down and bottom-up approaches, there is potential for a convergence of unifying explanatory constructs relating aetiology to brain dysfunction and treatment.	37,137
… information gathered in animal studies can be translated into clinical relevance and vice versa, thus providing a conceptual basis for developing better drugs.	
… the application of scientific tools and method to drug discovery and development … taking a pragmatic or operational rather than a definitional approach, a key to a successful translation of non-human research to human clinical trials lies in the choice of biomarkers.	32
… two-way communication between clinical and discovery scientists during the drug development process are likely to help in the development of more relevant, predictive preclinical models and biomarkers, and ultimately a better concordance between preclinical and clinical efficacy.	82

There are at least two aspects of translational research to be considered as a result of the definition proposed above. First is the concept of specific symptoms, or core features of the disorder to model. Attempts to simulate core disturbances in behavior formed the basis of early models of behavioral disorders. McKinney and Bunney, for example, describe how they sought to "translate" the clinically observed changes in human depressed behavior (secondary symptoms) with analogous changes in animals induced by environmental or pharmacological manipulations.[39]

Whereas modelers have traditionally referred to diagnostic criteria such as DSM-IV[40] or ICD-10[41] the consensus to be found in this book series and other sources is that these diagnostic criteria do not lend themselves easily to basic or applied research. The etiology of behavioral disorders is unclear, and there is considerable heterogeneity between patients with different disorders but similar symptoms. Nevertheless, attempts to model particular behavioral patterns have been and are being done. Thus, for example, the construct of anhedonia (the loss of ability to derive pleasure), or the construct of social withdrawal, may be diagnostic criteria for a number of behavioral disorders including depression, schizophrenia, as well as a number of other disorders (cf.,[42]). There is considerable momentum to establish a dimension – rather than diagnostic-based classification or to "deconstruct" syndromes into "symptom-related clusters" that would help guide neurobiological research.[ii 18,43,44] In order to define these "symptom-based clusters", however, the symptoms have to be defined. Previously, these were identified as behavioral patterns, though lately they have been referred to variously as behavioral endophenotypes or exophenotypes (e.g.,[45-49]). It is appropriate here to review the definitions of both. Exophenotype and endophenotypes have been defined by Gottesman and Shields[50] as:

> *John and Lewis (1966) introduced the useful distinction between* exophenotype (external phenotype) *and* endophenotype (internal), *with the latter only knowable after aid to the naked eye, e.g. a biochemical test or a microscopic examination of chromosome morphology (p. 19).*[iii]

Subsequently, endophenotypes have been more rigorously defined[51] as:

1. *The endophenotype is associated with illness in the population.*
2. *The endophenotype is heritable.*
3. *The endophenotype is primarily state-independent (manifests in an individual whether or not illness is active).*
4. *Within families, endophenotype and illness co-segregate.*
5. *The endophenotype found in affected family members is found in non-affected family members at a higher rate than in the general population. (p. 639)*

[ii] For reviews of the initiatives deconstructing a complex disorder like schizophrenia, the reader is invited to consult the following 2 issues of *Schizophrenia Bulletin*, where these initiatives are thoroughly discussed: *Schizophr Bull*, 2007, 33:1 and *Schizophr Bull*, 2007, 33:4.

[iii] See also Tannock *et al.*,[61] for definitions of endophenotypes and biomarkers.

And that "… The number of genes involved in a phenotype is theorized to be directly related to both the complexity of the phenotype and the difficulty of genetic analysis" (*op cit.*, p. 637). On the other hand, exophenotypes have been defined by Holzman[52] (and others) as:

> … *the external symptoms of a disorder that clinicians detect during an exami-nation. An endophenotype, on the other hand, is a characteristic that requires special tools, tests, or instruments for detection. (p. 300)*

It behooves the unwary researcher to be careful with terminology and thus not fall into the trap of pretending greater accuracy by changing the name of the phenom-enon being studied. Finally, to quote Hyman's *caveat,*[43]

> *The term "endophenotype" has become popular for describing putatively simpler or at least objectively measurable phenotypes, such as neuropsychological mea-sures that might enhance diagnostic homogeneity. I find this term less than ideal, because it implies that the current diagnostic classification is basically correct, and that all that is lacking is objective markers for these disorders. If, however, the lumping and splitting of symptoms that gave rise to the current classification was in error, then the search for biological correlates of these disorders will not prove fruitful. (p. 729)*

The second aspect to be considered in translational research is the concept of biomarkers. Biomarkers are crucial to translational research and serve as the inter-face between preclinical research, experimental medicine and clinical development. As with endophenotypes above, however, biomarkers also require some discussion. The FDA, NIH, and EMEA have been at the forefront in helping define and establish biomarkers, surrogate markers, and clinical endpoints[53-57] (http://ospp.od.nih.gov/ biomarkers/); an initiative now being carried out in partnership with private enter-prise[58] (http://ppp.od.nih.gov/pppinfo/examples.asp). Lesko and Atkinson have pro-vided summary definitions of various markers that are worth considering:[55]

> *A synthesis of some proposed working definitions is as follows: (a) biological marker (biomarker) - a physical sign or laboratory measurement that occurs in association with a pathological process and that has putative diagnostic and/or prognostic utility; (b) surrogate endpoint - a biomarker that is intended to serve as a substitute for a clinically meaningful endpoint and is expected to predict the effect of a therapeutic intervention; and (c) clinical endpoint - a clinically mean-ingful measure of how a patient feels, functions, or survives. The hierarchical distinction between biomarkers and surrogate endpoints is intended to indicate that relatively few biomarkers will meet the stringent criteria that are needed for them to serve as reliable substitutes for clinical endpoints (p. 348).*

An important characteristic of biomarkers is that they should also be capable of monitoring disease progression.[54] It is interesting more over that the establishment of biomarkers should also be subject to the same concepts of validity as defined by Willner initially for models of behavioral disorders, that is, face, construct and pre-dictive validity.[59] Lesko and Atkinson further indicate that biomarkers must be eval-uated and validated for (1) clinical relevance (face validity in being able to reflect physiologic/pathologic processes), (2) sensitivity and specificity (construct validity that it is capable to measure changes though a given mechanism in a target population) and (3) must ultimately be validated in terms of clinical change, that is, predictive validity. Biomarkers also have other criteria that they need to fulfill such as: their accuracy, precision and reproducibility; an estimated rate of false positive and false negative probability; and practicality and simplicity of use. In addition, pharmacological isomorphism is used to establish a biomarker's predictive validity where response to a known clinically effective standard is ultimately required, especially if drugs of different mechanisms of action produce the same response in the biomarker. These criteria are very familiar to the animal modeler and highlight the shared interests and expertise that the preclinical researcher brings to the clinical arena. Biomarkers for behavioral disorders thus share many of the problems inherent to their animal models.[60] Nevertheless, it is among the most active pursuits in Pharma today (*cf.*,[61-70]).

It is clear from the previous discussion that translational research demands the combined efforts of a number of participants, each of which contributes a particular expertise to achieve a common goal. Translational research cannot be done effectively using the "tried and true" process of compartmentalization prevalent up to the end of the last century, that is, the splitting of R from D, or maintaining the preclinical from clinical, academic from industrial divides. For the past decade Pharma has fostered cross-disciplinary collaboration with the creation of Project teams in which participants from preclinical, clinical and marketing sections of the Industry are brought together in relation to the maturity of the Project. The concept of "pitching the compound over the fence" is no longer tolerated, and preclinical participation even in mature Projects is expected. This creates a much more stimulating environment for all the participants, who not only learn from the experiences of others, but also maintain a sense of ownership even when their particular expertise is no longer required for a Project's core activities. Nevertheless, creation of and participation in Project teams is not always an easy task as group dynamics evolve. Team members are assigned to a Project by line managers, and can be removed depending on priorities. Some team members contribute more than their share, while others coast. The skills of the Project Leader must go beyond scientific expertise in order to forge an effective team and deliver a successful drug.

The use of animal models is an essential step in the drug discovery and indeed the translational research process. Use of appropriate models can minimize the number of drug candidates that later fail in human trials by accurately predicting the pharmacokinetic and dynamic (PK/PD) characteristics, efficacy and the toxicity of each compound. Selection of the appropriate models is critical to the process. Primary diseases such as those caused by infections, genetic disorders or cancers are less problematic to model using both *in vitro* and *in vivo* techniques. Similarly some aspects of degenerative diseases have also been successfully modeled. However, modeling of disorders with a strong behavioral component has been less successful. This is not to say that there are no models for various aspects of these disorders. Many models have been proposed, validated pharmacologically with standard, clinically effective drugs and extensively reviewed. Indeed, these models have become so standardized that their use to characterize mechanisms of action and lead novel compounds in CNS drug discovery projects is mandatory, and positive outcomes are required before these compounds are considered for further development. However, it has become clear that positive outcome in these models is no guarantee that these new compounds will be efficacious medicines in humans. Refinements of existing models and development of new models relevant to drug discovery and clinical outcome are being pursued and documented (e.g.,[71-74]). Advancements in genetic aspects of disease are also being aided through the development and use of genetically modified animals as model systems. However, even though these techniques are more precise in modeling aspects of a disease such as amyloid overexpression in Alzheimer's disease, the ability of procedures used to assess the changes in behavior, and relating them to altered human behavior remains uncertain.

Books on animal models of psychiatric and neurological diseases have tended to be compendia of so-called "standard" procedures developed over the years. Some of these books have formed part of classic reference texts for behavioral pharmacologists (e.g.,[75,76]). Others – more pragmatic in their approach – describe the application of these models and are useful as "cookbook" manuals (e.g.,[77,78]), while yet others have been very specific in their focus; for example, books entirely with models for a particular disorder, for example, depression or schizophrenia. It could be argued, however, that these books address a very circumscribed audience, and need not be necessarily so. Clinicians might and do claim that animal models are intellectually interesting, but of no relevance to their daily work of (1) demonstrating proof of concept, (2) showing efficacy or (3) treating their patients. Nevertheless, clinicians are constantly on the watch for potentially new pharmacological treatments with which to treat their patients, for example, new chemical entities that have reached their notice following extensive profiling in animal models. Academics develop a number of procedures or models to help them study neural substrates and disorders of behavior, and may use pharmacological compounds as tools to dissect behavior. The industrial scientist is charged with the application of these methods and models, establishing them in the lab at the request of the Project team and Leader. There is thus a shared interest in the development, use and ability of animal models to reflect the state of a disorder and predict changes in state following pharmacological manipulation. This shared interest has generated much collaboration between academics, clinicians and the industry (cf.,[79]).

Paradoxically in view of shared interest, close ties and general agreement on the need for bidirectional communication, the integration of the perspective and experience of the participants in the drug discovery and development process is not always apparent and is a source of concern (e.g.,[6,21,31,32,80-82]). Although we do not necessarily agree entirely with Horrobin's description of biomedical research scientists as latter day Castalians,[80] we suggest that there is a certain truth to the allusion that considerable segregation between the academic, clinician and industrial researcher exists (see also[21,81]). There have been numerous attempts to break down these barriers, such as having parallel sessions at conferences, or disorder-specific workshops organized by leading academics, clinicians and industrial scientists (e.g., *op. cit.*,[83]). With few exceptions, however, academics will talk to academics, clinicians to clinicians and industrial scientists will talk to either academics or clinicians; depending on at which stage their Project is. Willner's influential book,[84] "*Behavioral Models in Psychopharmacology: Theoretical, Industrial and Clinical Perspectives*" represents one of the first published attempts that brings together academics, pharmaceutical researchers and clinicians to discuss the various aspects of the animal models of behavioral disorders. Yet even in Willner's book with alternating chapters expounding the academic, industrial and clinical perspective on a subject, the temptation is always to go to the "more interesting", that is, directly relevant chapter and leave the others for later.

This three volume book series aims to bring objective and reasoned discussion of the relative utility of animal models to all participants in the process of discovery and development of new pharmaceuticals for the treatment of disorders with a strong behavioral component, that is, clearly psychiatric and reward deficits, but also neurodegenerative disorders in which changes in cognitive ability and mood are important characteristics. Participants include the applied research scientists in the Pharma industry as well as academics who carry out animal research, academic and industry clinicians involved in various aspects of clinical development, government officials and scientists setting funding priorities, and industrial, academic and clinical opinion leaders, who very clearly influence and help shape the decisions determining what therapeutic areas and molecular targets are to be pursued (or dropped) by Pharma. Rather than a catalog of existing animal models of behavioral disorders, the chapters of the book series seek to explore the role of these models within CNS drug discovery and development from the shared perspective of these participants in order to move beyond the concept of animal behavioral assays or "gut baths",[85,86] to stimulate the development of animal models to support present research of the genetic basis of behavioral disorders and to improve the ability to translate findings and concepts between animal research and clinical therapeutics.

As indicated, the aim and scope of this book series has been to examine the contribution of the animal models of behavioral disorders to the process of CNS drug discovery and development rather than a simple compendium of techniques and methods. This book goes beyond the traditional models book published in that it is more a considered review of *how* animal models of behavioral disorders are used rather than *what* they are. In order to achieve this goal, leading preclinical and clinical investigators from both Industry and Academia involved in translational research were identified and asked to participate in the Project. First, a single author was asked to write an introductory chapter explaining the role of animal and translational models for CNS drug discovery from their particular perspective. Each volume thus starts with an industry perspective from a senior Pharma research executive, which sets a framework. Considering the prominent role assumed by Governmental agencies such as the FDA or NIH in fostering translational research, NIH authors were asked to discuss animal and translational models from the perspective of the Government. A leading academic author was contacted to provide a general theoretical framework of how animal and translational models are evolving to provide the tools for the study of the neural substrates of behavior and how more efficient CNS drug discovery may be fostered. Finally, leading clinicians involved in the changing environment of clinical trial conductance and design were asked to discuss how issues in clinical trial design and conductance have affected the development and registration of CNS drugs in their area of specialty, and how changes are likely to affect future clinical trials.

Following these 4 introductory chapters, there are therapeutic area chapters in which a working party of at least 3 (industrial preclinical, academic and clinical) authors were identified and asked to write a consensual chapter that reflects the view of the role of animal models in CNS translational research and drug development in their area of expertise. We deliberately created our chapter teams with participants who had not necessarily worked together before. This was done for three reasons. First, we were anxious to avoid establishing teams with participants who had already evolved a conceptual framework *a priori*. Second, we felt that by forcing people to "brainstorm" and develop new ideas and concepts would be more stimulating both for the participants and the readers. Thirdly, we wanted to simulate the conditions of the creation of an industrial Project team, where participants need not know each other initially or indeed may not even like each other, but who are all committed to achieving the goals set out by consensus. We sought to draw upon the experiences of industrial and academic preclinical and clinical investigators who are actively involved in CNS drug discovery and development, as well as translational research. These therapeutic chapter teams have contributed very exciting chapters reflecting the state of animal models used in drug discovery in their therapeutic areas, and their changing roles in translational research. For many, this has been a challenging and exhilarating experience, forcing a paradigm shift from how they have normally worked. For some teams, the experience has been a challenge for the same reason. One is used to write for one's audience and usually on topics with which one is comfortable. For some authors, it was not easy to be asked to write with other equally strong personalities with different perspectives, and then to allow someone else to integrate this work into a consensual chapter. Indeed, some therapeutic area chapter teams were not able to establish an effective team. As a consequence, not all the therapeutic areas envisioned to be covered initially in this Project were possible. Nevertheless, as translational research becomes more established, what appears to be a novel and unusual way of working will become the norm for the benefit not only of science, but for the patient in need.

VOLUME OVERVIEW AND CHAPTER SYNOPSES

This volume comprises contributions by different authors on some psychiatric disorders, such as depression, bipolar disorders, anxiety, schizophrenia, attention deficit hyperactivity disorder (ADHD), autistic spectrum disorders (ASD), obsessive–compulsive disorders (OCD) and sleep disorders. A common theme that emerges from all of these chapters is the role played by stress, changes in the hypothalamic–pituitary–adrenal axis (HPA), and how the brain adapts to chronic stress through the process of allostasis (cf.,[87-89], and discussed more in detail by Koob in Volume 3, Reward Deficit Disorders of this book series[90]). Response to chronic stress and vulnerability to stress mediated by neurodevelopmental insults are key risk factors inherent in psychiatric disorders. As discussed above, dissatisfaction with DSM-IV or ICD-10 is leading to the "deconstruction" of syndromes and the classification of behavioral disorders in terms of clusters of symptoms, or phenotypes,[43] each of which are amenable to investigation. This shift away from viewing behavioral disorders as discrete syndromes has very much produced a conceptual change of viewing animal models from the traditional and unrealistic "of" to "for".[17,19,24,91] This is not only an important semantic change of emphasis, but one that (1) limits the expectations from positive results in one or more procedures or models to global changes in a heterogeneous patient population,[19,92]

(2) aligns academic, industrial and clinical uses of models to study the neurobiology of behavioral disorders,[18,61] and how new chemical entities and biological interact at a systems level to modulate those behaviors (e.g.,[5,17,24,93-97]).

Millan describes the issues regarding discovery and development of pharmacotherapy from an industrial point of view. While the development and implementation of animal models for aspects of abnormal behavior is crucial, this is not the only area in which animal models intervene in the drug discovery process. He discusses the importance of pharmacokinetic/pharmacodynamic approaches in defining the relationship drug exposure/drug effect, concluding that it is very difficult to define "therapeutic" doses of psychotropic drugs early in their pharmacological characterization. Correct PK/PD assessment in humans is crucial to determine whether the compound is present at the right receptors at a concentration sufficient to have the desired effect (see also[5,91,97-99] for further discussion on this theme). The author also points to the fact that there is a dearth of information on experiments addressing the consequences of stopping treatment, drug switching, drug combinations, comorbidity, and those with respect to age and gender. In addition to allostatic responses to chronic stress, Millan introduces the concept of epigenetics (*cf.*,[100,101]), which is later taken up by Jones *et al.*[18] and by Doran and colleagues.[96] Millan discusses epigenetic mechanisms, such as histone acetylation and methylation, meiotic imprinting, and how these can modify gene expression and could have behavioral consequences across generations. Brain imaging is far and beyond the most effective translational technique that is being used extensively in early development. This is, however, a very expensive technique, a factor that must be kept in mind. Notwithstanding the problems of adapting imaging techniques to animals, we can expect to see further developments in the future. Millan points to the fact that, in addition to animal models, complementary procedures (biochemical, electrophysiological, etc.) are necessary to validate models, targets and drugs, and points out that the true "predictive validity" of models really has not been put to the full test until a clinically effective drug; working through a novel mechanism is described. Finally, Millan introduces the importance of complementary non-pharmacological therapy in the treatment of behavioral disorders. These therapies, which include cognitive behavioral therapy, exercise, light exposure, phytotherapy, dietary supplements and even aromas are discussed by most authors in this Volume[18,61,97,102,103], as well as other chapters in the book series (e.g.,[95,104-106]).

Winsky *et al.* This chapter details the initiatives that the NIH has instituted to promote drug discovery and development, and model development for psychiatric disorders described previously above. Workshops are sponsored by the NIH that are tasked with identifying areas that allow for bidirectional translational work and to develop biologically based models to study psychopathology and to assess novel therapeutics. The NIH is also at the forefront of sponsoring initiatives such as the MATRICS and TURNS initiatives that aim to identify treatments of core features of a behavioral disorder such as cognition in schizophrenia and to provide the infrastructure of clinical development of such compounds (see also[18] for further discussion regarding these initiatives). The identification of endophenotypes and biomarkers is an important area of concern for the NIH. They are also concerned with genetic studies to identify genetic risk factors for complex disorders to facilitate new molecular target discovery for prevention, diagnosis and treatment. Development of novel models relies upon communications between clinicians and basic neuroscientists as well as improvements in clinical evaluation and application of basic science beyond translational boundaries.

McEvoy and Freudenreich Clinical trial design is undergoing major changes. McEvoy and Freudenreich present a very clear discussion of traditional clinical trial development from Phase 0 to Phase IV, and clinical trial design, and stress the need to keep the research questions of a trial as clear and simple as possible and avoid ambiguous outcomes. They stress the fact that diagnosis is syndrome based in psychiatry and, until more objective measurements can be found, the difficulty in assessing drug efficacy remains. Equally important is the need for strict patient selection in clinical trials. Heterogeneity in patient populations is starting to be controlled for genetically and more stringent selection criteria.[5,24,107] Adequate drug exposure is obviously a major concern in clinical development.[5,24,105] The incorporation of micro-dosing at Phase 0 for early human pharmacokinetic studies represents an innovation in clinical development (also discussed by Millan[24]). An important development in clinical trial design is the incorporation of adaptive design through which an ongoing trial may be monitored, and if needs be, changed, without compromising the statistical integrity of the study. The use of Bayesian statistics helps the investigator use ongoing information.[108] This statistical approach is discussed in other chapters of the book series[5,97,104]; including the use of Bayesian statistics to plan large scale preclinical studies with transgenic mice.[106] McEvoy and Freudenreich clearly distinguish between failed and negative results in clinical trials, as these are major issues affecting the outcomes of recent compounds with novel mechanisms of action that have not been approved (*cf.*, [91,109]). Effects of variability of the placebo response within and between studies are a major concern.[91,94,105,107,110] Finally, McEvoy and Freudenreich (as well as Schneider in Volume 2, Neurological Disorders[107]) discuss how the relationship between the sponsor and investigators has changed over the years; perhaps not for the better, as more responsibilities become relegated and additional factors such as language and/or culture differences in multi-country trials may compromise results.

Miczek discusses eight principles to guide the discussion of translation of preclinical findings into clinical applications, and vice versa. He emphasizes the importance of a sound conceptual basis for selecting core symptoms of psychiatric disorders when constructing experimental models. Miczek's first conceptual principle of translational psychopharmacology research, "*The translation of preclinical data to clinical concerns is more successful when the development of experimental models is restricted in their scope to a cardinal or core symptom of a psychiatric disorder*"[86] recalls the present phenotypic approach of conceptualizing the development and use of animals models discussed above, whereas his third principle, "*Preclinical data are more readily translated to the clinical situation when they are based on converging evidence from at least two, and preferably more, experimental procedures, each capturing cardinal features of the modeled disorder.*" Again reminds us of the need to bring together results from different sources – behavioral and otherwise – to approximate the clinical picture being studied. Finally, Miczek's eighth principle "*It is more productive to focus on behaviorally defined symptoms when translating clinical to preclinical measures, and vice versa. Psychological processes pertinent to affect and cognition are hypothetical constructs that need to be defined in behavioral and neural terms*" reminds us we are referring to hypothetical constructs when we talk about cognition, mood, affect, etc. (*cf.*,[110]). These may well be operationally defined in terms of changes in behavior, or electrical signals, but are still subject to philosophical debate (*cf.*,[111] and references within).

Steckler *et al.* make the distinction between models of a disorder and the tests used to measure the behavioral responses to conditions thought to provoke anxiety and recall Miczek's fifth conceptual principle of translational psychopharmacology research, "*The inducing conditions for modeling a cardinal symptom or cluster of symptoms may be environmental, genetic, physiological or a combination of these factors. The choice of the type of manipulation that induces the behavioral and physiological symptoms reveals the theoretical approach to the model construction.*" There has been considerable confusion between models and procedures that various authors of chapters in this book series have addressed (e.g.,[16,18,61,86, 90,91,94,97,98,102]). Pathological anxiety, for example, can be modeled chemically, through exposure to stress – especially developmental stress – and genetically. All three models have been successful in the study of the neurobiology of anxiety. Procedures such as the elevated plus maze, light-dark box, conditioned freezing, four-plates test, novelty-suppressed feeding, or Vogel conflict test, Geller-Seifter test are used to measure the effects of such models.

Anxiety is a very prevalent and devastating disorder for which pharmacological treatment is not optimal, and rather than producing a significant change in the treatment of anxiety, most efforts in the past 20 years have been to improve upon existing drugs. Part of this problem lies with the use of pharmacological isomorphism to validate models and procedures used in CNS drug discovery. According to Miczek's sixth principle, "*Preclinical experimental preparations can be useful screens that are often validated by predicting reliably treatment success with a prototypic agent. These screens detect 'me-too' treatments that are based on the same principle as an existing treatment that has been used to validate the screen.*" This real requirement to compare a novel compound's activity and potency against a clinical standard is paramount, but may be limiting to the discovery and exploitation of a truly novel mechanism of action.

As discussed above, model development of a disorder whose neurobiology is not clear is difficult. This difficulty is exacerbated through clinical diagnostic criteria (i.e., syndromal) that may change over time and are not exclusive. Moreover patient heterogeneity in behavioral disorders hampers unequivocal outcomes. FDA, academia and industry started initiatives to identify "core" constructs of disorders and use these as indicators of treatment outcome, as well as genomic stratification of patient samples are hoped to improve clinical trial outcome. Translational research in anxiety will greatly benefit by a better definition of psychiatric patient populations. Mechanistic or endophenotypic models are well suited for translational research and technology is also helping to develop translational models. Identification of patterns of behavior by measuring many variables simultaneously in rats and mice is a new direction. Another direction is back-translational, or from animal to human such as fMRI[112] and phMRI[113-115] are other methods being used and developed. However, all these techniques and approaches wait being pharmacologically validated.

Joel *et al.* Obsessive–compulsive disorders (OCD), shares many aspects with impulse control disorders, or obsessive–compulsive spectrum disorders, and illustrates some of the difficulty presented when considering behavioral disorders in terms of DSM-IV.[105] Indeed, there has been some debate whether OCD should be re-classified (cf.,[116,117]).

The authors consider OCD properly a disorder of anxiety, but indicate that genetic variation of cortico-striatal abnormalities may result in vulnerability to develop repetitive, non-functional behaviors, which underlie these phenomena. There is no unifying psychobiology of obsessive-spectrum disorders. However, a focus on endophenotypes and biomarkers to dissect elements of the spectrum rather than a syndromal approach would be more likely to advance not only of our understanding of OCD, but also to discover compounds effective in treating phenotypes common to these and other disorders such as stereotypy, mood and affect and cognition. A number of models for mania, depression, mood instability are presented. Some of these models and procedures are common for other psychiatric disorders considered in this Volume (e.g.,[18, 61, 97,102]). Rather than limiting the search for novel targets, the authors believe that the use of selective serotonin reuptake inhibitors (SSRIs) for pharmacological isomorphic validation of models is a necessary process, which will help differentiate treatment of OCD from other disorders. The standard treatment of OCD is with SSRIs, although treatment resistance is common (see also[61,91,97,118,119] for further discussion on treatment resistance). Recently, glutamatergic approaches are also being considered.

Cryan et al. point out that some endophenotypes or their relative stress-related biomarkers may be effective in studying the treatment of major unipolar depression. Among the endophenotypes being considered are anhedonia, cognitive function and sleep disturbances. However, no drug acting on the HPA stress system has so far has had antidepressant action confirmed in clinical Phase III trials; an outcome underlining that activity of a compound in current animal models is no guarantee of clinical success (please refer to the discussion on failed and negative trials above). Moreover, Cryan and colleagues bring up the very important point of the discrepancy between animal and human outcome measures (as do Steckler and colleagues). Whilst animal procedures typically measure changes in behavior such as, for example, immobility in forced swim or tail suspension tests (e.g.,[120]), sucrose consumption (e.g.,[90,121]), or rates of self-stimulation,[122] clinical trials outcome in psychiatry rely on subjective scales such as the Hamilton Rating Scale (depression), Positive and Negative Syndrome Scale (schizophrenia), Young Mania Rating Scale, or Liebowitz Social Anxiety Scale to mention a few.[19,97] Considering the variability of response in a heterogeneous patient population, with a considerable placebo response, it is clear that a re-alignment of human and animal outcome measures are needed (see Miczek's eighth principle discussed above as well as[6,123]).

Jones et al. Schizophrenia arguably is the behavioral disorder that has advanced further in terms of endophenotypes, "deconstruction", NIH initiatives and changes in clinical trial design, mostly through the NIH MATRICS, TURNS, initiatives reviewed by Jones and colleagues and by Winsky et al.[17] The treatment of schizophrenia has focussed primarily on the florid positive symptoms; although not without the serious side-effects produced by long-term neuroleptic treatment (cf.,[124]). Nevertheless, much of the present drug discovery effort is directed towards the treatment of negative and cognitive symptoms of schizophrenia.[125] The authors focus particularly on the development of appropriate animal models and translational approaches to aid in the understanding of the neurobiology of schizophrenia and to investigate the potential efficacy of compounds directed at novel pharmacological targets. There is considerable emphasis on investigations into susceptibility genes for schizophrenia and relationships between them and neurodevelopmental, environmental and epigenetic influences. Indeed, as indicated by Steckler and his colleagues previously,[110] new models based upon the combination of environmental stresses and/or neurodevelopmental insults on susceptible strains are being developed (see also[63,126]). Finally, the authors discuss how the most recent advances in understanding the disorder and the various academic/government/industry initiatives are likely to make a major impact upon drug discovery in this area in the near future.

Large *et al.* The dual nature of bipolar disorders (BPD) has encouraged the use of models for depressed-like and manic-like symptoms that stress the most superficial features of mania and depression, hyperactivity and immobility, respectively. However, bipolar depression, for example, should not be considered equivalent to unipolar depression, or mania as a special case of schizophrenia. BPD is best characterized by an allostatic process of periods of discrete episodes of poor functioning and normal functioning, symptom-free episodes,[127] and less attention has been placed on modeling the "recurrence" of episodes. Mood stabilizing drugs, such as lithium (Eskalith®/ Lithobid®), valproate (Depakote®), or lamotrigine (Lamictal®) are used to treat BPD as well as antipsychotics like olanzapine (Zyprexa®,[128]). Treatment resistance may develop to lithium as a function of previous manic or depressive episodes. Conversely, valproate efficacy may increase. The study of the mechanism of action of mood stabilizing drugs as well as anticonvulsants is helping to understand illness recurrence in BPD and other cyclic disorders, and identifying molecules such as protein kinase C (PKC), the Erk-MAP kinase pathway, GSK-3β, BCL-2, and mTOR; molecules related to cellular plasticity and resilience.

Miczek's third principle, "*Preclinical data are more readily translated to the clinical situation when they are based on converging evidence from at least two, and preferably more, experimental procedures, each capturing cardinal features of the modeled disorder*" can best be illustrated by the modeling approach taken in BPD, which is the establishment of a battery of tests with which putative endophenotypes for BPD can be further studied. Research is focusing on genetic associations and endophenotypes that may differentiate BPD from unipolar depression and schizophrenia. *Post hoc* genotyping is being carried out to identify alleles of candidate genes associated with treatment response as are whole genome.

Tannock *et al.* ADHD is one of the most studied childhood and adolescence behavioral disorders, which also affects adults. ADHD is characterized by large intra-individual variability and inconsistency in behavioral symptoms and task performance, which is now the focus of current theoretical and empirical work. Current theoretical frameworks for ADHD focus on neurodevelopmental, environmental and genetic influences on dysregulation of the prefrontal cortex and striatum and the dopaminergic and glutamatergic systems. The treatment of the symptoms of ADHD has traditionally been psychostimulants with their substance abuse potential, although the registration of the noradrenaline reuptake inhibitor atomoxetine (Strattera®) represents a major change in pharmacological treatment options.[iv] As discussed above in the context of BPD, ADHD is also characterized by a spectrum of behavioral abnormalities such as hyper-activity, impulsivity, impaired attention, etc., and procedures specifically measuring

---

[iv] See Rocha *et al.*,[16] for a comprehensive discussion on the Regulatory aspects and modeling of substance abuse liability.

changes in those behaviors have been adopted in ADHD drug discovery. Some of these procedures like the five-choice serial reaction time task or the continuous performance test, have human analogs, which facilitate translational initiatives in this and other therapeutic indications.[23,37] Tannock *et al.*, present a very thorough discussion of the search for and use of biomarkers in neuropsychiatric drug discovery and development, including imaging and physiological techniques. Equally important, the authors introduce the initiatives being carried out by experimental medicine such as the incorporation of a "virtual laboratory", where the effects of ADHD treatments are assessed in a controlled classroom setting, using both observational measures of behavior, as well as academic performance measures.

Bartz *et al.* Autism spectrum disorders (ASD) are a group of disorders characterized by three core symptom domains, namely social/social cognitive deficits, communication deficits, and/or repetitive and restricted behaviors and interests. Risk genes and/or pathophysiological mechanisms have been implicated in these disorders.[43] Like ADHD discussed above, these disorders are neurodevelopmental; they also share with ADHD symptomatic changes such as anxiety, hyperactivity, short attention span, irritability, mood instability, aggression, self-injurious behavior, and poor impulse control. The authors review the core ASD symptom domains and discuss how they are assessed in the clinic in response to treatment; in particular, subjective scales such as the Aberrant Behavior Checklist, Clinical Global Impressions Scale – Improvement, and the Yale-Brown Obsessive–Compulsive Scale are noted; this latter also being used to measure state and outcome in OCD.[103] Current pharmacological treatments are also reviewed; as in OCD discussed above, SSRIs and atypical antipsychotics are used in the treatment of ASD.[129,130] The authors then turn to animal model development in ASD. In particular model development in ASD has adopted an approach similar to that discussed above for OCD and ADHD, that is, the establishment of test batteries with which experimental changes in ASD-like behaviors or endophenotypes such as impaired motivation, social interaction, etc., particularly through genetic manipulation, can be assessed.[131,132] The authors emphasize that, to date, much of the drug development in ASD has been based on adopting treatments that have been successful in other psychiatric disorders; as a result, most available treatments target associated ASD symptoms. Indeed, no drugs are currently approved by the FDA for the treatment of core ASD symptoms. Animal models may be useful in this regard, especially in developing treatments for the social domain. An example of animal model driven drug intervention for ASD is presented in the case of oxytocin.

Doran *et al.* Sleep disorders are serious under-diagnosed and poorly treated allostatic pathologies that are also comorbid with many of the psychiatric, neurologic and reward deficit disorders discussed in this book series (e.g.,[91,99,107,133]) and although medications exist that promote sleep, there is a lack of drugs to promote sleep maintenance, and prevent rebound insomnia or next-day residual effects. Sleep research, however, has long since enjoyed recording techniques such as polysomnography that allows relatively close correspondence between responses in animals and humans, and is not so limited to inferences from changes in behavior, or subjective scales as in other disciplines. Furthermore, the discovery of the hypocretin/orexin system and its relationship to sleep and energy regulation[134,135] has opened up the study of genetic basis of sleep and increases our understanding of the functional links between sleep architecture and the effects on immune, CNS, mood and metabolic functions.

REFERENCES

1. Kline, N.S. (1958). Clinical experience with iproniazid (marsilid). *J Clin Exp Psychopathol*, 19(2, Suppl 1):72–78.
2. Selling, L.S. (1955). Clinical study of a new tranquilizing drug; use of miltown (2-methyl-2-n-propyl-1,3-propanediol dicarbamate). *JAMA*, 157(18):1594–1596.
3. Delay, J. and Deniker, P. (1955). Neuroleptic effects of chlorpromazine in therapeutics of neuropsychiatry. *J Clin Exp Psychopathol*, 16(2):104–112.
4. Kola, I. and Landis, J. (2004). Can the pharmaceutical industry reduce attrition rates? *Nat Rev Drug Discov*, 3(8):711–715.
5. Hunter, A.J. (2008). Animal and translational models of neurological disorders: An industrial perspective. In McArthur, R.A. and Borsini, F. (eds.), *Animal and Translational Models for CNS Drug Discovery: Neurologic Disorders*. Academic Press: Elsevier, New York.
6. McArthur, R. and Borsini, F. (2006). Animal models of depression in drug discovery: A historical perspective. *Pharmacol Biochem Behav*, 84(3):436–452.
7. FDA (2004). Innovation or Stagnation: Challenge and Opportunity on the Critical Path to New Medical Products. US Department of Health and Human Services, Food and Drug Administration, Washington, DC.
8. EMEA. (2005). *The European Medicines Agency Road Map to 2010: Preparing the Ground for the Future*. The European Medicines Agency, London.
9. Nestler, E.J., Gould, E., Manji, H., Buncan, M., Duman, R.S., Greshenfeld, H.K. *et al.* (2002). Preclinical models: Status of basic research in depression. *Biol Psychiatry*, 52(6):503–528.
10. Shekhar, A., McCann, U.D., Meaney, M.J., Blanchard, D.C., Davis, M., Frey, K.A. *et al.* (2001). Summary of a National Institute of Mental Health workshop: Developing animal models of anxiety disorders. *Psychopharmacology (Berl)*, 157(4):327–339.
11. Bromley, E. (2005). A Collaborative Approach to Targeted Treatment Development for Schizophrenia: A Qualitative Evaluation of the NIMH-MATRICS Project. Schizophr Bull, 31(4):954–961.
12. Winsky, L. and Brady, L. (2005). Perspective on the status of preclinical models for psychiatric disorders. *Drug Discov Today: Disease Models*, 2(4):279–283.
13. Stables, J.P., Bertram, E., Dudek, F.E., Holmes, G., Mathern, G., Pitkanen, A. *et al.* (2003). Therapy discovery for pharmacoresistant epilepsy and for disease-modifying therapeutics: Summary of the NIH/NINDS/AES models II workshop. *Epilepsia*, 44(12):1472–1478.
14. Stables, J.P., Bertram, E.H., White, H.S., Coulter, D.A., Dichter, M.A., Jacobs, M.P. *et al.* (2002). Models for epilepsy and epileptogenesis: report from the NIH workshop, Bethesda, Maryland. *Epilepsia*, 43(11):1410–1420.
15. McCann, D.J., Acri, J.B., and Vocci, F.J. (2008). Drug discovery and development for reward disorders. In McArthur, R.A. and Borsini, F. (eds.), *Animal and Translational Models for CNS Drug Discovery: Reward Deficit Disorders*. Academic Press: Elsevier, New York.
16. Rocha, B., Bergman, J., Comer, S.D., Haney, M., and Spealman, R.D. (2008). Development of medications for heroin and cocaine addiction and Regulatory aspects of abuse liability testing. In McArthur, R.A. and Borsini, F. (eds.), *Animal and Translational Models for CNS Drug Discovery: Reward Deficit Disorders*. Academic Press: Elsevier, New York.
17. Winsky, L., Driscoll, J., and Brady, L. (2008). Drug discovery and development initiatives at the National Institute of Mental Health: From cell-based systems to Proof-of-Concept. In McArthur, R.A. and Borsini, F. (eds.), *Animal and Translational Models for CNS Drug Discovery: Psychiatric Disorders*. Academic Press: Elsevier, New York.
18. Jones, D.N.C., Gartlon, J.E., Minassian, A., Perry, W., and Geyer, M.A. (2008). Developing new drugs for schizophrenia: From animals to the clinic. In McArthur, R.A. and Borsini, F. (eds.), *Animal and Translational Models for CNS Drug Discovery: Psychiatric Disorders*. Academic Press: Elsevier, New York.

19. McEvoy, J.P. and Freudenreich, O. (2008). Issues in the design and conductance of clinical trials. In McArthur, R.A. and Borsini, F. (eds.), *Animal and Translational Models for CNS Drug Discovery: Psychiatric Disorders.* Academic Press: Elsevier, New York.

20. Schuster, D.P. and Powers, W.J. (2005). *Translational and Experimental Clinical Research.* Lippincott Williams & Wilkins, Philadelphia, PA.

21. Mankoff, S.P., Brander, C., Ferrone, S., and Marincola, F.M. (2004). Lost in translation: Obstacles to translational medicine. *J Transl Med*, 2(1):14.

22. Littman, B.H. and Williams, S.A. (2005). The ultimate model organism: Progress in experimental medicine. *Nat Rev Drug Discov*, 4(8):631–638.

23. Robbins, T.W. (1998). Homology in behavioural pharmacology: An approach to animal models of human cognition. *Behav Pharmacol*, 9(7):509–519.

24. Millan, M.J. (2008). The discovery and development of pharmacotherapy for psychiatric disorders: A critical survey of animal and translational models, and perspectives for their improvement. In McArthur, R.A. and Borsini, F. (eds.), *Animal and Translational Models for CNS Drug Discovery: Psychiatric Disorders.* Academic Press: Elsevier, New York.

25. Domenjoz, R. (2000). From DDT to imipramine. In Healey, D. (ed.), *The Psychopharmacologists III: Interviews with David Healy.* Arnold, London, pp. 93–118.

26. Kuhn, R. (1999). From imipramine to levoprotiline: the discovery of antidepressants. In Healey, D. (ed.), *The Psychopharmacologists II: Interviews with David Healy.* Arnold, London, pp. 93–118.

27. Janssen, P. (1999). From haloperidol to risperidone. In Healy, D. (ed.), *The Psychopharmacologists II: Interviews by David Healy.* Arnold, London, pp. 39–70.

28. Almond, S. and O'Donnell, O. (2000). Cost analysis of the treatment of schizophrenia in the UK. A simulation model comparing olanzapine, risperidone and haloperidol. *Pharmacoeconomics*, 17(4):383–389.

29. Gasquet, I., Gury, C., Tcherny-Lessenot, S., Quesnot, A., and Gaudebout, P. (2005). Patterns of prescription of four major antipsychotics: A retrospective study based on medical records of psychiatric inpatients. *Pharmacoepidemiol Drug Safety*, 14(11):805–811.

30. Pizzo P. (2002). Letter from the Dean, *Stanford Medicine Magazine.* Stanford University School of Medicine.

31. Lerman, C., LeSage, M.G., Perkins, K.A., O'Malley, S.S., Siegel, S.J., Benowitz, N.L. *et al.* (2007). Translational research in medication development for nicotine dependence. *Nat Rev Drug Discov*, 6(9):746–762.

32. Horig, H. and Pullman, W. (2004). From bench to clinic and back: Perspective on the 1st IQPC Translational Research conference. *J Transl Med*, 2(1):44.

33. Beckmann, N., Kneuer, R., Gremlich, H.U., Karmouty-Quintana, H., Ble, F.X., and Muller, M. (2007). In vivo mouse imaging and spectroscopy in drug discovery. *NMR Biomed*, 20(3):154–185.

34. Risterucci, C., Jeanneau, K., Schoppenthau, S., Bielser, T., Kunnecke, B., von Kienlin, M. *et al.* (2005). Functional magnetic resonance imaging reveals similar brain activity changes in two different animal models of schizophrenia. *Psychopharmacology (Berl)*, 180(4):724–734.

35. Tamminga, C.A., Lahti, A.C., Medoff, D.R., Gao, X.-M., and Holcomb, H.H. (2003). Evaluating Glutamatergic Transmission in Schizophrenia. *Ann NY Acad Sci*, 1003(1):113–118.

36. Shah, Y.B. and Marsden, C.A. (2004). The application of functional magnetic resonance imaging to neuropharmacology. *Curr Opin Pharmacol*, 4(5):517–521.

37. Robbins, T.W. (2005). Synthesizing schizophrenia: A bottom-up, symptomatic approach. *Schizophr Bull*, 31(4):854–864.

38. Porrino, L.J., Daunais, J.B., Rogers, G.A., Hampson, R.E., and Deadwyler, S.A. (2005). Facilitation of task performance and removal of the effects of sleep deprivation by an ampakine (CX717) in nonhuman primates. *PLoS Biol*, 3(9):e299.

39. McKinney, W.T.J. and Bunney, W.E.J. (1969). Animal model of depression I: Review of evidence: implications for research. *Arch Gen Psychiatry*, 21(2):240–248.

40. American Psychiatric Association. (1994). Diagnostic and Statistical Manual of Mental Disorders, 4th edition. American Psychiatric Association, Washington, DC.

41. World Health Organization. (2007). International Statistical Classification of Diseases, 10th Revision, 2nd Edition. World Health Organization, Geneva.

42. Silverstone, P.H. (1991). Is anhedonia a good measure of depression? *Acta Psychiatr Scand*, 83(4):249–250.

43. Hyman, S.E. (2007). Can neuroscience be integrated into the DSM-V? *Nat Rev Neurosci*, 8(9):725–732.

44. Kupfer, D.J., First, M.B., and Regier, D.A. (eds.) (2002). *A Research Agenda for DSM-V*. American Psychiatric Association, Washington, DC.

45. Eisenberg, D.T., Mackillop, J., Modi, M., Beauchemin, J., Dang, D., Lisman, S.A. *et al.* (2007). Examining impulsivity as an endophenotype using a behavioral approach: A DRD2 TaqI A and DRD4 48-bp VNTR association study. *Behav Brain Funct*, 3:2.

46. Hasler, G., Drevets, W.C., Manji, H.K., and Charney, D.S. (2004). Discovering endophenotypes for major depression. *Neuropsychopharmacology*, 29(10):1765–1781.

47. Cannon, T.D. and Keller, M.C. (2006). Endophenotypes in the genetic analyses of mental disorders. *Ann Rev Clin Psychol*, 2(1):267–290.

48. Meehl, P.E. (1972). A critical afterword. In Gottesman, I.I. and Schields, J. (eds.), *Schizophrenia and Genetics: A Twin Study Vantage Point*. Academic Press, New York, pp. 367–415.

49. Breiter, H., Gasic, G., and Makris, N. (2006). Imaging the neural systems for motivated behavior and their dysfunction in neuropsychiatric illness. In Deisboeck, T.S. and Kresh, J.Y. (eds.), *Complex Systems Science in Biomedicine*. Springer, New York, pp. 763–810.

50. Gottesman, I.I. and Shields, J. (1973). Genetic theorizing and schizophrenia. *Br J Psychiatry*, 122(566):15–30.

51. Gottesman, I.I. and Gould, T.D. (2003/4/1). The endophenotype concept in psychiatry: Etymology and strategic intentions. *Am J Psychiatry*, 160(4):636–645.

52. Holzman, P.S. (2001). Seymour, S. Kety and the genetics of schizophrenia. *Neuropsychopharmacology*, 25(3):299–304.

53. Biomarkers Definitions Working Group. (2001). Biomarkers and surrogate endpoints: Preferred definitions and conceptual framework. *Clin Pharmacol Ther*, 69(3):89–95.

54. Katz, R. (2004). Biomarkers and surrogate markers: An FDA perspective. *NeuroRx*, 1(2):189–195.

55. Lesko, L.J. and Atkinson, A.J.J. (2001). Use of biomarkers and surrogate endpoints in drug development and regulatory decision making: Criteria, validation, strategies. *Ann Rev Pharmacol Toxicol*, 41:347–366.

56. De Gruttola, V.G., Clax, P., DeMets, D.L., Downing, G.J., Ellenberg, S.S., Friedman, L. *et al.* (2001). Considerations in the evaluation of surrogate endpoints in clinical trials. Summary of a National Institutes of Health workshop. *Control Clin Trials*, 22(5):485–502.

57. EMEA. (2007). *Innovative Drug Development Approaches: Final Report from the EMEA/ CHMP-Think-Tank Group on Innovative Drug Development*. The European Medicines Agency, London.

58. Zerhouni, E.A., Sanders, C.A., and von Eschenbach, A.C. (2007). The biomarkers consortium: Public and private sectors working in partnership to improve the public health. *Oncologist*, 12(3):250–252.

59. Willner, P. (1991). Methods for assessing the validity of animal models of human psychopathology. In Boulton, A., Baker, G., and Martin-Iverson, M. (eds.), *Neuromethods Vol 18: Animal Models in Psychiatry I*. Humana Press, Inc., pp. 1–23.

60. Kraemer, H.C., Schultz, S.K., and Arndt, S. (2002). Biomarkers in psychiatry: Methodological issues. *Am J Geriatr Psychiatry*, 10(6):653–659.

61. Tannock, R., Campbell, B., Seymour, P., Ouellet, D., Soares, H., Wang, P. *et al.* (2008). Towards a biological understanding of ADHD and the discovery of novel therapeutic approaches.

In McArthur, R.A. and Borsini, F. (eds.), *Animal and Translational Models for CNS Drug Discovery: Psychiatric Disorders*. Academic Press: Elsevier, New York.

62. Gordon, E., Liddell, B.J., Brown, K.J., Bryant, R., Clark, C.R., Das, P. *et al.* (2007). Integrating objective gene-brain-behavior markers of psychiatric disorders. *J Integr Neurosci*, 6(1):1–34.

63. Turck, C.W., Maccarrone, G., Sayan-Ayata, E., Jacob, A.M., Ditzen, C., Kronsbein, H. *et al.* (2005). The quest for brain disorder biomarkers. *J Med Invest*, 52(Suppl):231–235.

64. Gomez-Mancilla, B., Marrer, E., Kehren, J., Kinnunen, A., Imbert, G., Hillebrand, R. *et al.* (2005). Central nervous system drug development: an integrative biomarker approach toward individualized medicine. *NeuroRx*, 2(4):683–695.

65. Javitt, D.C., Spencer, K.M., Thaker, G.K., Winterer, G., and Hajos, M. (2008). Neurophysiological biomarkers for drug development in schizophrenia. *Nat Rev Drug Discov*, 7(1):68–83.

66. Cho, R.Y., Ford, J.M., Krystal, J.H., Laruelle, M., Cuthbert, B., and Carter, C.S. (2005). Functional neuroimaging and electrophysiology biomarkers for clinical trials for cognition in schizophrenia. *Schizophr Bull*, 31(4):865–869.

67. Choi, D.W. (2002). Exploratory clinical testing of neuroscience drugs. *Nat Neurosci*, 5(Suppl):1023–1025.

68. Pien, H.H., Fischman, A.J., Thrall, J.H., and Sorensen, A.G. (2005 Feb 15). Using imaging biomarkers to accelerate drug development and clinical trials. *Drug Discov Today*, 10(4):259–266.

69. Thal, L.J., Kantarci, K., Reiman, E.M., Klunk, W.E., Weiner, M.W., Zetterberg, H. *et al.* (2006). The role of biomarkers in clinical trials for Alzheimer disease. *Alzheimer Dis Assoc Disord*, 20(1):6–15.

70. Phillips, M.L. and Vieta, E. (2007). Identifying functional neuroimaging biomarkers of bipolar disorder: toward DSM-V. *Schizophr Bull*, 33(4):893–904.

71. Schaller, B. (ed.) (2004). *Cerebral Ischemic Tolerance: From Animal Models to Clinical Relevance*. Nova Science Publishers, Hauppauge, NY.

72. Carroll, P.M. and Fitzgerald, K. (eds.) (2003). *Model Organisms in Drug Discovery*. John Wiley and Sons, Chichester, UK.

73. Offermanns, S. and Hein, L. (eds.) (2003). *Transgenic Models in Pharmacology (Handbook of Experimental Pharmacology)*. Springer, Heidelberg, Germany.

74. Levin, E.D. and Buccafusco, J.J. (eds.) (2006). *Animal Models of Cognitive Impairment*. Taylor & Francis CRC Press.

75. Boulton, A.A., Baker, G.B., and Martin-Iverson, M.T. (eds.) (1991). *Neuromethods: Animal Models in Psychiatry I*. The Humana Press, Clifton, New Jersey.

76. Olivier, B., Mos, J., and Slangen, J.L. (eds.) (1991). *Animal Models in Psychophramacology*. Birkhaüser-Verlag, Basel.

77. Myers, R.D. (ed.) (1971). *Methods in Psychobiology: Laboratory Techniques in Neuropsychology and Neurobiology*. Academic Press, New York.

78. Svartengren, J., Modiri, A.-R., and McArthur, R.A. (2005). Measurement and characterization of energy intake in the mouse. *Curr Protocols Pharmacol*, 5(Supplement 28). 5.40.1–5..19.

79. Chin-Dusting, J., Mizrahi, J., Jennings, G., Fitzgerald, D. (2005). Finding improved medicines: The role of academic–industrial collaboration, *Nat Rev Drug Discov*, 4(11):891–7.

80. Horrobin, D.F. (2003). Modern biomedical research: An internally self-consistent universe with little contact with medical reality? *Nat Rev Drug Discov*, 2(2):151–154.

81. FitzGerald, G.A. (2005). Anticipating change in drug development: The emerging era of translational medicine and therapeutics, *Nat Rev Drug Discov* 4(10):815–8.

82. Pangalos, M.N., Schechter, L.E., and Hurko, O. (2007). Drug development for CNS disorders: Strategies for balancing risk and reducing attrition. *Nat Rev Drug Discov*, 6(7):521–532.

83. Agid, Y., Buzsaki, G., Diamond, D.M., Frackowiak, R., Giedd, J., Girault, J.-A. *et al.* (2007). How can drug discovery for psychiatric disorders be improved? *Nat Rev Drug Discov*, 6(3):189–201.

84. Willner, P. (ed.) (1991). *Behavioural Models in Psychopharmacology: Theoretical, Industrial and Clinical Perspectives*. Cambridge University Press, Cambridge.

85. Willner, P. (1991). Behavioural models in psychopharmacology. In Willner, P. (ed.), *Behavioural models in psychopharmacology: theoretical, industrial and clinical perspectives*. Cambridge University Press, Cambridge, pp. 3–18.

86. Miczek, K.A. (2008). Challenges for translational psychopharmacology research – the need for conceptual principles. In McArthur, R.A. and Borsini, F. (eds.), *Animal and Translational Models for CNS Drug Discovery: Psychiatric Disorders*. Academic Press: Elsevier, New York.

87. Korte, S.M., Koolhaas, J.M., Wingfield, J.C., and McEwen, B.S. (2005). The Darwinian concept of stress: Benefits of allostasis and costs of allostatic load and the trade-offs in health and disease. *Neurosci Biobehav Rev*, 29(1):3–38.

88. McEwen, B.S. and Seeman, T. (1999). Protective and Damaging Effects of Mediators of Stress: Elaborating and Testing the Concepts of Allostasis and Allostatic Load. *Ann NY Acad Sci*, 896(1):30–47.

89. Sterling, P. and Eyer, J. (1988). Allostasis: A new paradigm to explain arousal pathology. In Fisher, S. and Reason, J. (eds.), *Handbook of Life Stress, Cognition and Health*. John Wiley & Sons, New York, pp. 629–649.

90. Koob, G.F. (2008). The role of animal models in reward deficit disorders: Views from Academia. In McArthur, R.A. and Borsini, F. (eds.), *Animal and Translational Models for CNS Drug Discovery: Reward Deficit Disorders*. Academic Press: Elsevier, New York.

91. Cryan, J.F., Sánchez, C., Dinan, T.G., and Borsini, F. (2008). Developing more efficacious antidepressant medications: Improving and aligning preclinical and clinical assessment tools. In McArthur, R.A. and Borsini, F. (eds.), *Animal and Translational Models for CNS Drug Discovery: Psychiatric Disorders*. Academic Press: Elsevier, New York.

92. Lindner, M.D. (2007). Clinical attrition due to biased preclinical assessments of potential efficacy. *Pharmacol Ther*, 115(1):148–175.

93. Dourish, C.T., Wilding, J.P.H., and Halford, J.C.G. (2008). Anti-obesity drugs: From animal models to clinical efficacy. In McArthur, R.A. and Borsini, F. (eds.), *Animal and Translational Models for CNS Drug Discovery: Reward Deficit Disorders*. Academic Press: Elsevier, New York.

94. Lindner, M.D., McArthur, R.A., Deadwyler, S.A., Hampson, R.E., and Tariot, P.N. (2008). Development, optimization and use of preclinical behavioral models to maximise the productivity of drug discovery for Alzheimer's Disease. In McArthur, R.A. and Borsini, F. (eds.), *Animal and Translational Models for CNS Drug Discovery: Neurologic Disorders*. Academic Press: Elsevier, New York.

95. Shilyansky, C., Li, W., Acosta, M., Elgersma, Y., Hannan, F., Hardt, M. *et al.* (2008). Molecular and cellular mechanisms of learning disabilities: A focus on neurofibromastosis type I. In McArthur, R.A. and Borsini, F. (eds.), *Animal and Translational Models for CNS Drug Discovery: Neurologic Disorders*. Academic Press: Elsevier, New York.

96. Doran, S.M., Wessel, T., Kilduff, T.S., Turek, F.W., and Renger, J.J. (2008). Translational models of sleep and sleep disorders. In McArthur, R.A. and Borsini, F. (eds.), *Animal and Translational Models for CNS Drug Discovery: Psychiatric Disorders*. Academic Press: Elsevier, New York.

97. Large, C.H., Einat, H., and Mahableshshwarkar, A.R. (2008). Developing new drugs for bipolar disorder (BPD): From animal models to the clinic. In McArthur, R.A. and Borsini, F. (eds.), *Animal and Translational Models for CNS Drug Discovery: Psychiatric Disorders*. Academic Press: Elsevier, New York.

98. Markou, A., Chiamulera, C., and West, R.J. (2008). Contribution of animal models and preclinical human studies to medication development for nicotine dependence. In McArthur, R.A. and Borsini, F. (eds.), *Animal and Translational Models for CNS Drug Discovery: Reward Deficit Disorders*. Academic Press: Elsevier, New York.

99. Merchant, K.M., Chesselet, M.-F., Hu, S.-C., and Fahn, S. (2008). Animal models of Parkinson's Disease to aid drug discovery and development. In McArthur, R.A. and Borsini, F. (eds.),

Animal and Translational Models for CNS Drug Discovery: Neurologic Disorders. Academic Press: Elsevier, New York.

100. Bird, A. (2007). Perceptions of epigenetics. *Nature*, 447(7143):396-398.

101. Jablonka, E.V.A. and Lamb, M.J. (2002). The changing concept of epigenetics. *Ann NY Acad Sci*, 981(1):82-96.

102. Bartz, J., Young, L.J., Hollander, E., Buxbaum, J.D., and Ring, R.H. (2008). Preclinical animal models of Autistic Spectrum Disorders (ASD). In McArthur, R.A. and Borsini, F. (eds.), *Animal and Translational Models for CNS Drug Discovery: Psychiatric Disorders.* Academic Press: Elsevier, New York.

103. Joel, D., Stein, D.J., and Schreiber, R. (2008). Animal models of obsessive-compulsive disorder: From bench to bedside via endophenotypes and biomarkers. In McArthur, R.A. and Borsini, F. (eds.), *Animal and Translational Models for CNS Drug Discovery: Psychiatric Disorders.* Academic Press: Elsevier, New York.

104. Gardner, T.J., Kosten, T.A., and Kosten, T.R. (2008). Issues in designing and conducting clinical trials for reward disorders. In McArthur, R.A. and Borsini, F. (eds.), *Animal and Translational Models for CNS Drug Discovery: Reward Deficit Disorders.* Academic Press: Elsevier, New York.

105. Heidbreder, C. (2008). Impulse and reward deficit disorders: Drug discovery and development. In McArthur, R.A. and Borsini, F. (eds.), *Animal and Translational Models for CNS Drug Discovery: Reward Deficit Disorders.* Academic Press: Elsevier, New York.

106. Wagner, L.A., Menalled, L., Goumeniouk, A.D., Brunner, D.P., and Leavitt, B.R. (2008). Huntington disease. In McArthur, R.A. and Borsini, F. (eds.), *Animal and Translational Models for CNS Drug Discovery: Neurologic Disorders.* Academic Press: Elsevier, New York.

107. Schneider, L.S. (2008). Issues in design and conduct of clinical trials for cognitive-enhancing drugs. In McArthur, R.A. and Borsini, F. (eds.), *Animal and Translational Models for CNS Drug Discovery: Neurologic Disorders.* Academic Press: Elsevier, New York.

108. Berry, D.A. (2006). Bayesian clinical trials, *Nat Rev Drug Discov*, 5(1):27-36.

109. Rupniak, N.M. (2003). Animal models of depression: challenges from a drug development perspective. *Behav Pharmacol*, 14(5-6):385-390.

110. Steckler, T., Stein, M.B., and Holmes, A. (2008). Developing novel anxiolytics: Improving preclinical detection and clinical assessment. In McArthur, R.A. and Borsini, F. (eds.), *Animal and Translational Models for CNS Drug Discovery: Psychiatric Disorders.* Academic Press: Elsevier, New York.

111. Kandel, E.R. (2006). *In search of memory: The emergence of a new science of mind.* W.W. Norton & Company, New York.

112. Borsook, D., Becerra, L., and Hargreaves, R. (2006). A role for fMRI in optimizing CNS drug development. *Nat Rev Drug Discov*:1-14.

113. Wise, R.G. and Tracey, I. (2006). The role of fMRI in drug discovery. *J Magn Reson Imaging*, 23(6):862-876.

114. Tracey, I. (2001). Prospects for human pharmacological functional magnetic resonance imaging (phMRI). *J Clin Pharmacol*(Suppl):21S-28S.

115. Steward, C.A., Marsden, C.A., Prior, M.J., Morris, P.G., and Shah, Y.B. (2005). Methodological considerations in rat brain BOLD contrast pharmacological MRI. *Psychopharmacology (Berl)*, 180(4):687-704.

116. Bartz, J.A. and Hollander, E. (2006). Is obsessive-compulsive disorder an anxiety disorder? *Prog Neuropsychopharmacol Biol Psychiatry*, 30(3):338-352.

117. Nutt, D. and Malizia, A. (2006). Anxiety and OCD – the chicken or the egg? *J Psychopharmacol*, 20(6):729-731.

118. Klitgaard, H., Matagne, A., Schachter, S.C., and White, H.S. (2008). Animal and translational models of the epilepsies. In McArthur, R.A. and Borsini, F. (eds.), *Animal and Translational Models for CNS Drug Discovery: Neurologic Disorders.* Academic Press: Elsevier, New York.

119. Montes, J., Bendotti, C., Tortarolo, M., Cheroni, C., Hallak, H., Speiser, Z. *et al.* (2008). Translational research in ALS. In McArthur, R.A. and Borsini, F. (eds.), *Animal and Translational Models for CNS Drug Discovery: Neurologic Disorders*. Academic Press: Elsevier, New York.

120. Cryan, J.F. and Holmes, A. (2005). Model organisms: The ascent of mouse: advances in modelling human depression and anxiety. *Nat Rev Drug Discov*, 4(9):775–790.

121. Willner, P. (1997). The chronic mild stress procedure as an animal model of depression: Valid, reasonably reliable, and useful. *Psychopharmacology (Berl)*, 134(4):371–377.

122. Moreau, J.L., Jenck, F., Martin, J.R., Mortas, P., and Haefely, W.E. (1992). Antidepressant treatment prevents chronic unpredictable mild stress-induced anhedonia as assessed by ventral tegmentum self-stimulation behavior in rats. *Eur Neuropsychopharmacol*, 2(1):43–49.

123. Matthews, K., Christmas, D., Swan, J., and Sorrell, E. (2005). Animal models of depression: Navigating through the clinical fog. *Neurosci Biobehav Rev*, 29(4–5):503–513.

124. NICE (2002). *NICE technology appraisal guidance 43. Guidance on the use of newer (atypical) antipsychotic drugs for the treatment of schizophrenia*. National Institute for Health and Clinical Excellence, London.

125. Carpenter, W.T. and Koenig, J.I. (2007). The evolution of drug development in schizophrenia: Past issues and future opportunities. *Neuropsychopharmacology*.

126. Ditzen, C., Jastorff, A.M., Kessler, M.S., Bunck, M., Teplytska, L., Erhardt, A. *et al.* (2006). Protein biomarkers in a mouse model of extremes in trait anxiety. *Mol Cell Proteomics*, 5(10):1914–1920.

127. Kapczinski, F., Vieta, E., Andreazza, A.C., Frey, B.N., Gomes, F.A., Tramontina, J. *et al.* (2008). Allostatic load in bipolar disorder: Implications for pathophysiology and treatment. *Neurosci Biobehav Rev*, 32(4):675–692.

128. Moller, H.J. and Nasrallah, H.A. (2003). Treatment of bipolar disorder. *J Clin Psychiatry*, 64(Suppl 6):9–17.

129. Morgan, S. and Taylor, E. (2007). Antipsychotic drugs in children with autism. *BMJ*, 334(7603):1069–1070.

130. Bethea, T.C. and Sikich, L. (2007). Early pharmacological treatment of autism: a rationale for developmental treatment. *Biol Psychiatry*, 61(4):521–537.

131. Moy, S.S., Nadler, J.J., Magnuson, T.R., and Crawley, J.N. (2006). Mouse models of autism spectrum disorders: the challenge for behavioral genetics. *Am J Med Genet C Semin Med Genet*, 142(1):40–51.

132. Moy, S.S., Nadler, J.J., Young, N.B., Perez, A., Holloway, L.P., Barbaro, R.P. *et al.* (2006). Mouse behavioral tasks relevant to autism: Phenotypes of 10 inbred strains. *Behav Brain Res*.

133. Little, H.J., McKinzie, D.L., Setnik, B., Shram, M.J., and Sellers, E.M. (2008). Pharmacotherapy of alcohol dependence: Improving translation from the bench to the clinic. In McArthur, R.A. and Borsini, F. (eds.), *Animal and Translational Models for CNS Drug Discovery: Reward Deficit Disorders*. Academic Press: Elsevier, New York.

134. Sakurai, T. (2007). The neural circuit of orexin (hypocretin): Maintaining sleep and wakefulness. *Nat Rev Neurosci*, 8(3):171–181.

135. Knutson, K.L., Spiegel, K., Penev, P., and Van Cauter, E. (2007). The metabolic consequences of sleep deprivation. *Sleep Med Rev*, 11(3):163–178.

136. Marincola, F.M. (2003). Translational Medicine: A two-way road. *J Transl Med*, 1(1):1.

137. Fray, P.J., Robbins, T.W., and Sahakian, B.J. (1996). Neuropsychiatric applications of CANTAB. *Int J Geriatr Psychiatry*, 11(4):329–336.

Acknowledgements

We would like to thank our many colleagues who have pooled their knowledge and who have contributed to the creation of this book. We have enjoyed this experience of working with them on a "Global Project Team." Hopefully this sharing of our experiences will "translate" into a more efficient and fruitful use of animals to model the devastating disorders we are trying to understand, and to help us discover and develop the drugs needed to alleviate them.

We would especially like to thank Stephanie Diment, Keri Witman, Kirsten Funk and Renske van Dijk of Elsevier for their cheerful encouragement throughout this project, and without their help this book would have never been completed. We thank as well the members of our "advisory board": Professors Trevor Robbins, Tamas Bartfai, Bill Deakin; and Doctors Danny Hoyer, David Sanger, Julian Gray and Markus Heilig for their productive interventions and thoughtful discussions at various times over the past 18 months.

Finally we would like to thank all those who provided the space and opportunity so that this book could become a reality. You know who you are....

List of Contributors

Jennifer A. Bartz, PhD Seaver and New York Autism Center of Excellence, Department of Psychiatry, Mount Sinai School of Medicine, 1 Gustave L. Levy Place, Box 1230, New York, NY 10029, USA

Franco Borsini, PhD Sigma-tau Industrie Farmaceutiche Riunite S.p.A., Via Pontina km 30,400, 00040 Pomezia (Rome), Italy

Linda Brady, PhD Division of Neuroscience and Basic Behavioral Science, NIMH, NIH, 6001 Executive Blvd MSC 9641, Bethesda, MD 20892-9641, USA

Joseph D. Buxbaum, PhD Laboratory of Molecular Neuropsychiatry, Department of Psychiatry, Mount Sinai School of Medicine, 1 Gustave L. Levy Place, Box 1668, New York, NY 10029, USA

Brian Campbell, PhD Pfizer Global Research and Development, Eastern Point Road, MS 8220-4012, Groton, CT 06340, USA

Phillip Chappell, MD Pfizer Global Research and Development, MS 8260-1538, Eastern Point Road, Groton, CT 06340, USA

John F. Cryan, PhD University College Cork, School of Pharmacy, Cavanagh Pharmacy Building, Room UG06, College Road, Cork, Ireland

Timothy G. Dinan, MD, PhD, DSc Department of Psychiatry, Cork University Hospital, University College Cork, Cork, Ireland

Scott M. Doran, PhD Merck Research Laboratories, West Point, PA 19486, USA

Jamie Driscoll, BS Division of Neuroscience and Basic Behavioral Science, NIMH, NIH, 6001 Executive Blvd MSC 9641, Bethesda, MD 20892-9641, USA

Haim Einat, PhD College of Pharmacy, University of Minnesota, 123 Life Science, 1110 Kirby Drive, Duluth, MN 55812, USA

Oliver Freudenreich, MD First Episode and Early Psychosis Program, Massachusetts General Hospital, Harvard Medical School, Boston, MA 02114, USA

Jane E. Gartlon, BMedSci New Frontiers Science Park, GlaxoSmithKline, Harlow, Essex, CM19 5AW, UK

Mark A. Geyer, PhD University of California School of Medicine, Department of Psychiatry, 9500 Gilman Dr, MC 0603, La Jolla, CA 92037-0603, USA

Eric Hollander, MD Seaver and New York Autism Center of Excellence, Mount Sinai School of Medicine, Chair of Psychiatry, 1 Gustave L. Levy Place, Box 1230, New York, NY 10029, USA

Andrew Holmes, PhD NIAA, Section on Behavioral Science and Genetics, 5625 Fishers Lane, Room 2N09, Rockville, MD 20892-9411, USA

Daphna Joel, PhD Department of Psychology, Tel Aviv University, Ramat-Aviv, Tel Aviv, 69978, Israel

Declan N.C. Jones, PhD New Frontiers Science Park, GlaxoSmithKline, Harlow, Essex, CM19 5AW, UK

Thomas S. Kilduff, PhD SRI International, 333 Ravenswood Avenue, Menlo Park, CA 94025, USA

Charles H. Large, PhD Psychiatry CEDD, GlaxoSmithKline S.p.A., Via A. Fleming 4, 37135 Verona (VE), Italy

Atul R. Mahableshwarkar, MD Neurosciences Medical Development Center, GlaxoSmithKline Research and Development, Five Moore Drive, MAI-C2421, Research Triangle Park, NC 27709, USA

Robert A. McArthur, PhD McArthur and Associates, GmbH, Ramsteinerstrasse 28, CH-4052, Basel, Switzerland

Joseph P. McEvoy, MD John Umstead Hospital, Clinical Research Service, 1003 12th Street, Butler, NC 27509, USA

Klaus A. Miczek, PhD Department of Psychology, Tufts University, Bacon Hall 530 Boston Avenue, Medford, MA 02155, USA

Mark J. Millan, PhD Institut de Recherche SERVIER, Centre de Recherches de Croissy, 125 Chemin de Ronde, 78290 Croissy Sur Seine, France

Arpi Minassian, PhD Department of Psychiatry, University of California, San Diego, 200 West Arbor Drive, Mail code 8620, San Diego, CA 92103-8620, USA

Daniele Ouellet, PhD Clinical Pharmacokinetics/Modeling & Simulation, GlaxoSmithKline, Five Moore Drive, (Mailstop 17.2227), Research Triangle Park, NC 27709–3398, USA

William Perry, PhD Department of Psychiatry, University of California at San Diego, 9500 Gilman Drive, San Diego, CA 92093-8218, USA

John J. Renger, PhD Sleep Research, Merck Research Laboratories, 770 Sumneytown Pike, West Point, PA 19486, USA

Robert H. Ring, PhD Molecular Neurobiology, Depression and Anxiety Disorders, Discovery Neuroscience, Wyeth Research, CN 8000, Princeton, NJ 08543-8000, USA

Connie Sánchez, PhD Neuroscience, Lundbeck Research USA, Inc, 215 College Road, Paramus, NJ 07652, USA

Rudy Schreiber, PhD Sepracor, Inc., 84 Waterford Drive, 3-North, Marlborough, MA 01752, USA

Patricia Seymour, PhD Pfizer Global Research and Development, Eastern Point Road, Groton, CT 06340, USA

Holly Soares, PhD Pfizer Global Research and Development, Eastern Point Road, Groton, CT 06340, USA

Thomas Steckler, MD, PhD   Psychiatric Therapeutic Area, Janssen Pharmaceutica NV, Turnhoutseweg 30, 2340 Beerse, Belgium

Murray B. Stein, MD, FRCP(C) MPH   La Jolla Village Professional Center, 8960 Villa La Jolla Drive, Ste. 2243, La Jolla, CA 92037-0603, USA

Dan J. Stein, MD, PhD, FRCP   Department of Psychiatry, University of Cape Town, Groote Schuur Hospital J-2, Anzio Road, Observatory 7925, Cape Town, South Africa

Rosemary Tannock, PhD   Human Development and Applied Psychology, The Ontario Institute for Studies in Education, University of Toronto, Room 9-288, 252 Bloor Street West, Toronto, ON M5S 1V6, Canada; Neurosciences and Mental Health Research Program, Research Institute of the Hospital for Sick Children, 555 University Avenue, Toronto, Ontario M5G 1X8, Canada

Fred Turek, PhD   Center for Sleep and Circadian Biology, Northwestern University, Evanston, IL 60208, USA

Paul Wang, MD   Pfizer Global R&D, MS 8260-140, Eastern Point Road, Groton, CT 06340, USA

Paul Willner, PhD, DSC   Department of Psychology, University of Swansea, Singleton Park, Swansea, Wales SA2 8D, UK

Thomas Wessel, MD   Sepracor, Inc., 84 Waterford Drive, 3-North, Marlborough, MA 01752, USA

Lois Winsky, PhD   Molecular, Cellular and Genomic Research Branch, Division of Neuroscience and Basic Behavioral Science, NIMH, NIH, 6001 Executive Blvd MSC 9641, Bethesda, MD 20892-9641, USA

Larry J. Young, PhD   Emory University, Yerkes Research Center, 954 Gatewood Dr, Atlanta, GA 30322, USA

The Discovery and Development of Pharmacotherapy for Psychiatric Disorders: A Critical Survey of Animal and Translational Models and Perspectives for Their Improvement

Mark J. Millan

Institut de Recherches Servier, 125 chemin de Ronde, 78290 Croissy/Seine, France

Animal and Translational Models for CNS Drug Discovery,
Vol. 1 of 3: Psychiatric Disorders
Robert McArthur and Franco Borsini (eds), Academic Press, 2008

1

INTRODUCTION: PSYCHIATRIC DISORDERS, COMMON FEATURES, AND COMMON CHALLENGES

In view of the huge global burden of psychiatric disorders and the inadequacy of current treatment, intensive efforts are being made to improve their management and prevention.[1,4] While alternative therapies as diverse as deep brain stimulation (DBS) and cognitive behavioral therapy (CBT) are attracting serious attention,[5,6] pharmacotherapy is likely to remain of central importance. In the search for better drugs, it is essential to: (1) improve our understanding of the causes of psychiatric disorders, (2) clarify how currently available drugs act, and (3) identify novel treatment targets and concepts. Animal models fulfill vital roles both in realizing these goals and in determining the therapeutic potential of novel pharmacotherapy, the core concern of drug discovery. It is crucial to integrate findings from animal models with human observations in volunteers and patients: this process has been ongoing since the very advent of drug discovery and has recently been re-baptized "translational" research. The present commentary, which focuses in particular on antidepressants and antipsychotics, comprises a brief overview of the use of animal and translational models for identifying improved psychotropic drugs. Further, it emphasizes their limitations and outlines some perspectives for their amelioration. Finally, animal and translational models are placed into the broader and complex context of "R and D" (Research and Development, [Figure 1.1]).

Despite obvious differences amongst psychiatric disorders, it is worth pointing out several communalities in terms of: (1) multiple categories of symptoms and pronounced co-morbidity (Figure 1.2); (2) diverse genetic, developmental and environmental triggers differing amongst sub-populations of patients and amongst sub-sets of symptoms; (3) the implication of overarching cerebral circuits rather than any circumscribed neuronal lesion; and (4) distinctly "human" features that are difficult if not impossible to reproduce in animals, such as perturbation of language, insight, "theory of mind," social cognition, and verbal memory.[7,8] These points have important implications for the modeling and management of psychiatric states. For example, it would be foolhardy to try to develop an animal model *of* a disease as complex as schizophrenia, and a catchall paradigm reflecting all causes, reproducing all symptoms and detecting all classes of antipsychotic agent will likely never exist. Accordingly, it is more realistic to focus on models *for* particular risk factors or symptoms, and responsiveness to specific mechanisms of drug action or other treatment modes.[9-14]

ANIMAL MODELS FOR, NOT OF, PSYCHIATRIC DISORDERS: BASIC GOALS

Understanding Pathogenesis: Finding New Targets for Improved Management

Numerous animal models are available for analysing risk factors for psychiatric disorders and the pathological mechanisms underlying specific symptoms.[13,15-19] Taking schizophrenia as an example, these can be illustrated as follows: *First*, environmental: such as administration of psychostimulants, cannabinnoids, or hallucinogens.[16]

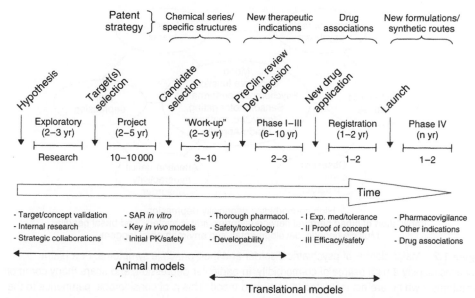

Figure 1.1   Animal and translational models as key elements of the complex process of psychotropic drug discovery and development. Animal models are crucial throughout drug discovery and development, in particular during pre-clinical phases of target validation, drug selection and characterization. Translational models bi-directionally bridge pre-clinical and clinical studies in exploiting common parameters and techniques like measures of cognitive function. "R and D" time-scales vary hugely as a function of the target, drug, therapeutic orientation – and luck. Nonetheless, from "hypothesis to launch," a core period of 15 years is incompressible, and generally things take much longer. Once a patent is taken, the clock starts to run seriously and loss of time can be costly: hence the tendency (despite the risk) to delay a patent covering the drug structure as long as possible. Subsequently, companion patents can enhance protection. During the project phase, high-throughout chemistry (HTS) may examine innumerable (mostly useless) structures, but medicinal chemistry focuses on a smaller array of relevant structures (often *not* derived from HTS). Relevant structures are characterised *in vitro* and *in vivo* in a limited set of core procedures, but more complex animal models will only be applied in the "work-up" of serious candidates. This occurs in parallel with the evaluation of safety and metabolic profiles, including occupation of drug targets in the brain. SAR, structure-activity relationships and PK, pharmacokinetics.

Second, developmental: such as post-weaning isolation, neonatal damage to the hippo-campus, or chronic exposure of young rats to the glutamatergic antagonist and "pro-psychotic" agent, phencyclidine.[20-23] *Third*, genetic: such as deletion/over-expression of specific susceptibility genes like Disrupted in Schizophrenia-1 (DISC-1), and use of mice strains with inherited alterations in behavior; including the "DBA/2J" strain that displays sensorimotor gating deficits.[24,25] In view of the multiplicity of interacting fac-tors implicated in psychiatric states, models where several factors are concomitantly manipulated are of particular pertinence; pursuing the examples above, exposure to stress of adolescent rats neonatally lesioned in the ventral hippocampus, or adminis-tration of cannabinoids to mice with genetically knocked-down N-Methyl-D-Asparate (NMDA) receptors-which are known to be dysfunctional in schizophrenia.[26,27]

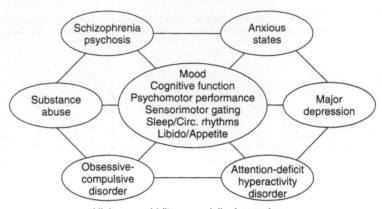

High co-morbidity: especially depression
Implication of broad cerebral networks: cortex, limbic system, and basal ganglia
Multiple genetic, developmental, and environmental triggers

Figure 1.2   Major classes of psychiatric disorder and their principle symptoms. Psychiatric diseases display a high degree of co-morbidity, in particular depression, and share many common symptoms – which are not restricted to perturbed mood. This is of considerable pertinence to the characterization of animal models, treatment concepts and drugs.

Clearly, there is also enormous scope for exploiting genetically manipulated mice, selective pharmacological agents, and technologies such as RNA silencing in characterizing the roles of cerebral modulators, and in elaborating innovative treatment strategies. However, studies of genetically modified mice are not without their problems, and there is a need for caution when extrapolating findings to the clinic.[27-31] Even if a gene (product) is implicated in the induction of a disorder, it is not necessarily a target for its treatment; causal is not synonymous with curative. Thus, a susceptibility gene may only be developmentally expressed in the young, transiently active, and/or provoke a cascade of downstream events de-coupled from the original trigger. Moreover, analogous problems are faced in deciphering the clinical relevance of targets pinpointed by use of another popular experimental strategy. Where a change in gene expression accompanies a model of, say, depression, "correlated" should not be conflated with causal.[32-34] The change may not actually underlie but rather *counter* depressed affect, or merely be an epiphenomenon. Direct intervention is required to distinguish these possibilities, since the consequences of therapeutic manipulation are radically different. Moreover, a gene can yield multiple proteins with diverse functions.[32,35-37]

Characterizing Mechanisms of Action of Clinically Effective Drugs

A further strategy for identifying novel targets lies in evaluation of the mechanisms of action of established agents. This is a far from completed task since, despite more than 20 years of intensive efforts, the therapeutic codes of selective serotonin (5-HT) reuptake inhibitors (SSRIs) and clozapine (Clozaril®) remain to be cracked.[32,38-40] As concerns the former, 5-HT$_{2C}$ receptors have been incriminated in several of their side effects (acute nervousness, nausea, decreased appetite, and sexual dysfunction), and 5-HT$_{1A}$ sites may mediate insomnia.[32,41,42] By contrast, there is still no consensus as to which transduce their beneficial actions: 5-HT$_{2C}$ sites are a controversial candidate to which may be added 5-HT$_{1A}$, 5HT$_{1B}$, 5-HT$_{2A}$, 5-HT$_4$, and 5-HT$_6$ receptors.[32,39,43,44] Very probably, as a function of the parameter under study (e.g., improved affect versus neurogenesis), several different subtypes and cerebral populations are implicated. Thus, there is no unitary, simple answer and, rather than "a" key mechanism, we should be looking for multiple components of action. Improved knowledge of how SSRIs – as well as tricyclics – act would bring us closer to the goal of concocting an ideal monoaminergic antidepressant from the diverse palette of G-protein coupled receptors (GPCRs) (29 cloned to date!), transporters and enzymes of synthesis and metabolism.[32,45-48] Similarly, if we could at last decipher the mechanism of action of clozapine, it should be possible to develop "selectively non-selective," multi-target successors sharing its beneficial actions yet divested of its undesirable side effects.[49]

Predicting Clinical Efficacy and Safety: The Core Concern of Drug Discovery

The primordial concern of R and D is to transform improved knowledge of psychiatric disorders and their causes into better pharmacotherapy. Correspondingly, the major use of animal models in an industrial context is in predicting the therapeutic efficacy of new drugs, as well as their propensity to elicit side effects. For example, determining the therapeutic margin between doses of (and exposure to) antipsychotics controlling psychosis as compared to those eliciting an extrapyramidal syndrome (EPS).[15,49,50] Predicting clinical activity is arguably the most challenging objective of animal models since, as emphasized below; the only real answers come from the clinic, providing a retrospective substantiation of the model and mechanism under study. Moreover, validation of models and drugs is very much a reciprocal affair. Drugs are vital for characterizing models that, in turn, are essential for evaluating actions of drugs; clearly, the potential danger of circular arguments must be avoided. In any case, interpretation is rarely simple. If a new drug is effective in a standard model, then it may have a profile not better than (or distinct to) that of available drugs. Yet, if inactive, it may well differ, but other arguments will be needed to push it into the clinic for proof of concept testing. Indeed, there is invariably a need to look at overall drug profiles across numerous procedures (see below).

Rather than examining the effects of drugs under baseline conditions, it is instructive to evaluate their actions in models of pathological states. For example, reversal by antidepressants of the decreased neurogenesis associated with chronic social stress, or normalization of the decreased sucrose appetite of rats exposed to chronic mild stress (CMS).[51,52] This CMS procedure has the merit of both "face" (anhedonia) and "construct" (compromised dopaminergic transmission) value, but exemplifies those complex models that cannot be employed routinely for screening large numbers of ligands: it is generally reserved for "work-up" of serious candidates. On the other hand, "high-throughput" behavioral screens of vast numbers of agents are generally inappropriate since automated procedures run the risk of error and information loss; moreover, we should be looking to *reduce* animal use where possible.[53-55] Thus, a balance between efficiency and rigor must be found in behavioral drug characterization, and rapid and simple models are needed for evaluating quite large numbers of drugs in a precocious phase of development. Hence, the continued use of the forced-swim test for antidepressants, despite notorious risk of false negatives, not least SSRIs.[56,57] In addition, empirical procedures may be used that have no major etiological relevance, but which offer a quick primary screen for *in vivo* activity as, for example, suppression of marble burying behavior in mice by antidepressants at doses that do not affect motor behavior.[58-60] Used in isolation, such "noddy" models can be misleading, but when employed in parallel with other measures, or as a precursor to more sophisticated procedures like neurochemistry, they are a useful point of departure. Moreover, they are helpful in guiding the choice of doses for more onerous protocols.

In addition to the preference for straightforward models in early screening, mice are popular in view of the small quantities of drug available and the possibility of (subsequently) integrating studies of genetically modified animals. The subcutaneous route is also often prioritized since it bypasses pharmacokinetic complications like absorption and hepatic passage during the characterization of structure–activity relationships for new chemical series. Nonetheless, at some point, data for oral (po) administration becomes essential in assessing pharmacokinetic parameters in relation to drug activity; ideally, using a quantitative "PK/PD" (pharmacokinetic/pharmacodynamic) approach to define the relationship between drug exposure (in specific compartments and tissues) to drug effect.[61] Such information is important when translating experimental observations into clinical studies (see below). Further, in addition to direct measures of drug exposure, po routes are usually preferred when estimating therapeutic margins between desirable and untoward actions. In any case, wherever possible, it is advisable to be consistent in this regard with respect to species, age, and gender as well as mode of administration. Deleterious drug actions seen upon acute, cumulative, rapid, bolus intravenous (iv) injection to anesthetized animals (though mechanistically informative) are of dubious relevance when making comparisons to effects expressed upon long-term po administration in another species (like humans). Further, it is very difficult to define "therapeutic" doses of psychotropic drugs early in their pharmacological characterization. Even at the completion of testing, one should be very prudent in specifying active doses and therapeutic margins. Not least since doses *lower* than those anticipated are often found to be effective in patients, who generally tolerate drugs better than their healthy counterparts. As pointed out below, translational research is important in addressing such issues.

COMPLEMENTARY EXPERIMENTAL PROCEDURES FOR VALIDATION OF MODELS, TARGETS, AND DRUGS

Much of the discussion above was articulated around the behavioral actions of drugs, and such information remains quintessential for new agents irrespective of their mechanisms of action. Nonetheless, a spectrum of complementary measures is best exploited in evaluating the actions of drugs in experimental models and, *ipso facto*, in characterizing the models themselves. These are schematically summarized in Figure 1.3.

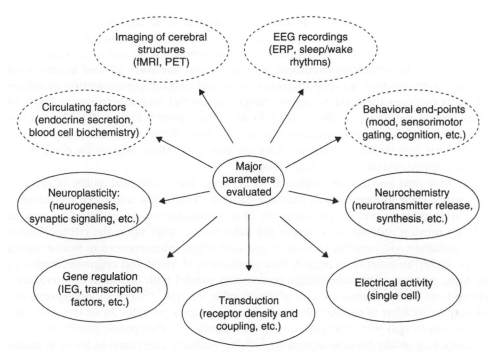

Figure 1.3 Complementary read-outs exploited in animal models of psychiatric states and the evaluation of drugs and other therapies. Though behavioral end-points remain indispensable, they should be complemented by other strategies for phenotyping animal models and evaluating the actions of drugs (see text for details). Note that certain parameters (indicated in italics and surrounded by dotted ovals) can be measured in human volunteers and patients ("translation"). Further, as detailed in the text, using Mass Resonance Spectroscopy, neurogenesis can now be tracked in the human brain and the levels of glutamate, GABA and other neuromodulators quantified. EEG, electroencephalographic; fMRI, functional magnetic resonance imaging; PET, positron emission tomography; ERP, event-related potential and IEG, immediate early gene.

At the cellular level, traditional studies of the effects of long-term drug administration on GPCR coupling and density, such as 5-HT$_{2A}$ receptor down-regulation by antidepressants, have now been expanded to their influence on markers of neuronal activity. These include transcription factors like "CREB," Immediate Early Genes like "c-fos," and Immediate Early Effector genes like "Arc".[62-65] Specific drug classes and mechanisms of action are associated with distinctive patterns of effect across discrete brain regions though there remains a need to: (1) focus more on the corresponding proteins and (2) to establish the significance of such changes in relation to changes in mood using selective inhibitors, small interfering RNA (siRNA) and genetically modified mice. This should help more clearly identify and interpret cellular fingerprints of the acute and chronic administration of drugs in relation to their behavioral actions in animal models and their clinical profiles in human.

Likewise as determined by cellular markers, there is intense current interest in the influence of drugs upon "neuronal plasticity," a seductive but somewhat nebulous term which could refer to practically anything that happens in the CNS. Likewise, though the term "neuronal resilience" is currently fashionable, it has never been clearly defined (see further below). Despite these reservations, the following observations are of note. Animal models of depression are accompanied by reduced cellular proliferation and neurogenesis (neuronal generation and survival), as well as structural changes from dendritic atrophy to axonal retraction: chronic administration of antidepressants opposes these pathological changes in parallel with alterations in levels of brain-derived neurotrophic factor (BDNF) and other growth factors.[66,67] Though the interrelationships between alterations in neurogenesis, BDNF levels and mood are still contentious, this should not distract from the utility of cellular signals for characterizing antidepressants (and other drug classes).[68,69]

An additional mechanistic approach to assessing the therapeutic utility of drugs is to examine their influence upon neuronal pathways employing single cell recording of their firing patterns and dialysis measures of neurotransmitters in discrete CNS regions of freely moving rodents. For example, the influence of drugs upon the electrical activity of glutamatergic pyramidal neurones and GABAergic interneurones in frontal cortex can be highly informative as regards their modulation of mood and cognition. Studies of the firing patterns of monoaminergic perikarya in parallel with measures of monoamine release from their terminals are also of considerable interest.[70-72] For antidepressants like SSRIs, quantification of extracellular levels of monoamines provides an *in vivo* correlate of their interaction with transporters, and an indication of therapeutic activity every bit as compelling as any behavioral read-out.[32,45,46,70] Similarly, alterations in levels of monoamines and other transmitters are highly informative in assessing the therapeutic potential of antipsychotics and anxiolytics. Interest in the influence of psychotropic drugs upon glutamate and γ-amino-butyric acid (GABA) mediated transmission is underpinned by their key importance in psychiatric states,[26,32,73-75] and by the increasing precision with which glutamate and GABA levels can be quantified in human brain (see below).

In evoking read-outs in animals common to translational models in human, the continuing significance of endocrine secretion should be emphasized, not least since many hormones act in the brain to affect mood.[32,76,77] For example, the impact of drugs upon the hypothalamo-pituitary-adrenal (HPA) axis, both basally and in interaction with stress, is a crucial variable for antidepressants and anxiolytics – and such information should arguably be generated for all drug classes.[78-81] Further, growth hormone (GH) and prolactin (PRL) release are useful signals for monitoring the functional status of specific sub-classes of monoaminergic receptor and, in the latter case, represent an essential element in the characterization of antipsychotics.[32,76,82] In a different context, diurnal scheduling of melatonin secretion provides insights into the influence of drugs upon circadian rhythms and sleep, which are profoundly perturbed in depression and other psychiatric disorders.[32,83]

A quite different, but likewise translatable, approach to monitoring the influence of drugs upon circadian rhythms, wake-sleep patterns, and sleep architecture is represented by quantitative electroencephalography (EEG). Spectral analysis can yield otherwise unaccessible information on sleep characteristics. This is important in drug development in view of: (1) the virtually universal disruption of sleep-wake scheduling in psychiatric patients and (2) the modulation of sleep and circadian rhythms by antidepressants.[32,41,84-86] The downside of comprehensive EEG recording is the complexity and lengthiness of analyses. This tends to push back EEG studies until the conclusion of preclinical studies – with the exception of drugs for treating insomnia (and epilepsy), for which EEG output is obviously the key parameter.[87,88 i] Nonetheless, rodent studies have attempted to define characteristic EEG profiles of antipsychotics, anxiolytic agents, and other classes of psychotropic drug.[50,89,90]

Finally as discussed below, driven by spectacular advances in human, techniques of neuroimaging (detailed below) are being incrementally applied to rats to characterize cerebral structures, neuronal circuits, GPCRs and transporters impacted by antipsychotics, antidepressants, and other classes of psychotropic drug.[91-96] This "reverse" translational approach should eventually switch directions. Once sufficient experience and technical expertise have been acquired, it should be possible to assimilate neuroimaging into preclinical programs of research and, in parallel with other measures summarized above, optimize the transition from animals to human.

Thus, there is an impressive variety of complementary end-points available for characterization of new models, rigorous verification of novel targets, and definition of the functional profiles and therapeutic potential of innovative drugs.

THE IMPACT OF "RATIONAL" DRUG DISCOVERY ON THE USE OF ANIMAL MODELS

Sequencing the human genome neatly demolished the naïve and anthropocentric vision that human would possess a uniquely vast genome.[97,98] Correspondingly, optimistic forecasts that several thousand high-quality drug targets would be rapidly identified evaporated to yield more well-founded and sober estimates.[99-101] Further, there is no reason why genome-derived targets should be fundamentally "superior" to others, nor why there should be a pre-programmed, streamlined route from the genome to an improved drug.[32,102,103] This has not, of course, hindered the designation of genome-driven drug discovery-aided and abetted by virtual screening, high-throughout screening (HTS) and combinatorial chemistry (CC) – as "rational," as if R and D had hitherto been *irrational*.[32,104-106] In fact, rational drug discovery by no means side steps all the usual challenges of R and D and adds some particular problems of its own (Figures 1.1 and 1.4). For example, despite progress, HTS/CC strategies are still geared toward selectivity and tend to yield structures far removed from real psychotropic drugs with required galenic, safety, pharmacokinetic, and pharmacological properties.[107-110] Further, despite some interesting findings, the huge resources invested in efforts to identify genes "for" psychiatric disorders have proven of limited, if any, relevance to the identification of novel *targets* for *drug discovery*: reliability and reproducibility of data also remains key issues.[111-113] Moreover, single gene-driven notions of psychiatric disorders and their treatment neglects the fact that: (1) mood is an *emergent* property of networks of interacting genes and neurones, not of individual proteins; (2) that essentially all genes/proteins have multiple functions, of which modulation can be beneficial and/or deleterious; and (3) multiple and variable genetic, epigenetic, developmental, and/or environmental factors account for heterogeneous psychiatric states.[32,36,114-118] As regards consequences for the use of animal models, there has

---

[i]For further discussion of measurement techniques of sleep and the effects of drugs upon sleep architecture, please refer to Doran *et al.*, Translational models of sleep and sleep disorders, in this Volume.

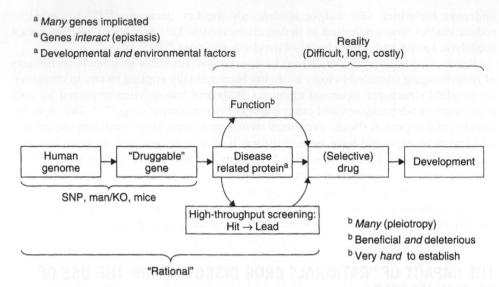

ª *Many* genes implicated
ª Genes *interact* (epistasis)
ª Developmental *and* environmental factors

Reality
(Difficult, long, costly)

Function^b

| Human genome | → | "Druggable" gene | → | Disease related protein^a | → | (Selective) drug | → | Development |

SNP, man/KO, mice

High-throughput screening:
Hit → Lead

^b *Many* (pleiotropy)
^b Beneficial *and* deleterious
^b Very *hard* to establish

"Rational"

Figure 1.4   The "rational" and the reality of genome-driven drug discovery. This dogma of "rational" drug discovery (a misnomer) from the genome to a selective drug is only part of the challenge of "R and D." It can be straightforward to find chemical "hits" but transformation of leads into real drugs is difficult, expensive and time-consuming. Genomic approaches – like single nucleotide polymorphism (SNP) studies and knockout (KO) mice – to elucidate the therapeutic relevance of gene targets are of limited power. Further, psychiatric disorders are triggered and controlled by multiple genetic, as well as developmental and environmental factors. In any case, gene function is hard to elucidate since – almost always – individual genes have several (pleiotropic) effects expressed in interaction with other genes (epistatis) and associated with both beneficial and deleterious actions. An over-emphasis on "rational" discovery of highly-selective drugs is one (though not the only) reason why the last decade has not been terribly productive for drug discovery, in particular for psychiatric disorders.

been a heavy emphasis on genetic models of target validation, all too often with little independent supporting evidence – in some cases owing to dissuasive (and ethically dubious) patents on the mice themselves.[19,31,119] Indeed, despite increasing awareness of the constraints of genetic models (see above), there has been a general tendency to neglect standard *in vivo* pharmacological approaches of drug characterization.

In its focus on "new" targets, genome-driven rational drug discovery has tended to ignore conventional, clinically validated (like monoaminergic) mechanisms despite their unfulfilled scope for improvement.[45-48] This exploration of potentially innovative mechanisms of psychotropic drug action is indisputably to be welcomed. However, a less favorable aspect has been the extreme focus on highly selective agents: despite the fact that they are *not* inherently more efficacious, rapidly active, or better tolerated than drugs acting at *several* relevant targets. Moreover, though useful against subsets of symptoms and in sub-groups of patients (see below), in contrast to multi-target drugs, selective agents are unlikely to permit broad control of the cardinal and co-morbid symptoms of psychiatric disorders.[32,102,103,105,106,120] One solution is to pursue a balanced portofolio of: (1) agents acting selectively at unexploited targets and

(2) multi-target drugs with combined actions at new *and* clinically validated targets. For example, selective neurokinin (NK$_3$) and mixed NK$_3$/D$_2$ dopamine receptor antagonists for schizophrenia. This strategy is beginning to assert itself as part of a reaction against the excessive zeal (and disappointing productivity) of genome-driven, selective drug discovery (*op. cit.*). Moreover, complementary therapies acting at higher levels of integration, from electroconvulsive therapy (ECT) to CBT may also be considered as functionally equivalent to multi-target agents.[5,6,32]

As alluded to above, the issue of multi-target versus selective drugs has repercussions for the use of animal models. Innovative classes of selective drug may require the setting-up of new animal models for their characterization and, in any case, they are likely to be effective in a more confined range of models than multi-target drugs. Accordingly, it will be more difficult to generate reliable estimations of their activity. For example, highly selective NK$_1$ or NK$_2$ receptor antagonists versus tricyclic antidepressants like clomipramine (Anafranil®), and selective D$_3$ antagonists versus atypical multireceptorial antipsychotics like olanzapine (Zyprexa®[16,121]). On the other hand, it can be difficult to pinpoint the contribution of various components of activity to the overall profiles of multi-target agents. For example, the roles of 5-HT versus noradrenaline (NA) reuptake in the actions of tricyclics and of 5-HT$_{2A}$ versus D$_2$/D$_3$ receptor blockade in the clinical actions of olanzapine still remain uncertain.[32,38,40,122]

TRANSLATIONAL MODELS: LINKING PRECLINICAL AND CLINICAL STUDIES

Revising a Paradigm: New Procedures and New Possibilities

The current search for improved animal models is one encouraging expression of renewed interest in *non*-reductionist approaches to improving the treatment of psychiatric disorders, though the much-abused terms "Systems Biology" and "Paradigm Shift" now bestowed on the (*traditional*) study of intact systems appear somewhat portentous for this welcome shift in emphasis. By analogy, the current penchant for the term "translational" (be it models, research, medicine, science, etc.) seems more to reflect the use of an *en vogue* buzz-word than a radical shift in thinking, while the embarrassingly trite and essentially meaningless turn-of-phrase, "from bench to bed-side" would best be eschewed. Indeed, the notion of "integrating preclinical information to inform human pharmacology" – a contemporary definition of translational science – is surely what we have been doing for decades: improving the link between experimental and clinical research, including measurement (where feasible) of the *same* actions of drugs in human subjects as in animals (Figure 1.5). Accordingly, today's preoccupation with translational research is less of a conceptual revolution than a procedural amendment, inasmuch as we can now appeal to hitherto-unavailable techniques like imaging. In any case, the goal of improving the transition from basic research to the clinic is crucial and, coupled to more adventurous therapeutic trials, should lead to reduced attrition in drug development, superior treatment, and better understanding of psychiatric disorders.

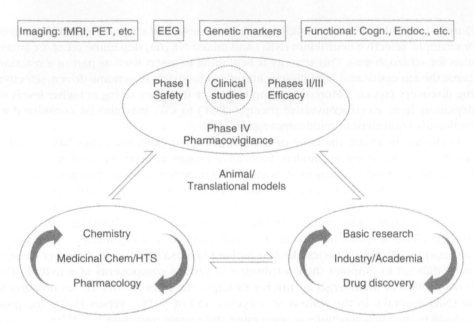

Figure 1.5 The central role of translational models in the synergistic process of "R and D" for finding improved psychotropic drugs. Basic research drives drug discovery, which reciprocally favors research in providing improved pharmacological tools. Further, the progressive improvement of new chemical structures by chemists depends upon feedback from pharmacologists who, conversely, require new drugs to refine cellular and animal models. Together these pre-clinical activities comprise one axis of synergy that is interlinked by translational models to the clinical characterisation of drugs. Further, data from human subjects is critical in comprising the only real validation of animal models, treatment strategies and novel drugs. Two-way traffic between animals and man encompasses a broad range of techniques such as neuroimaging, measures of cognition function and endocrine secretion, as well as genetic markers. PET, positron emission tomography; fMRI, functional magnetic resonance imaging and EEG, electroencephalography.

The reciprocal (and bidirectional) nature of this translational (clinical–preclinical) exchange is underscored by the current importance of imaging techniques. Their development has progressed with break-neck speed in human and they are now being applied to the rodent CNS. Though much groundwork still remains to be done (and should not be taken for granted), neuroimaging should help more effectively interlink preclinical and clinical research by: (1) providing biomarkers of prodromal psychiatric states as yet undiagnosed by clinical criteria – this would permit trials of preventative treatments; (2) improving the stratification of patients for inclusion of more homogeneous and appropriate groups into clinical studies; (3) complementary to ineluctable – but restrictive – rating-scales, evaluating (potentially throughout the course of treatment) beneficial and/or undesirable actions of drugs;[ii] (4) demonstrating drug entry into the

---

[ii] Please refer to McEvoy and Freudenreich, Issues in the design and conductance of clinical trials, or Jones *et al.*, Developing new drugs for schizophrenia: from animals to the clinic, in this Volume, or Schneider, Issues in design and conduct of clinical trials for cognitive-enhancing drugs, in Volume 2, *Neurologic Disorders* for further discussion on the use of rating scales to chart disease state and progression in clinical trials.

CNS over defined dose-ranges; and (5) characterizing neuronal networks modulated by drugs, visualizing their sites of action, and non-invasively monitoring cerebral levels of the transmitters that they affect.

Relating Drug Exposure to Drug Doses and Actions

The most obvious place to start "translating" experimental data into human is with the drug itself. Levels should be carefully quantified in the circulation and exposure related to drug doses and effects, ideally by PK/PD, Bayesian and like analyses.[61,123-125] Recently, there has been interest in Phase "Zero" studies where administration of sub-pharmacological "micro-doses" of drugs (some 100-fold lower than those predicted to be effective) can be performed even before Phase I studies.[iii] This may provide an early appreciation of pharmacokinetics; perhaps, pharmacodynamics – detection of potent and unsuspected drug actions.[126] Such information may indeed help the choice of Phase I doses and variables to be measured, but findings should be interpreted cautiously since drug exposure at minuscule doses may follow very different rules and patterns than therapeutic doses where other factors (like enzyme saturation, induction, etc.) intervene.

Circulating Biomarkers: From Hormones to Genes

Long before the now rampant marketing of the term "translational," astute clinical investigators had realized that vast amounts of information could be gleaned from blood samples in the course of early Phase I and II trials. In a few cases, measures of a neuromodulator itself can prove useful in tracking drug actions. For example, plasma levels of D-serine – a co-agonist at NMDA receptors – appear to be in equilibrium with CSF pools, so their elevation may provide an index of antipsychotic activity for certain drug classes.[26,127] Plasma levels of tryptophan, transformed centrally into 5-HT, may also be a useful marker of drug actions; notably, for a β_3-adrenoceptor agonist and antidepressant that enhances tryptophan provision to the brain (wherein β_3 sites, rather awkwardly, are barely detectable).[128] Of course, measures of transmitters and proteins in the CSF could yield important information relative to potential drug actions and psychiatric states – as recently demonstrated for Alzheimer's disease,[129,130] – but little information is as yet available and such samples can rarely be acquired.[iv]

As concerns hormonal read-outs, GH provides an index of activity at α_2-adrenoceptors while PRL secretion, under the control of D_2 and a variety of serotonergic receptors (such as $5-HT_{1A}$ and $5-HT_{2C}$), is useful in characterizing the acute and long-term actions of antidepressants and antipsychotics.[78,131,132] A critical question to be addressed for essentially all antidepressants and anxiolytics is how they affect basal and stress-induced

---

[iii] Please refer to McEvoy and Freudenreich, Issues in the design and conductance of clinical trials, in this Volume for further discussion of early Phase studies.

[iv] Please refer to Large *et al.*, Developing therapeutics for bipolar disorder: from animal models to the clinic in this Volume; Lindner *et al.*, Development, optimization and use of preclinical behavioral models to maximize the productivity of drug discovery for Alzheimer's disease, in Volume 2, *Neurologic Disorders*; Dourish *et al.*, Anti-obesity drugs: from animal models to clinical efficacy, in Volume 3, *Reward Deficit Disorders*; and others in the series for further discussion of biomarkers and their use.

activity of the HPA axis, for which determination of both adrenocorticotrophin (ACTH) and corticosterone levels provides complementary data sets.[78,79,131] Further, the dexamethasone suppression test (though not invariably reliable) has long been used as a biomarker of depression, while generally low and high (resting) levels of corticosteroids are characteristic of "atypical" and psychotic depression, respectively.[79-81,131,133] Moreover, ACTH and corticosterone are critical parameters in the clinical development of corticotrophin releasing factor (CRF) and vasopressin$_{1B}$ antagonists for anxiodepressive states.[32,77,134] For antipsychotics, induction of PRL secretion by blockade of D$_2$ receptors in lactotrophs is an important early measure of activity in human,[49,82] and can be compared to central D$_2$ receptor occupation quantified by imaging (see below). Though hyperprolactinaemia can be problematic, a more pressing concern with newer antipsychotics is their inclination to provoke obesity and diabetes: a preliminary appraisal can be derived from measures of plasma glucose in parallel with hormones like insulin and leptin.[49,135,136]

For many years, 5-HT transporters on platelets have served as surrogates for their cerebral counterparts in permitting an evaluation of the influence of SSRIs upon 5-HT reuptake in human, and in preparing the way for subsequent visualization of their occupation by imaging.[137,138] Platelets also bear 5-HT$_{2A}$ receptors with binding and coupling properties similar to those in the brain. Their functional status is possibly related to the response of negative symptoms to atypical antipsychotics, as well as providing a proxy for down-regulation of central 5-HT$_{2A}$ sites by antidepressants.[139,140] Interestingly, immunocompetent cells bear similarities to neurones, not least in their complement of diverse monoaminergic receptors and transporters.[141,142] For example, peripheral D$_3$ receptors on lymphocytes have been evoked as a putative biomarker for schizophrenia and their functional status may be related to the central actions of antipsychotic drugs.[143,144] More recently, D$_3$ sites on (T)-lymphocytes were found to control their migration, a process involving molecular substrates similar to those engaged by neurones.[145] The influence of antipsychotics on lymphoblast migration may provide insights into their modulation of neuronal migration and development, processes implicated in the induction of schizophrenia.[146,147]

Pharmacogenomic screening of blood samples (nucleated cells) for distinct isoforms of cytochromes, like 2D6, can simplify pharmacokinetic and functional studies in providing a more homogeneous group of subjects for study.[123,148,149,418] Correspondingly, variability in the exposure to and actions of drugs acting as their substrates can be reduced. While cytochromes modify drug availability, their actions may also be conditioned by the presence (and expression level) of specific alleles of target proteins.[150,151] Such information can also be derived from genetic profiling of blood cells. For example, the possession of long as compared to short forms of the 5-HT transporter has been related to mood status and sensitivity to antidepressants.[32,150,152] However, this example also illustrates the huge difficulties faced in using genetic markers to predict drug responsiveness and to select patients for trials: 5-HT$_{1A}$ receptor and BDNF genotype is likewise related to differential responsiveness to SSRIs.[32,153] Indeed, quite apart from isoforms of cytochromes, actions of psychotropic drugs are influenced by multiple genetic factors of individually minor impact.[32,153-155] Thus, despite much hope (and far too much hype), and irrespective of financial, organizational and ethical concerns, the notion of genotyping patients (volunteers) before inclusion into drug trials remains largely elusive.[123,156] Further, though subgroups of patients may show contrasting and measurable features at least partially related to genetic risk factors ("endophenotypes"), there is to date insufficient evidence that patients can be reliably identified and stratified by genetic markers alone.[10-12,157] Clinical diagnostic criteria still appear indispensable.

Sensorimotor Gating, Cognitive Performance, and Motor Behavior

Psychiatric disorders like schizophrenia and bipolar depression are characterized by interference with information processing and sensory gating. These processes can be monitored in humans by a number of procedures. Notably, pre-Pulse Inhibition (PPI) refers to the blunting of the startle reflex (eye blink) to an auditory stimulus caused by pre-exposure to a sub-threshold stimulus ~100 msec previously. On the other hand, the reduced "event-related potential" triggered by the second (500 msec later) of two clicks, termed P50 in human, is related to the "P20-N40" (N40) response in rats. Interestingly, neural substrates underpinning the P50 response and its disruption *differ* to PPI.[20,24,87,158-160] Atypical antipsychotics usually restore PPI gating deficits in schizophrenic patients and in volunteers treated with psychomimetic agents. Testing of novel agents in human can be guided by preclinical studies of their influence upon the disruption of PPI in rodents (whole body startle reflex) by pro-psychotic agents like ketamine (Ketanest®), and by developmental isolation.[161-163] Further, clozapine both counters P50 auditory deficits in patients and reduces the spontaneous N40 gating deficits (hippocampal evoked potentials) displayed by DBA/2J mice. Nicotinic modulators and histamine H_3 receptor antagonists mimic the above actions of clozapine in rodents, so these procedures should prove useful in the experimental and early-clinical evaluation of antipsychotics displaying such novel mechanisms of action.[163-166] v

Though certain components of cognition, like verbal memory, cannot be reproduced in rodents, animal models of working memory, attention and executive function, and so on provide a foundation for evaluating the actions of novel drugs upon cognition in healthy and psychiatrically ill subjects: both baseline performance and interactions with amnesic agents.[18,167-169] Such studies can most profitably be coupled to EEG and imaging.[170-173] The above-mentioned cognitive domains are of special interest since they recruit the pre-frontal cortex, a structure markedly perturbed in schizophrenia – though recent work emphasizes that the traditional notion of "hypo-frontality" is a misleading simplification[174,175,204] (see below). Improved treatment of poorly controlled cognitive symptoms of schizophrenia is a major thrust of current R and D programs.[167,175,176] This has been formally recognized by the FDA/industry/NIMH ("MATRICS/TURNS/CNTRICS") collaboration to facilitate the clinical evaluation of drugs for restoring cognitive function in psychosis.[177] However, it is important not to neglect the significance of cognitive impairment and prefrontal dysfunction in other psychiatric disorders, notably depression.[32,114,178] There is an urgent need

---

v See also Jones *et al.,* Developing new drugs for schizophrenia: from animals to the clinic, in this volume.

likewise to detect and clinically translate drugs for enhancing mnemonic function in depressed patients: this should facilitate their social and occupational re-integration.

For appropriate interpretation of studies of sensorimotor gating and cognition, it is necessary to determine the influence of drugs on general motor function, usually monitored from the very onset of human testing. This is of particular relevance to agents known to perturb motor performance, like antipsychotics (D_2 receptor antagonism) and antidepressants possessing high affinity for Histamine H_1, muscarinic and α_1-adrenoceptors, blockade of which is sedating and impairs arousal and psychomotor function.[179,180] Curiously, despite the impact of these and other drugs upon psychomotor status, which can be profoundly modified in psychiatric disorders (e.g., agitation, retardation, or disorganization), little progress has been made in quantifying complex motor behavior in humans. Nonetheless, a multivariate procedure for monitoring motor patterns both in bipolar depression *and* in a rodent model of this disorder was recently described: this would be instructive for translating actions of drugs into humans.[181]

Quantitative Electroencephalography

As pointed out above, in parallel with behavioral measures, EEG monitoring can provide complementary information on the influence of drugs on cognition and information processing.[169,171] Quantitative EEG coupled to spectral analysis has also assumed a more global role in early psychiatric drug evaluation by virtue of its ability to probe *directly* electrical events in the human brain with pronounced temporal resolution.[182,183] Its use for monitoring patterns of activity in specific (primarily hippocampal and/or cortical) cerebral circuits is of great interest since alterations in synchronization and connectivity are fundamental features of psychiatric states.[32,159,184,185]

Generally speaking, power spectra are partitioned into distinct frequency bands like delta (≤ 3 Hz), theta (4–8 Hz), beta (12–30 Hz), and gamma ($\sim$30–80 Hz): differential changes can be related to the contrasting influence of drugs upon cognition, sensorimotor integration, voluntary movement, mood, arousal, and sleep-wake cycles.[159,168,182,183,186] Rodent work has prompted the suggestion that reduced and augmented hippocampal theta rhythms may be correlated with pro-cognitive and anxiolytic properties, respectively.[90] This remains to be confirmed. In any case, several attempts have been made to correlate the influence of drugs upon EEG recordings in psychiatric patients with their clinical efficacy.[183,187] For example, EEG signals in the theta band range appear to reflect activity in cortical-hippocampal-subcortical networks incorporating the anterior cingulate cortex, a structure implicated in the control of affect. Mimicking PET studies of cingulate activity,[188] low theta power at baseline and 1 week into treatment was correlated with long-term responsiveness to SSRIs – but *not* placebo.[183,189] Assuming that such findings prove reproducible and can be extended to other classes of antidepressant agent,[183,190] EEG monitoring may become a useful guide in patient recruitment for drug trials. Similarly, asynchrony of cortical gamma oscillations, perhaps due to deficient GABAergic interneurone function, may be a biomarker of the cognitive deficits of schizophrenia – and their control.[191]

Much EEG work has been performed to quantify the influence of drugs upon circadian and sleep-wake cycles in human and rodents.[84,85,192] It still contentious whether decreased rapid eye-movement (REM) sleep is *causally* related to improved affect in depression. Nonetheless, in parallel with subjective measures of sleep and motor function, polysomnographic EEG recording early in development fulfils an important role in characterizing the impact of drugs upon arousal, sleep architecture, onset, continuity, and quality.[32,193-195] This is critical information since a favorable (or unfavorable) influence upon sleep and/or arousal has major repercussions for clinical testing and for the use of drugs in essentially all psychiatric disorders.

It should briefly be mentioned that two related techniques can add complementary information concerning the influence of drugs on electrical activity in the human brain. Magnetoencephalography, which picks up magnetic fields generated by intra-neuronal currents,[196] and Low Resolution Magnetic Imaging ("LORETA") which provides three-dimensional information on electrical activity in the brain.[197] These nascent techniques can amplify EEG studies in characterizing the effects of drugs upon neuronal oscillations, connectivity and firing patterns of neural circuits related to perturbed mood, cognition, and sleep.

Finally, diffusion tensor imaging is a fascinating counterpart to EEG in visualizing white matter tracts in the brain.[198] Its use supports the notion of disrupted connectivity in schizophrenia, depression, and OCD. However, its application to early-clinical testing is unclear since long-term exposure to drugs may be required to yield robust changes in dysfunctional circuits detectable by this procedure.[199]

Functional Magnetic Resonance Imaging (fMRI)

The (non-ionizing) technique of fMRI exploits the differential paramagnetic properties of oxy and deoxyhaemoglobin to determine local cerebral blood oxygenation level ("BOLD") dependent activity: this is considered as proportional to neuronal activity.[170,182,200,201] A further contrast to EEG is the high spatial but less pronounced temporal resolution of fMRI. Thus, fMRI and EEG have complementary roles in identifying neuronal circuits affected in psychiatric disorders and by the administration of drugs.[182,200,420] In fact, fMRI studies, performed under conditions of cognitive challenge or exposure to some other task/stimulus, have ballooned to spectacular proportions over the last few years. For example, as compared to haloperidol, atypical antipsychotics exert a more pronounced impact upon frontocortical versus striatal function in subjects undergoing cognitive tasks.[202] This is of importance in view of overwhelming evidence that a dysfunction of the frontal cortex is related to cognitive and affective symptoms of schizophrenia.[204] Further, recent work showing acute effects of antipsychotics on cerebral activation during cognitive tasks in first-episode patients underpins argument that fMRI may be useful in translational studies of new drugs.[203] However, the traditional notion that psychotic patients display "hypofrontality" (generally speaking, reduced dorsolateral prefrontal cortex activation during a working memory or executive task) appears to be an over-simplification. Recent fMRI and other studies suggest that a network of cortical and sub-cortical structures are implicated, with a complex pattern of regional-dependent hypo or hyperactivation dependent upon the precise region imaged, the cognitive load and other variables.[168,174,175,204,205] Thus, a definitive fMRI marker for schizophrenia is awaited.

Inasmuch as fMRI has progressed rapidly in humans and is now being increasingly applied to small animals, it exemplifies the notion of a "reverse" translational model.[91,94,206] Currently, the aim is to move in the opposite direction with new drugs, in comparing the "fingerprint" of their influence upon neural networks in rodents to their actions in human subjects, which can hopefully be determined early in development. Indeed, fMRI studies in humans may provide information on centrally active drug doses, as well as insights into their potential therapeutic and undesirable effects as a function of the circuits activated. For innovative mechanisms, hitherto-unsuspected sites of action and clinical indications may be revealed (at defined drug doses) early in development.[200,207,420] Moreover, the possibility of predicting drug actions on the basis of functional (and structural) MRI scans has also been evoked. For example, antidepressant efficacy of SSRIs is predicted to be faster in patients showing more marked fMRI activation of the anterior cingulate cortex by "sad" faces.[208,421] Further, antidepressants modify the fMRI response of depressed subjects to emotionally negative and positive stimuli, providing a potentially useful early marker of efficacy.[209,210]

However, the assertion that fMRI gives an "objective" read-out of brain function (whatever that means?) remains largely unsubstantiated. It is worth briefly considering certain limitations of the current use of fMRI in "R and D" in view of its status as *the* prototypical translational model; its prospective use as a biomarker for the segmentation of patient populations; and the impending application of pharmacological fMRI to the therapeutic classification and orientation of drugs early in development.

First, questions still remain concerning the reproducibility and comparability of observations within individuals (do consecutive scans over periods of days to weeks generate similar data?), between individuals (is it possible to define the fMRI "signature" of drugs in reasonably-sized groups of patients?), and across scanners and imaging centers (test conditions vary and there is as yet no real common database).[211,212]

Second, fMRI can give an early indication of centrally active drug doses, but few studies have as yet examined dose-dependent actions in relation to drug exposure.[123,124]

Third, interpretation of data remains challenging.[170,201,213] The BOLD signal is an indirect measure of a combination of excitatory and inhibitory neuronal influences quantified in a defined volume of tissue. "False negatives" may reflect changes that cancel out, while some "false positive" findings may be epiphenomena of alterations in cerebral vasculature or systemic haemodynamic variables. Though neuronal circuits affected by mood states and drugs may be identifiable, despite advances in time-resolution,[214] the temporal sequence of activation of discrete structures generally remains undefined in human studies. Further, local and remote effects of drugs cannot usually be distinguished.

Fourth, fMRI is responsive to an astonishingly wide range of natural stimuli from body shape satisfaction, tickling and trust to romantic love.[215-218] All very amusing, but some legitimate doubts are permitted as to what exactly changes in fMRI signals mean. Indeed, the very versatility and responsiveness of fMRI might be a disadvantage. This is exemplified by the influence of placebo, underpinning the need for thorough proof of the specificity of drug actions.[219,427]

Fifth, within the framework of translational use, despite a few exceptions, experimental fMRI work in rats is undertaken in anesthetized and behaviorally inactive subjects, in contrast to conscious humans performing cognitive or other tasks.[220,221] The issue of comparability arises.

Sixth, the (human) brain appears to have a "default" mode of baseline activity.[182,222,223] Interestingly, resting-state fMRI signals from the cortex appear to correlate with EEG-characterized oscillations in the low frequency delta-band as compared to evoked responses which mainly relate to gamma frequencies.[224] This suggests that their neuronal bases *differ* so more attention must be devoted to the as yet poorly studied baseline actions of drugs. The observation of increased resting state activity in the subgenual cingulate in depression (mimicking PET findings) supports this contention.[225] However, it is uncertain whether drugs exert baseline effects robust and consistent enough for systematic evaluation, reinforcing interest in studies of their influence upon signals elicited during cognitive testing, psychostimulant administration, or exposure to emotionally loaded stimuli. In this regard, issues of standardization and comparability arise – as well as the complexity of studies[200] Mathews *et al.*, 2006. Currently, there is still no well-defined fMRI response in healthy volunteers that can unambiguously predict therapeutic actions of drugs.

Finally, can we afford it? Scientific arguments for allocating resources to the preclinical/therapeutic neuroimaging of *innovative* drugs by fMRI are compelling and, at least in the long term, such information is likely to yield major insights and significant economies. However, the cost–benefit ratio is unclear today and the current environment is not exactly propitious for increasing investment in new drugs early in their clinical development.

To summarize, fMRI exemplifies the promise and pitfalls of neuroimaging in the translation of findings from animals to human, in the development of novel psychotropic agents, and in understanding the causes of psychiatric disorders. Control studies with complementary techniques like "deoxyglucose" measures of brain metabolism (see below), EEG in conscious subjects, and cellular markers of drug actions in rats can be helpful in interpreting data generated by fMRI. Nonetheless, pharmacological MRI as an approach for defining the clinical profiles of drugs remains in its infancy. Much work remains to be done with animal and translational models for its enormous potential to be realized.

Proton Magnetic Resonance Spectroscopy

Dependent on the ion imaged, Magnetic Resonance Spectroscopy (MRS) can be exploited for quantification of cerebral levels of drugs, neurotransmitters, and/or metabolites.[226-228] For example, ^{7}Li is used to detect central levels of Lithium, ^{19}F to quantify cerebral exposure to Fluorine-bearing antidepressants, and ^{P}31 for measures of phosphor-containing molecules like phosphodiesterases and phosphoinositides. Nevertheless, in the characterization of psychiatric disorders and the actions of psychotropic agents, most attention has focused to date on proton (^{1}H)MRS.[226-228] Using this technique, a very recent study detected a distinctive spectral peak of fatty acids characteristic of progenitor neuronal cells in human and rodent brain.[229] This signal may constitute a long-sought means of monitoring the influence of drugs upon neurogenesis in humans. MRS has been more widely used to determine levels of *N*-acetyl-aspartate (NAA), a mitochondrial marker for neuronal energy turnover and integrity. Though its levels do not seem to be markedly affected by antipsychotics, there is evidence for an early-onset reduction of NAA levels in frontal and other cortical regions in schizophrenia that is correlated with cognitive impairment.[230,231] NAA reductions may be a useful biomarker for precocious detection of psychotic states and instigation of therapy.

Proton MRS is also being exploited to determine cerebral levels of GABA, and of glutamate and its precursor, glutamine, which are frequently read as a composite "glx" signal. This is important since glutamatergic and GABAergic transmission is markedly affected in psychiatric disorders and modulated by many classes of psychotropic agent.[26,75,228,230,232] Thus, proton MRS provides a tool for tracking the influence of drugs upon GABAergic and glutamatergic signaling in human, and relating these effects to actions measured in rats by electrochemistry and microdialysis.[32,75,232,422] For example, metabotropic (2/3) agonists attenuate glutamatergic transmission and are attracting interest as potential antipsychotics and/or anxiolytics: in parallel with fMRI analysis of neuronal circuits, their neurochemical effects in human could be evaluated by MRS.[233,234]

MRS analyses of schizophrenia suggest elevated hippocampal and frontocortical levels of glx (likely glutamate) in young and asymptomatic, high-risk subjects, indicating its pertinence as a biomarker of the prodrome.[235-237] This change may be regionally selective and/or time-dependent since lower levels were seen in the anterior cingulate cortex in chronic schizophrenia, while data were contradictory for the frontal cortex.[238,239] Changes in chronic schizophrenia may reflect an influence of treatment, but to date there is little concrete information from MRS concerning the effects of antipsychotics upon glutamatergic and GABAergic transmission in psychotic patients (above citations). Nonetheless, the pro-psychotic agent, ketamine, rapidly increases glutamate levels in cingulate cortex.[240] Consequently, MRS studies of the effects of antipsychotics should be feasible early in development, though much work remains to define their basic patterns of effect.

Proton MRS studies in human gel well with findings from animal models suggesting a glutamatergic excess and a GABAergic underactivity in anxious states.[74,241,242] Further, probably related to a disruption of glial function, there is convincing evidence from proton MRS for a GABAergic deficit in depression, and for a suppressed glx signal in the cortex of melancholic depressives.[75,243,244] Supporting the role of MRS in drug characterization, SSRIs and ECT both elevate levels of GABA in the occipital cortex of depressed patients and, like transcranial magnetic stimulation, they have been reported to increase glx levels in volunteers.[228,245,424,426] MRS suggests that cortical levels of glutamate and glx are augmented in bipolar depression, together with reductions of NAA. Intriguingly, opposite changes appear to be induced by lamotrigine (Lamictal®) and/or lithium, at least in volunteers.[246-248]

Clearly, despite technical challenges, MRS complements EEG and fMRI in its potential for detecting *neurochemical* biomarkers of psychiatric states and for characterizing the actions of novel psychotropic drugs early in development.

Positron Emission Tomography and Single Photon Emission Computerized Tomography

By analogy to fMRI, the nuclear imaging (gamma ray emitting) technique of positron emission tomography (PET) can indirectly provide insights into neuronal activity and synaptic transmission, but by use of a complementary approach.[249-251] Cerebral blood flow can be measured using ^{15}O-H_2O with good temporal resolution in view of its short half-life, while "FDG-PET" exploits a ^{18}F-tagged, stable analog of glucose, ^{18}F-2 fluoro-2-deoxyglucose, to monitor cellular metabolism. As compared to ^{15}O-H_2O PET and fMRI, FDG-PET is less easily influenced by haemodynamic factors.[249,252] Many studies have found altered metabolic rates of glucose use in the prefrontal and cingulate cortex of depressed patients. Though it is not clear exactly how these findings relate to the perturbed neuronal activity detected by fMRI (*vide supra*), changes may provide a predictor or marker of responsiveness to treatment.[253,254] Accordingly, in parallel with fMRI imaging, FDG-PET is instructive for comparing the influence of antidepressants to other therapies (like CBT and sleep deprivation) upon cerebral patterns of glucose utiliation.[253-255] Though the effects of various treatments are not identical, several studies suggest that antidepressants reduce glucose metabolism in sub-territories of the frontal cortex, and possibly increase metabolism in the temporal cortex.[254-256] Thus, such approaches may offer an early indication of therapeutic activity and, perhaps, help identify sub-sets of patients.

PET imaging also mirrors fMRI in that much progress was initially made in human. This has subsequently been "reverse" translated into small animals for which (microPET) techniques are progressing rapidly, despite the obvious need to keep the subject immobile *without* stress or discomfort which implies anesthesia since asking nicely is seldom sufficient.[91,94,129]

A further important analogy to fMRI is quite simply the enormous significance of PET to translational research. Where possible, a Phase I PET study of dose (exposure) and time-dependent occupation of specific populations of cerebral target(s) is an indispensable point of departure for translational and clinical evaluation of new ligands. Accordingly, despite the inherent difficulties of finding PET ligands with appropriate characteristics (and the need for their generation in close proximity to scanners owing to short half lives of ^{11}C, ^{18}F, ^{15}O, and ^{13}N), a whole succession of PET ligands are emerging for determining the interaction of new glutatamergic, cholinergic, GABAergic, adenosinergic, and so on drugs with their targets – usually GPCRs, transporters and channels.[249,257,428] In such PET studies, the key variable is the "Binding Potential" which corresponds to the Bmax/Kd *in vitro* and is determined by the distribution volume of the specially bound radiotracer, in turn equivalent to the ratio of tissue concentration to free concentration in plasma (proxy for the brain) at equilibrium.[249,258] The following examples exemplify the broad utility of PET studies, as well as certain limitations.

Of PET labels available for monoamine reuptake sites, several highly selective agents that specifically label sub-cortical populations of 5-HT transporters (SERTs) have been described though, despite intensive efforts, cortical SERTs remain less accessible.[257,259,260,428] PET quantification of SERT availability has been used to relate the functional status of limbic serotonergic transmission to the response to emotional stimuli. Such measures may be useful in the characterization of anxiety-related traits and in the incorporation of patients genotyped for short versus long alleles of the 5-HT transporter into clinical trials.[152,261] PET has also been extensively used in the evaluation of antidepressant agents. A good correlation has been found between plasma levels of antidepressants and occupation of cerebral SERTs, with 80–85%

needed for robust efficacy.[259,262,428] Thus, in parallel with studies of platelet 5-HT reuptake and endocrine read-outs, PET labeling of central 5-HT transporters was invaluable in the clinical evaluation of drugs like the SSRI, escitalopram (Lexapro®/Cipralex®).[260] A further target of putative antidepressants, NK_1 receptors,[32,263] are also privileged by the availability of excellent PET ligands. Their application has been made in rather different, though equally instructive, circumstances. Despite encouraging results in early-clinical trials, NK_1 antagonists like MK869 (aprepitant, Emend®) proved disappointing in the treatment of depression. This led to a meticulously designed study where it was demonstrated that, despite dose-dependent and pronounced occupation of central NK_1 sites, the therapeutic activity of a novel NK_1 receptor antagonist was insufficient – though equivalent data for MK869 itself are unavailable.[264,265]

PET studies of D_2 receptor occupation have proven informative both in quantifying their occupation by drugs and in determining their degree of occupation by endogenous ligands (mainly dopamine), basally and in response to psychostimulants.[266] Under resting conditions, there is significant baseline occupation of D_2 sites that is increased (reflected in the reduced binding potential of PET radioligands) upon administration of amphetamine. Though the possibility of D_2 receptor internalization should not be ignored,[267] this method has shown that mesolimbic dopaminergic pathways are overactive and/or hyper-responsiveness in schizophrenics – a useful marker of psychotic states.[250] Further, there is much current interest in putative antipsychotic agents that moderate the hyperactivity of mesolimbic dopaminergic projections, like $5\text{-}HT_{2C}$ agonists.[268] Their actions could be evaluated early in human by PET estimations of D_2 receptor availability.

This therapeutic strategy is an alternative to the more conventional approach of directly blocking postsynaptic D_2 receptors by antipsychotic agents like haloperidol and clozapine. Following on from imaging and functional studies in animal models, PET imaging is a quasi-obligatory step upon their introduction into the clinic inasmuch as essential information on CNS entry and occupation of central D_2 receptors at defined times and doses can be generated with a variety of excellent, radiolabeled antagonists. PET quantification suggests that 65–75% of D_2 sites need to be blocked for efficacy against positive symptoms, while a greater magnitude of occupation (~80–90%) may evoke an EPS[249,266,269] (Note that beneficial actions are likely mediated in limbic and associative regions, in contrast to EPS effects induced in motor-striatal structures, though this has not as yet been directly shown by PET). Such PET studies can complement clinical and experimental data in differentiating various classes of drug. Thus, aripiprazole (Abilify®) can occupy a higher proportion of sites without the risk of EPS due to its partial agonist properties.[270,271] Further, clozapine may exert antipsychotic actions at lower levels of D_2 receptor occupation, possibly due to its rapid dissociation kinetics,[272] but also reflecting its actions at other PET-imaged sites like $5\text{-}HT_{1A}$, $5\text{-}HT_{2A}$, and D_1 receptors.[249,273]

More recently, newer radiotracers like ^{11}C-FLB-457 and ^{18}F-fallypride have rendered it possible to visualize anatomically and functionally distinct sub-populations of D_2 sites in striatal, limbic, and cortical regions of human and primates: this should yield additional insights into the potential effects of new antipsychotics when adopted precociously in their development.[274-276] In fact, these and other radiolabeled receptor antagonists, like all clinically exploited antipsychotics themselves, fail to discriminate D_2 from D_3 sites for which their affinities are essentially identical. Inasmuch as the significance of D_3 versus D_2 receptor occupation for treating schizophrenia (and other disorders) is still uncertain,[121] it is of some importance that the preferential D_3 versus D_2 radiolabeled receptor agonist, [^{11}C] "PHNO," appears to label cerebral D_3 sites, notably in the (primate) globus pallidus, part of a circuit implicated in the control of mood and cognition.[277-279] [^{11}C]PHNO should prove of considerable utility in characterizing psychotic states, and in comparing the actions of antipsychotics at D_3 versus D_2 sites in humans. Anticipating clinical evaluation of selective D_3 ligands, this could help decipher the genuine role of D_3 versus D_2 receptors in CNS disorders and their management.[121,280]

Finally, it is important to evoke the issue of radioligand "asymmetry." While receptor antagonists effectively displace both agonist and antagonist radioligands, receptor agonists tend to poorly displace antagonists. This can have implications for the interpretation of PET observations. For example, D_2/D_3 receptor agonists may be more susceptible to displacement by endogenous dopamine than their antagonist counterparts.[266,278,279,281,282] Further emphasizing this point, drugs acting as 5-HT$_{1A}$ receptor agonists like the antipsychotic, ziprasidone (Geodon®), are weakly effective in displacing the radiolabeled antagonist, [^{11}C]WAY100,635, in PET studies of cerebral 5-HT$_{1A}$ receptors.[249,283] The probable explanation is not insufficient potency, or that agonists only need a low degree of 5-HT$_{1A}$ receptor occupation for functional actions (huge receptor reserve). Rather, agonists and antagonists may interact with contrasting binding sites on 5-HT$_{1A}$, – as well as D_2 and other classes of GPCRs.[32] Ideally, then, as for binding studies *in vitro*, agonists and an antagonists should ideally be available for PET imaging. This is quite a challenge, but efforts to generate newer and more specific PET ligands are justified in view of the importance of PET data in the translational evaluation of new drugs.

Like PET, the related technique of single photon emission computerized tomography (SPECT) generates 3D images of the brain using a radioactive label. Since SPECT nuclei have longer half-lives than their PET counterparts, accelerators do not have to be located close to scanners and SPECT is less expensive, though spatial resolution is usually less impressive than PET.[226,249,251,254] A good example is the use of SPECT to visualize central 5-HT transporters with high specificity and sensitivity.[259] Further, [^{123}I]epidepride has been used to compare the preferential occupation of limbic and cortical versus striatal populations of D_2/D_3 receptors by atypical antipsychotics like amisulpride (Solian®).[284] Finally, the SPECT label,^{123}I-CNS-1261, is a NMDA antagonist of use for evaluating the influence of drugs upon the occupation of NMDA receptors, which are thought to be hypoactive in schizophrenia.[26,285,286] Thus, SPECT also has its role to play in the translational characterization of new ligands.

ANIMAL AND TRANSLATIONAL MODELS FOR PSYCHIATRIC DISORDERS: SCOPE FOR REFINEMENT

Modeling New Targets: Glia, Intracellular Proteins, Neuronal Plasticity, and Epigenesis

As routinely trotted out in all discussions of this genre, we likely need improved models for psychiatric disorders; and we definitely need a clearer idea of just how well the ones we already have predict drug efficacy, the overriding preoccupation of "R and D".[9,15,17,57,419] However, this will not be easy to acquire since: (1) false negatives do not generally make it into humans and (2) it takes time to generate really solid data in therapeutic trials. In any case, as pointed out above, it would be futile to attempt to fully reproduce a truly human disease like schizophrenia, with all its perturbation of thought, language, insight, and theory of mind, in an animal. Irrespective of the clinical pertinence of models, there is a need to identify novel mechanisms for treating and preventing psychiatric disorders. Thus, as we are likewise regularly reminded (*op. cit.*, other chapters), we will likely need new procedures responsive to *innovative* drug mechanism of actions. In this regard, the following broad lines of research deserve mention.

One intriguing piste would be to devise models for characterizing more directly the significance of glial and microglial cells in the pathogenesis and modulation of psychiatric states, and to elucidate their potential as targets for innovative drugs.[26,287,288]

A further idea would be to find new procedures for evaluating the utility (and safety) of drugs acting at targets downstream of and/or interacting with membrane-localized transporters, channels, and GPCRs: for example, intracellular proteins regulating their localization and signaling, modulating synaptic structure and transmission, and controlling gene transcription[66,100,289] (Figure 1.6). Nonetheless, despite massive interest, nobody really knows how to manipulate such targets selectively in specific CNS structures (which is exactly what channel, GPCR, and transporter-directed drugs so effectively do!), nor how best to apply and monitor such mechanisms clinically.[32,46]

One promising line of research in this context focuses on neuronal plasticity, and the prevention (or reversal) of structural-functional alterations provoked by chronic stress and neurodevelopmental insults.[2,66,67,289] However, the term "neuronal plasticity" remains very vague and, to the skeptic, covers virtually anything and everything that happens in the brain (19 850 hits in Medline as of February 2008!). There is, thus, a need for clearer conceptual and operational definitions of what exactly is meant if we wish: (1) to develop drugs for enhancing "neuronal plasticity" and improving "neuronal resilience" and (2) to show such effects in animal models, translational research, and clinical trials. One source of ideas might be the original engineering and ecological definitions.[290–293] The former refers to the time needed to get back to the original condition (equilibrium) after disturbance. The latter relates to the degree of disruption tolerated before a shift to an alternative state. In the former case, coping will have succeeded and permanent damage has not been sustained; for example, the return of the HPA axis to quiescence following a severe threat. In the latter case, a threshold will have been transgressed, resilience overcome, and damage has ensued; for example, permanent excitotoxic damage to hippocampal cells following chronic stress.[80,81,294] Recurrent and multiple stressors are the most dangerous (like excess glutamate plus corticosteroids), and there may be several cycles of attack and recovery followed by relapse. An encouraging trend in studies of plasticity is the recent crystallization of methods for evaluating the influence of antidepressants upon hippocampal neurogenesis[67,68] and, very recently, a procedure appropriate to its translational tracking in human was revealed (see above).

Though still very fashionable and not just pertinent to depression,[69] neurogenesis has recently been "out-cooled" by a yet trendier focus of animal models: epigenetics. This refers to mechanisms for transmission of information during cell division other

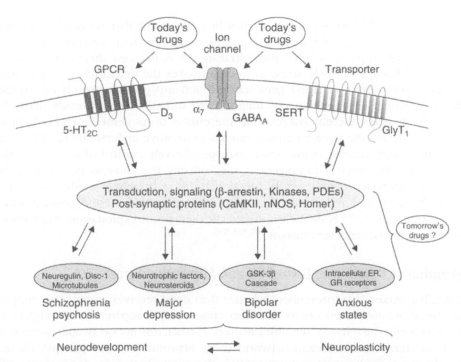

Figure 1.6   Putative drug targets for the future treatment of psychiatric disorders. With a few
exceptions, such as monoamine oxidase inhibitors, currently available drugs act at proteins
localized on the neuronal plasma membrane, like G-protein coupled receptors (GPCR),
monoamine transporters and ion channels. Many such targets, and combinations thereof,
still await clinical exploitation, but there is increasing interest in novel, downstream targets: in
particular, proteins related to susceptibility genes and developmentally incriminated in the genesis
of psychiatric disorders. However, it is unclear how these targets can be specifically, safely
and effectively exploited, and how their modulation can be monitored in patients. Animal and
translational models should help answer these questions. SERT, 5-HT transporter; GlyT, glycine
transporter; $\alpha 7$, $\alpha 7$-nicotinic; PDE, phosphodiesterase; CaMKII, calmodulin kinase II;
nNos, neuronal nitric oxide synthase; ER/GR, estrogen/glucocorticoid receptor; GSK, glycogen
synthase kinase; and DISC, dysregulated in schizophrenia.

than *via* the DNA sequence itself. Though small species of RNA are involved, epigenetics generally relates to histone acetylation, methylation and other changes that
modify gene expression (access to transcription factors), and to altered methylation
of DNA itself.[295,296] Meiotic imprinting is important since it implies that the emotional status and stress sensitivity of the parents (especially the mother) can have epigenetic – not just "environmental" – consequences for offspring.[297-299] On the other
hand, mitotic epigenetic changes concern life-long (and tissue-specific) alterations in
gene transcription (a form of phenotypical plasticity). Factors suspected to trigger
trait changes in mood include negative experiences as an infant, and hypoxia during birth, a risk factor for schizophrenia.[300,301] Illustrating the interest of epigenetics,
prefrontal dysfunction in schizophrenia may involve chromatin modification.[302] As a
further example, a down-regulation of reelin and GABA synthesis has been reported
in cortical interneurones, and reelin knockout mice display behaviors reminiscent of

psychosis.[232,301,303,304] Experimental studies in rats suggest that reduced reelin and GABA levels reflect hypermethylation of the promoters for their synthesis, and pharmacological interruption of DNA methyltransferase re-induced their expression.[305] As a second example, chronic stress in mice provokes the demethylation of histone H3 leading to repression of BDNF gene transcription and, possibly, associated changes in mood. Chronic administration of imipramine (Tofranil®) de-represses BDNF by hyperacetylating H3, thereby overcoming the effects of its demethylation.[306] These examples underpin the need for animal models to improve understanding of the role of epigenetic mechanisms in the onset and, speculatively, control of psychiatric disorders. Supporting interest in epigenetic mechanisms, the anti-epileptic/anti-bipolar agent, valproate (Depacon®), exerts functional effects in animal models of schizophrenia that appear to reflect modification of histone acetylation and, possibly, other epigenetic actions.[307-309] Nonetheless, systematic therapeutic exploitation of epigenetic mechanisms would seem very distant.[301,303,304]

Prevention of Psychiatric Disorders and Alleviating Stress

The familiar maxim that "prevention is better than cure" receives unexpected support from the above-mentioned observations on epigenetics – apparently, this applies to parents as well, which hardly simplifies matters. Further, this notion is underpinned by models of complex, non-random networks (from neurones to social groups). Though networks are generally resistant to disruption, damage to key nodes (or multiple, secondary nodes) can provoke widespread disorganization and a phase-shift to an alternative and pathological attractor that is hard to lever back to the original condition (see further below).[32,102,310,311] Indeed, though one should not be fatalistic (there are exceptions), well-established psychiatric states like severe, relapsing depression, panic attacks, and schizophrenia often prove to be life-long affairs;[3] hence, the importance of precocious intervention. For example, exposure of children and adolescents to social and other forms of stress can induce permanent alterations in neural and neuroendocrine function associated with changes in emotionality, cognition, and vulnerability to psychiatric problems as an adult.[312-316] Wait and see strategies may appear sensible but can be ill advised. It is unfortunate if pharmacotherapy is belatedly introduced essentially as a "last resort" when it could have more effectively been adopted earlier.[32]

These comments accentuate the need to use animal models for more intensive study of the early phases of psychiatric disorders in the hope, together with translational work in humans, of finding genetic, endocrine and cognitive biomarkers, and of designing effective pro-active treatments. However, biomarkers will need to be highly reliable and well validated, and the question arises of how to apply them, a hornet's nest of ethical, socioeconomic, and scientific challenges.[317,318] At-birth genomic sequencing aside, one can hardly imposes universal screening on all 14-year olds in an attempt to identify the 1% or so at high risk for schizophrenia. Further, biomarkers assume that the vulnerable individuals *wish* to be identified, which may be unlikely if appropriate prophylactic treatment is not available – something of a "Catch-22." Despite these *caveats*, animal models should focus on broadly relevant triggers of psychiatric states such as drug abuse, social isolation and excessive stress,[294,319,320] and on the development of therapies for early intervention once the diagnosis is quasi-certain and the need for treatment undisputed.

In focusing on risk factors for psychiatric disorders, the issue of stress is inescapable: both in the young (as mentioned above) and in the adult. Indeed, it might be argued that stress (disruption of homeostasis) is something of a Lowest Common Denominator – and symptom – of virtually all psychiatric states.[80,81,131,294,314] Further, there is increasing evidence for the broad disruptive impact of aversive stimuli upon glial, immune, and neuronal function in the brain,[287,288] while HPA axis overdrive coupled to CRF hyperactivation has been incriminated in the deleterious effects of uncontrolled stress.[77,79,131,314] There is a need to exploit animal models for a better understanding of the effects of stress, in particular low level and recurrent, unpredictable, and uncontrolled stress. This should help us devise concepts for countering its extreme and negative consequences, while respecting the positive attributes of stress when controlled and of limited duration and intensity.[131,294,314] For example, the HPA axis is modulated around a set point: pathological and prolonged hyperactivity should not be moderated at the price of compromised baseline circadian secretion.

Modeling Non-pharmacotherapeutic Strategies

In exploiting animal models of stress and other factors favoring psychiatric disorders, it is important to remember that pharmacotherapy is *not* the only solution adopted for their *prevention* and control.

The term "alternative" therapy is perhaps inappropriate, and it should not be construed as pejorative inasmuch as "complementary" approaches to countering stress and maintaining psychological equilibrium fulfill important roles in the lives of many people.[321,322] Indeed, approaches other than pharmacotherapy are often preferred for the alleviation of (at least minor) states of low mood, anxiety, and heightened stress-sensitivity.[323-327] Though it is premature to conclude, several complementary procedures are currently undergoing controlled therapeutic evaluation – alone or as adjunctive therapy – for the amelioration of mood disorders, including yoga,[328] aromatherapy,[329] light exposure,[330] exercise,[331] and meditation.[332] As can be gauged from these examples, some interventions cannot be modeled in animals, and neither can (somewhat disconcerting) attempts to affect "psychotherapy"*via* the internet and e-mails.[333-335] Nonetheless, certain complementary strategies can, at least partially, be reproduced in animals such as the influence of exercise, light exposure, defined herbal treatments (phytotherapy), dietary supplements and even aromas.[336,337,338,416] This is of some consequence for several reasons. *First*, complementary treatments may be combined with drugs – even during clinical trials without the investigator being aware. More generally, it should be possible to harmonize positive effects of complementary interventions with those of drugs.[326,339,340] *Second*, though "natural" treatments like plant extracts are often considered inherently safer than drugs, the modest examples of morphine, digitalis, aspirin, and penicillin tend to suggest otherwise. For example, omega-3 fatty acids were recently reported to possess immunosuppressive properties at high doses.[336,341,342] Thus, possible risks should be evaluated. *Third*, phytotherapy still holds many secrets, and insights into the mechanisms of (beneficial and undesirable) actions of specific plants constituents may provide leads toward novel classes of pharmacological agent.[337]

In the same spirit, there is a need further to develop animal models of other modes of potential therapy that tend to be instituted late in the course of disorders – generally in the wake of unsatisfactory response to drugs. These include: (1) ECT, which can be highly effective in otherwise refractory depression; (2) DBS of the subgenual cortex, effective even where ECT fails, but still at the experimental phase; (3) vagal nerve stimulation, likewise for resistant mood disorders; and (4) transcranial magnetic stimulation, which is under investigation both in depression and in schizophrenia.[5,32,34,343,344] All these interventions – and sleep deprivation which can rapidly (*albeit* transiently) improve affect – harness broad neural circuits and mobilize a variety of neurochemical substrates. That is, they exert network-coordinated (multi-target) actions very different from those of highly selective drugs. Ideally, the goal is their "transformation" into more accessible pharmacotherapy.

Finally, inter-personal therapy, CBT, behavioral activation and related techniques are attracting increasing attention for the control, prevention and perhaps (at least for CBT) *durable* treatment of depression and anxiety both alone[6,345-347] and – likely most effectively – in combination with pharmacotherapy.[326,348-350] Ongoing studies are also evaluating the utility of CBT in the treatment of other disorders like OCD and schizophrenia.[55,345,351,352,423] Despite encouraging findings, it would be premature to conclude concerning long-term efficacy, cost-effectiveness, practicability, and overall patterns of therapeutic effects across large and heterogeneous populations of (often co-morbid) patients. Moreover, the relationship of psychotherapeutic approaches to placebo arms of clinical trials is an important question,[219,349,350] and both psychological and social support is an important part of any drug treatment program.[294,324,353] Nonetheless, procedures like CBT are focused and specific techniques (which should be) practiced by specialists.[6,352] Though they cannot realistically be modeled in animals, translational techniques of imaging are providing important insights into their mechanisms of action. Of considerable interest are studies comparing the neuronal and neurochemical substrates recruited by CBT to those engaged by conventional antidepressants, inasmuch as there appear to be both common and distinct substrates.[255,256,354,355] The pursuit of such investigations may yield insights into novel mechanisms for the control of psychiatric disorders (translatable back into animal models) and, hence, improved classes of psychotropic agent – though CBT "in a pill" may be a logical impossibility.

Modeling Long-term and Unwanted Drug Actions

For practical reasons, most preclinical screening is undertaken with acute administration. Clinical candidates are also usually evaluated upon chronic treatment bearing in mind that they will be used in this way in patients, and in light of the regulatory requirement for showing long-term therapeutic activity of drug classes like antidepressants. Nonetheless, there is a need for more systematic and broad-based evaluation of the actions of drugs upon prolonged administration: both in "acute" animal models like inhibition of amphetamine-locomotion (for an antipsychotic) and in developmental models like post-weaning isolation where both short and long-term actions should be measured – in the latter case, in the above-evoked context of preventative therapy. One obvious issue is to show that drug actions are maintained and that there is no major problem of tolerance (progressive loss of efficacy).[32,356]

Moreover, animal models should also directly address the issue of what happens upon stopping treatment. Remarkably little is known for most drugs, despite the fact that discontinuation frequently occurs in patients due to a variety of causes – either autonomously or upon consulting a doctor: unacceptable side effects, unsatisfactory efficacy, poor compliance, involuntary failure to take medication and the conviction that one is cured.[32,326,355,357,358] Questions of tolerance, dependence and withdrawal need to be examined in a drug-by-drug and class-by-class manner. For example, the effects of long-term administration then discontinuation of a benzodiazepine are likely to be very different to those of a CRF_1 antagonist in the treatment of anxiety.[359,360] The same holds true for a β_3-adrenoceptor agonist for treating depression compared to a SSRI.[361,362] The latter agents also illustrate the importance of kinetics. Due to its short half-life, paroxetine (Seroxat®/Paxil®) is more likely to be accompanied by a discontinuation syndrome (and rapid recrudescence of symptoms) than fluoxetine (Prozac®), which possesses an active metabolite (nor-fluoxetine) with a very long elimination time: "tapering" of doses is recommended at the end of treatment for the former agent.[362,363]

However, precisely for this reason, the issue of substitution (owing to tachyphylaxis, irresponsiveness, or poor tolerance, etc.) can be problematic for drugs like fluoxetine. Irrespective of pharmacokinetic factors, there is a dearth of information from animal models on drug switching. This is surprising in view of the substantial proportion of patients who fail to react sufficiently to a first choice antidepressant or antipsychotic.[355,357,364,365,429] Evaluation in animal models of how a new drug acts in the wake of a standard agent is important, not least for early-clinical studies where patient selection is crucial. (Further, the less agreeable question of switching treatment when one's *own* drug is inadequate should not be neglected.) A good clinical example is provided by 5-HT_{1A} agonists for anxiety. Following pre-treatment with benzodiazepines, anxiolytic properties of the partial 5-HT_{1A} agonist, buspirone (Buspar®), are initially compromised.[359,366] On the other hand, illustrating a positive aspect of studying actions of a drug after long-term exposure to another class, animal models suggest that CRF_1 antagonists are still effective following benzodiazepines and that they suppress withdrawal symptoms.[367] Moreover, CRF_1 antagonists likewise attenuate undesirable consequences of stopping chronic treatment with other drug classes like nicotine and opioids, and there is currently much interest in drugs that reduce the risk of relapse in drug-seeking behavior.[368,369] By analogy to buspirone, it is likely that the impact of novel, non-sedating antipsychotics will differ in patients accustomed to drugs like haloperidol (Haldol®) and quetiapine (Seroquel®) as compared to naïve subjects whom have never been treated. Quite apart from animal models, there is no reason why translational approaches like imaging should not explore how drugs with novel mechanisms of action behave in naïve patients as compared to subjects pre-treated (successfully or unsuccessfully) with other drug classes.

As pointed out above, imaging and other translational paradigms are also useful for revealing potentially undesirable effects of drugs; in certain cases, based on pre-clinical work, and in others based on clinical experience with a specific drug class (like hyperprolactinaemia with antipsychotics). However, for drugs with innovative mechanisms, there can be relatively few "guide-lines" as to what to look for. This partly reflects the greater motivation of focusing in pre-clinical work on target-mediated *efficacy* rather than untoward effects.

Moreover, this tendency has perhaps been reinforced by the mind-set of rational drug discovery that tends to consider highly *selective* drugs as inherently safer than their multi-target counterparts. Yet, quite apart from unpleasant *off*-target surprises reflecting unfamiliar chemical structures and idiosyncratic drug reactions, this is not necessarily true. For example, highly selective drugs are more likely than polyvalent drugs to provoke an imbalance (one thinks of rofecoxib [Vioxx®], a selective COX 1 versus COX 2 inhibitor) and to disrupt the equilibrium of complex circuits (like haloperidol versus clozapine).[32,106] Furthermore, the adding-in of complementary components of activity can *counter* side effects and *improve* tolerance; for example, 5-HT_{1A}, 5-HT_{2A}, or D_3 receptor antagonism for opposing D_2 receptor blockade-mediated EPS, and 5-HT_{2C} receptor blockade for reducing SSRI-elicited sexual dysfunction and anxiety.[38,50,121] Finally, as exemplified by adjunctive use of H_3 and α_7-nicotinic ligands for improving cognition in schizophrenia, many selective agents are intended for co-administration, so the issue of interaction with other drugs must be thoroughly addressed.[32,165,166,370]

Though unpopular, more attention needs to be devoted with animal models to the question of unwanted pharmacological effects of new mechanisms of action, and to the elaboration of strategies for their translational appraisal and, hopefully, limitation.

Modeling Drug Combinations

Apart form the use of highly selective drugs alone in sub-populations of patients with relevant pathologies and/or symptoms; they are often candidates for adjunctive use. Indeed, drug associations are (despite certain intrinsic drawbacks) one valid strategy for mimicking the benefits of multi-target drugs.[32,49,370,371] Their utility is illustrated by the variety of mechanistically distinct drugs used for improving the treatment of refractory depression, from lithium to antipsychotics to thyroxine.[32,370] This logic could also offer an escape-hatch for selective NK_1 antagonists, since their co-administration with SSRIs for resistant depression may enhance efficacy, reduce the delay to action, and improve tolerance, a seductive hypothesis convincingly underpinned by studies in animal models.[32,372] Clearly, then, there is a need to intensify experimental studies of drug associations well before their use in the clinic. This should prepare the way for more focused translational clinical trials, help explore multi-target concepts, and offer therapeutically relevant data for validating new animal procedures. Indeed, it is surprising how little data for drug combinations is available for animal models.

Finally, other than controlled clinical trials of drug associations and validated use of drug combinations in patients, polypharmacy can be common in the treatment of schizophrenia and other psychiatric disorders – generally prescribed, but also patient-inspired.[373-375] Self-medication can alter the actions of psychotropic drugs. At least some core information from animal models on the likely consequences of association (such as co-use of benzodiazepines) with new agents might be helpful prior to encountering such situations in patients.

Modeling Drug Actions in Specific Populations

Apart from drug combinations, highly selective agents at specific targets may find use in sub-populations of patients. Current reasoning decrees that they should present the relevant pathology ("genetic risk factor") to be identified by genotyping or other approaches.[9-12,14] Animal models based on the genetic manipulation of mice are instructive in the elaboration of such agents, but have their limitations. For optimizing the clinical orientation of selective drugs, a broad range of animal models should be used to explore their therapeutic potential (see above).

Notwithstanding a plethora of studies on subtle genetic differences at the allelic level of single nucleotide polymorphisms, it is surprising how little attention has been paid to a further and not entirely irrelevant genetic distinction between XX and XY chromosomes. Males and females differ dramatically (especially from the adolescent onslaught of "sex" hormones) in their emotional status, response to stress, predisposition to and profiles of psychiatric disorders, and response to drugs.[241,376-378] Despite this dichotomy, animal models are almost invariably undertaken in males.[379] More work needs to be done on the – arguably more challenging – female gender and such observations translated into clinical work in (wo)man.

A further crucial issue is age. Despite many cognitive studies on aged mice and primates, remarkably little is known concerning the actions of psychotropic agents in aged subjects – placebo-controlled psychotropic drug trials in the elderly are uncommon.[380-382] This is unfortunate, since the pathological bases and co-morbidity of psychiatric disorders, as well as their treatment and drug acceptability, can radically differ in the elderly: in particular, as regards depression and antidepressants, while imaging studies confirm long-suspected differences between chronic and first-episode schizophrenia (see above).[32,383,384] Such features need to be captured and studied in animal – and translational – models. One pragmatic reason for doing this is the regulatory requirement (in Europe) of demonstrating efficacy of new antidepressants in the elderly (>65-years old): experimental work may help orient such clinical investigations. At the opposite scale of the spectrum, one is also concerned with the young. The above insistence on preventative strategies evidently implies greater emphasis on studying therapeutic actions in immature and young subjects and, again, more animal work is needed in this respect. Apart from attention deficit hyperactivity disorder (ADHD), few new drugs are likely to be specifically oriented towards (first) use in children and adolescents. Nonetheless, in view of: (1) the distinctive characteristics of psychiatric states in the young; (2) the importance of pre-emptive treatment of incipient disorders; and (3) inadequacies in the current control (pharmacotherapy and other) of depressed and anxious states in juveniles, the need for improved modeling of psychiatric disorders in young animals is evident.[55,331,345,347,385,386]

Finally, a more general point of concern is that conventional models tend not to embrace the issue of co-morbidity, such as cardiovascular disease, cancer, and epilepsy.[4,32,383] Further work on the mood effects of psychotropic agents in models of other disease states would appear desirable.

NEW CONCEPTS FOR UNDERSTANDING PSYCHIATRIC DISORDERS AND FACILITATING DRUG DISCOVERY

In focusing on animal models, it seems not unreasonable to raise the question of the species.[387] In a sense, one fundamental message of translational research is that the definitive experimental species should be human. However, not surprisingly, use of *Homo sapiens* is only envisable after extensive studies in other animal species. The overwhelming majority are performed in rodents but other candidates should perhaps be considered.

Gerbils, hamsters, and guinea pigs all have their uses; for example, in characterizing drugs acting at NK_1 receptors, which (unfortunately for them) are far closer to human than NK_1 sites in rats or mice.[263] Voles have proven useful to examine the control of social behavior by oxytocin and would surely be of use in future studies of schizophrenia, ADHD, social phobia, and autism, which are epitomized by perturbations of social cognition and behavior[388,389] (see other chapters). In the aquatic realm, zebrafish are great favorites of developmental biologists and studies of Wnt, GSK-3β and other (orthologous and homologous) genes may provide insights into early events triggering schizophrenia: though zebrafish are of limited use for studies of behavior, motor function (swimming), and cognitive performance are open to study.[390-393] Dolphins and whales, despite their imposing brains and intellectual gifts, are rather impractical laboratory animals and it is depressing enough to see them reduced to the status of entertainers in "sea-worlds."[394] Accordingly, in the search for higher cognitive function, the move is generally to primates. However, ethical issues apart (the desire to minimize the use of higher primates is paramount), their cognitive powers may be less impressive and relevant than sometimes thought. Not even chimps and bonobos can master a level of language superior to that of the average toddler and their problem-solving abilities are unremarkable.[394,395] One surprising alternative may be birds.

Reflecting evolutionary convergence, there are remarkable functional and organizational homologies between the brain of humans and those of parrots, owls, and crows.[394,396] Further, avian brains are left-right assymetric, regulated neurogenesis is well established in birds, and avian centers of song learning display pronounced expression of the celebrated Fox-2 gene.[397,398] This may not permit the full gamut of language, but there are amazing parallels between processes of bird song acquisition and the learning of human language.[399,400] Most strikingly, it was recently shown that starlings (relegating apes to a distant second place) can handle recursion, one quintessential element of human language.[7,401] Studies of nutcrackers (which have formidable powers of spatial memory) suggest that birds have an at least rudimentary Theory of Mind: they re-locate nuts upon realizing that they have been observed during their hiding.[394] Finally, New Caledonian crows out-class chimps in their ability to design and modify tools, and to use them creatively to solve problems like access to food.[402,403] In view of their powers of "language," their causal reasoning, their foresight, their behavioral flexibility, and their social intelligence, behavioral observations of "higher" birds could provide important insights into some features of psychiatric disorders that are poorly modeled in other species.[404,405]

Finally, though reductionist molecular approaches to understanding psychiatric disorders can tell us much, they cannot teach us everything. Moving up in scale may also be instructive, as exemplified by imaging techniques revealing features of neuronal circuits affected by psychiatric states and their treatment. From a theoretical perspective, it is of particular interest to consider mathematical models of non-random networks, including protein clusters in neurones, neural circuits, and the brain as whole.[32,310,311,406] Networks are comprised of inter-linked nodes organized in functional modules and operating at several temporal and spatial scales. They can be highly resistant to minor and transient (internal and external) perturbation, but are disrupted under conditions of severe and protected stress, reflecting failure of multiple weak links or key hubs. Further, disruption can be associated with a phase-shift into an alternative pathological and sometimes irreversible state (hysteresis), underpinning as accentuated above the importance of biomarkers for early detection and prevention.

By analogy to the brain, ecosystems are composed of heterogeneous networks possessing characteristics that generally enhance stability in the face of threats to homeostasis: diversity (species and individuals), redundancy (guilds with similar functional roles), and contrasting responsiveness to stress.[407-409] In general, species-rich systems are more resilient to perturbation than species-poor ecosystems like the Arctic and Antarctic dominated by polar bears and penguins as key predators, respectively. One example, and a genuine animal model (!), is provided by coral reefs. When exposed to multiple and repetitive, anthropogenic and natural stressors, such as hurricanes, pollution, climatic warning and predation, they can collapse and flip (phase-shift) from a coral to an algal-dominated state. This notoriously happened in the Caribbean in the 1980s when, in the wake of several hurricanes, over-fished algovorous parrotfish could not compensate for decimation of urchins by disease.[410-412,430] Restoration of degraded coral reefs is difficult, mimicking the challenge of achieving full recovery in patients with established psychiatric disorders, and likewise emphasizing the need for prevention. Indeed, by analogy to psychiatric disorders, early warning biomarkers of reef collapse are being actively sought for translation into preventative measures.[411-415,417,431]

While hardly advocating coral reefs as experimental platforms, they can indirectly teach us much about the principles of complex networks like the brain, its dysfunction and its treatment. These principles can then be applied to animal and translational research and communicated to vulnerable individuals and their carers: improved comprehension of psychiatric disorders (facilitated by the coral reef metaphor) is itself a step on the path to prevention and better treatment. Moreover, if we fail urgently to preserve coral reefs, other ecosystems and indeed the entire planet from environmental stress, then the consequences for mental health will be dire – and likely refractory to an entire pharmacy of psychotropic drugs.

CONCLUDING COMMENTS

Animal models are indispensable for improving our understanding of psychiatric disorders, identifying innovative targets for pharmacotherapy, and characterizing the actions (beneficial and deleterious) of drugs. Currently available models are far from ideal and there is a particular need to improve procedures for the validation of novel targets and concepts. In this regard, there has perhaps been too much reliance on (sometimes) unconfirmed data from studies of genetically manipulated mice. In any case, it is naïve to imagine that one could perfectly reproduce the emotional, psychological, cognitive, and other facets of complex disorders like schizophrenia or OCD in a rat or mouse, and map their progression across the entire life span. In this respect, the search for models *of* psychiatric disorders *per se* is an illusory goal and, even if we knew exactly which set of genes (proteins) triggered a disorder, the functional consequences of their manipulation in animals would be very different from human. In any case, in modeling specific symptoms of psychiatric disorders and the underlying genetic, developmental, and environmental factors, it is preferable to manipulate several vulnerability factors in combination since this corresponds more closely to the real world of psychiatric disorders.

From the perspective of R and D, the most distinctive and crucial consideration regarding animal models (irrespective of their construct, face, and what-have-you value) is the rapid and reliable characterization of desirable and undesirable effects of new drugs that act via known or novel mechanisms. Here, a compromise needs to be found between output and quality of information, and it is indispensable to exploit multiple measures in working-up serious candidates for clinical development. Within this industrial framework, despite decades of hand wringing, it is important not to make the issue of animal models a "straw man." Standard paradigms are just not that bad for drugs with conventional (generally monoaminergic and, perhaps, glutamatergic) mechanisms of action. Further, much of the agonizing about whether models are good, poor, or indifferent rings hollow: we do not actually know since it is so incredibly difficult to get novel drugs into the clinic and acquire solid clinical feedback on their therapeutic efficacy. The predictive power of animal models may be a lot better (or worse!) than we think. Moreover, they are just one of several no less major concerns including: draconian safety criteria; limited patent life coupled to the threat of generics; the excessive length and expense of clinical testing; and most critically, therapeutic trials themselves. Notably, high-placebo responses, antiquated rating-scales, and straight-jacketed designs poorly suited to new mechanisms of action and to drugs acting against specific symptoms or in discrete sub-populations. Hopefully, in combination with the rigorous exploitation of experimental models, translational research will improve the chances of success in: (1) characterizing genetic, cognitive, imaging, and other biomarkers of incipient psychiatric disorders; (2) identifying appropriate patient sub-populations for pharmacotherapy and other modes of treatment; (3) optimizing the choice and dose-regimes of drugs; (4) elucidating their modes and sites of action; and (5) providing complementary measures of treatment efficacy and side effects.

Nonetheless, the fundamental issue remains of "translating" translational research. If its promise is to be fulfilled, imaginative and well-designed clinical trials rather than standard and conventional protocols are needed to explore rigorously the therapeutic efficacy and potential of psychotropic agents possessing novel mechanisms of action.

Finally, no psychotropic drug, nor any "alternative" mode of treatment, will ever provide a panacea. Pharmacotherapy is, and will likely remain, a core and central strategy for treating serious psychiatric disorders. However, optimal therapeutic benefit will often require the association of pharmacotherapy with psychological, somatic, and other strategies. Experimental and translational models still have much to achieve in resolving the very real issue of how best to integrate the use of drugs with complementary approaches for the prevention and management of psychiatric states.

ACKNOWLEDGEMENTS

The author would like to thank T. Branchek, S. Kapur and K. Fone for helpful comments, M. Soubeyran for secretarial assistance, and M. Brocco and A. Gobert for logistical help.

REFERENCES

1. The Who World Mental Health Survey Consortium (2004). Prevalence, severity, and unmet need for treatment of mental disorders in the world health organization world mental health surveys. *JAMA*, 291:2581–2590.

2. Agid, Y., Buzsäki, G., Diamond, D.M., Frackowiak, R., Giedd, J., Girault, J.A., Grace, A., Lambert, J.J., Manji, H., Mayberg, H. *et al.* (2007). How can drug discovery for psychiatric disorders be improved? *Nat Rev*, 6:189–201.

3. Kessler, R.C., Amminger, G.P., Aguilar-Gaxiola, S., Alonso, J., Lee, S., and Bedirhan Ustün, T. (2007). Age of onset of mental disorders: A review of recent literature. *Curr Opin Psychiatry*, 20:359–364.

4. Merikangas, K.R. and Kalaydjian, A. (2007). Magnitude and impact of comorbidity of mental disorders from epidemiologic surveys. *Curr Opin Psychiatry*, 20:353–358.

5. Eitan, R. and Lerer, B. (2006). Nonpharmacological, somatic treatments of depression: Electroconvulsive therapy and novel brain stimulation modalities. *Dialogues Clin Neurosci*, 8:241–258.

6. Hollon, S.D., Stewart, M.O., and Strunk, D. (2006). Enduring effects for cognitive behavior therapy in the treatment of depression and anxiety. *Annu Rev Psychol*, 57:285–315.

7. Hauser, M.D., Chomsky, N., and Tecumseh-Fitch, W. (2002). The faculty of language: What is it, who has it, and how did it evolve? *Science*, 298:1569–1579.

8. Penn, D.C. and Povinelli, D.J. (2007). On the lack of evidence that non-human animals possess anything remotely resembling a "theory of mind". *Philos Trans R Soc Lond B Biol Sci*, 362:731–744.

9. Bakshi, V.P. and Kali, N.H. (2002). Animal models and endophenotypes of anxiety and stress disorders. *Neuropsychopharmacology*, 62:883–900.

10. Gottesman, I.I. and Gould, T.D. (2003). The endophenotype concept in psychiatry: Etymology and strategic intentions. *Am J Psychiatry*, 160:636–645.

11. Hasler, G., Drevets, W.C., Manji, H.K., and Charney, D.S. (2004). Discovering endophenotypes for major depression. *Neuropsychopharmacology*, 29:1765–1781.

12. Bearden, C.E. and Freimer, N.B. (2006). Endophenotypes for psychiatric disorders: Ready for primetime? *Trends Gen*, 22:306–313.

13. Anders, H.J. and Vielhauser, V. (2007). Identifying validating novel targets with in vivo disease models: Guidelines for study design. *Drug Discov Today*, 12:446–451.

14. Thaker, G.K. (2007). Schizophrenia endophenotypes as treatment targets. *Expert Opin Ther Targets*, 11:1189–1206.

15. Geyer, M.A. and Markou, A. (2002). The role of preclinical models in the development of psychotropic drugs. *Neuropsychopharmacology*, 33:445–455.

16. Geyer, M.A. and Ellenbroek, B. (2003). Animal behavior models of the mechanisms underlying antipsychotic atypicality. *Prog Neuropsychopharmacol Biol Psychiatry*, 27:1071–1079.

17. Deussing, J.M. (2006). Animal models of depression. *Drug Discov Today Dis Models*, 3(4):375–383.

18. Powell, C.M. and Miyakawa, T. (2006). Schizophrenia-relevant behavioral testing in rodent models: A uniquely human disorder? *Biol Psychiatry*, 59:1198–1207.

19. Cryan, J.F. and Slattery, D.A. (2007). Animal models of mood disorders: Recent developments. *Curr Opin Psychiatry*, 20:1–7.

20. Weiss, I.C. and Feldon, J. (2001). Environmental animal models for sensorimotor gating deficiencies in schizophrenia: A review. *Psychopharmacology*, 156:305–326.

21. Lapiz, M.D.S., Fulford, A., Muchimapura, S., Mason, R., Parker, T., and Marsden, C.A. (2003). Influence of postweaning social isolation in the rat on brain development, conditioned behavior, and neurotransmission. *Neurosci Behav Physiol*, 33:13–22.

22. Lipska, B.K. (2004). Using animal models to test a neurodevelopmental hypothesis of schizophrenia. *J Psychiatry Neurosci*, 29:282–286.

23. Rasmussen, B.A., O'Neil, J., Manaye, K.F., Perry, D.C., and Tizabi, Y. (2007). Long-term effects of developmental PCP administration on sensorimotor gating in male and female rats. *Psychopharmacology*, 190:43–49.

24. Braff, D.L. and Light, G.A. (2004). Preattentional and attentional cognitive deficits as targets for treating schizophrenia. *Psychopharmacology*, 174:175–185.

25. Matsuzaki, S. and Tohyama, M. (2007). Molecular mechanism of schizophrenia with reference to disrupted-in-schizophrenia 1 (DISC1). *Neurochem Int*, 51:165–172.

26. Millan, M.J. (2005). N-methyl-D-aspartate receptors as a target for improved antipsychotic agents: Novel insights and clinical perspectives. *Psychopharmacology*, 179:30–53.

27. O'Tuathaigh, C.M.P., Babovic, D., O'Meara, G., Clifford, J.J., Croke, D.T., and Waddington, J.L. (2007). Susceptibility genes for schizophrenia: Characterisation of mutant mouse models at the level of phenotypic behavior. *Neurosci Biobehav Rev*, 31:60–78.

28. Dunn, D.A., Kooyman, D.L., and Pinkert, C.A. (2005). Foundation review: Transgenic animals and their impact on the drug discovery industry. *Drug Discov Today*, 10:757–767.

29. Kafkafi, N., Benjamini, Y., Sakov, A., Elmer, G.I., and Golan, I. (2005). Genotype-environment interactions in mouse behavior: A way out of the problem. *Proc Natl Acad Sci USA*, 102:4619–4624.

30. Van der Staay, F.J. (2006). Animal models of behavioral dysfunctions: Basic concepts and classifications, and an evaluation strategy. *Brain Res Rev*, 52:131–159.

31. Yoshiki, A. and Moriwaki, K. (2006). Mouse phenome research: Implications of genetic background. *ILAR J*, 47:94–102.

32. Millan, M.J. (2006). Multi-target strategies for the improved treatment of depressive states: Conceptual foundations and neuronal substrates, drug discovery and therapeutic application. *Pharmacol Ther*, 110:135–370.

33. Yanai, I., Korbel, J.O., Boue, S., McWeeney, S.K., Bork, P., and Lercher, M.J. (2006). Similar gene expression profiles do not imply similar tissue functions. *Trends Genet*, 22:132–138.

34. Conti, B., Maier, R., Barr, A.M., Morale, M.C., Lu, X., Sanna, P.P., Bilbe, G., Hoyer, D., and Bartfai, T. (2007). Region-specific transcriptional changes following the three antidepressant treatments electroconvulsive therapy, sleep deprivation and fluoxetine. *Mol Psychiatry*, 12:167–189.

35. Lee, C.J. and Irizarry, K. (2003). Alternative splicing in the nervous system: An emerging source of diversity and regulation. *Biol Psychiatry*, 54:771–776.

36. Jeffery, C.J. (2004). Moonlighting proteins: Complications and implications for proteomics research. *Drug Discov Today Targets*, 3:71–78.

37. Stetefeld, J. and Ruegg, M.A. (2005). Structural and functional diversity generated by alternative mRNA splicing. *Trends Biochem Sci*, 30:515–521.

38. Meltzer, H.Y., Li, Z., Kaneda, Y., and Ichikawa, J. (2003). Serotonin receptors: Their key role in drugs to treat schizophrenia. *Prog Neuropsychopharmacol Biol Psychiatry*, 27:1159–1172.

39. Cryan, J.F., Valentino, R.J., and Lucki, I. (2005). Assessing substrates underlying the behavioral effects of antidepressants using the modified rat forced swimming test. *Neurosci Biobehav Rev*, 29:547–569.

40. Horacek, J., Bubenikova-Valesova, V., Kopecek, M., Palenicek, T., Dockery, C., Mohr, P., and Höschl, C. (2006). Mechanisms of action of atypical antipsychotic drugs and the neurobiology of schizophrenia. *CNS Drugs*, 20:389–409.

41. Monaca, C., Boutrel, B., Hen, R., Hamon, M., and Adrien, J. (2003). 5-HT$_{1A}$/$_{1B}$ receptor-mediated effects of the selective serotonin reuptake inhibitor, citalopram, on sleep: Studies in 5-HT$_{1A}$ and 5-HT$_{1B}$ knockout mice. *Neuropsychopharmacology*, 28:850–856.

42. Millan, M.J. (2005). Serotonin 5-HT$_{2C}$ receptors as a target for the treatment of depressive and anxious states: Focus on novel therapeutic strategies. *Thérapie*, 60:441–460.

43. Lucas, G., Rymar, V.V., Du, J., Mnie-Filali, O., Bisgaard, C., Manta, S., Lambas-Senas, L., Wiborg, O., Haddjeri, N., Pineyro, G. *et al.* (2007). Serotonin($_4$) (5-HT($_4$)) receptor agonists are putative antidepressants with a rapid onset of action. *Neuron*, 55:712–725.

44. Svenningsson, P., Tzavara, E.T., Qi, H., Carruthers, R., Witkin, J.M., Nomikos, G.G., and Greengard, P. (2007). Biochemical and behavioral evidence for antidepressant-like effects of 5-HT$_6$ receptor stimulation. *J Neurosci*, 27:4201–4209.

45. Bymaster, F.P., McNamara, R.K., and Tran, P.V. (2003). New approaches to developing antidepressants by enhancing monoaminergic neurotransmission. *Expert Opin Invest Drugs*, 12:531–543.

46. Millan, M.J. (2004). The role of monoamines in the actions of established and "novel" antidepressant agents: A critical review. *Eur J Pharmacol*, 500:371–384.

47. Morilak, D.A. and Frazer, A. (2004). Antidepressants and brain monoaminergic systems: A dimensional approach to understanding their behavioral effects in depression and anxiety disorders. *Int J Neuropsychopharmacol*, 7:193–218.

48. Skolnick, P. and Basile, A.S. (2006). Triple reuptake inhibitors as antidepressants. *Drug Discov Today Therap Strategies*, 3:489–494.

49. Roth, B.L., Shefflet, D.J., and Kroeze, W.K. (2004). Magic shotguns versus magic bullets: Selectively non-selective drugs for mood disorders and schizophrenia. *Nat Rev Drug Discov*, 3:353–359.

50. Millan, M.J., Schreiber, R., Dekeyne, A., Rivet, J.-M., Bervoets, K., Mavridis, M., Sebban, C., Maurel-Remy, S., Newman-Tancredi, A., Spedding, M., *et al.* (1998). S16924 ((R)-2-[1-[2-(2,3-dihydro-benzo[1,4]dioxin-yloxy)-ethyl]-pyrrolidin-3yl]-1-(4-fluoro-phenyl)ethanone), a novel, potential antipsychotic with marked serotonin (5-HT)$_{1A}$ agonist properties: II. Functional profile in comparison to clozapine and haloperidol. *J Pharmacol Exp Ther*, 286:1356–1373.

51. Willner, P. (2005). Chronic mild stress (CMS) revisited: Consistency and behavioral-neurobiological concordance in the effects of CMS. *Neuropsychobiology*, 52:90–110.

52. Czeh, B., Müller-Keuker, J.I.H., Rygula, R., Abumaria, N., Hiemke, C., Domenici, E., and Fuchs, E. (2007). Chronic social stress inhibits cell proliferation in the adult medial prefrontal cortex: Hemispheric asymmetry and reversal by fluoxetine treatment. *Neuropsychopharmacology*, 32:1490–1503.

53. Brunner, D., Nestler, E., and Leahy, E. (2002). In need of high-throughput behavioral systems. *Drug Discov Today*, 7:S107–S112.

54. Crowley, J.J., Jones, M.D., O'Leary, O.F., and Lucki, I. (2004). Automated tests for measuring the effects of antidepressants in mice. *Pharmacol Biochem Behav*, 78:269–274.

55. Pogorelov, V.M., Lanthorn, T.H., and Savelieva, K.V. (2007). Use of a platform in an automated open-field to enhance assessment of anxiety-like behaviors in mice. *J Neurosci Methods*, 162:222–228.

56. Conn, P.J. and Roth, B.L. (2008). Oppportunities and challenges of psychiatric drug discovery: roles for scientists in academic, industry, and government settings, *Neuropsychopharmacology*

57. McArthur, R. and Borsini, F. (2006). Animal models of depression in drug discovery: A historical perspective. *Pharmacol Biochem Behav*, 84:436–452.

58. Millan, M.J., Dekeyne, A., Papp, M., La Rochelle, C.D., MacSweeny, C., Peglion, J.-L., and Brocco, M. (2001). S33005, a novel ligand at both serotonin and norepinephrine transporters: II. Behavioral profile in comparison with venlafaxine, reboxetine, citalopram, and clomipramine. *J Pharmacol Exp Ther*, 298:581–591.

59. Deacon, R.M. (2006). Digging and marble burying in mice: Simple methods for in vivo identification of biological impacts. *Nat Protoc*, 1:122–124.

60. Nicolas, L.B., Kolb, Y., and Prinssen, E.P. (2006). A combined marble burying-locomotor activity test in mice: A practical screening test with sensitivity to different classes of anxiolytics and antidepressants. *Eur J Pharmacol*, 547:106–115.

61. Csajka, C. and Verotta, D. (2006). Pharmacokinetic-pharmacodynamic modeling: History and perspectives. *J Pharmacokin Pharmacodyn*, 33:227–279.
62. Clayton, D.F. (2000). The genomic action potential. *Neurobiol Learn Mem*, 74:185–216.
63. Grande, C., Zhu, H., Martin, A.B., Lee, M., Ortiz, O., Hiroi, N., and Moratalla, R. (2004). Chronic treatment with atypical neuroleptics induces striosomal FosB/DeltaFosB expression in rats. *Biol Psychiatry*, 55:457–463.
64. Pei, Q., Sprakes, M., Millan, M.J., Rochat, C., and Sharp, T. (2004). The novel monoamine reuptake inhibitor and potential antidepressant, S33005, induces Arc gene expression in cerebral cortex. *Eur J Pharmacol*, 489:179–185.
65. Blendy, J.A. (2006). The role of CREB in depression and antidepressant treatment. *Biol Psychiatry*, 59:1144–1150.
66. Berton, O. and Nestler, E.J. (2006). New approaches to antidepressant drug discovery: Beyond monoamines. *Nat Rev Neurosci*, 7:37–151.
67. Duman, R.S. and Monteggia, L.M. (2006). A neurotrophic model for stress-related mood disorders. *Biol Psychiatry*, 59:1116–1127.
68. Morse, A.C. and Barlow, C. (2006). Unraveling the complexities of neurogenesis to guide development of CNS therapeutics. *Drug Discov Today Therap Strategies*, 3:495–501.
69. Toro, C.T. and Deakin, J.F.W. (2007). Adult neurogenesis and schizophrenia: A window on abnormal early brain development? *Schizophr Res*, 90:1–14.
70. Millan, M.J., Lejeune, F., and Gobert, A. (2000). Reciprocal autoreceptor and heteroceptor control of serotonergic, dopaminergic and noradrenergic transmission in the frontal cortex: Relevance to the actions of antidepressant agents. *J Psychopharmacol*, 14:114–138.
71. Westerink, B.H.C. (2002). Can antipsychotic drugs be classified by their effects on a particular group of dopamine neurons in the brain? *Eur J Pharmacol*, 455:1–18.
72. Celada, P., Puig, M.V., Armagos-Bosch, M., Adell, A., and Artigas, F. (2004). The therapeutic role of 5-HT$_{1A}$ and 5-HT$_{2A}$ receptors in depression. *Rev Psychiatr Neurosci*, 29:252–265.
73. Zarate, C.A., Quiroz, J., Payne, J., and Manji, H.K. (2002). Modulators of the glutamatergic system: Implications for the development of improved therapeutics in mood disorders. *Psychopharmacol Bull*, 36:35–83.
74. Millan, M.J. (2003). The neurobiology and control of anxious states. *Prog Neurobiol*, 70:83–244.
75. Sanacora, G., Rothman, D.L., Mason, G., and Krystal, J.H. (2003). Clinical studies implementing glutamate neurotransmission in mood disorders. *Ann N Y Acad Sci*, 1003:292–308.
76. Dinan, T.G. (1998). Psychoneuroendocrinology of depression: Growth hormone. *Psychiatr Clin North Am*, 21:325–339.
77. Arzt, E. and Holsboer, F. (2006). CRF signalling: Molecular specificity for drug targeting the CNS. *Trends Pharmacol*, 27:531–538.
78. Carrasco, G.A. and Van de Kar, L.D. (2003). Neuroendocrine pharmacology of stress. *Eur J Pharmacol*, 463:235–272.
79. Gold, P.W. and Chrousos, G.P. (2002). Organization of the stress system and its dysregulation in melancholic and atypical depression: High versus low CRH/NE states. *Mol Psychiatry*, 7:254–275.
80. De Kloet, E.R., Joels, M., and Holsboer, F. (2005). Stress and the brain: From adaption to disease. *Nat Rev Neurosci*, 6:463–475.
81. De Kloet, E.R., Sibug, R.M., Helmerhorst, F.M., Schmidt, M.V., and Schmidt, M. (2005). Stress, genes and the mechanism of programming the brain for later life. *Neurosci Biobehav Rev*, 29:271–281.
82. Byerly, M., Suppes, T., Tran, Q.V., and Baker, R.A. (2007). Clinical implications of antipsychotic-induced hyperprolactinemia in patients with schizophrenia spectrum or bipolar spectrum disorders: Recent development and current perspectives. *J Clin Psychopharmacol*, 27:639–661.

83. Borjigin, J., Li, X., and Snyder, S.H. (1999). The pineal gland and melatonin: Molecular and pharmacologic regulation. *Annu Rev Pharmacol Toxicol*, 39:53–65.

84. Cespuglio, R., Rousset, C., Debilly, G., Rochat, C., and Millan, M.J. (2005). Acute administration of the novel serotonin and noradrenaline reuptake inhibitor, S33005, markedly modifies sleep-wake cycle architecture in the rat. *Psychopharmacology*, 181:639–652.

85. Kantor, S., Jakus, R., Bodizs, R., Halasz, P., and Bagdy, G. (2002). Acute and long-term effects of the 5-HT$_2$ receptor antagonist ritanserin on EEG power spectra, motor activity, and sleep: Changes at the light-dark phase shift. *Brain Res*, 943:105–111.

86. Sanchez, C., Brennum, L.T., Storustovu, S., Kreilgard, M., and Mork, A. (2007). Depression and poor sleep: The effect of monoaminergic antidepressants in a pre-clinical model in rats. *Pharmacol Biochem Behav*, 86:468–476.

87. Patterson, J.V., Hetrick, W.P., Boutros, N.N., Jin, Y., Sandman, C., Stern, H., Potkin, and S., Bunney, W.E. (2008). P50 sensory gating ratios in schizophrenics and controls: A review and data analysis. *Psychiatry Res*. 158:226–247.

88. Van Lier, H., Drinkenburg, W.H.I.M., van Eeten, Y.J.W., and Coenen, A.M.L. (2004). Effects of diazepam and zolpidem on EEG beta frequencies are behavior-specific in rats. *Neuropharmacology*, 47:163–174.

89. Sebban, C., Zhang, X.Q., Tesolin-Decros, B., Millan, M.J., and Spedding, M. (1999). Changes in EEG spectral power in the prefrontal cortex of conscious rats elicited by drugs interacting with dopaminergic and noradrenergic transmission. *Br J Pharmacol*, 128:1045–1054.

90. McNaughton, N., Kocsis, B., and Hajos, M. (2007). Elicited hippocampal theta rhythm: A screen for anxiolytic and precognitive drugs through changes in hippocampal function? *Behav Pharmacol*, 18:329–346.

91. Sossi, V. and Ruth, T.J. (2005). Micropet imaging: In vivo biochemistry in small animals. *J Neural Transm*, 112:319–330.

92. Easton, N., Marshall, F.H., Fone, K.C., and Marsden, C.A. (2007). Atomoxetine produces changes in cortico-basal thalamic loop circuits: Assessed by phMRI BOLD contrast. *Neuropharmacology*, 52:812–826.

93. Easton, N., Shah, Y.B., Marshall, F.H., Fone, K.C., and Marsden, C.A. (2006). Guanfacine produces differential effects in frontal cortex compared to striatum: Assessed by phMRI BOLD contrast. *Psychopharmacology*, 189:369–385.

94. Beckmann, N., Kneuer, R., Gremich, H.U., Karmouty-Quintana, H., Blé, F.X., and Müller, M. (2007). In vivo mouse imaging and spectroscopy in drug discovery. *NMR Biomed*, 20:154–185.

95. Nordquist, R.E., Risterucci, C., Moreau, J.L., von Kienlin, M., Künnecke, B., Maco, M., Freichel, C., Riemer, C., and Spooren, W. (2008). Effects of aripiprazole/OPC-14597 on motor activity, pharmacological models of psychosis, and brain activity in rats. *Neuropharmacology*, 54:405–416.

96. Stark, J.A., McKie, S., Davies, K.E., Williams, S.R., and Luckman, S.M. (2008). 5-HT$_{2C}$ antagonism blocks blood oxygen level-dependent pharmacological-challenge magnetic resonance imaging signal in rat brain areas related to feeding. *Eur J Neurosci*, 27:457–465.

97. Su, A.I., Wiltshire, T., Batalov, S., Lapp, H., Ching, K.A., Block, D., Zhang, J., Soden, R., Hayakawa, M., Kreiman, G., Cooke, M.P., Walker, J.R., and Hogenesch, J.B. (2004). A gene atlas of the mouse and human protein-encoding transcriptomes. *Proc Natl Acad Sci USA*, 101:6062–6067.

98. Gerstein, M.B., Bruce, C., Rozowsky, J.S., Zheng, D., Du, J., Korbel, J.O., Emanuelsson, O., Zhang, Z.D., Weissman, S., and Snyder, M. (2007). What is a gene, post-encode? History and updated definition. *Genome Res*, 17:669–681.

99. Zambrowicz, B.P. and Sands, A.T. (2003). Knockouts model: The 100 best-selling drugs, will they model the next 100? *Nat Rev Drug Discov*, 2:38–51.

100. Zheng, C.J., Han, L.Y., Yap, C.W., Xie, B., and Chen, Y.Z. (2005). Trends in exploration of therapeutic targets. *Drug News Perspect*, 18:109–127.

101. Overington, J.P., Al-Lazikani, B., and Hopkins, A.L. (2006). How many drug targets are there? *Nat Rev Drug Discovery*, 5:993–996.

102. Csermely, P., Agoston, V., and Pongor, S. (2005). The efficiency of multi-target drugs: The network approach might help drug design. *Trends Pharmacol Sci*, 26:180–182.

103. Hopkins, A.L., Mason, J.S., and Overington, J.P. (2006). Can we rationally design promiscuous drugs? *Curr Opin Structural Biol*, 16:127–136.

104. Wermuth, C.G. (2004). Selective optimization of side activities: Another way for drug discovery. *J Med Chem*, 47:1303–1314.

105. Morphy, R. and Rankovic, Z. (2007). Fragments, network biology and designing multiple ligands. *Drug Discov Today*, 12:156–160.

106. Wong, E.H.F., Nikam, S.S., and Shahid, M. (2008). Multi- and single-target agents for major psychiatric diseases: Therapeutic opportunities and challenges. *Curr Opin Invest Drugs*, 9:28–36.

107. Oprea, T.I., Davis, A.M., Teague, S.J., and Leeson, P.D. (2001). Is there a difference between leads and drugs? A historical perspective. *J Chem Inf Comput*, 41:1308–1315.

108. Bleicher, K.H., Böhm, H.-J., Müller, K., and Alanine, A.I. (2003). Hit and lead generation: Beyond high-throughput screening. *Nat Rev Drug Discov*, 2:369–378.

109. Walters, W.P. and Namchuk, M. (2003). Designing screens: How to make your hits a hit. *Nat Rev Drug Discov*, 2:259–266.

110. Gribbon, P. and Sewing, A. (2005). High-throughput drug discovery: What can we expect from HTS? *Drug Discov Today*, 10:17–22.

111. Munafo, M.R. and Flint, J. (2004). Meta-analysis of genetic association studies. *Trends Genet*, 20:439–444.

112. Chanock, S.D. and Manolio, T. (2007). Replicating genotype-phenotype associations. *Nature*, 447:655–659.

113. Sullivan, P.F. (2007). Spurious genetic associations. *Biol Psychiatry*, 61:1121–1126.

114. Stahl, S.M., Zhang, L., Damatarca, C., and Grady, M. (2003). Brain circuits determine destiny in depression: A novel approach to the psychopharmacology of wakefulness, fatigue, and executive dysfunction in major depressive disorder. *J Clin Psychiatry*, 64:6–17.

115. Solé, R.V., Ferrer-Cancho, R., Montoya, J.M., and Valverde, S. (2003). Selection, tinkering, and emergence in complex networks. *Complexity*, 8:20–33.

116. Castren, E. (2005). Is mood chemistry? *Nat Rev Neurosci*, 6:241–246.

117. Ford, J.M., Krystal, J.H., and Mathalon, D.H. (2007). Neural synchrony in schizophrenia: From networks to new treatments. *Schizophr Bull*, 33:848–852.

118. Jaffee, S.R. and Price, T.S. (2007). Gene-environment correlations: A review of the evidence and implications for prevention of mental illness. *Mol Psychiatry*, 12:432–442.

119. El Yacoubi, M. and Vaugeois, J.-M. (2007). Genetic rodent models of depression. *Curr Opin Pharmacol*, 7:3–7.

120. Youdim, M.B. and Buccafusco, J.J. (2005). Multi-functional drugs for various CNS targets in the treatment of neurodegeneration disorders. *Trends Pharmacol Sci*, 26:27–35.

121. Joyce, J.N. and Millan, M.J. (2005). Dopamine D_3 receptor antagonists as therapeutic agents. *Drug Discov Today*, 10:917–925.

122. Papakostas, G.I., Thase, M.E., Fava, M., Nelson, J.C., and Shelton, R.C. (2007). Are antidepressant drugs that combine serotonergic and noradrenergic mechanisms of action more effective than the selective serotonin reuptake inhibitors in treating major depressive disorder? A meta-analysis of studies of newer agents. *Biol Psychiatry*, 62:1217–1227.

123. Eap, C.B., Jaquenoud Sirot, E., and Baumann, P. (2004). Therapeutic monitoring of antidepressant in the era of pharmacogenetics studies. *Ther Drug Monit*, 26:152–155.

124. Lotrich, F.E., Bies, R.R., Smith, G.S., and Pollock, B.G. (2006). Relevance of assessing drug concentration exposure in pharmacogenetic and imaging studies. *J Psychopharmacol*, 20:33–40.

125. Mauri, M.C., Volonteri, L.S., Colasanti, A., Fiorentini, A., De Gaspari, I.F., and Bareggi, S.R. (2007). Clinical pharmacokinetics of atypical antipsychotics: A critical review of the relationship between plasma concentrations and clinical response. *Clin Pharmacokinet*, 46:359-388.

126. Lappin, G., Kuhnz, W., Jochemsen, R., Kneer, J., Chaudhary, A., Oosterhuis, B., Drijfhout, W.J., Rowland, M., and Garner, R.C. (2006). Use of microdosing to predict pharmacokinetics at the therapeutic dose: Experience with 5 drugs. *Clin Pharmacol Ther*, 80:203-215.

127. Grant, S.L., Shulman, Y., Tibbo, P., Hampson, D.R., and Baker, G.B. (2006). Determination of D-serine and related neuroactive amino acids in human plasma by high-performance liquid chromatography with fluorimetric detection. *J Chromotography B*, 844:278-282.

128. Stemmelin, J., Cohen, C., Terranova, J.-P., Lopez-Grancha, M., Pichat, P., Bergis, O., Decobert, M., Santucci, V., Françon, D. *et al.* (2007). Stimulation of the β_3-adrenoceptor as a novel treatment strategy for anxiety and depressive disorders. *Neuropsychopharmacology*, 33:574-587.

129. Bieck, P.R. and Potter, W.Z. (2005). Biomarkers in psychotropic drug development: Integration of data across multiple domains. *Annu Rev Pharmacol Toxicol*, 45:227-246.

130. Ray, S., Britschgi, M., Herbert, C., Takeda-Uchimura, Y., Boxer K. Blennow, A., Friedman, L.F., Galasko, D.R., Jutel, M., Karydas, A., Kaye, J.A. *et al.* (2007). Classification and prediction of clinical Alzheimer's diagnosis based on plasma signalling proteins. *Nat Med*, 13:1359-1364.

131. Wolkowitz, O.M., Epel, E.S., and Reus, V.I. (2001). Stress hormone-related psychopathology: Pathophysiological and treatment implications. *World J Biol Psychiatry*, 2:115-143.

132. Schüle, C. (2007). Neuroendocrinological mechanisms of actions of antidepressant drugs. *J Neuroendocrinol*, 19:213-226.

133. Contreras, F., Menchon, J.M., Urretavizcaya, M., Navarro, M.A., Vallejo, J., and Parker, G. (2007). Hormonal differences between psychotic and non-psychotic melancholic depression. *J Affect Disord*, 100:64-73.

134. Griebel, G., Stemmelin, J., Gal, C.S., and Soubrié, P. (2005). Non-peptide vasopressin V1b receptor antagonists as potential drugs for the treatment of stress-related disorders. *Curr Pharm Des*, 11:1549-1559.

135. Matsui-Sakata, A., Ohtani, H., and Sawada, Y. (2005). Receptor occupancy-based analysis of the contributions of various receptors to antipsychotic-induced weight gain and diabetes mellitus. *Drug Metab Pharmacokinet*, 20:368-378.

136. Newcomer, J.W. (2005). Second-generation (atypical) antipsychotics and metabolic effects: A comprehensive literature review. *CNS Drugs*, 19:1-93.

137. Rao, M.L., Frahnert, C., and Zagorski, O. (2002). Initial serotonin transport into viable platelets and imipramine binding to platelet membranes. *J Neural Transm*, 109:547-556.

138. Fisar, Z., Anders, M., and Kalisova, L. (2005). Effect of pharmacologically selective antidepressants on serotonin uptake in rat platelets. *Gen Physiol Biophys*, 24:113-128.

139. Arranz, B., Rosel, P., San, L., Ramirez, N., Duenas, R.M., Salavert, J., Centeno, M., and del Moral, E. (2007). Low baseline serotonin-$_{2A}$ receptors predict clinical response to olanzapine in first-episode schizophrenia patients. *Psychiatry Res*, 153:103-109.

140. Padin, J.F., Rodriguez, M.A., Dominguez, E., Dopeso-Reyes, I.G., Buceta, M., Cano, E., Sotelo, E., Brea, J., Caruncho, H.J., Isabel Cadavid, M. *et al.* (2006). Parallel regulation by olanzapine of the patterns of expression of 5-HT$_{2A}$ and D$_3$ receptors in rat central nervous system and blood cells. *Neuropharmacology*, 51:923-932.

141. Barkan, T., Gurwitz, D., Levy, G., Weizman, A., and Rehavi, M. (2004). Biochemical and pharmacological characterization of the serotonin transporter in human peripheral blood lymphocytes. *Eur Neuropsychopharmacol*, 14:237-243.

142. Barnes, N.M. and Gordon, J. (2008). Harnessing serotonergic and dopaminergic pathways for lymphoma therapy: Evidence and aspirations. *Semin Cancer Biol*. 18:218-225.

143. Ilani, T., Strous, R.D., and Fuchs, S. (2004). Dopaminergic regulation of immune cells via D$_3$ dopamine receptor; a pathway mediated by activated T cells. *FASEB J*, 18:1600-1617.

144. Boneberg, E.M., von Seydlitz, E., Pröpster, K., Watzl, H., Rockstroh, B., and Illges, H. (2006). D_3 dopamine receptor mRNA is elevated in T cells of schizophrenic patients whereas D_4 dopamine receptor mRNA is reduced in CD4+ -T cells. *J Neuroimmunol*, 173:180–187.

145. Watanabe, Y., Nakayama, T., Nagakubo, D., Hieshima, K., Jin, Z., Katou, F., Hashimoto, K., and Yoshie, O. (2006). Dopamine selectively induces migration and homing of naïve CD8 + T cells via dopamine D_3 receptors. *J Immunol*, 176:848–856.

146. Benzel, I., Bansal, A., Browning, B.L., Galwey, N.W., Maycox, P.R., McGinnis, R., Smart, D., St Clair, D., Yates, P., and Purvis, I. (2007). Interactions among genes in the ErbB-neuregulin signalling network are associated with increased susceptibility to schizophrenia. *Behav Brain Functions*, 3:1–11.

147. Sei, Y., Ren-Patterson, R., Li, Z., Tunbridge, E.M., Egan, M.D., Klachana, B.S., and Weinberger, D.R. (2007). Neuregulin$_1$-induced cell migration is impaired in schizophrenia: Association with neurogulin$_1$ and catechol-o-methyltransferase gene polymorphisms. *Mol Psychiatry*, 12:946–957.

148. Phillips, K.A. and Van Bebber, S.L. (2005). Measuring the value of pharmacogenomics. *Nat Rev Drug Discov*, 4:500–509.

149. Ingelman-Sundberg, M., Sim, S.C., Gomez, A., and Rodriguez-Antona, C. (2007). Influence of cytochrome P450 polymorphisms on drug therapies: Pharmacogenetic, pharmacoepigenetic and clinical aspects. *Pharmacol Ther*, 116:496–526.

150. Malhotra, A.K., Murphy, G.M., and Kennedy, J.L. (2004). Pharmacogenetics of psychotropic drug response. *Am J Psychiatry*, 161:780–796.

151. Bondy, B. (2005). Pharmacogenomics in depression and antidepressants. *Dialogues Clin Neurosci*, 7:223–230.

152. Lotrich, F.E. and Pollock, B.G. (2004). Meta-analysis of serotonin transporter polymorphisms and affective disorders. *Psychiatr Genet*, 14:121–129.

153. Arias, B., Catalan, R., Gasto, C., Gutierrez, B., and Fananas, L. (2005). Evidence for a combined genetic effect of the 5-HT$_{1A}$ receptor and serotonin transporter genes in the clinical outcome of major depressive patients treated with citalopram. *J Psychopharmacol*, 19:166–172.

154. Prathikanti, S. and Weinberger, D.R. (2005). Psychiatric genetics-the new era: Genetic research and some clinical implications. *Br Med Bull*, 73–74:107–122.

155. Kato, T. (2007). Molecular genetics of bipolar disorder and depression. *Psychiatry Clin Neurosci*, 61:3–19.

156. Arranz, M.J., Collier, D., and Kerwin, R.W. (2001). Pharmacogenetics for the individualization of psychiatric treatment. *Am J Pharmacogenomics*, 1:3–10.

157. Preston, G.A. and Weinberger, D.R. (2005). Intermediate phenotypes in schizophrenia: A selective review. *Dialogues Clin Neurosci*, 7:165–179.

158. Adler, L.E., Olincy, A., Cawthra, E.M., McRae, K.A., Harris, J.G., Magamoto, H.T., Waldo, M.C., Hall, M.H., Bowles, A., Woodward, L. *et al.* (2004). Varied effects of atypical neuroleptics on P50 auditory gating in schizophrenia patients. *Am J Psychiatry*, 161:1822–1828.

159. Hajos, M. (2006). Targeting information-processing deficit in schizophrenia: A novel approach to psychotherapeutic drug discovery. *Trends Pharmacol Sci*, 27:391–398.

160. Swerdlow, N.R., Geyer, M.A., Shoemaker, J.M., Light, G.A., Braff, D.L., Stevens, K.E., Sharp, R., Breier, M., Neary, A., and Auerbach, P.P. (2006). Convergence and divergence in the neurochemical regulation of prepulse inhibition of startle and N40 suppression in rats. *Neuropsychopharmacology*, 31:506–515.

161. Braff, D.L., Geyer, M.A., and Swerdlow, N.R. (2001). Human studies of prepulse inhibition of startle: Normal subjects, patient groups, and pharmacological studies. *Psychopharmacology*, 156:234–258.

162. Geyer, M.A., Krebs-Thomson, K., Braff, D.L., and Swerdlow, N.R. (2001). Pharmacological studies of prepulse inhibition models of sensorimotor gating deficits in schizophrenia: A decade in review. *Psychopharmacology*, 156:117–154.

163. Cilia, J., Hatcher, P.D., Reavill, C., and Jones, D.N. (2005). Long-term evaluation of isolation-rearing induced prepulse inhibition deficits in rats: An update. *Psychopharmacology*, 180:57–62.

164. Cilia, J., Cluderay, J.E., Robbins, M.J., Reavill, C., Southam, E., Kew, J.N., and Jones, D.N. (2005). Reversal of isolation-rearing-induced PPI deficits by an α_7 nicotinic receptor agonist. *Psychopharmacology*, 82:214–219.

165. Fox, G.B., Esbenshade, T.A., Pan, J.B., Radek, R.J., Krueger, K.M., Yao, B.B., Browman, K.E., Buckley, M.J., Ballard, M.E., Komater, V.A. *et al.* (2005). Phamacological properties of ABT-239 [4-(2-{2-[2R)-2-methylpyrrolidinyl]ethyl}-benzofuran-5-yl)benzonitriels]: II. Neuro-physiological characterization and broad preclinical efficacy in cognition and schizophrenia of a potent and selective histamine H_3 receptor antagonist. *J Pharmacol Exp Ther*, 313:176–190.

166. Olincy, A. and Stevens, K.E. (2007). Treating schizophrenia symptoms with an alpha$_7$ nicotinic agonist, from mice to men. *Biochem Pharmacol*, 74:1192–1201.

167. Peuskens, J., Demily, C., and Thibaut, F. (2005). Treatment of cognitive dysfunction in schizophrenia. *Clin Ther*, 27:25–S37.

168. Ehlis, A.-C., Herrmann, M.J., Pauli, P., Stoeber, G., Pfuhlmann, B., and Fallgatter, A.J. (2007). Improvement of prefrontal brain function in endogenous psychoses under atypical antipsychotic treatment. *Neuropsychopharmacology*, 32:1669–1677.

169. Gilles, C. and Luthringer, R. (2007). Pharmacological models in healthy volunteers: Their use in the clinical development of psychotropic drugs. *J Pharmacol*, 21(3):272–282.

170. Honey, G. and Bullmore, E. (2004). Human pharmacological MRI. *Trends Pharmacol Sci*, 25:366–374.

171. Schmiedt, C., Brand, A., Hildebrandt, H., and Basar-Eroglu, C. (2005). Event-related theta oscillations during working memory tasks in patients with schizophrenia and healthy controls. *Cognitive Brain Res*, 25:936–947.

172. Cropley, V.L., Fujita, M., Innis, R.B., and Nathan, P.J. (2006). Molecular imaging of the dopaminergic system and its association with human cognitive function. *Biol Psychiatry*, 59:898–907.

173. Poldrack, R.A. (2006). Can cognitive processes be inferred from neuroimaging data? *Trends Cognitive Sci*, 10:59–63.

174. Glahn, D.C., Ragland, J.D., Abramoff, A., Barrett, J., Laird, A.R., Bearden, C.E., and Velligan, D.I. (2005). Beyond hypofrontality: A quantitative meta-analysis of functional neuroimaging studies of working memory in schizophrenia. *Hum Brain Mapping*, 25:60–69.

175. McGuire, P., Howes, O.D., Stone, J., and Fusar-Poli, P. (2008). Functional neuroimaging in schizophrenia: Diagnosis and drug discovery. *Trends Pharmacol Sci*, 29:91–98.

176. Hagan, J.J. and Jones, D.N. (2005). Predicting drug efficacy for cognitive deficits in schizophrenia. *Schizophr Bull*, 31:830–853.

177. Buchanan, R.W., Davis, M., Goff, D., Green, M.F., Keefe, R.S., Leon, A.C., Nuechterlein, K.H., Laughren, T., Levin, R., Stover, E. *et al.* (2005). A summary of the FDA-NIMH-MATRICS workshop on clinical trial design for neurocognitive drugs for schizophrenia. *Schizophr Bull*, 31:5–19.

178. Austin, M.P., Mitchell, P., and Goodwin, G.M. (2001). Cognitive deficits in depression: Possible implications for functional neuropathology. *Br J Psychiatry*, 178:200–206.

179. Tsujii, T., Yamamoto, E., Ohira, T., Saito, N., and Watanabe, S. (2007). Effects of sedative and non-sedative H_1 antagonists on cognitive tasks: Behavioral and near-infrared spectroscopy (NIRS) examinations. *Psychopharmacology*, 194:83–91.

180. Wezenberg, E., Sabbe, B.G., Hulstijn, W., Ruigt, G.S., and Verkes, R.J. (2007). The role of sedation tests in identifying sedative drug effects in healthy volunteers and their power to dissociate sedative-related impairments from memory dysfunctions. *J Psychopharmacol*, 21:579–587.

181. Young, J.W., Minassian, A., Paulus, M.P., Geyer, M.A., and Perry, W. (2007). A reverse-translational approach to bipolar disorder: Rodent and human studies in the behavioral pattern monitor. *Neurosci Biobehav Rev*, 31:882–896.

182. Menon, V. and Crottaz-Herbette, S. (2005). Combined EEG and fMRI studies of human brain function. *Int Rev Neurobiol*, 66:291–321.

183. Hunter, A.M., Cook, I.A., and Leuchter, A.F. (2007). The promise of the quantitative electro-encephalogram as a predictor of antidepressant treatment outcomes in major depressive disorder. *Psychiatric Clin N Am*, 30:105–124.

184. Friston, K.J. (2002). Dysfunctional connectivity in schizophrenia. *World Psychiatry*, 1:66–81.

185. Uhlhaas, P.J. and Singer, W. (2006). Neural synchrony in brain disorders: Relevance for cognitive dysfunctions and pathophysiology. *Neuron*, 52:155–168.

186. Mizuhara, H. and Yamaguchi, Y. (2007). Human cortical circuits for central executive function emerge by theta phase synchronization. *Neuroimage*, 36:232–244.

187. Gross, A., Joutsiniemi, S.L., Rimon, R., and Appelberg, B. (2004). Clozapine-induced QEEG changes correlate with clinical response in schizophrenic patients: A prospective, longitudinal study. *Phamacopsychiatry*, 37:119–122.

188. Smith, G.S., Ma, Y., Dhawan, V., Gunduz, H., Carbon, M., Kirshner, M., Larson, J., Chaly, T., Belakhleff, A., Kramer, E. *et al.* (2002). Serotonin modulation of cerebral glucose metabolism measured with positron emission tomography (PET) in human subjects. *Synapse*, 45:105–112.

189. Leuchter, A.F., Cook, I.A., Witte, E.A., Morgan, M., and Abrams, M. (2002). Changes in brain function of depressed subjects during treatment with placebo. *Am J Psychiatry*, 159:122–129.

190. Bares, M., Brunovsky, M., Kopecek, M., Stopkova, P., Novak, T., Kozeny, J., and Höschl, C. (2007). Changes in QEEG prefrontal cordance as a predictor of response to antidepressants in patients with treatment resistant depressive disorder: A pilot study. *J Psychiatr Res*, 41:319–325.

191. Daskalakis, Z.J., Fitzgerald, P.B., and Christensen, B.K. (2007). The role of cortical inhibition in the pathophysiology and treatment of schizophrenia. *Brain Res Rev*, 56:427–442.

192. Vyazovskiy, V.V. and Tobler, I. (2005). Theta activity in the waking EEG is a marker of sleep propensity in the rat. *Brain Res*, 1050:64–71.

193. Sharpley, A.L. and Cowen, P.J. (1995). Effect of pharmacologic treatments on the sleep of depressed patients. *Biol Psychiatry*, 37:85–98.

194. Rijnbeek, B., de Visser, S.J., Franson, K.L., Cohen, A.F., and van Gerven, J.M. (2003). REM sleep effects as a biomarker for the effects of antidepressants in healthy volunteers. *J Psychopharmacol*, 17:196–203.

195. Wilson, S. and Argyropoulos, S. (2005). Antidepressants and sleep: A qualitative review of the literature. *Drugs*, 65:927–947.

196. Reite, M., Teale, P., and Rojas, D.C. (1999). Magnetoencephalography: Applications in psychiatry. *Biol Psychiatry*, 45:1553–1563.

197. Saletu, B., Anderer, P., and Saletu-Zyhlarz, G.M. (2006). EEG topography and tomography (LORETA) in the classification and evaluation of the pharmacodynamics of psychotropic drugs. *Clin EEG Neurosci*, 37:66–80.

198. Le Bihan, D., Mangin, J.F., Poupon, C., Clark, C.A., Pappata, S., Molko, N., and Chabriat, H. (2001). Diffusion tensor imaging: Concepts and applications. *J Magn Reson Imaging*, 13:534–546.

199. Yoo, S.Y., Jang, J.H., Shin, Y.W., Kim, D.J., Moon, W.J., Chung, E.C., Lee, J.M., Kim, I.Y., Si, K., and Kwon, J.S. (2007). White matter abnormalities in drug-naïve patients with obsessive-compulsive disorder: A diffusion tensor study before and after citalopram treatment. *Acta Psychiatr Scand*, 116:211–219.

200. Borsook, D., Becerra, L., and Hargreaves, R. (2006). A role for fMRI in optimizing CNS drug development. *Nat Rev Drug Discov*, 5:411–424.

201. Iannetti, G.D. and Wise, R.G. (2007). BOLD functional MRI in disease and pharmacological studies: Room for improvement? *Magn Reson Imaging*, 25:978–988.

202. Lahti, A.C., Holcomb, H.H., Weiler, M.A., Medoff, D.R., Frey, K.N., Hardin, M., and Tamminga, C.A. (2004). Clozapine but not haloperidol re-establishes normal task-activated rCBF patterns in schizophrenia within the anterior cingulate cortex. *Neuropsychopharmacology*, 29:171–178.

203. Fusar-Poli, P., Broome, M.R., Matthiasson, P., Williams, S.C.R., Brammer, M., and McGuire, P.K. (2007). Effects of acute antipsychotic treatment on brain activation in first episode psychosis: An fMRI study. *Eur Neuropsychopharmacol*, 17:492–500.

204. Manoach, D.S. (2003). Prefrontal cortex dysfunction during working memory performance in schizophrenia: Reconciling discrepant findings. *Schizophr Res*, 60:285–298.

205. Morey, R.A., Inan, S., Mitchell, T.V., Perkins, D.O., Lieberman, J.A., and Belger, A. (2005). Imaging frontostriatal function in ultra-high-risk, early, and chronic schizophrenia during executive processing. *Arch Gen Psychiatry*, 62:254–262.

206. Shah, Y.B. and Marsden, C.A. (2004). The application of functional magnetic resonance imaging to neuropharmacology. *Curr Opin Pharmacol*, 4:517–521.

207. Paulus, M.P. and Stein, M.B. (2007). Role of functional magnetic resonance imaging in drug discovery. *Neuropsychol Rev*, 17:179–188.

208. Chen, C.-H., Ridler, K., Suckling, J., Williams, S., Fu, C.H.Y., Merlo-Pich, E., and Bullmore, E. (2007). Brain imaging correlates of depressive symptom severity and predictors of symptom improvement after antidepressant treatment. *Biol Psychiatry*, 62:407–414.

209. Davidson, R.J., Irwin, W., Anderle, M.J., and Kalin, N.H. (2003). The neural substrates of affective processing in depressed patients treated with venlafaxine. *Am J Psychiatry*, 160:64–75.

210. Fu, C.H., Williams, S.C., Brammer, M.J., Suckling, J., Kim, J., Walsh, A.J., Cleare, N.D., Mitterschiffthaler, M.T., Andrew, C.M., Pich, E.M. *et al.* (2007). Neural responses to happy facial expressions in major depression following antidepressant treatment. *Am J Psychiatry*, 164:599–607.

211. Casey, B.J., Cohen, J.D., O'Craven, K., Davidson, R.J., Irwin, W., Nelson, C.A., Noll, D.C., Hu, X., Lowe, M.J., Rosen, B.R. *et al.* (1998). Reproducibility of fMRI results across four institutions using a spatial working memory task. *Neuroimage*, 8:249–261.

212. Wei, X., Yoo, S.-S., Dickey, C.C., Zou, K.H., Guttmann, C.R.G., and Panych, L.P. (2004). Functional MRI of auditory verbal working memory: Long-term reproducibility analysis. *Neuroimage*, 21:1000–1008.

213. Brett, M., Johnsrude, I.S., and Owen, A.M. (2002). The problem of functional localization in the human brain. *Nature Rev Neurosci*, 3:245–249.

214. Ploran, E.J., Nelson, S.M., Velanova, K., Donaldson, D.I., Petersen, S.E., and Wheeler, M.E. (2007). Evidence accumulation and the moment of recognition: Dissociating perceptual recognition processes using fMRI. *J Neurosci*, 27:11912–11924.

215. Carlsson, K., Petrovic, P., Skare, S., Petersson, K.M., and Ingvar, M. (2000). Tickling expectations: Neural processing in anticipation of a sensory stimulus. *J Cogn Neurosci*, 12:691–703.

216. Bartels, A. and Zeki, S. (2004). The neural correlates of maternal and romantic love. *Neuroimage*, 21:1155–1166.

217. Friederich, H.-C., Uher, R., Brooks, S., Giampietro, V., Brammer, M., Williams, S.C.R., Herzog, W., Treasure, J., and Campbell, I.C. (2007). I'm not as slim as that girl: Neural bases of body shape self-comparison to media images. *NeuroImage*, 37:674–681.

218. Krueger, F., McCabe, K., Moll, J., Kriegeskorte, N., Zahn, R., Strenziok, M., Heinecke, A., and Grafman, J. (2007). Neural correlates of trust. *Proc Natl Acad Sci USA*, 104:20084–20089.

219. Beauregard, M. (2007). Mind does really matter: Evidence from neuroimaging studies of emotional self-regulation, psychotherapy, placebo effect. *Progress Neurobiol*, 81:218–236.

220. Febo, M., Segarra, A.C., Tenney, J.R., Brevard, M.E., Duong, T.Q., and Ferris, C.F. (2004). Imaging cocaine-induced changes in the mesocorticolimbic dopaminergic system of conscious rats. *J Neurosci Methods*, 139:167–176.

221. Hildebrandt, I.J., Su, H., and Weber, W.A. (2008). Anesthesia and other considerations for in vivo imaging of small animals. *ILAR J*, 49:17–26.

222. Raichle, M.E., MacLeod, A., Snyder, A.Z., Powers, W.J., Gusmard, D.A., and Shulman, G.L. (2001). A default mode of brain function. *Proc Natl Acad Sci USA*, 98:676–682.

223. De Luca, M., Beckmann, C.F., De Stefano, N., Mathews, P.M., and Smith, S.M. (2006). fMRI resting state networks define distinct modes of long-distance interactions in the human brain. *Neuroimage*, 29:1359–1367.

224. Lu, H., Zuo, Y., Gu, H., Waltz, J.A., Zhan, W., Scholl, C.A., Rea, W., Yang, Y., and Stein, E.A. (2007). Synchronized delta oscillations correlate with the resting-state functional MRI signal. *Proc Natl Acad Sci*, 104:18265–18269.

225. Greicius, M.D., Flores, B.H., Menon, V., Glover, G.H., Solvason, H.B., Kenna, H., Reiss, A.L., and Schatzberg, A.F. (2007). Resting-state functional connectivity in major depression: Abnormally increased contributions from subgenual cingulate cortex and thalamus. *Biol Psychiatry*, 62:429–437.

226. Broderick, D.F. (2005). Neuroimaging in neuropsychiatry. *Psychiatr Clin North Am*, 28:549–566.

227. Lyoo, I.K. and Renshaw, P.F. (2002). Magnetic resonance spectroscopy: Current and future applications in psychiatric research. *Biol Psychiatry*, 51:195–207.

228. Mason, G.F. and Krystal, J.H. (2006). MR spectroscopy: It's potential role for drug development for the treatment of psychiatric diseases. *NMR Biomed*, 19:690–701.

229. Manganas, L.N., Zhang, X., Li, Y., Hazel, R.D., Smith, S.D., Wagshul, M.E., Henn, F., Benveniste, H., Djuric, P.M., Enikolopov, G. *et al.* (2007). Magnetic resonance spectroscopy identifies neural progenitor cells in the live human brain. *Science*, 318:980–985.

230. Abbott, C. and Bustillo, J. (2006). What have we learned from proton magnetic resonance spectroscopy about schizophrenia? A critical update. *Curr Opin Psychiatry*, 19:135–139.

231. Jessen, F., Scherk, H., Träber, F., Theyson, S., Berning, J., Tepest, R., Falkai, P., Schild, H.H., Maier, W., Wagner, M. *et al.* (2006). Proton magnetic resonance spectroscopy in subjects at risk for schizophrenia. *Schizophr Res*, 87:81–88.

232. Lewis, D.A. and Hashimoto, T. (2007). Deciphering the disease process of schizophrenia: The contribution of cortical gaba neurons. *Int Rev Neurobiol*, 78:109–131.

233. Dunayevich, E., Erickson, E.J., Levine, L., Landbloom, R., Schoepp, D.D. and Tollefson, G.D. (2007). Efficacy and tolerability of an mGlu2/3 agonist in the treatment of generalized anxiety disorder. *Neuropsychopharmacology*.

234. Patil, S.T., Zhang, L., Martenyi, F., Lowe, S.L., Jackson, K.A., Andreev, B.V., Avedisova, A.S., Bardenstein, L.M., Gurovich, I.Y., Morozova, M.A. *et al.* (2007). Activation of mGlu2/3 receptors as a new approach to treat schizophrenia: A randomized phase 2 clinical trial. *Nat Med*, 13:1102–1107.

235. Tibbo, P., Hanstock, C., Valiakalayil, A., and Allen, P. (2004). 3-T proton MRS investigation of glutamate and glutamine in adolescents at high genetic risk for schizophrenia. *Am J Psychiatr*, 161:1116–1118.

236. Van Elst, L.T., Valerius, G., Büchert, M., Thiel, T., Rüsch, N., Bubl, E., Hennig, J., Ebert, D., and Olbrich, H.M. (2005). Increased prefrontal and hippocampal glutamate concentration in schizophrenia: Evidence from a magnetic resonance spectroscopy study. *Biol Psychiatry*, 58:724–730.

237. Olbrich, H.M., Valerius, G., Rüsch, N., Büchert, M., Thiel, T., Hennig, J., Ebert, D., and Van Elst, L.T. (2007). Frontolimbic glutamate alterations in first episode schizophrenia: Evidence from a magnetic resonance spectroscopy study. *World J Biol Psychiatry*, 5:1-5.

238. Ohrmann, P., Siegmund, A., Suslow, T., Pedersen, A., Spitzberg, K., Kersting, A., Rothermundt, M., Arolt, V., Heindel, W., and Pfleiderer, B. (2007). Cognitive impairment and in vivo metabolites in first-episode neuroleptic-naive and chronic medicated schizophrenic patients: A proton magnetic resonance spectroscopy study. *J Psychiatr Res*, 41:625-634.

239. Théberge, J., Al-Semaan, Y., Williamson, P.C., Menon, R.S., Neufeld, R.W., Rajakumar, N., Schaefer, B., Densmore, M., and Drost, D.J. (2003). Glutamate and glutamine in the anterior cingulate and thalamus of medicated patients with chronic schizophrenia and healthy comparison subjects measured with 4.0-T proton MRS. *Am J Psychiatry*, 160:2231-2233.

240. Rowland, L.M., Bustillo, J.R., Mullins, P.G., Jung, R.E., Lenroot, R., Landgraf, E., Barrow, R., Yeo, R., Lauriello, J., and Brooks, W.M. (2005). Effects of ketamine on anterior cingulate glutamate metabolism in healthy humans: A 4-T proton MRS study. *Am J Psychiatry*, 162:394-396.

241. Grachev, I.D. and Apkarian, A.V. (2000). Chemical mapping of anxiety in the brain of healthy humans: An in vivo 1H-MRS study on the effects of sex, age, and brain region. *Hum Brain Mapp*, 11:261-272.

242. Chang, L., Cloak, C.C., and Ernst, T. (2003). Magnetic resonance spectroscopy studies of GABA in neuropsychiatric disorders. *J Clin Psychiatry*, 64:7-14.

243. Ende, G., Demirakca, T., and Tost, H. (2006). The biochemistry of dysfunctional emotions: Proton MR spectroscopic findings in major depressive disorder. *Prog Brain Res*, 156:481-501.

244. Yikdiz-Yesiloglu, A. and Ankerst, D.P. (2006b). Review of 1H magnetic resonance spectroscopy findings in major depressive disorder: A meta-analysis. *Psychiatry Res*, 147:1-25.

245. Luborzewski, A., Schubert, F., Seifert, F., Danker-Hopfe, H., Brakemeier, E.-L., Schlattmann, P., Anghelescu, I., Colla, M., and Bajbouj, M. (2007). Metabolic alterations in the dorsolateral prefrontal cortex after treatment with high-frequency repetitive transcranial magnetic stimulation in patients with unipolar major depression. *J Psychiatric Res*, 41:606-615.

246. Frye, M.A., Watzl, J., Banakar, S., O'Neill, J., Mintz, J., Davanzo, P., Fischer, J., Chirichigno, J. W., Ventura, J., Elman, S. *et al.* (2007). Increased anterior cingulate/medial prefrontal cortical glutamate and creatine in bipolar depression. *Neuropsychopharmacology*, 32:2490-2499.

247. Shibuya-Tayoshi, S., Tayoshi, S.Y., Sumitani, S., Ueno, S.-I., Harada, M., and Ohmori, T. (2008). Lithium effects on brain glutamatergic and GABAergic systems of healthy volunteers as measured by proton magnetic resonance spectroscopy. *Prog Neuropsychopharmacol Biol Psychiatry*, 32:249-256.

248. Yikdiz-Yesiloglu, A. and Ankerst, D.P. (2006). Neurochemical alterations of the brain in bipolar disorder and their implications for pathophysiology: A systematic review of the in vivo proton magnetic resonance spectroscopy findings. *Prog Neuropsychopharmacol Biol Psychiatry*, 30:969-995.

249. Frankle, W.G. (2007). Neuroreceptor imaging studies in schizophrenia. *Harv Rev Psychiatry*, 15:212-232.

250. Laruelle, M. (2000). Imaging synaptic neurotransmission with in vivo binding competition techniques: A critical review. *J Cereb Blood Flow Metab*, 20:423-451.

251. Zipursky, R.B., Meyer, J.H., and Verhoeff, N.P. (2007). PET and SPECT imaging in psychiatric disorders. *Can J Psychiatry*, 52:146-157.

252. Geday, J., Hermansen, F., Rosenberg, R., and Smith, D.F. (2005). Serotonin modulation of cerebral blood flow measured with positron emission tomography (PET) in humans. *Synapse*, 55:224-229.

253. Drevets, W.C., Bogers, W., and Raichle, M.E. (2002). Functional anatomical correlates of anti-depressant drug treatment assessed using PET measures of regional glucose metabolism. *Eur Neuropsychopharmacol*, 12:527–544.

254. Konarski, J.Z., McIntyre, R.S., Soczynska, J.K., and Kennedy, S.H. (2007). Neuroimaging approaches in mood disorders: Technique and clinical implications. *Annals Clin Psychiatr*, 19:265–277.

255. Kennedy, S.H., Konarski, J.Z., Segal, Z.V., Lau, M.A., Bieling, P.J., McIntyre, R.S., and Mayberg, H.S. (2007). Differences in brain glucose metabolism between responders to CBT and venlafaxine in a 16-week randomized controlled trial. *Am J Psychiatry*, 164:778–788.

256. Brody, A.L., Saxena, S., Mandelkern, M.A., Fairbanks, L.A., Ho, M.L., and Baxter, L.R. (2001). Brain metabolic changes associated with symptom factor improvement in major depressive disorder. *Biol Psychiatry*, 50:171–178.

257. Meyer, J.H. (2007). Imaging the serotonin transporter during major depressive disorder and antidepressant treatment. *J Psychiatry Neurosci*, 32:86–102.

258. Innis, R.B., Cunningham, V.J., Delforge, J., Fujita, M., Gjedde, A., Gunn, R.N., Holden, J., Houle, S., Huang, S.-C., Ichise, M. *et al.* (2007). Consensus nomenclature for in vivo imaging of reversibly binding radioligands. *J Cerebral Blood Flow Metab*, 27:1533–1539.

259. Moresco, R.M., Matarrese, M., and Fazio, F. (2006). PET and SPET molecular imaging: Focus on serotonin system. *Curr Top Med Chem*, 6:2027–2034.

260. Lundberg, J., Christophersen, J.S., Petersen, K.B., Loft, H., Halldin, C., and Farde, L. (2007). PET measurement of serotonin transporter occupancy: A comparison of escitalopram and citalopram. *Int J Neuropsychopharmacol*, 10:777–785.

261. Rhodes, R.A., Venkatesha Murthy, N., Dresner, M.A., Selvaraj, S., Stavrakakis, N., Babar, S., Cowen, P.J., and Grasby, P.M. (2007). Human 5-HT transporter availability predicts amygdala reactivity in vivo. *J Neurosci*, 27:9233–9237.

262. Voineskos, A.N., Wilson, A.A., Boovariwala, A., Sagrati, S., Houle, S., Rusjan, P., Sokolov, S., Spencer, E.P., Ginovart, N., and Meyer, J.H. (2007). Serotonin transporter occupancy of high-dose selective serotonin reuptake inhibitors during major depressive disorder measured with [^{11}C]DASB positron emission tomography. *Psychopharmacology*, 193:539–545.

263. Herpfer, I. and Lieb, K. (2005). Substance P receptor antagonists in psychiatry. *CNS Drugs*, 19:275–293.

264. Bergström, M., Hargreaves, R.J., Burns, H.D., Goldberg, M.R., Sciberras, D., Reines, S.A., Petty, K.J., Ogren, M., Antoni, G., Langström, B. *et al.* (2004). Human positron emission tomography studies of brain neurokinin1 receptor occupancy by aprepipant. *Biol Psychiatry*, 55:1007–1012.

265. Keller, M., Montgomery, S., Ball, W., Morrison, M., Snavely, D., Liu, G., Hargreaves, R., Hietala, J., Lines, C., Beebe, K. *et al.* (2006). Lack of efficacy of the substance P (neurokinin$_1$ receptor) antagonist aprepitant in the treatment of major depressive disorder. *Biol Psychiatry*, 59:216–223.

266. Guillin, O., Abi-Dargham, A., and Laruelle, M. (2007). Neurobiology of dopamine in schizophrenia. *Int Rev Neurobiol*, 78:1–39.

267. Goggi, J.L., Sardini, A., Egerton, A., Strange, P.G., and Grasby, P.M. (2007). Agonist-dependent internalization of D$_2$ receptors: Imaging quantification by confocal microscopy. *Synapse*, 61:231–341.

268. Siuciak, J.A., Chapin, D.S., McCarthy, S.A., Guanowsky, V., Brown, J., Chiang, P., Marala, R., Patterson, T., Seymour, P.A., Swick, A. *et al.* (2007). CP-809,101, a selective 5-HT$_{2C}$ agonist, shows activity in animal models of antipsychotic activity. *Neuropharmacology*, 52:279–290.

269. Kapur, S., Zipursky, R., Jones, C., Remington, G., and Houle, S. (2000). Relationship between dopamine D_2 occupancy, clinical response, and side effects: A double-blind PET study of first-episode schizophrenia. *Am J Psychiatry*, 157:514–520.

270. Yokoi, F., Gründer, G., Biziere, K., Stephane, M., Dogan, A.S., Dannals, R.F., Ravert, J., Siro, A., Bramer, S., and Wong, D.F. (2002). Dopamine D2 and D3 receptor occupancy in normal humans treated with the antipsychotic drug aripiprazole (OPC 14597): A study using positron emission tomography and [^{11}C] raclopride. *Neuropsychopharmacology*, 27:248–259.

271. Novi, F., Millan, M.J., Corsini, G.U., and Maggio, R. (2007). Partial agonist actions of aripiprazole and the candidate antipsychotics S33592, bifeprunox, N-desmethylclozapine and preclamol at dopamine D2L receptors are modified by co-transfection of D_3 receptors: Potential role of heterodimer formation. *J Neurochem*, 102:1410–1424.

272. Kapur, S. and Seeman, P. (2001). Does fast dissociation from the dopamine D_2 receptor explain the action of atypical antipsychotics? A new hypothesis. *Am J Psychiatry*, 158:360–369.

273. Mamo, D., Graff, A., Mizrahi, R., Shammi, C.M., Romeyer, F., and Kapur, S. (2007). Differential effects of aripiprazole on D_2, 5-HT$_2$, and 5-HT$_{1A}$ receptor occupancy in patients with schizophrenia: A triple tracer PET study. *Am J Psychiatry*, 164:1411–1417.

274. Slifstein, M., Narendran, R., Hwang, D.R., Sudo, Y., Talbot, P.S., Huang, Y., and Laruelle, M. (2004). Effect of amphetamine on [$^{(18)}$F]fallypride in vivo binding to D_2 receptors in striatal and extrastriatal regions of the primate brain: Single bolus and bolus plus constant infusion studies. *Synapse*, 54:46–63.

275. Riccardi, P., Baldwin, R., Salomon, R., Anderson, S., Ansari, M.S., Li, R., Dawant, B., Bauernfeind, A., Schmidt, D., and Kessler, R. (2008). Estimation of baseline dopamine D_2 receptor occupancy in striatum and extrastriatal regions in humans with positron emission tomography with [^{18}F]fallypride. *Biol Psychiatry*, 63:241–244.

276. Agid, O., Mamo, D., Ginovart, N., Vitcu, I., Wilson, A.A., Zipursky, R.B., and Kapur, S. (2007). Striatal vs extrastriatal dopamine D_2 receptors in antipsychotic response-a double-blind PET study in schizophrenia. *Neuropsychopharmacology*, 32:1209–1215.

277. Narendran, R., Slifstein, M., Guillin, O., Hwang, Y., Hwang, D.-R., Scher, E., Reeder, S., Rabiner, E., and Laruelle, M. (2006). Dopamine $D_{2/3}$ receptor agonist positron emission tomography radiotracer [^{11}C]-(+)-PHNO is a D_3 receptor preferring agonist in vivo. *Synapse*, 60:485–495.

278. Ginovart, N., Willeit, M., Rusjan, P., Graff, A., Bloomfield, P.M., Houle, S., Kapur, S., and Wilson, A.A.J. (2007). Positron emission tomography quantification of [^{11}C]-(+)-PHNO binding in the human brain. *Cereb Blood Flow Metab*, 27:857–871.

279. Willeit, M., Ginovart, N., Graff, A., Rusjan, P., Vitcu, I., Houle, S., Seeman, P., Wilson, A.A., and Kapur, S. (2008). First human evidence of d-amphetamine induced displacement of a $D_{2/3}$ agonist radioligand: A [^{11}C](+)-PHNO positron emission tomography study. *Neuropsychopharmacology*, 33:79–289.

280. Sokoloff, P., Diaz, J., Le Foll, B., Guillin, O., Leriche, L., Bezard, E., and Gross, C. (2006). The dopamine D_3 receptor: A therapeutic target for the treatment of neuropsychiatric disorders. *CNS Neurol Disord Drug Targets*, 5:25–43.

281. Narendran, R., Hwang, D.R., Slifstein, M., Talbot, P.S., Erritzoe, D., Huang, Y., Cooper, T.B., Martinez, D., Kegeles, L.S., Abi-Dargham, A. *et al.* (2004). In vivo vulnerability to competition by endogenous dopamine: Comparison of the D_2 receptor agonist radiotracer (-)-N-[^{11}C] propylnorapomorphine [^{11}C]NPA) with the D_2 receptor antagonist radiotracer [^{11}C]-raclopride. *Synapse*, 52:188–208.

282. Seneca, N., Finnema, S.J., Farde, L., Gulyas, B., Wikström, H.V., Halldin, C., and Innis, R.B. (2006). Effect of amphetamine on dopamine D_2 receptor binding in nonhuman primate

brain: A comparison of the agonist radioligand [^{11}C]MNPA and antagonist [^{11}C]raclopride. *Synapse*, 59:260–269.

283. Bantick, R.A., Rabiner, E.A., Hirani, E., de Vries, M.H., Hume, S.P., and Grasby, P.M. (2004). Occupancy of agonist drugs at the 5-HT$_{1A}$ receptor. *Neuropsychopharmacology*, 29:847–859.

284. Bressan, R.A., Erlandsson, K., Jones, H.M., Mulligan, R., Flanagan, R.J., Ell, P.J., and Pilowsky, L. S. (2003). Is regionally selective D$_2$/D$_3$ dopamine occupancy sufficient for atypical antipsychotic effect? An in vivo quantitative [^{123}I]epidepride SPET study of amisulpride-treated patients. *Am J Psychiatry*, 160:1413–1420.

285. Bressan, R.A., Erlandsson, K., Stone, J.M., Mulligan, R.S., Krystal, J.H., Ell, P.J., and Pilowsky, L.S. (2005). Impact of schizophrenia and chronic antipsychotic treatment on [^{123}I]CNS-1261 binding to N-methyl-D-aspartate receptors in vivo. *Biol Psychiatry*, 58:41–46.

286. Stone, J.M., Erlandsson, K., Arstad, E., Bressan, R.A., Squassante, L., Teneggi, V., Ell, P.J., and Pilowsky, L.S. (2006). Ketamine displaces the novel NMDA receptor SPET probe [(^{123})I]CNS-1261 in humans in vivo. *Nucl Med Biol*, 33:239–243.

287. Schiepers, O.J.G., Wichers, M.C., and Maes, M. (2005). Cytokines and major depression. *Prog NeuroPsychopharmacol Biol Psychiatry*, 29:201–217.

288. Rajkowska, G. and Miguel-Hidalgo, J.J. (2007). Gliogenesis and glial pathology in depression. *CNS Neurol Disord Drug Targets*, 6:219–233.

289. Manji, H.K., Quiroz, J.A., Sporn, J., Payne, J.L., Denicoff, K., Gray, A.N., Zarate, C.A., and Charney, D.S. (2003). Enhancing neuronal plasticity and cellular resilience to develop novel, improved therapeutics for difficult-to-treat depression. *Biol Psychiatry*, 53:707–742.

290. Holling, C.S. (1973). Resilience and stability of ecological systems. *Ann Rev Ecol Syst*, 4:1–23.

291. Gunderson, L.H. (2000). Ecological resilience in theory and application. *Annu Rev Ecol Syst*, 31:425–439.

292. Carpenter, S., Walker, B., Anderies, J.M., and Abel, N. (2001). From metaphor to measurement: Resilience of what to what? *Ecosystems*, 4:765–781.

293. Loreau, M., Naeem, S., Inchausti, P. (Eds.). (2002). *Biodiversity and Ecosystems Functioning: Synthesis and Perspectives*, Oxford University Press, Oxford, UK, p. 289.

294. McEwen, B.S. (2007). Physiology and neurobiology of stress and adaptation: Central role of the brain. *Physiol Rev*, 87:873–904.

295. Feinberg, A.P. (2007). Phenotypic plasticity and the epigenetics of human disease. *Nature*, 447:433–440.

296. Mill, J. and Petronis, A. (2007). Molecular studies of major depressive disorder: The epigenetic perspective. *Mol Psychiatry*, 12:799–814.

297. Meaney, M.J. (2001). Maternal care, gene expression, and the transmission of individual differences in stress reactivity across generations. *Annu Rev Neurosci*, 24:1161–1192.

298. Calatayud, F., Coubard, S., and Belzung, C. (2004). Emotional reactivity in mice may not be inherited but influenced by parents. *Physiol Behav*, 80:465–474.

299. Rakyan, V.K. and Beck, S. (2006). Epigenetic variation and inheritance in mammals. *Curr Opin Genet Dev*, 16:573–577.

300. Perkins, D.O., Jeffries, C., and Sullivan, P. (2005). Expanding the "central dogma": The regulatory role of nonprotein coding genes and implications for the genetic liability to schizophrenia. *Mol Psychiatry*, 10:69–78.

301. Sharma, R.P. (2005). Schizophrenia, epigenetics and ligand-activated nuclear receptors: A framework for chromatin therapeutics. *Schizophr Res*, 72:79–90.

302. Akbarian, S., Ruehl, M.G., Bliven, E., Luiz, L.A., Peranelli, A.C., Baker, S.P., Roberts, R.C., Bunney, W.E., Conley, R.C., Jones, E.G. *et al.* (2005). Chromatin alterations associated with

down-regulated metabolic gene expression in the prefrontal cortex of subjects with schizophrenia. *Arch Gen Psychiatry*, 62:829–840.

303. Grayson, D.R., Chen, Y., Costa, E., Dong, E., Guidotti, A., Kundakovic, M., and Sharma, R.P. (2006). The human reelin gene: Transcription factors (+), repressors (−) and the methylation switch (+/−) in schizophrenia. *Pharmacol Ther*, 111:272–286.

304. Levenson, J.M. (2007). DNA (cytosine-5) methyltransferase inhibitors: A potential therapeutic agent for schizophrenia. *Mol Pharmacol*, 71:635–637.

305. Kundakovic, M., Chen, Y., Costa, E., and Grayson, D.R. (2007). DNA methyltransferase inhibitors coordinately induce expression of the human reelin and GAD67 genes. *Mol Pharmacol*, 71:644–653.

306. Tsankova, N., Renthal, W., Kumar, A., and Nestler, E.J. (2007). Epigenetic regulation in psychiatric disorders. *Nat Rev Neurosci*, 8:355–367.

307. Detich, N., Bovenzi, V., and Szyf, M. (2003). Valproate induces replication-independent active DNA demethylation. *J Biol Chem*, 278:27586–27592.

308. Tremolizzo, L., Doueiri, M.S., Dong, E., Grayson, D.R., Davis, J., Pinna, G., Tueting, P., Rodriguez-Menendez, V., Costa, E., and Guidotti, A. (2005). Valproate corrects the schizophrenia-like epigenetic behavioral modifications induced by methionine in mice. *Biol Psychiatry*, 57:500–509.

309. Jessberger, S., Nakashima, K., Clemenson, G.D., Mejia, E., Mathews, E., Ure, K., Ogawa, S., Sinton, C.M., Gage, F.H., and Hsieh, J. (2007). Epigenetic modulation of seizure-induced neurogenesis and cognitive decline. *J Neurosci*, 27:5967–5975.

310. Newman, M.E.J. (2003). The structure and function of complex networks. *SIAM Rev*, 45:167–256.

311. Barabasi, A.L. and Oltvai, Z.N. (2004). Network biology: Understanding the cell's functional organization. *Nat Rev Genet*, 5:101–113.

312. Heim, C. and Nemeroff, C.B. (2001). The role of childhood trauma in the neurobiology of mood and anxiety disorders: Preclinical and clinical studies. *Biol Psychiatry*, 49:1023–1039.

313. Pine, D.S., Cohen, P., Johnson, J.G., and Brook, J.S. (2002). Adolescent life events as predictors of adult depression. *J Affect Disord*, 68:49–57.

314. Bale, T.L. (2006). Stress sensitivity and the development of affective disorders. *Hormones Behav*, 50:529–533.

315. Spauwen, J., Krabbendam, L., Lieb, R., Wittchen, H.U., and van Os, J. (2006). Impact of psychological trauma on the development of psychotic symptoms: Relationship with psychosis proneness. *Br J Psychiatry*, 188:527–533.

316. Carpenter, L.L., Carvalho, J.P., Tyrka, A.R., Wier, L.M., Mello, A.F., Mello, M.F., Anderson, G.M., Wilkinson, C.W., and Price, L.H. (2007). Decreased adrenocorticotropic hormone and cortisol responses to stress in healthy adults reporting significant childhood maltreatment. *Biol Psychiatry*, 62:1080–1087.

317. Addington, J., Cadenhead, K.S., Cannon, T.D., Cornblatt, B., McGlashan, T.H., Perkins, D.O., Seidman, L.J., Tsuang, M., Walker, E.F., Woods, S.W. *et al.* (2007). North American Prodrome Longitudinal Study. *Schizophr Bull*, 3:665–672.

318. Young, A.R. and McGorry, P.D. (2007). Prediction of psychosis: Setting the stage. *Br J Psychiatry*, 51:S1–S8.

319. Linszen, D. and van Amelsvoort, T. (2007). Cannabis and psychosis: An update on course and biological plausible mechanisms. *Curr Opin Psychiatry*, 20:116–120.

320. Morgan, C., Burns, T., Fitzpatrick, R., Pinfold, V., and Priebe, S. (2007). Social exclusion and mental health. *Br J Psychiatry*, 191:477–483.

321. Cuijpers, P., Smit, F., and Van Straten, A. (2007). Psychological treatments of subthreshold depression: A meta-analytic review. *Acta Psychiatr Scand*, 115:434–441.

322. Khan, N., Bower, P., and Rogers, A. (2007). Guided self-help in primary care mental health. *Br J Psychiatry*, 191:206–211.

323. Wong, A.H., Smith, M., and Boon, H.S. (1998). Herbal remedies in psychiatric practice. *Arch Gen Psychiatry*, 55:1033–1044.

324. Southwick, S., Vythilingam, M., and Charney, D.S. (2005). The psychobiology of depression and resilience to stress: Implications for prevention and treatment. *Annu Rev Clin Psychol*, 1:255–291.

325. Badger, F. and Nolan, P. (2007). Use of self-chosen therapies by depressed people in primary care. *J Clin Nurs*, 16:1343–1352.

326. Baghai, T.C., Grunze, H., and Sartorius, N. (2007). Antidepressant medications and other treatments of depressive disorders: A CINP task force report based on a review of evidence. *Int J Neuropsychopharmacol*, 10:S1–S207.

327. Thachil, A.F., Mohan, R., and Bhugra, D. (2007). The evidence base of complementary and alternative therapies in depression. *J Affect Disorders*, 97:23–35.

328. Pilkington, K., Kirkwood, G., Rampes, H., and Richardson, J. (2005). Yoga for depression: The research evidence. *J Affect Disorder*, 89:13–24.

329. Perry, N. and Perry, E. (2006). Aromatherapy in the management of psychiatric disorders: Clinical and neuropharmacological perspectives. *CNS Drugs*, 20:257–280.

330. Aan het Rot, M., Benkelfat, C., Boivin, D.B., and Young, S.N. (2008). Bright light exposure during acute tryptophan depletion prevents a lowering of mood in mildly seasonal women. *Eur Neuropsychopharmacol*, 18:14–23.

331. Larun, L., Nordheim, L.V., Ekeland, E., Hagen, K.B., and Heian, F. (2006). Exercise in prevention and treatment of anxiety and depression among children and young people. *Cochrane Database Syst Rev*, 193:CD004691.

332. Tang, Y.-Y., Ma, Y., Wang, J., Fan, Y., Feng, S., Lu, Q., Yu, Q., Sui, D., Rothbart, M.K., Fan, M. *et al.* (2007). Short-term meditation training improves attention and self-regulation. *Proc Natl Acad Sci USA*, 104:17152–17156.

333. Marks, I.M., Cavanagh, K., and Gega, L. (2007). Computer-aided psychotherapy: Revolution or bubble? *Br J Psychiatry*, 191:471–473.

334. Ruwaard, J., Lange, A., Bowman, M., Broeksteeg, J., and Schriekin, B. (2007). E-mailed standardized cognitive behavioral treatment of work-related stress: A randomized controlled trial. *Cogn Behav Ther*, 36:179–192.

335. Spek, V., Cuijpers, P., Nyklicek, I., Riper, H., Keyzer, J., and Pop, V. (2007). Internet-based cognitive behavior therapy for symptoms of depression and anxiety: A meta-analysis. *Psychol Med*, 37:319–328.

336. Logan, A.C. (2003). Neurobehavioral aspects of omega-3 fatty acids: Possible mechanisms and therapeutic value in major depression. *Altern Med Rev*, 8:410–425.

337. O'Connor, K.A. and Roth, B.L. (2005). Screening the receptorome for plant-based psychoactive compounds. *Life Sci*, 78:506–511.

338. Bradley, B.F., Starkey, N.J., Brown, S.L., and Lea, R.W. (2007). The effects of prolonged rose odor inhalation in two animal models of anxiety. *Physiol Behav*, 92:931–938.

339. Marder, S.R. (2000). Integrating pharmacological and psychosocial treatments of schizophrenia. *Acta Psychiatr Scand*, 102:87–90.

340. POTS (Pediatric OCD Treatment Study) Team (2004). Cognitive-behavior therapy, sertraline, and their combination for children and adolescents with obsessive-compulsive disorder: The Pediatric OCD treatment Study (POTS) randomized controlled trial. *JAMA*, 292:1969–1976.

341. Bush, T.M., Rayburn, K.S., Holloway, S.W., Sanchez-Yamamoto, D.S., Allen, B.L., Lam, T., So, B.K., Trand de, H., Greyber, E.R., Kantor, S., and Roth, L.W. (2007). Adverse interactions between herbal and dietary substances and prescription medications: A clinical survey. *Altern Ther Health Med*, 13:30–35.

342. Maes, M., Mihaylova, I., Kubera, M., and Bosmans, E. (2007). Why fish oils may not always be adequate treatments for depression or other inflammatory illnesses: Docosahexaenoic acid, an omega-3 polyunsaturated fatty acid, induces a Th-1-like immune response. *NeuroEndocrinol Lett*, 28:875–880.

343. O'Reardon, J.P., Brent Solvason, H., Janicak, P.G., Sampson, S., Isenberg, K.E., Nahas, Z., McDonald, W.M., Avery, D., Fitzgerald, P.B., Loo, C. *et al.* (2007). Efficacy and safety of transcranial magnetic stimulation in the acute treatment of major depression: A multisite randomized controlled trial. *Biol Psychiatry*, 62:1208–1216.

344. Stanford, A.D., Sharif, Z., Corcoran, C., Urban, N., Malaspina, D., and Lisanby, S.H. (2008). rTMS strategies for the study and treatment of schizophrenia: A review. *Int J Neuropsychopharmacol*, 1:1–14.

345. James, A., Soler, A., and Weatherall, R. (2005). Cognitive behavioral therapy for anxiety disorders in children and adolescents. *Cochrane Database Syst Rev*, 4:CD004690.

346. Luty, S.E., Carter, J.D., McKenzie, J.M., Rae, A.M., Frampton, C.M., Mulder, R.T., and Joyce, P.R. (2007). Randomised controlled trial of interpersonal psychotherapy and cognitive-behavioral therapy for depression. *Br J Psychiatry*, 190:496–502.

347. March, J.S., Silva, S., Petrycki, S., Curry, J., Wells, K., Fairbank, J., Burns, B., Domino, M., McNulty, S., Vitiello, B. *et al.* (2007). The Treatment for Adolescents with Depression Study (TADS): Long-term effectiveness and safety outcomes. *Arch Gen Psychiatry*, 64:1132–1143.

348. De Maat, S.M., Dekker, J., Schoevers, R.A., and de Jonghe, F. (2007). Relative efficacy of psychotherapy and combined therapy in the treatment of depression: A meta-analysis. *Eur Psychiatry*, 22:1–8.

349. Furukawa, T.A., Watanabe, N., and Churchill, R. (2007). Combined psychotherapy plus antidepressants for panic disorder with or without agoraphobia. *Cochrane Database Systematic Rev*, 1:CD004364.

350. Furukawa, T.A., Watanabe, N., Omori, I.M., and Churchill, R. (2007). Can pill placebo augment cognitive-behavior therapy for panic disorder? *BMC Psychiatry*, 7:1–5.

351. Turkington, D., Kingdon, D., and Weiden, P.J. (2006). Cognitive behavior therapy for schizophrenia. *Am J Psychiatry*, 163:365–373.

352. Jackson, H.J., McGorry, P.D., Killackey, E., Bendall, S., Allott, K., Dudgeon, P., Gleeson, J., Johnson, T., and Haffigan, S. (2007). Acute-phase and 1-year follow-up results of a randomized controlled trial of CBT versus befriending for first-episode psychosis: The ACE project. *Psychol Med*, 16:1–11.

353. Eisenberger, N.I., Taylor, S.E., Gable, S.L., Hilmert, C.J., and Lieberman, M.D. (2007). Neural pathways link social support to attenuated neuroendocrine stress responses. *Neuroimage*, 35:1601–1612.

354. Siegle, G.J., Carter, C.S., and Thase, M.E. (2006). Use of fMRI to predict recovery from unipolar depression with cognitive behavior therapy. *Am J Psychiatry*, 163:735–738.

355. Thase, M.E., Friedman, E.S., Biggs, M.M., Wisniewsk, S.R., Trivedi, M.H., Luther, J.F., Fava, M., Nierenberg, A.A., McGrath, P.J., Warden, D. *et al.* (2007). Cognitive therapy versus medication in augmentation and switch strategies as second-step treatments: A STAR*D report. *Am J Psychiatry*, 164:739–752.

356. Samaha, A.N., Seeman, P., Stewart, J., Rajabi, H., and Kapur, S. (2007). "Breakthrough" dopamine supersensitivity during ongoing antipsychotic treatment leads to treatment failure over time. *J Neurosci*, 14:2979–2986.

357. Stroup, T.S., Lieberman, J.A., McEvoy, J.P., Swartz, M.S., Davis, S.M., Rosenheck, R.A., Perkins, D.O., Keefe, R.S., Davis, C.E., Severe, J. CATIE Investigators. *et al.* (2006). Effectiveness of olanzapine, quetiapine, risperidone, and ziprasidone in patients with chronic schizophrenia following discontinuation of a previous atypical antipsychotic. *Am J Psychiatry*, 163:611–622.

358. Kilzieh, N., Todd-Stenberg, J.A., Kennedy, A., Wood, A.E., and Tapp, A.M. (2008). Time to discontinuation and self-discontinuation of olanzapine and risperidone in patients with schizophrenia in a naturalistic outpatient setting. *J Clin Psychopharmacol*, 28:74–77.

359. Denis, C., Fatséas, M., Lavie, E., and Auriacombe, M. (2006). Pharmacological interventions for benzodiazepine mono-dependence management in outpatient settings. *Cochrane Database Syst Rev*, 3:CD005194.

360. Voshaar, R.C., Couvée, J.E., can Balkom, A.J., Mulder, P.G., and Zitman, F.G. (2006). Strategies for discontinuing long-term benzodiazepine use: Meta-analysis. *Br J Psychiatry*, 189:213–220.

361. Black, K., Shea, C., Dursun, S., and Kutcher, S. (2000). Selective serotonin reuptake inhibitor discontinuation syndrome: Proposed diagnostic criteria. *J Psychiatry Neurosci*, 25:255–261.

362. Judge, R., Parry, M.G., Quail, D., and Jacobson, J.G. (2002). Discontinuation symptoms: Comparison of brief interruption in fluoxetine and paroxetine treatment. *Int Clin Psychopharmacol*, 17:217–225.

363. Van Geffen, E.C., Hugtenburg, J.G., Heerdink, E.R., van Hulten, R.P., and Egberts, A.C. (2005). Discontinuation symptoms in users of selective serotonin reuptake inhibitors in clinical practice: Tapering versus abrupt discontinuation. *Eur J Clin Pharmacol*, 61:303–307.

364. Ruhé, H.G., Huyser, J., Swinkels, J.A., and Schene, A.H. (2006). Switching antidepressants after a first selective serotonin reuptake inhibitor in major depressive disorder: A systematic review. *J Clin Psychiatry*, 67:1836–1855.

365. Suzuki, T., Uchida, H., Watanabe, J.K., Nomura, K., Takeuchi, H., Tomita, K., Tsunoda, K., Nio, S., Den, R., Manki, H., Tanabe, A., Yagi, G., and Kashima, H. (2007). How effective is it to sequentially switch among olanzapine, quetiapine and risperidone? A randomized, open-label study of algorithm-based antipsychotic treatment to patients with symptomatic schizophrenia in the real-world clinical setting. *Psychopharmacology*, 195:285–295.

366. DeMartinis, N., Rynn, M., Rickels, K., and Mandos, L. (2000). Prior benzodiazepine use and buspirone response in the treatment of generalized anxiety disorder. *J Clin Psychiatry*, 61:91–94.

367. Skelton, K.H., Gutman, D.A., Thrivikraman, K.V., Nemeroff, C.B., and Owens, M.J. (2007). The CRF$_1$ receptor antagonist R121919 attenuates the neuroendocrine and behavioral effects of precipitated lorazepam withdrawal. *Psychopharmacology*, 192:385–396.

368. Heidbreder, C.A., Gardner, E.L., Xi, Z.X., Thanos, P.K., Mugnaini, M., Hagan, J.J., and Ashby, C.R. (2005). The role of central dopamine D$_3$ receptors in drug addiction: A review of pharmacological evidence. *Brain Res Rev*, 49:77–105.

369. Bruijnzeel, A.W., Zislis, G., Wilson, C., and Gold, M.S. (2007). Antagonism of CRF receptors prevents the deficit in brain reward function associated with precipitated nicotine withdrawal in rats. *Neuropsychopharmacology*, 32:955–963.

370. McIntyre, M. and Moral, A.M. (2006). Augmentation in treatment-resistant depression. *Drugs of the Future*, 31:1069–1081.

371. Zimmermann, G.R., Lehar, J., and Keith, C.T. (2007). Multi-target therapeutics: When the whole is greater that the sum of the parts. *Drug Discov Today*, 12:34–42.

372. Chenu, F., Guiard, B.P., Bourin, M., and Gardier, A.M. (2006). Antidepressant-like activity of selective serotonin reuptake inhibitors combined with a NK$_1$ receptor antagonist in the mouse forced swimming test. *Behav Brain Res*, 172:256–263.

373. Stahl, S.M. and Grady, M.M. (2004). A critical review of atypical antipsychotic ulilisation: Comparing monotherapy with polypharmacy and augmentation. *Curr Med Chem*, 11:313–327.

374. Chakos, M.H., Glick, I.D., Miller, A.L., Hamner, M.B., Miller del, D., Patel, J.K., Tapp, A., Keefe, R.S., and Rosenheck, R.A. (2006). Baseline use of concomitant psychotropic medications to treat schizophrenia in the CATIE trial. *Psychiatr Serv*, 57:1094–1101.

375. Lin, D., Mok, H., and Yatham, L.N. (2006). Polytherapy in bipolar disorder. *CNS Drugs*, 20:29–42.

376. Bell, E.C., Willson, M.C., Wilman, A.H., Dave, S., and Silverstone, P.H. (2006). Males and females differ in brain activation during cognitive tasks. *Neuroimage*, 30:529–538.

377. Becker, J.B., Monteggia, L.M., Perrot-Sinal, T.S., Romeo, R.D., Taylor, J.R., Yehuda, R., and Bale, T.L. (2007). Stress and disease: Is being female a predisposing factor? *J Neurosci*, 27:11851–11855.

378. Jovanovic, H., Lundberg, J., Karlsson, P., Cerin, A., Saijo, T., Varrone, A., Halldin, C., and Nordström, A.L. (2008). Sex differences in the serotonin1A receptor and serotonin transporter binding in the human brain measured by PET. *Euroimage*, 39:1408–1419.

379. Hughes, R.N. (2007). Sex does matter: Comments on the prevalence of male-only investigations of drug effects on rodent behavior. *Behav Pharmacol*, 18:583–589.

380. Gareri, P., Falconi, U., De Fazio, P., and De Sarro, G. (2000). Conventional and new antidepressant drugs in the elderly. *Prog Neurobiol*, 61:353–396.

381. Smith, G.S., Gunning-Dixon, F.M., Lotrich, F.E., Taylor, W.D., and Evans, J.D. (2007). Translational research in late-life mood disorders: Implications for future intervention and prevention research. *Neuropsychopharmacology*, 32:1857–1875.

382. Taylor, W.D. and Doraiswamy, P.M. (2004). A systematic review of antidepressant placebo-controlled trials for geriatric depression: Limitations of current data and directions for the future. *Neuropsychopharmacology*, 29:2285–2299.

383. Alexopoulos, G.S., Kiosses, D.N., Murphy, C., and Heo, M. (2004). Executive dysfunction, heart disease burden, and remission of geriatric depression. *Neuropsychopharmacology*, 29:2278–2284.

384. Blazer, D.G. and Hybels, C.F. (2005). Origins of depression in later life. *Psychol Med*, 35:1241–1252.

385. Papanikolaou, K., Richardson, C., Pehlivanidis, A., and Papadopoulou-daifoti, Z. (2006). Efficacy of antidepressants in child and adolescent depression: A meta-analytic study. *J Neural Transm*, 113:399–415.

386. Vasa, R.A., Carlino, A.R., and Pine, D.S. (2006). Pharmacotherapy of depressed children and adolescents: Current issues and potential directions. *Biol Psychiatry*, 59:1021–1028.

387. Insel, T.R. (2007). From animal models to model animals. *Biol Psychiatry*, 62:1337–1339.

388. Storm, E.E. and Tecott, L.H. (2005). Social circuits: Peptidergic regulation of mammalian social behavior. *Neuron*, 47:483–486.

389. Lim, M.M. and Young, L.J. (2006). Neuropeptide regulation of affiliative behavior and social bonding in animals. *Horm Behav*, 50:506–517.

390. Buckles, G.R., Thorpe, C.J., Ramel, M.C., and Lekven, A.C. (2004). Combinatorial Wnt control of zebrafish midbrain-hindbrain boundary formation. *Mech Dev*, 121:437–447.

391. Amoyel, M., Cheng, Y.C., Jiang, Y.J., and Wilkinson, D.G. (2005). Wnt1 regulates neurogenesis and mediates lateral inhibition of boundary cell specification in the zebrafish hindbrain. *Development*, 132:775–785.

392. Panula, P., Sallinen, V., Sundvik, M., Kolehmainen, J., Torkko, V., Tiittula, A., Moshnyakov, M., and Podlasz, P. (2006). Modulatory neurotransmitter systems and behavior: Towards zebrafish models of neurogenerative diseases. *Zebrafish*, 3:235–247.

393. Sutton, L.P., Honardoust, D., Mouyal, J., Rajakumar, N., and Rushlow, W.J. (2007). Activation of the canonical Wnt pathway by the antipsychotics haloperidol and clozapine involves dishevelled-3. *J Neurochem*, 102:153–169.

394. Striedter, G.E. (ed.). (2005). *Principles of Brain Evolution*. Sinauer Associates, Inc. Publishers, Sunderland, MA.

395. Fitch, W.T. and Hauser, M.D. (2004). Computational constraints on syntactic processing in a nonhuman primate. *Science*, 303:377–380.

396. Lefebvre, L., Reader, S.M., and Sol, D. (2004). Brains, innovations and evolution in birds and primates. *Brain Behav Evol*, 63:233-246.

397. Teramitsu, I., Kudo, L.C., London, S.E., Geschwind, D.H., and White, S.A. (2004). Parallel FoxP1 and FoxP2 expression in songbird and human brain predicts functional interaction. *J Neurosci*, 24:3152-3163.

398. Vargha-Khadem, R., Gadian, D.G., Copp, A., and Mishkin, M. (2005). FOXP2 and the neuro-anatomy of speech and language. *Nat Rev Neurosci*, 6:131-138.

399. Doupe, A.J. and Kuhl, P.K. (1999). Birdsong and human speech: Common themes and mechanisms. *Annu Rev Neurosci*, 22:567-631.

400. White, S.A., Fisher, S.E., Geschwind, D.H., Scharff, C., and Holy, T.E. (2006). Singing mice, songbirds, and more: Models for FOXP2 function and dysfunction in human speech and language. *J Neurosci*, 26:10376-10379.

401. Gentner, T.Q., Fenn, K.M., Margoliash, D., and Nusbaum, H.C. (2006). Recursive syntactic pattern learning by songbirds. *Nature*, 440:1204-1207.

402. Weir, A.A. and Kacelnik, A. (2006). A new caledonian crow (corvus moneduloides) creatively re-designs tools by bending or unbending aluminium strips. *Anim Cogn*, 9:317-334.

403. Taylor, A.H., Hunt, G.R., Holzhaider, J.C., and Gray, R.D. (2007). Spontaneous metatool use by new Caledonian crows. *Curr Biol*, 17:1504-1507.

404. Templeton, J.J., Kamil, A.C., and Balda, R.P. (1999). Sociality and social learning in two species of corvids: The pinyon jay (Gymnorhinus cyanocephalus) and the Clark's nutcracker (Nucifraga columbiana). *J Comp Psychol*, 113:450-455.

405. Bond, A.B., Kamil, A.C., and Balda, R.P. (2007). Serial reversal learning, the evolution of behavioral flexibility in three species of North American corvids (Gymnorhinus, cyanocephalus, Nucifraga columbiana, Aphelocoma californica). *J Comp Psychol*, 121:372-379.

406. May, R.M. (2006). Network structure and the biology of populations. *Trends Ecol Evol*, 21:394-399.

407. McCann, K.S. (2000). The diversity-stability debate. *Nature*, 405:228-234.

408. Hooper, D.U., Chapin, F.S., Ewel, J.J., Hector, A., Inchausti, P., Lavorel, S., Lawton, J.H., Lodge, D.M., Loreau, M., Nabem, S. *et al.* (2005). Effects of biodiversity on ecosystem functioning: A consensus of current knowledge. *Ecological Monographs*, 75:3-35.

409. Proulx, S.R., Promislow, D.E., and Phillips, P.C. (2005). Network thinking in ecology and evolution. *Trends Ecol Evol*, 20:345-353.

410. McCook, L.J. (1999). Macroalgae, nutrients and phase shifts on coral reefs: Scientific issues and management consequences for the great barrier reef. *Coral Reefs*, 18:357-367.

411. Mumby, P.J., Hastings, A., and Edwards, H.J. (2007). Thresholds and the resilience of Caribbean coral reefs. *Nature*, 450:98-101.

412. Knowlton, N. and Jackson, J.B.C. (2008). Shifting baselines, local impacts, and global change on coral reefs. *PLOS Biol*, 6:0215.

413. Rapport, D.J., Regier, H.A., and Hutchinson, T.C. (1985). Ecosystem behavior under stress. *Am Nat*, 125:617-640.

414. Hughes, T.P., Bellwood, D.R., Folke, C., Steneck, R.S., and Wilson, J. (2005). New paradigms for supporting the resilience of marine ecosystems. *Trends Ecol Evol*, 20:380-386.

415. Graham, N.A.J., Wilson, S.K., Jennings, S., Polunin, N.V.C., and Bijoux, J.P. (2006). Dynamic fragility of oceanic coral reef ecosystems. *Proc Natl Acad Sci USA*, 103:8425-8429.

416. Brené, S., Bjornebekk, A., Aberg, E., Mathé, A.A., Olson, L., and Werme, M. (2007). Running is rewarding and antidepressive. *Physiol Behav*, 92:136-140.

417. Folke, C., Carpenter, S., Walker, B., Scheffer, M., Elmqvist, T., Gunderson, L., and Holling, C.S. (2004). Regime shifts, resilience, and biodiversity in ecosystem management. *Annu Res Ecol Evol Syst*, 35:557-581.

418. Ingelman-Sundberg, M., Oscarson, M., and McLellan, R.A. (1999). Polymorphic human cytochrome P450 enzymes: An opportunity for individualized drug treatment. *Trends Pharmacol Sci*, 20:342–349.

419. Matthews, K., Christmas, D., Swan, J., and Sorrell, E. (2005). Animal models of depression: Navigating through the clinical fog. *Neurosci Biobehav Rev*, 29:503–513.

420. Matthews, P.M., Honey, G.D., and Bullmore, E.T. (2006). Applications of fMRI in translational medicine and clinical practice. *Nat Rev Neurosci*, 7:732–744.

421. Mayberg, H.S., Brannan, S.K., Mahurin, R.K., Jerabek, P.A., Brickman, J.S., Tekell, J.L., Silva, J.A., McGinnis, S., Glass, T.G., Martin, C.C. *et al.* (1997). Cingulate function in depression: A potential predictor of treatment response. *NeuroReport*, 8:1057-1061.

422. Millan, M.J., Panayi, F., Rivet, J.-M., Di Cara, B., Cistarelli, L., Billiras, R., Girardon, S., and Gobert, A. (2007). The role of microdialysis in drug discovery: Focus on antipsychotic agents. In Westerink B.H.C. and Cremers T.I.F.H. (eds.), *Handbook of Microdialysis*, Vol. 16, pp. 485-511, Elsevier, Amsterdam.

423. Morrison, A.P., French, P., Parker, S., Roberts, M., Stevens, H., Bentall, R.P., and Lewis, S.W. (2007). Three-year follow-up of a randomized controlled trial of cognitive therapy for the prevention of psychosis in people at ultrahigh risk. *Schizophre Bull*, 33:682–687.

424. Sanacora, G., Mason, G.F., Rothman, D.L., Ciarcia, J.J., Ostroff, R.B., and Krystal, J.H. (2003a). Increased cortical GABA concentrations in depressed patients receiving ECT. *Am J Psychiatry*, 160:577–579.

425. Tardito, D., Perez, J., Tiraboschi, E., Musazzi, L., Racagni, G., and Popoli, M. (2006). Signaling pathways regulating gene expression, neuroplasticity, and neurotrophic mechanisms in the action of antidepressants: A critical overview. *Pharmacol Rev*, 58:115-134.

426. Taylor, M., Murphy, S.E., Selvaraj, S., Wylezinska, M., Jezzard, P., Cowen, P.J., and Evans, J. (2008). Differential effects of citalopram and reboxetine on cortical Glx measured with proton MR spectroscopy. *J Psychopharmacol*.

427. Mayberg, H.S., Silva, J.A., Brannan, S.K., Tekell, J.L., Mahurin, R.K., McGinnis, S., and Jerabek, P.A. (2002). The functional neuroanatomy of the placebo effect. *Am J Psychiatry*, 59:728-737.

428. Smith, G.S., Koppel, J., and Goldberg, S. (2003). Applications of neuroreceptor imaging to psychiatry research. *Psychopharmacol Bull*, 37:26-65.

429. Weiden, P.J. (2007). Discontinuing and switching antipsychotic medications: understanding the CATIE schizophrenia trial. *J Clin Psychiatr*, 68:Suppl 1, 12-19.

430. Mora, C. (2008). A clear human footprint in the coral reefs of the Caribbean. *Proc Biol Sci.*, 275:767-773.

431. Scheffer, M., Carpenter, S., Foley, J.A., Folke, C., and Walker, B. (2001). Catastrophic shifts in ecosystems. *Nature*, 413:591-596.

CHAPTER 2

Drug Discovery and Development Initiatives at the National Institute of Mental Health: From Cell-Based Systems to Proof of Concept

Lois Winsky, Jamie Driscoll and Linda Brady

Division of Neuroscience and Basic Behavioral Science NIMH NIH, 6001 Executive Blvd. MSC 9641, Bethesda, MD 20892-9641, USA

Animal and Translational Models for CNS Drug Discovery,
Vol. 1 of 3: Psychiatric Disorders
Robert McArthur and Franco Borsini (eds), Academic Press, 2008

59

The mission of the National Institute of Mental Health (NIMH) is to reduce the burden of mental illness and behavioral disorders through research. Toward this goal, the NIMH promotes the development of novel models as an integral part of a larger effort aimed at understanding the neurobiological mechanisms responsible for both normal and disrupted cognitive and emotional control and toward the development of new mechanism of action therapeutics. This chapter presents an overview of NIMH efforts to stimulate treatment discovery and development through support of basic research, targeted drug discovery programs, translational research support, and facilitation of communication between public, private, and government agencies.

THE NEED FOR NEW TREATMENTS FOR MENTAL DISORDERS

Neuropsychiatric disorders have devastating impact for individuals and communities and are among five of the top ten causes of disability worldwide.[1] Available medications and non-pharmaceutical treatments are effective in treating specific symptoms for subsets of affected individuals. However, a significant proportion of individuals with mental disorders do not demonstrate considerable life improvement with available treatments. In addition, serious side effects limit the use of some otherwise effective medications. Finally, specific domains of function, such as cognitive deficits in schizophrenia, are only poorly treated by available psychotherapeutics.

Tremendous advances have been made in the past few decades toward understanding the neurobiology of cognition and emotional regulation. However, these basic science discoveries have not yielded parallel advances in the treatment of mental disorders. Indeed, most of the classes of drugs currently used to treat neuropsychiatric disorders were identified well before much of our current knowledge of brain biology was established.[2,3] Drugs more recently marketed for the treatment of psychosis, mood, and anxiety disorders represent predominantly variations of existing compounds that presumably act through similar mechanisms.[4] Many factors contribute to the absence of novel mechanism of action drugs for treating mental disorders including the staggering cost of bringing drugs to market, and the high attrition rate of candidate therapeutics during development and clinical testing. The inability of preclinical screens to predict potential clinical efficacy accurately and adverse effects contributes to the high rate of failure of new compounds in clinical trials.[5]

MODELS IN DRUG DISCOVERY OF NEUROPSYCHIATRIC DISORDERS

Mental disorders are diagnosed and treatment effectiveness in patients is assessed through behavioral measures, usually as self-reports. While the DSM and ICD-10 diagnostic manuals produce reliable diagnoses,[i] they do not weigh the relative disability imparted by specific clinical features and the symptom profile of some individuals may qualify them for multiple diagnoses.[6] As a result, it is accepted that individuals with the same diagnosis may have different underlying pathology within the brain resulting from different causes.[7] While promising avenues are under investigation, the development of a reliable bioassay for diagnostic purposes is at this point only a goal. Thus, it is not surprising that preclinical screens for the potential effectiveness of new candidate therapeutics rely on assessment of drug effects in behavioral models that are intended to measure changes in function within core domains such as cognitive and emotional processes associated with disorders. It is also not surprising that the match between the preclinical models and measures and clinical diagnoses is generally poor. Since potentially effective drugs may not produce behavioral effects against a normal background, much of the preclinical screening is performed against a genetic and/or environmental (e.g., stressor) manipulation meant to mimic some component of underlying pathology in an animal. The failure of a screen to predict efficacy may thus be due to the use of a manipulation that does not adequately model the neuropathology of a disorder, or only does so for a small percentage of patients. While the target behavioral effects of a new compound in preclinical screens may represent the best estimate of efficacy available, it is difficult to assess if the measures tap into key deficit areas of function for mental disorders. Finally, the predictive validity of many preclinical screens is based on the degree to which the models detect drugs of known clinical efficacy. This requirement may inadvertently limit the ability to detect truly novel mechanism of action compounds.

Models typically employ syndromal or parallel measures approaches. Syndromal models attempt to emulate, through some manipulation, an array of deficits with characteristics indicative of diagnostic criteria for a specific mental disorder. It is presently not possible to assess whether any syndrome model is truly analogous to a mental disorder. Such verification must wait for the availability of reliable and specific non-verbal assessment tools (biomarkers) that are similarly affected in both humans and models. However, the use of a battery of measures to examine the effect of a presumed contributor to the pathology of a disorder, such as a gene defect, may help to identify the aspects of the disorder most affected by the perturbation.

The parallel measures approach involves investigation of a key area of deficit that may be present in more than one mental disorder. Typically, these measures are objective and well-defined behavioral or physiological indices that may be validated as disrupted in both animal models as well as in patients. For example, sensory gating deficits have been demonstrated in both schizophrenic patients and in animal

---

[i] Please refer to the Diagnostic and Statistical Manual of Mental Disorders, Fourth Edition – Text Revision (DSM-IV-TR), or The International Statistical Classification of Diseases and Related Health Problems 10th Revision, published by the American Psychiatric Association and the World Health Organization, respectively, for current diagnostic criteria manuals in use.

models emulating the dopaminergic or glutamatergic dysregulation of this disorder.[8] The advantage of this approach is that it is amenable to neurobiological investigation and the application of knowledge of underlying brain processes and regulatory systems may suggest new avenues for therapeutic target development. Depending on how well linked the measure is to a key area of deficit in a disorder, this parallel measure approach may provide a reasonable model for screening novel mechanism of action drugs. An example of how this approach is being applied toward measuring cognitive function and response to novel drug treatments for schizophrenia is presented later in this chapter.

NIMH SUPPORT FOR DISCOVERY SCIENCE AND BASIC NEUROSCIENCE RESEARCH

The NIMH supports a wide breadth of research spanning from basic molecular neuroscience and behavioral science through clinical trials testing the effectiveness of therapeutics for treating mental disorders. Support of basic neuroscience is critical for placing newly identified brain changes associated with mental disorders and treatment targets within a functional context. Discovery science and neuroscience research are supported predominantly through the funding of investigator-initiated grants. Funding decisions are based on the merit of proposed work as well as relevance to the goals of the NIMH.

The NIMH engages in periodic review of the portfolio of basic research support in order to identify potential new opportunities for expanding basic knowledge and increasing the potential impact of basic research findings toward treatment development (Breaking Ground, Breaking Through: The Strategic Plan for Mood Disorders Research, Setting Priorities for Basic Brain and Behavioral Research at NIMH, http:// www.nimh.nih.gov/strategic/stplan_mooddisorders.cfm). These reviews provide guidance and recommendations of areas for research advancement relevant to mental disorders. For example, the NIMH National Advisory Council workgroup review of the basic behavioral and neuroscience grant support concluded that the NIMH had a strong and impressive portfolio but suggested that more emphasis could be placed in support of research spanning across levels of analysis including the support for refined animal models. NIMH also conducts workshops, aimed at identifying areas of specific need or interest and developing strategies to address them.[9]

ROLE OF NIMH IN DRUG DISCOVERY AND MODEL DEVELOPMENT

In addition to its traditional role of evaluating the efficacy and effectiveness of currently available medications, the NIMH has launched a broad network of programs and initiatives aimed at increasing the likelihood and speed of developing novel treatments for mental disorders. This new effort resulted from the recognized public health need for a new generation of innovative therapeutics for the most prevalent disorders and a first generation of medications for orphan diseases, including developmental disorders. In addition to new NIMH initiatives, the Institute is highly invested in larger scale National Institutes of Health (NIH) efforts related to both the NIH Roadmap for

Biomedical Research and NIH Blueprint for Neuroscience Research, ⟨http://neurosci-enceblueprint.n ih.gov/⟩.The following section outlines the breadth of NIMH programs and initiatives spanning from drug and target discovery through first in human studies. A description of ongoing and recently completed large clinical trials supported by NIMH can be found at the NIMH: Clinical Trials ⟨http://www.nimh.nih.gov/studies/index.cfm⟩.

GRANT SUPPORT FOR DRUG DISCOVERY AND MECHANISM OF ACTION STUDIES

Basic research pertinent to drug discovery and model development is supported within defined programmatic areas.These programs house most of the NIMH funded basic research aimed at developing and characterizing both novel ligands and approved drug treatments across levels of analyses from design, synthesis, and molecular characterization through identification of effects within relevant signaling pathways and cells, identification of mechanism of behavioral action in intact systems, to first in human studies. These efforts are further supported through specific funding initiatives identified below. A complete listing of programs is available at the NIMH website ⟨http://www.nimh.nih.gov/researchfunding/index.cfm⟩.

NIMH Resource Support for Drug Discovery

The NIMH has identified several opportunities for linking molecular neuroscience with efforts to facilitate both drug and tool discovery relevant to mental disorders. In order to address the needs of a diverse set of researchers interested in advancing the study of novel compounds toward these goals, the NIMH has established contract services for drug screening, synthesis, and preclinical toxicology studies ⟨http://www.nimh.nih.gov/research-funding/grants/biological-and-technical-resources-for-research.shtml⟩.

The *NIMH Psychoactive Drug Screening Program* is a resource program that provides screening of novel psychoactive compounds for pharmacological and functional activity at cloned human or rodent CNS receptors, channels, and transporters.The contract also provides assays for predicting bioavailability and cardiovascular toxicity and supports a Ki database ⟨http://pdsp.med.unc.edu/pdsp.php⟩ of affinity constants for ligand binding.

The *NIMH Chemical Synthesis and Drug Supply Program* synthesizes and distributes novel research chemicals, psychoactive drugs, and compounds unavailable to the scientific community from commercial sources.The program also supports radio-synthesis and Good Manufacturing Practice (GMP) synthesis of promising candidate compounds for use in clinical studies.

The *NIMH Toxicological Evaluation of Novel Ligands Program* provides toxicology and safety assessment of promising, target-selective compounds for use as imaging ligands in human studies, and limited assessment of novel psychoactive agents for clinical research and as potential therapeutics.Toxicology and safety data generated by the program can be used to support an Investigational New Drug (IND) application to the Food and Drug Administration (FDA), and for Radioactive Drug Research Committee (RDRC) evaluation of a compound for human studies.

NIH Resource Support for Drug Discovery

The goal of the *Molecular Libraries and Imaging Roadmap* (http://nihroadmap.nih.gov/molecularlibraries) initiative is to establish a national high throughput screening (HTS) resource in the academic environment to improve the understanding of biology and disease mechanisms. At the core of this initiative is the Molecular Libraries Screening Centers Network (MLSCN, http://www.mli.nih.gov). The MLSCN optimizes and performs HTS for the identification of small biologically active molecules. While the focus of the MLSCN is not explicitly geared toward any disease, many of the assays would detect current treatments for mental disorders through their effects on, for example, G-protein coupled receptors (GPCRs), transporters, ion channels, protein kinases, and other enzymes. Compounds screened by the MLSCN are maintained within the Small Molecule Repository (http://mlsmr.glpg.com/) that was established in 2004 and currently has a set of approximately 300,000 compounds of specified purity, quantity, and solubility. Data generated by the MLSCN centers including assay descriptions, chemical structures, and results for individual compounds is stored in a publicly accessible database maintained by the National Library of Medicine (PubChem, http://pubchem.ncbi.nlm.nih.gov/). Investigators may access the MLSCN resources through the submission of assays for optimization and HTS development, by submitting compounds into the Small Molecule Repository for screening, and through PubChem. For more information on this effort, see recent review.[10]

NIH-RAID (Rapid Access to Interventional Development) is an NIH Roadmap Pilot program intended to reduce some of the common barriers between laboratory discoveries and clinical trails of new therapeutic entities (http://nihroadmap.nih.gov/raid/). The goal of the NIH-RAID Pilot is to make available, on a competitive basis, certain critical resources needed for the development of new small molecule therapeutic agents. Potentially available services by the NIH-RAID program include production, bulk supply, GMP manufacturing, formulation, development of an assay suitable for pharmacokinetic testing, and animal toxicology. The NIH-RAID Pilot is not a grant program. The funds to support individual projects are provided by Roadmap funds and individual Institutes. NIH-RAID projects of interest to the NIMH involve the development of novel small molecule therapeutics for mental disorders.

NIMH Initiatives Supporting Drug Discovery and Target Identification

The NIMH complements support of investigator-initiated grants in the area of treatment research through specific initiatives developed to stimulate and facilitate drug discovery and development efforts. These initiatives are intended to encourage investigators interested in developing new therapeutics or novel ways to test candidate compounds, including new assays or model systems to evaluate potential efficacy and utility in the treatment of mental disorders. The initiatives span the breadth of the drug development process, from target identification and ligand discovery, to preclinical development and clinical testing, through effectiveness trials.

Preclinical CNS Drug Discovery

To maximize the potential for translating basic molecular science into treatment and tool discoveries, the NIMH created this initiative specifically to encourage the submission of applications aimed at drug discovery and early preclinical testing of compounds with therapeutic potential (http://grants.nih.gov/grants/guide/pa-files/ PAR-07–048.html). The initiative encourages studies aimed at design, synthesis, and preclinical testing of compounds, development of novel delivery systems, and cell-based assays for screening of candidate compounds for efficacy and/or toxicity. The announcement also encourages the development of novel assays using model organisms or behavioral systems for preliminary screening or further evaluation of candidate compounds, including *in vivo* models that emulate critical features of specific CNS disorders. Model development must be directed toward assessing potential efficacy rather than elucidating disease mechanisms. Applications submitted in response to this announcement are directed to a Drug Discovery Special Emphasis Review Panel convened by the Center for Scientific Review.

PET and SPECT Ligand Imaging

This initiative encourages applications aimed at developing novel radioligands for positron emission tomography (PET) or single photon emission computed tomography (SPECT) imaging in human brain, and that incorporate pilot or clinical feasibility evaluation in preclinical studies, model development, or clinical studies. The long-term goal of this initiative is to facilitate the broad application of neuroimaging probes in pathophysiological studies, drug discovery/development research, and in biomarker development/qualification studies as quantifiable indicators of disease progression and treatment efficacy (http://grants.nih.gov/grants/guide/pa-files/PA-06–461.html).

Small Business Innovation Research (SBIR)

Small businesses play an increasingly important role in drug discovery and development (http://www.nimh.nih.gov/research-funding/small-business/index.shtml). The NIMH supports small business involvement in drug discovery through the publication of several targeted initiatives that support the development of novel pharmacologic treatments for mental disorders (http://grants.nih.gov/grants/guide/pa-files/PA-06-027.html), including novel screening assays from molecular/cellular screens to whole animal tests, the commercial development of novel radioligands for PET and SPECT imaging in human brain (http://grants.nih.gov/grants/guide/pa-files/PA-06-017.html), the development of biomarkers, and high throughput tools for brain research at any level of analysis from molecules through behavior (http://www.nimh.nih.gov/research-funding/small-business/index.shtml).

Developmental Psychopharmacology

Developmental psychopharmacology solicits applications to examine the neurobiological impact of psychotherapeutic medications upon the immature brain. Investigations in model organisms that examine molecular, genetic, neurochemical, physiological, and behavioral effects of early drug administration in both juvenile and adolescent animals are encouraged (http://grants.nih.gov/grants/guide/pa-files/PA-07-084.html).

Neurodevelopmental and Neuroendocrine Signaling in Adolescence: Relevance to Mental Health

This program encourages submission of applications aimed at the identification of neurodevelopmental and neuroendocrine mechanisms that impact emotional and cognitive development and emerging psychopathology during adolescence, using animal models and human studies (http://grants1.nih.gov/grants/guide/pa-files/PA-07-208.html).

Women's Mental Health and Sex/Gender Differences Research

This program invites applications targeting the development of models to examine sex differences and the impact of hormonal transitions across the lifespan of females on brain physiology and function, including, for example, neural plasticity, cognition, and mood (http://grants.nih.gov/grants/guide/pa-files/PA-07-164.html).

Women's Mental Health in Pregnancy and the Postpartum Period

Women's mental health in pregnancy and the postpartum period encourages the development of appropriate models of the peripartum period combining genetic and environmental influences on postpartum hormonal status, emotionality, and/or maternal behavior, which will be essential for understanding the neurobiology of perinatal mood disorders (http://grants.nih.gov/grants/guide/pa-files/PA-07-081.html).

Functional Links Between the Immune System, Brain Function and Behavior

This program targets the development and refinement of animal models of immune signaling in brain, including models examining the effects of pre- and post-natal infection on brain development and behavior, models of the effects of acute and chronic immune challenge on brain function and behavior, and models of the role of the blood–brain barrier in neuroimmune responses (http://grants.nih.gov/grants/guide/pa-files/PA-07-088.html).

NIMH Initiatives for Drug Development: Preclinical, First in Human, and Clinical Studies

The NIMH participates in several large grant and cooperative agreement mechanisms aimed at fostering partnerships between NIMH, academia, and industry to advance the development and testing of fundamentally new, rationally designed medications, and treatments for mental disorders. These initiatives provide a vehicle for industry and academic scientists to pool intellectual and material resources for the translation of basic science findings into the conceptualization, discovery, and evaluation of new chemical entities in preclinical, first in human, and proof of concept studies in the treatment of mental disorders. Below are descriptions of translational programs, active in 2007, which have been an effective means for NIMH to assist the academic and private sector efforts to fill the drug discovery pipeline with novel mechanism of action compounds for the treatment of mental disorders.

National Cooperative Drug Discovery Group Program

The goal of the National Cooperative Drug Discovery Group (NCDDG) program (http://grants.nih.gov/grants/guide/pa-files/PAR-07-159.html) is to accelerate innovative drug discovery, the development of pharmacologic tools for basic and clinical research on mental disorders, drug or alcohol addiction, and the development and validation of models for evaluating novel therapeutics for mental disorders through encouraging scientific collaborations between academia and the private sector. The NIMH supports NCDDG studies of molecular targets in two or more of the following areas:

1. ligand discovery for therapeutics development and as research tools (e.g., imaging probes) for novel molecular targets implicated in mental illnesses;
2. preclinical testing of novel compounds in disease-based models;
3. development and validation of novel, disease-based genetic models combined with environmental or behavioral manipulations for evaluating therapeutic compounds;
4. initial Good Laboratory Practice (GLP) toxicology, safety pharmacology, and pharmacokinetics to support IND application to the FDA to begin human clinical testing; and/or
5. limited Phase I studies.

The program also supports the goal of developing and evaluating new cellular, circuit, genetic, or pathophysiology based models for validation of novel targets for mental disorders.

Cooperative Drug Development Group

As with the NCDDG, grants funded under the Cooperative Drug Development Group (CDDG) program are intended to foster long-term partnerships between NIMH, academia, and industry aimed at advancing the development and testing of new medications and treatments for serious mental disorders (http://grants1.nih.gov/grants/guide/pa-files/PAR-05-010.html). However, in contrast with the NCDDG, which is aimed at more preclinical discovery, the principal aim of the CDDG program has been the testing in humans of novel mechanism therapeutics, with testing of new IND-ready pharmacological agents or approved agents in clinical populations as a mandatory element. As such, the grants funded under the CDDG program help fill the gap between preclinical drug discovery efforts and clinical effectiveness trials networks also supported by the NIMH.

Centers for Intervention Development and Applied Research

The Centers for Intervention Development and Applied Research (CIDAR) program encourages interdisciplinary teams of leading basic, applied, and clinical investigators to engage in a focused research program targeting a specific problem in the diagnosis or treatment of mental illness. The program focuses on research to (1) define predictors and understand the mechanism of treatment response in major mental disorders; (2) create and refine biomarkers to assess the presence and/or extent of mental illness; and/or (3) hasten the development of novel treatments for mental disorders. The goal of CIDAR is to support the translation of basic and clinical research into innovations in clinical assessment and therapeutics (this program is currently not accepting new applications).

FACILITATING THE DEVELOPMENT AND EVALUATION OF PRECLINICAL MODELS FOR THERAPEUTIC DISCOVERY

Many of the programs and initiatives described above incorporate within them requests for the development of novel models capable of reliably detecting clinical efficacy of new mechanism of action compounds. Not included in this list are previous targeted and time-limited funding initiatives. For example, a specific request for applications was issued in 2003 to request proposals aimed at developing new models relevant to bipolar disorder, based on the recognized need in this difficult to study area. It is too early to assess the success of this specific request. In general, the success of such initiatives is likely to depend on the state of both clinical and basic research at the time of the request and the ability to translate information into relevant neurobiological questions. Through support of a strong portfolio of basic neuroscience research and efforts aimed at increasing the communication between clinical and basic researchers, the NIMH is well poised to translate novel clinical neuroscience findings toward the development of novel models.

Workshops Addressing Barriers in Treatment Development

The NIMH has conducted several workshops and workgroups to evaluate the status of preclinical models as used for understanding psychopathology and for novel treatment development.[9] These workgroups customarily task groups of clinical and basic researchers to identify areas of opportunity with maximal traction for expanding bidirectional translational work toward the development of novel, biologically based models for understanding psychopathology, and for assessing novel therapeutics. Common themes expressed during these workshops include the need to develop parallel measures in model systems that emulate core deficits in mental disorders, the value of identifying appropriate quantifiable behavioral and physiological cross-species measures to assess key neurobiological deficits, the need to expand basic neurobiological studies of circuits contributing to pathology, and complementary efforts to determine how and when specific susceptibility factors contribute to the etiology of specific disorders and the expression of symptoms.

IDENTIFICATION OF KEY MEASURES OF CLINICAL EFFICACY: THE EXAMPLE OF COGNITIVE DEFICITS IN SCHIZOPHRENIA

Assessment of the usefulness of new models and screens for testing potential therapeutics is typically based on the ability of the new model to identify medications having efficacy for treating disorders (predictive validity). However, this approach is not available in drug discovery for new indications where effective treatments are not yet available. For example, while currently available models may sufficiently identify treatments for psychotic symptoms of schizophrenia, other areas of deficit that significantly impact function are only beginning to be modeled for treatment development.

Cognitive deficits are core and enduring features of schizophrenia and the extent of cognitive deficits is considered a key predictor of outcome and quality of life for patients with schizophrenia. Unfortunately, existing antipsychotic medications are relatively ineffective in improving cognitive function, strongly indicating the need for new mechanism of action drugs targeting these deficits. The programs elaborated below are examples of collaborative efforts focusing on this problem and involving broad participation of NIMH, FDA, academia, and the pharmaceutical/biotechnology sector. This model approach could be applied to identify clinical targets in other disease areas where broad input is needed, such as social cognition in autism, impulse control in ADHD or bipolar disorder, or anhedonia and sleep disturbances in mood disorders.

Measurement and Treatment Research to Improve Cognition in Schizophrenia

The Measurement and Treatment Research to Improve Cognition in Schizophrenia (MATRICS) program was designed by the NIMH to support the development of pharmacological agents for improving the neurocognitive impairments that are a core feature of schizophrenia (http://www.matrics.ucla.edu/). The goals of the NIMH MATRICS program were to catalyze regulatory acceptance of cognition in schizophrenia as a target for drug registration, promote development of novel compounds to enhance cognition in schizophrenia, leverage economic research power of industry to focus on important but neglected clinical targets, and identify lead compounds that support proof of concept trials for cognitive enhancement in schizophrenia. A series of conferences were held as part of the MATRICS process to assess what is known about cognitive deficits in schizophrenia, develop a consensus on the promising targets for intervention and the most promising models (animal and human) for use in drug development for this indication, identify a core battery of cognitive assessment tests, and identify the most appropriate clinical trials design. These conferences included participants from NIMH, the FDA, academia, and industry. The major outcome of these conferences was the identification of key domains of cognitive function that are disrupted in schizophrenia and the development of a consensus test battery to assess those domains for use in clinical trials of procognitive medications for schizophrenia. For a recent review of the program and targets for cognitive enhancement in schizophrenia, see[11-14].

NIMH Workshops on Developing Assessment Tools for Cognitive Functioning

NIMH has recently supported a new series of workshops as a continuation of MATRICS. The goal of these workshops is to develop measures for use in clinical trials further. The current clinical tests used to assess cognition in schizophrenic patients and the effects of therapeutics on ameliorating cognitive deficits were developed before basic research in cognitive neuroscience identified specific neural circuits and systems potentially involved in cognitive processes. Cognitive neuroscientists have developed animal models and testing paradigms that tap into the basic neural mechanisms believed to underlie cognition; however, these paradigms have not, for the most part, been used in the drug development process and have not been translated to the clinical setting. The workshops are intended to help develop tests that are more specific measures of brain functions related to cognitive function in schizophrenia and to assure that these measures are validated for use in clinical trials.

Treatment Units for Research on Neurocognition and Schizophrenia

The Treatment Units for Research on Neurocognition and Schizophrenia (TURNS) initiative is another component of the NIMH effort to stimulate academic and industry sponsored research focused on cognitive deficits in schizophrenia. It follows completion of MATRICS described above (http://www.turns.ucla.edu/). The TURNS program is an NIMH-supported network that provides an infrastructure for clinical studies of pharmacological agents for enhancing neurocognition in patients with schizophrenia. The TURNS clinical research network evaluates the safety, efficacy, pharmacokinetics, and pharmacodynamics of new agents for the treatment of cognitive deficits of schizophrenia. The TURNS program also aims to further characterize and define key aspects of cognition in schizophrenia as potential treatment targets.[ii]

FUTURE OPPORTUNITIES FOR MODEL DISCOVERY

The NIMH has adapted a broad strategy of support ranging from basic neuroscience through clinical research toward the goal of improving outcomes for individuals with mental disorders. This includes the recognized need to identify model systems and measures that more closely predict clinical benefit or adverse effects of new drug entities for the treatment of mental disorders. Below are some areas of promise and opportunity for facilitating this effort.

Development of Biomarkers for Mental Disorders

As previously discussed, the greatest impediment in the development of reliable animal models for drug discovery relevant to psychiatric disorders is the inherent discontinuity between models and the use of imprecise diagnostic methods that are not based on the neurobiology of the disorders. The development of endophenotypes or biomarkers that reliably identify individuals with specific deficits is expected to be a major advance for both clinical research and treatment development. The biomarkers may arise from efforts to develop well-defined psychometric measures, neuroimaging, genetics, proteomics, and other approaches supported through NIMH. In addition, the Foundation for NIH, a non-profit organization that complements NIH efforts, recently announced support for an extension of the NIMH-supported STAR*D depression trials to identify biomarkers associated with effective treatment response (Whole Genome Association in Major Depressive Disorder: Identifying Genomic Biomarkers for Treatment Response; WGA), through the Biomarkers Consortium (http://www.fnih.org/news/news_events_Oct.shtml).[iii]

[ii] Please refer to Jones *et al.*, Developing new drugs for schizophrenia: From animals to the clinic, in this volume for further discussion on modeling cognitive disorders in schizophrenia as well as the MATRICS and TURNS initiatives.

[iii] For more information about the Biomarkers Consortium, see http://www.fnih.org/Biomarkers%20Consortium/Biomarkers_home.shtml.

Modeling Genetic, Developmental, and Environmental Risk Factors

Additional large efforts to identify genes associated with mental disorders are being supported by NIH and other agencies. For example, through the Autism Consortium, NIH is supporting studies aimed at identifying genes associated with autism spectrum disorders (http://www.nimh.nih.gov/press/autismconsortiumgrants.cfm). NIH funds whole genome association studies to identify genetic factors influencing risk for complex diseases in order to facilitate discovery of new molecular targets for prevention, diagnosis, and treatment through the Genetic Association Information Network (GAIN, http://www.fnih.org/GAIN/GAIN_home.shtml) and genotyping and other genomic research methodologies to identify the major susceptibility and etiologic factors for complex diseases of significant public health impact through the Genes and Environment Initiative (GEI, http://www.genome.gov/19518663). These efforts are complimentary to private efforts. For example, the Broad Institute of MIT and Harvard University recently announced the application of a sizable gift fund from the Stanley Medical foundation primarily to identify and characterize risk genes for psychiatric diseases through linkage and association studies in the human population, with additional efforts to develop animal and cellular models to investigate the function of candidate genes and pathways, to develop sophisticated imaging techniques for elucidating brain-based phenotypes in clinical disease, and to design high throughput chemical screens for identifying molecules that modulate important cellular targets related to neural function (see http://www.broad.mit.edu/psych/).

Functional genomics approaches are beginning to identify risk factors in humans that may offer valuable insights into the molecular, cellular, and systems-level pathogenesis of mental disorders and potentially new targets for therapeutic development. Translational strategies such as a convergent functional genomics approach used by Le-Niculescu and colleagues[15] to identify schizophrenia candidate genes by integration of brain gene expression data from pharmacogenetic mouse models with human genetic linkage and postmortem brain data hold promise for identifying risk alleles in other mental disorders. As results of genetic studies in clinical populations begin to identify potential risk factors, it will be important to follow up these results with functional studies in basic neurobiological systems to identify how identified genes impact brain function. In addition, as we discover risk genes in humans we may, by the creation of transgenic mice, expressing one or more human risk alleles, begin to understand how disease-associated gene alterations impact brain signaling within circuits contributing to the core symptoms of mental disorders and use this information to develop at least partial animals models of pathology. Understanding where, when, and how these genes affect normal brain function will likely lead to new model systems, perhaps even cell-based models, that may be applied toward the development and testing of new potential therapeutics in an efficient manner.

Genetic analysis of behavioral domains is another example of a promising approach to develop models of genetic, developmental, and environmental risk factors for psychiatric disorders. The behavioral domain approach of Kas and colleagues[16] focuses on understanding the genetics of naturally occurring behaviors such as social interaction, appetitive motivation, activity, and cognitive function that cut across DSM-IV diagnostic boundaries of mental disorders. The approach depends on conserved gene function, the presence of functional polymorphism(s) in the gene or set of genes across species, and is critically dependent on the choice of an analogous phenotype in both humans and the model species. The combined use of genetically tractable model organisms and behavioral measures of disease domains will be crucial to understanding the mechanisms by which gene–environment, genotype–phenotype relationships, and gene-by-sex interactions influence susceptibility to mental disorders.

MODELING KEY DEFICITS IN MENTAL DISORDERS

Mental disorders are heterogeneous, with significant differences in the patterns of emotional, cognitive, and physiological symptoms that may be present in affected individuals as well as age of onset and precipitating factors. Focused efforts aimed at identifying core deficits of these disorders, such as the MATRICS and TURNS initiatives described above, serve as a model for programs aimed at exploring new opportunities for targeting endophenotypes or key symptoms as therapeutic targets. These initiatives encourage greater collaboration between clinical researchers and basic scientists toward identification of areas for targeting treatment development and assessment of efficacy.

APPLICATION OF DATA-MINING TECHNOLOGY IN MODEL EVALUATION AND DRUG DISCOVERY

While novel pharmacological treatments have not yet been approved for treating mental disorders, several new mechanism of action compounds are in the pipeline for potential drug discovery for major mental disorders targeting, for example, NMDA, GABA, and peptide systems.[12,17] Early trials of novel compounds will present an opportunity to evaluate the predictive validity of existing preclinical models for their potential to identify new mechanism of action drugs. Informatics efforts linking results of preclinical tests with clinical effectiveness for promising new treatments in trials could illuminate which currently used models best predict efficacy, and could also elaborate the clinical characteristics or patient populations with the greatest treatment response. Success of this type of endeavor would require increased communication and sharing of preclinical data between industry, academia, and government motivated by the understanding that such data could ultimately reduce the time and cost of bringing new drugs to market. Furthermore, as efforts such as the NIH Molecular Libraries continue to collect data on the chemical structure and functional activity of a broad range of small molecules, they are creating a large searchable database (PubChem) that links structure to functional assay analyses. These databases may suggest not only new lead structures for drug development but may also identify structures conferring potential adverse effects. For example, recent evaluation of drugs inducing valvular heart dysfunction revealed common binding of a diverse series of drugs with this effect on serotonin 5-HT_{2B} receptors suggesting that activity of a new chemical entity at this receptor might be a strong indicator of an adverse effect on heart function.[18]

CONCLUSIONS

The NIMH encourages the development and refinement of preclinical models through investigator-initiated research support and by targeted efforts addressing the need for novel mechanism of action treatments. The potential for success in developing new models that reliably predict clinical efficacy or adverse effects relies ultimately on improvements in both clinical evaluation and the application of basic science toward translational boundaries. Communication between clinicians and clinical and basic neuroscientists is essential for this synthesis. Support for basic science is critical for understanding the underlying biological mechanisms and functional significance of newly identified clinical indicators (e.g., genetic, neuroimaging) of risk, pathology, or treatment response. As pathways are identified and linked, new molecular and cellular targets for treatment development are likely to emerge from this translational discovery science. These discoveries will need to be adapted into cellular, circuit-based, physiological, and/or behavioral models to allow screening and efficacy testing of candidate therapeutic compounds. Similarly, the identification of core deficits in psychiatric disorders with significant negative impact on the health and functioning of patients, such as the recognition of cognitive deficits as a treatment development target in schizophrenia, also has potential to improve the predictive validity of preclinical models. Efforts to increase the concordance between the measures of the clinical condition and the models will likely improve the utility of models for identifying truly novel medications.

REFERENCES

1. Lopez, A.D. and Murray, C.C. (1998). The global burden of disease, 1990–2020. *Nat Med*, 4(11):1241–1243.
2. Spedding, M., Jay, T., Costa e Silva, J., and Perret, L. (2005). A pathophysiological paradigm for the therapy of psychiatric disease. *Nat Rev Drug Discov*, 4(6):467–476.
3. Spedding, M. (2006). New directions for drug discovery. *Dialog Clin Neurosci*, 8(3):295–301.
4. Insel, T.R. and Scolnick, E.M. (2006). Cure therapeutics and strategic prevention: raising the bar for mental health research. *Mol Psychiatry*, 11(1):11–17.
5. Duyk, G. (2003). Attrition and translation. *Science*, 302(5645):603–605.
6. Hyman, S.E. and Fenton, W.S. (2003). Medicine. What are the right targets for psychopharmacology?. *Science*, 299(5605):350–351.
7. Agid, Y., Buzsaki, G., Diamond, D.M., Frackowiak, R., Giedd, J., Girault, J.A. *et al.* (2007). How can drug discovery for psychiatric disorders be improved?. *Nat Rev Drug Discov*, 6(3):189–201.
8. Braff, D.L., Geyer, M.A., and Swerdlow, N.R. (2001). Human studies of prepulse inhibition of startle: Normal subjects, patient groups, and pharmacological studies. *Psychopharmacology (Berl)*, 156(2–3):234–258.
9. Winsky, L. and Brady, L. (2005). Perspective on the status of preclinical models for psychiatric disorders, *Drug Discovery Today: Disease Models*, 30(20):1–5.
10. Lazo, J.S., Brady, L.S., and Dingledine, R. (2007). Building a pharmacological lexicon: Small molecule discovery in academia. *Mol Pharmacol*, 72(1):1–7.
11. Gray, J.A. and Roth, B.L. (2007). Molecular targets for treating cognitive dysfunction in schizophrenia. *Schizophrenia Bull*, 33(5):1100–1119.

12. Roth, B.L. (2006). Contributions of molecular biology to antipsychotic drug discovery: Promises fulfilled or unfulfilled? *Dialog Clin Neurosci*, 8(3):303–309.

13. Stover, E.L., Brady, L. and Marder, S.R. (2007). New paradigms for treatment development. *Schizophrenia Bull*, 33(5):1093–1099.

14. Tamminga, C.A. (2006). The neurobiology of cognition in schizophrenia. *J Clin Psychiatry*, 67(9):e11.

15. Le-Niculescu, H., Balaraman, Y., Patel, S., Tan, J., Sidhu, K., Jerome, R.E. *et al.* (2007). Towards understanding the schizophrenia code: An expanded convergent functional genomics approach. *Am J Med Genet B Neuropsychiatr Genet*, 144(2):129–158.

16. Kas, M.J., Fernandes, C., Schalkwyk, L.C., and Collier, D.A. (2007). Genetics of behavioural domains across the neuropsychiatric spectrum; of mice and men. *Mol Psychiatry*, 12(4):324–330.

17. Norman, T.R. and Burrows, G.D. (2007). Emerging treatments for major depression. *Expert Rev Neurother*, 7(2):203–213.

18. Roth, B.L. (2007). Drugs and valvular heart disease. *N Engl J Med*, 356(1):6–9.

CHAPTER 3

Issues in the Design and Conductance of Clinical Trials

Joseph P. McEvoy[1] and Oliver Freudenreich[2]

[1]Duke Clinical Research Service, John Umstead Hospital, 1003 12th Street Building 32, Butner, NC 27509, USA
[2]First Episode and Early Psychosis Program, Massachusetts General Hospital, Harvard Medical School, Boston, MA 02114, USA

INTRODUCTION

Clinical trials are conducted to determine the therapeutic efficacy, effectiveness, safety, and tolerability of interventions for clinical disorders. The best clinical trials are designed to do this efficiently with minimal potential for bias. In this chapter, we will focus on trials of pharmacological interventions for psychiatric disorders, in particular, how translational models can improve the quality of these trials.

Animal and Translational Models for CNS Drug Discovery,
Vol. 1 of 3: Psychiatric Disorders
Robert McArthur and Franco Borsini (eds), Academic Press, 2008

Animal and translational models that closely recapitulate aspects of the patho-physiology of psychiatric disorders will improve the processes for selecting candidate compounds for further development. Translational models will also help to identify the most appropriate patients for trial participation and permit sub-typing of patients into groups with greater or lesser likelihoods of response to specific pharmacological actions. Translational models of therapeutic action can provide markers to assure that adequate doses of investigational compounds are used in pivotal clinical trials, and can provide independent, objective measures of change. Translational models of toxicity can help to approximate the maximum tolerated doses of investigational compounds.

NEW DRUG DEVELOPMENT

The first clinically available antipsychotic, antidepressant, and mood-stabilizing compounds were identified by serendipitous clinical observations of therapeutic effects from agents administered for other indications. As the pharmacological actions of these initial compounds became better understood, "me, too" candidate compounds were developed through medicinal chemistry to recapitulate the therapeutic actions of the original compounds and limit their associated side effects. These "me, too" compounds were screened in animal and laboratory models for pharmacological actions expected to predict therapeutic effects in humans. The more promising compounds then underwent comprehensive testing in animal species to determine their toxicities, metabolism, pharmacokinetics, and pharmacodynamics prior to extensive testing in humans.

The pharmaceutical industry now faces growing pressure on drug pricing; in particular, there is declining willingness to support "me, too" compounds that offer little, if any, advantage over very good and now generic, existing drugs. Improving methods in molecular biology, including genomics, proteomics, and others, have identified thousands of *new* potential targets for pharmaceutical compounds.[1] Improving methods in combinatorial chemistry and high throughput analyses can rapidly provide numerous compounds that bind *in vitro* with these potential molecular targets. Unfortunately, the relationships between these novel molecular targets and clinical disease are uncertain. Classical animal models of therapeutic action that do not include sites of action for novel compounds offer no guidance prior to clinical testing in humans. It is not surprising that lack of efficacy now accounts for approximately half of the attrition of novel compounds entering clinical testing.[2] It is expected that many investigational compounds with unproven mechanisms of action will prove to be inefficacious; the key now is to identify inefficacious compounds early, before the great expense of an extended Phase II program, and certainly before Phase III.

Humans have become the ultimate "model organism" in which to determine efficacy.[3] Experimental medicine is a conceptual framework that attempts to amass evidence of mechanism and evidence of efficacy in late Phase I and as early as possible in Phase II in humans.[i] Experimental medicine also expects to find that the clinical manifestations

---

[i] Please refer to Large *et al.*, Developing therapeutics for bipolar disorder: from animal models to the clinic or Tannock *et al.*, Towards a biological understanding of ADHD and the discovery of novel therapeutic approaches, in this Volume, for further discussion regarding initiatives in experimental medicine biomarkers and surrogate markers in psychiatric drug development.

of chronic psychiatric syndromes (psychosis, anxiety, depression, etc.) are the common results of multiple different pathophysiological mechanisms, as are shortness of breath or fever. Parsing and explicating these mechanisms may lead to treatments that are specific to individual mechanisms, to biomarkers that identify a patient as a candidate for a specific treatment or that indicate the efficacy of that treatment.[ii] Clinical models of disease developed through experimental medicine will feed information back to preclinical researchers that will help them to develop and refine new animal models for therapeutic mechanisms first identified in humans. Drug development has traditionally been divided in phases with relatively standardized goals and activities comprising each phase. New developments, including micro-dosing and adaptive trial designs, have blurred distinctions between the traditional clinical trial phases.[iii]

Phase 0

Phase 0 micro-dosing involves administering very tiny single doses of an investigational compound to humans before extensive testing in animals with the goal of culling early those compounds with problematic bioavailability or pharmacokinetics. These doses are well below those expected to have any pharmacological effect in humans, but permit evaluation of the absorption, distribution, metabolism, and excretion of the investigational compound via accelerator mass spectrometry (AMS), an ultra-sensitive bio-analytical platform capable of quantifying C^{14} labeled compounds with attamole (10^{-18}) sensitivity.[4] When combined with positron-emission tomography (PET) or gamma-scintigraphy, micro-dosing can also provide early evidence that the investigational compound reaches the brain. The European Medicines Agency (EMEA) and the US Food and Drug Administration (FDA) have issued guidelines encouraging the exploration of micro-dosing as a means to improve the efficiency of lead compound selection.[4,5]

Micro-doses are so low, and the associated risk is so small that only limited animal testing is required prior to micro-dosing studies. Only a single mammalian animal species need be studied with increasing single doses administered via the expected clinical route until a pharmacological effect is detectable. Body weight, clinical signs, hematology, and histopathology are assessed at 2 and 14 days. No genetic toxicology is required. This animal testing, along with studies in tissue culture and computer modeling, help to establish what the micro-dose is for the compound; usually 1/100th the dose expected to produce any pharmacological effect in humans, or 100 µm, whichever is smaller, is selected. Animal testing also protects against compounds that could be fatal even at minute doses, for example, ricin.

[ii] Please refer to Tannock *et al.*, Towards a biological understanding of ADHD and the discovery of novel therapeutic approaches, in this Volume and Lindner *et al.*, Development, optimization and use of preclinical behavioral models to maximize the productivity of drug discovery for Alzheimer's Disease, in Volume 2, *Neurologic Disorders*, for further discussion regarding biomarkers and surrogate markers in experimental medicine.

[iii] Please refer to Winsky *et* al., Drug discovery and development initiatives at the National Institute of Mental Health: From cell-based systems to proof of concept in this volume and to Wilding *et al.*, Anti-obesity drugs: From animal models to clinical efficacy, in Volume 3, *Reward Deficit Disorders*, for description and discussion of preclinical strategies in drug discovery programs prior to drug entry into humans.

It was estimated that in the 1990s, up to 40% of investigational compounds failed during early clinical trials because of problematic bioavailability or pharmacokinetics.[3] Micro-dosing studies have the potential to identify some of these failures early, thus avoiding wasted time and money in extensive animal testing. Traditional comprehensive animal testing, building to first-in-human exposure of an investigational compound, costs $1.5–3.0 million, and requires more than 18 months to complete. Micro-dosing studies can be completed in less than 6 months at a cost less than $500 000.[4] Currently, bioavailability or pharmacokinetic problems account for only 10% of drug attrition in human development.[3]

Micro-doses are specifically selected to not have pharmacological effects. The focus of micro-dosing studies is on pharmacokinetics. Many, but not all, of the processes controlling the pharmacokinetics of a compound are independent of the dose level. Investigational compounds with obvious pharmacokinetic problems (e.g., exceptionally rapid clearance) can be culled early. However, if the pharmacokinetics of a compound involves transporters, enzymes, or binding sites that can become saturated at higher therapeutic doses, its clinical pharmacokinetics may turn out to be very different from those predicted by micro-dosing studies.

Phase I

Phase I trials comprise the initial exposure of an investigational compound to humans (if micro-dosing studies were not previously done) and are only begun after demonstration of minimal toxicity during extensive exposures of the compound in a variety of animal species. The goals of Phase I trials include: (1) exploring the safety of the investigational compound carefully and progressively through gradually increasing doses and durations of exposure; (2) determining the absorption/bioavailability, pharmacokinetics, metabolism, and excretion of the compound; and (3) delineating the pharmacodynamic actions of the investigational compound, first in normal volunteers, and later in patients with the target indication.[7,8]

Phase I trials focus primarily on safety and the distribution of the investigational drug throughout the human body, not on potential therapeutic actions on the target indication. Therefore, the participants in early Phase I trials are usually normal volunteers who can be efficiently recruited and studied. Phase I trials are usually undertaken in dedicated trial centers with established protocols for multifaceted safety monitoring and repeated blood sampling. Normal volunteers are housed in these centers for the duration of the trials, with emergency personnel constantly available.

Single-dose studies begin at a small fraction, for example, 1/100th, of the maximum dose that produced no pharmacological effects in large animal species. Dose increments, made only after all data from initial doses are reviewed by safety monitors, are determined based on pharmacokinetic and pharmacodynamic data from prior animal studies. Doses are gradually increased until some evidence of dose-limiting intolerance is detected. Single dose pharmacokinetic blood sampling is done on at least a portion of participating subjects.[9,10]

After careful review of all safety data from single-dose studies, repeated-dose studies begin. Dosing intervals are determined based on pharmacokinetic data and the duration of pharmacodynamic effects from the single-dose studies. Repeated-dose studies are usually done for 10–14 days. Pharmacokinetic data are obtained during repeated-dose studies in at least a portion of participating subjects. Participants are usually monitored closely for 4–5 times the elimination half-life after the last dose of the investigational drug was received, and again 30 days after the last dose. Any adverse events occurring during this period must be included in the study report.

In the interests of safety, the sequence of progressively administering higher doses to successive subjects cannot be altered. However, interpolated, random, and blinded administration of placebo to ~25% of subjects at each dose level will result in more objective evaluation of the safety and tolerability data obtained.

The investigational drug is usually administered in the fasting state initially to avoid any potential variability in absorption associated with food intake. Later studies directly examine the effects on absorption of food or agents that change stomach pH (e.g., antacids), and the effects on blood levels of the investigational of drugs that affect protein binding or common pathways of drug metabolism (e.g., the cytochromes). Metabolic disposition of the investigational drug is explored through preparations of the compound containing radioactive isomers of constituent elements. The handling of the investigational drug by volunteers with renal or hepatic impairment is examined. Establishing full and complete dose- or plasma concentration-effect curves for wanted and unwanted drug effects is very helpful in guiding design specifics for later studies.[7]

Patients with psychiatric disorders may tolerate higher doses of some drugs than can normal volunteers. Late in Phase I, single- and multiple-dose studies exploring the safety and tolerability of higher doses in patients with the target indication are undertaken. Translational models may suggest chemical, physiological, or behavioral measures that can be monitored during these early dosing studies that can guide Phase II studies toward earliest determinations of therapeutic efficacy, or the lack thereof, for the investigational compound.[7,10]

Phase II

Phase II trials represent the first administration of the investigational compound to patients with the primary expressed purpose of detecting therapeutic activity of the investigational compound for the target indication, if such activity exists. A proof of concept study is done early in Phase II to test the fundamental question: does the investigational compound have therapeutic activity for the target indication? Pharmaceutical management often bases the decision whether to continue clinical development of the investigational compound on the results of a proof of concept study. Finding evidence of a dose–response relationship, as well as superiority over a comparator (usually placebo), in a proof of concept study provides early confidence in the compound. By the end of Phase II, it is crucial to have approximated the optimal therapeutic dose range to be used in pivotal Phase III trials. Phase II trials also expand the safety and tolerability data on the investigational compound. Because of the limited prior experience with the investigational compound in humans, risk is inherent in Phase II trials; safety monitoring must be comprehensive and in real time so that exposure of patients can be halted immediately if toxicity is detected.

Prior to a proof of concept study, single- and multiple-dose-rising studies should proceed to identify the maximum tolerated dose of the investigational compound in patients with the target indication (if this was not done late in Phase I). It is desirable that experienced investigators who see participating patients themselves conduct these trials, both for the safety of participating patients and for the best selection of investigational compound doses in the proof of concept study. A proof of concept study usually includes a dose close to the maximum tolerated dose in patients with the target indication.[11,12]

Proof of concept studies usually focus on the treatment of acute exacerbations of chronic illnesses (e.g., schizophrenia or recurrent depression) since patients in acute exacerbations can be expected to show a large therapeutic benefit from an efficacious compound and little effect from placebo, providing statistically significant evidence of efficacy. Relapse-prevention studies, studies of the investigational compound as an add-on to other treatments, and studies of the investigational compound in patients unresponsive to other treatments usually come later.

A proof of concept study is usually a relatively large, blinded, randomized, fixed-dose trial that has the potential to bracket the optimal range for the pivotal Phase III trials; in particular, fixed-dose trials are particularly effective in approximating the lowest effective dose of an investigational compound. Concurrent placebo-control is essential. Regulatory agencies expect placebo control as a key component of the scientific quality of trials throughout development.[11] In addition, placebo control can provide preliminary evidence of therapeutic benefit (if at least one dose of the investigational compound proves superior to placebo on the primary outcome measure); once preliminary evidence of therapeutic benefit is provided, regulatory agencies may relax restrictions on the enrollment of women of child-bearing potential and on the duration of treatment with the investigational compound for future studies[7] A standard comparator control is highly desirable in early trials. The presence of a placebo-standard comparator difference assures that the study was done well enough to detect a therapeutic effect if it is present (assay sensitivity). If an investigational drug is superior to placebo, but inferior to existing treatments in therapeutic efficacy (without a large tolerability advantage), it is useful to learn this early before embarking on an expensive full development program.

> *"Adaptive design is a trial design that allows modifications to some aspects of the trial after its initiation without undermining the validity and integrity of the trial. Adaptive design makes it possible to discover and rectify inappropriate assumptions in trial designs, lower development costs, and reduce the time to market".[13]*

Only limited information is available about the optimal dose range, the optimal patient population, the variability in measurement of the primary outcome measure, etc. before initiating a proof of concept study. The trial may have been set up suboptimally, in ways that only become apparent after the data become unblinded. Staged protocol or group-sequential designs give investigators more opportunities for decision points as the trial is in progress, rather than waiting to see the whole picture at the end. An early look at unblinded data may lead investigators to re-estimate sample size requirements, to adapt randomization so that more successful treatment assignments receive disproportionately higher allotments of patients, to drop inferior treatment assignments, or to stop the study early due to established efficacy or futility.[13]

Proposed biomarkers of likelihood of response can be examined in an early look, and patient selection criteria can be adapted to enrich the population with patients most likely to favorably respond to the investigational compound.[iv]

Outcomes that are apparent early, and quick and reliable electronic data collection, are mandatory for an adaptive trial design that is dependent on mid-study updating. Bayesian statistical methods were developed to incorporate new data as they come in and to update the probabilities under investigation.[12] Unlike traditional statistical approaches, Bayesian methods make use of the results of previous information from the ongoing experiment to assign probabilities to all remaining unknowns. The Bayesian approach exploits the results, as the trial is ongoing and adapts the design based on interim information. Endpoints and sample size have to be chosen to ensure that sufficient statistical power is available to answer the questions posed at each decision point. Finding analytical solutions for adaptive designs is theoretically challenging and usually involves large numbers of computer simulations.[13]

Substantial variability across patients in the absorption, pharmacodynamic response, and clearance of any investigational compound is to be expected. The goal of Phase II is not to identify a single optimal dose for all patients, but rather to bracket a range across which the majority of patients will find the investigational compound tolerable, and many will display whatever therapeutic benefit it offers.[7]

Continued blood sampling for population pharmacokinetics is desirable throughout the Phase II studies (and continuing in Phase III) in the effort to delineate important relationships between plasma levels of the investigational compound and therapeutic effects and/or important adverse effects. Blood sampling also provides information about treatment compliance.[15]

Once preliminary (but compelling) evidence of therapeutic benefit, extended evidence of safety, and a confident approximation of the optimal dose range of the investigational compound have been obtained, the sponsor can formulate a plan for full development of the investigational compound and approach regulatory agencies for their input and approval.

Phase III

Phase IIIa trials are done to provide convincing evidence, to be used in the New Drug Application (NDA) to regulatory agencies, that the investigational compound is safe and has substantial therapeutic efficacy for the target indication. Convincing evidence consists of at least two high quality, clearly positive pivotal efficacy trials that are part of an overall pattern of results supporting the safety and efficacy of the investigational compound.[7]

The established and preferred experimental design for Phase IIIa pivotal efficacy trials is the randomized, double blind, 3-5 arms, parallel trial (including placebo, a standard comparator, and 1-3 doses of the investigational compound). Data from Phases 1 and 2 guide dose selection for these trials. In at least one trial, a "no effect" dose expected to be below the optimal therapeutic dose range should be included.

[iv] Please refer to Gardener *et al.*, Issues in designing and conducting clinical trials for reward disorders: a clinical view in Volume 3, *Reward Deficit Disorders*, for further discussion of patient selection in clinical trials.

In another trial, a dose approaching the maximum tolerated dose should be included. Doses believed to be in the optimal therapeutic and tolerability ranges should be duplicated across two or more of the trials. Adaptive design approaches may be considered in Phase III if uncertainty about the optimal dose range persists, or if developing knowledge in translational models provides potential biomarkers for use in patient selection or outcome measurement.

It is not uncommon to have *failed* (no difference between the placebo and standard comparator arms) or *negative* (a difference between the placebo and standard comparator arms, but not between the placebo and investigational compound arms) psychopharmacology trials, even with an investigational compound that will ultimately prove to be a useful therapeutic agent. It is therefore wise to undertake 3–4 potentially pivotal trials in order to have a high likelihood of having two successful positive trials (differences between the placebo and standard comparator arms and between the placebo and investigational drug arms) for submission to regulatory agencies.[7,11]

Regulatory agencies require safety experience over at least 12 months of exposure to the investigational compound, preferably with several hundred patients, prior to NDA approval.[16] Therefore, patients who achieve therapeutic benefit during pivotal acute treatment trials should be invited to remain on treatment with their assigned medication with a least safety follow-up until the NDA is approved or abandoned. Alternatively, or in addition, separate long-term maintenance trials can be initiated once an optimal dose range can be offered with confidence. Relapse-prevention trials can also be considered. These trials may continue through Phase IIIb.

Phase IIIb trials are undertaken after submission of an NDA application to expand practical clinical experience with the investigational compound. Trials may be done in new populations, such as those experiencing their first episode of illness or the elderly, to investigate more aggressive initial dosing strategies of the investigational compound (in particular, if rapid management of acute illness is desirable), or to explore the safety, tolerability, and efficacy (perhaps additive) of co-prescription of the investigational compound with other medications used for the target indication. The utility of the investigational compound in patients receiving minimal therapeutic benefit from available treatments may be examined.

Phase IV

Phase IV trials serve to widen the breadth and duration of experience with the investigational compound in clinical settings. Sponsors use Phase IV trials to position the investigational drug best for marketing if the NDA is approved.[7] Large numbers of non-research clinicians may be offered the investigational compound for use in their patients without charge, with the requirement that they will collect simple outcome data regarding duration of treatment, acceptability to patients, doses used, and ongoing safety. Cost-effectiveness studies may be done, and broader measures of outcome such as quality of life and functioning may be addressed. Additional randomized, blinded trials involving different standard comparators than were used in Phases II and III may be undertaken in order to differentiate the investigational drug further from other agents prescribed for the target indication. Different drug-delivery systems, for example, a once-daily sustained release preparation or an injectable preparation may be studied.

PRAGMATIC EVALUATION OF APPROVED DRUGS

When an NDA is approved, much remains to be learned about the new drug. Clinicians will use the new drug in patients excluded from the sponsored clinical trials done for regulatory approval (e.g., patients with comorbid medical conditions or substance-use disorders, children and the elderly) unless specifically prohibited. Clinicians will combine the new drug with adjunctive and concomitant medications excluded from the regulatory trials, and use the new drug at doses above those addressed in the regulatory trials. Clinicians initiate the new drug at higher doses and at different dosing intervals than those supported by the regulatory trials. Safety monitoring of the worldwide use of a new drug may detect problems with these new use patterns, and reveal rare but important safety risks that could not be detected in the small sample of selected patients comprising the pre-marketing database.[16,17]

Sponsors develop an investigational compound at enormous cost, with the hope of garnering substantial profit from its clinical use. Conscious or unconscious bias can be expected in the design of development trials that can give advantages to the "home team".[17,18] For this reason, independent granting agencies sponsor later trials that attempt to "level the playing field" for the new drug and its comparators. These trials may evaluate untested patterns of use of the drug that unfold in clinical practice, may compare the new drug to other drugs prescribed for the target indication at optimal doses of all treatments, and may examine the effectiveness of the drug in the hands of practicing clinicians treating "real world" patient populations with few if any exclusion criteria. Commonly, these trials temper enthusiasm generated by the marketing wing of the pharmaceutical sponsor. For example, the recent Clinical Antipsychotic Trials of Intervention Effectiveness (CATIE) Schizophrenia trials found little evidence for greater effectiveness of the newer atypical antipsychotic medications relative to proper doses of an older, generic conventional antipsychotic, perphenazine (Trilafon®).[19]

March and colleagues[20] proposed key characteristics of practical clinical trials in psychiatry: they should address a straightforward, clinically relevant question; they should include representative samples of patients and practice settings; they should have sufficient power to identify statistically modest but clinically relevant effects; they should be randomized to protect against bias and blinded if logistically possible; there should be uncertainty among knowledgeable clinicians regarding the outcome of treatment at the patient level; the assessment and treatment protocols should enact best clinical practices; there should be simple and clinically relevant outcomes, and limited subject and investigator burden. We believe that, in addition, these trials should be sponsored by public funds.

CLINICAL TRIAL DESIGN AND IMPLEMENTATION

The central question asked in a clinical trial determines the trial design and the method of data analysis. Early in the development of an investigational compound the central question is whether the investigational compound offers more therapeutic efficacy than placebo (with acceptable safety and tolerability). In individual early developmental trials, the question becomes whether the investigational compound (at doses x, y, and z) produces greater reductions in psychopathology (as measured by a particular instrument) in patients (characterized by a specific diagnosis, level of acuity, etc.) over a given period of time, relative to placebo. A standard comparator is included for assay sensitivity, that is, to document that the study procedures were implemented well enough to demonstrate the superior efficacy of the standard comparator relative to placebo. Later in development, maintenance trials compare the durability of the investigational compound over time, relative to placebo and an active comparator, as the patient attempts to live his or her life in the community as successfully as possible. Patients may begin maintenance trials in either an acutely ill or a stabilized state. The initial goal is to transition patients successfully to the assigned treatments. The later goal is to observe how well therapeutic benefit and tolerability endure over time, and how well patients in each treatment group function across broad measures of outcome. An argument can be made to not include a placebo arm in maintenance trials for patients with severe and persistent mental illnesses; relapse can severely disrupt the lives of patients and their families, and may be dangerous. Recovery from a relapse cannot be guaranteed, even if previously effective treatments are re-instituted.

It is best to ask only one or two primary questions in any clinical trial, and to answer these correctly. Multiple measures of efficacy will be highly inter-correlated, and for probabilistic reasons may provide contradictory results. Prolonged series of assessments can be wearisome and irritating for patients with psychiatric disorders, leading to inattentive or unmotivated participation, or to withdrawal of consent for participation. Harried research assistants, struggling to complete multiple assessments, may value all assessments equally and have less time and care than is necessary for those that are most important. As stated by Wooding, "large numbers of required responses usually contribute little to the fundamental objective, may be detrimental to careful and precise work, and may introduce needless statistical problems even when they produce positive results",[11] (p. 63).

Randomization, concurrent controls, and blinding are fundamental for limiting bias in clinical trials. Random assignment of treatments implies that it is a matter of pure chance which treatment assignment will be made next, and "assures lack of bias in the distribution of the treatments to the sample",[11] (p. 34). Concurrent controls are "included in the experiment and tested at the same time and in the same way as the other treatments",[11] (p. 35). Blinding may not be perfect, but must be sufficient to make raters uncertain as to what treatment assignment each patient has received.

Patient Populations

In early efficacy trials, the patients most likely to demonstrate a difference in outcome between treatment with an active comparator and treatment with placebo are treatment-responsive patients who have not recently been receiving treatment (either because this is their first episode or because they have discontinued their prescribed medications against the advice of their treating clinicians), and who have experienced an acute, *unmedicated* exacerbation of their illness.

Such patients cannot be defined solely by a severity rating on a rating scale. Patients who have been reliably taking prescribed medications can have acute, *medicated* exacerbations (with substantial increases in psychopathology ratings) related to psychosocial stressors or substance use. Such exacerbations have different clinical dynamics than unmedicated exacerbations and may resolve spontaneously with support and removal from stress or the abused substance, irrespective of treatment with an active comparator or placebo. Patients with *treatment non-responsive illness*[v] may maintain high psychopathology ratings and have little potential for demonstrating a difference between placebo and an active comparator. Investigators that have a good understanding of the dynamics of the target indication, and a commitment to the integrity of the trial, must presently be relied on to select appropriate patients. Better biomarkers for diagnosis and the activity state of psychiatric illnesses or centralized ratings of televised patient interviews may lead to more objective determination of patients' appropriateness for participation in early efficacy trials in the future.

For maintenance trials, it is important to exclude patients with little likelihood of complying with assigned treatments, such as patients with known histories of non-compliance or patients who have comorbid attributes associated with non-compliance (e.g., substance use disorders).

Inclusion criteria are an effort to ensure that all participating patients have the disease that is the target indication, and that the disease is in the state designated best to address the central study question. An age range is selected; most early studies are done in adults 18–65 years of age. Early studies exclude women of childbearing potential; only after initial evidence of efficacy is demonstrated are women of childbearing potential included, and then only if they maintain acceptable birth control methods. Only after efficacy and safety are strongly supported are the effects of the investigational compound explored in children and adolescents and in older individuals.

Exclusion criteria are an effort to limit confounding effects on the key comparisons of the trial, and to protect the safety of participants. For safety reasons, patients with comorbid illnesses that could be exacerbated by participation, or who must take medications with potential interactions with any of the study medications should be excluded. Patients taking medications with lingering effects that could interfere with assessment of primary outcomes should be excluded.

Duration of Trials

Shorter efficacy trials, for example, 4 rather than 8 weeks of comparative treatment duration, are more likely to result in complete data on the largest percentage of participating patients. Patients drop out of trials for a wide range of reasons, including reasons having little directly to do with the primary outcomes (efficacy and safety). Progressively more patients drop out the longer studies endures.[21,22]

Studies of treatments for acute exacerbations of schizophrenia or bipolar disorder are usually done in the inpatient setting and are expensive because of "bed costs" for the inpatient stay. In addition to providing a safety net for participating patients who may be randomized to placebo or ineffective treatments, the inpatient setting permits

---

[v] Please refer to Klitgaard *et al.*, Animal and translational models of the epilepsies, in Volume 2, Neurological Disorders, for further discussion on treatment resistance.

support for treatment compliance, provides consistent low levels of stress, and limits confounding substance use. Duration of 4 weeks is presently considered adequate, if treatment responsive patients in an unmedicated exacerbation comprise the great majority of the patient sample. If the majority of participating patients were stable outpatients before entering hospital, recruited by advertisement to participate in the trial, differences between placebo and an active comparator may not become apparent until 6–8 weeks; in fact, this represents a variant of a relapse-prevention study rather than an acute treatment study, it will be more expensive to do, and the likely placebo-active comparator differences will be smaller.

Maintenance trials usually last at least 6 months; trials of 2 years or more provide valuable safety information and may be necessary to distinguish differences in the effectiveness of treatments, as manifest in social relationships, employment, and other complex outcomes that unfold slowly.[23,24]

Sample Size and Statistical Power

The null hypothesis in early efficacy trials is that the investigational compound has no therapeutic efficacy for the target disorder, that is, that it is no better than placebo.[7,11] Type I error is to conclude incorrectly that the investigational compound has therapeutic efficacy when it does not, that is, to reject a true null hypothesis. The purpose of a placebo control is to signal the risk for a Type I error (all treatment groups do well). Appropriately selected patients assigned to placebo should do poorly, and patients assigned to the active comparator should do significantly better.

Type II error is to conclude incorrectly that the investigational compound does not have therapeutic efficacy when it does, that is, to accept a false null hypothesis. The purpose of an active comparator is to signal the risk for a Type II error (all treatment groups do badly). Appropriately selected patients assigned to the active comparator should do well, and patients assigned to placebo should do poorly. Power (calculated as 1 – the probability of a Type II error) is defined as the probability of rejecting the null hypothesis when it should be rejected, that is, when the null hypothesis is indeed false.

Simply put, power is the likelihood that investigators will detect a difference between the efficacy of the investigational compound and the efficacy of placebo when such a difference exists. Less variance in the assessment of the primary outcome measure and larger sample sizes (of appropriately selected patients) increase power.

Many trials in psychiatry are underpowered to answer research questions.[25,26] Pilot studies notoriously overestimate effect sizes, leading to inadequately powered trials. Cost-conscious limitation of sample size can prove disastrous if differences in key measures only approach significant difference at trial's end. Adaptive designs that focus on re-estimation of sample size requirements after the trial is underway allow for adjustment in sample size, and the possibility of dropping unproductive treatment arms. Always err is in the direction of excess power. The risks of potentially exposing a few additional patients to an investigational compound to determine that compound's worth definitively are less than the risks of wasting the exposures of all participating patients in a non-definitive underpowered study.

Pharmacological Treatments

Packaging of study medications in as simple a manner as possible is highly desirable. Patients with psychiatric illnesses may be impatient, cognitively impaired or suspicious. They may balk at being asked to take 6–8 capsules daily, or several from one bottle and several more from another. Blister packs that are completely obvious to pharmacists can be completely confusing to non-guild members. Licensed practical nurses in hospitals are accustomed to administering 1–2 tablets or capsules from a bottle at each dosing interval; complicated packaging leads to medication errors. Every effort should be made to achieve simplicity and clarity in the delivery of the assigned treatments.

A drug that must be titrated over 7–10 days to therapeutic doses will not be an acceptable alternative for acute disorders characterized by agitation or distress. As development proceeds, exploring ways to reach therapeutic doses as quickly as possible becomes a priority. Limitations of dose escalation seen in normal volunteers should be challenged in patients who may be far more tolerant. If a drug cannot be brought to a therapeutic dose rapidly enough for use in acute treatment but is well tolerated and effective once it reaches an adequate dose, it may still have a role in maintenance treatment, for example, lamotrigine for the treatment of bipolar depression (see below). This option can be studied in patients initially stabilized with other treatments.[vi]

Adjunctive medications are those that treat some aspect of psychopathology not directly addressed by the active comparator or investigational compound, for example, insomnia in a study of antidepressant medications or depression in a study of antipsychotic medications. It is foolish to lose patients from a trial because they cannot sleep before a potential antidepressant has the opportunity to demonstrate efficacy. It is foolish to allow a patient recovering nicely from a psychotic episode to suffer depression during a maintenance trial of antipsychotic medications. Careful thought must be given regarding every excluded treatment alternative because of potential loss of otherwise highly appropriate patients for testing the central question of the trial. Only those likely to clearly make testing of the central hypothesis more difficult should be excluded.

Concomitant medications are those prescribed to treat a side effect of the active comparator or investigational drug (e.g., anticholinergic anti-Parkinson medications prescribed to relieve extrapyramidal side effects) or to treat a comorbid medical condition (e.g., oral hypoglycemic medications for diabetes mellitus). Again, only those that directly confound the primary study question should be excluded.

All adjunctive and concomitant medications should be recorded during a clinical trial, along with the clinical indication for their use, and comparisons made in the rates of their use across the treatment groups. Such analyses may point out that an antidepressant is prescribed at greater frequency with the active comparator relative to the investigational compound.

[vi] Please refer to Large *et al.*, Developing therapeutics for bipolar disorder (BPD): From animal models to the clinic, in this Volume for a discussion of the use of lamotrigine for the treatment of bipolar disorder.

Outcomes

A fundamental requirement for answering that question is the certainty that patients assigned to treatment with the investigational compound and patients assigned to placebo or the active comparator were receiving their assigned treatments and no confounding treatments. Sponsors or investigators should *always* measure compliance with medication, preferably by means of blood levels. Assays for the investigational compound, the active comparator, and all other agents prescribed for the target indication should be done on blood samples from all patients participating in registration trials. Medication errors by staff, surreptitious non-compliance or self-medication by patients, and other errors can lead to patients not getting their assigned medication or taking confounding medication.

Duration in treatment (survival in trial) is a summary measure that integrates efficacy and tolerability. At each assessment point, the participating patient and the treating clinician must decide whether the assigned treatment is demonstrating sufficient efficacy and is tolerable enough to continue. The percent of patients successfully completing a trial tells much about the future clinical acceptability of an investigational compound. Even if discontinuation from treatment is not a primary measure, it should be included in all study reports.

It is important to keep psychopathology outcome measures limited and focused. Careful consideration has to be given preferably to one well-chosen outcome measure or study endpoint.[vii] The best available measure, usually a rating scale (see below) is completed at baseline, repeatedly over the course of treatment, and at the end of study; the treatment groups are compared on rates or amounts of change. It is highly desirable to have the same rater assess the patient at each assessment point and to have substantial experience with patients with the target indication. Rating scales that have clear item descriptors and anchor point descriptors and initial and continuing training of raters will assist in maintaining the reliability of ratings.[27]

The particular choice of a rating scale of psychopathology depends on the disorder under investigation. Well-validated scales are available for the major psychiatric syndromes (e.g., the Positive and Negative Syndrome Scale (PANSS) for schizophrenia[28] or the Young Mania Rating Scale (YMRS) for mania.[29] There is no benefit to having additional assessments that get at the same psychopathology constructs. As previously mentioned these will be highly correlated with the primary rating, add useless burden to participating patients and research staff, and are likely to complicate the interpretation of results.

An effort should be made to distinguish changes in the core features of target illness psychopathology from non-specific agitation or withdrawal. It can be hoped that biomarkers from translational models will provide consistent correlates with such core psychopathological features.

Tolerability assessments should be comprehensive at first, but become more focused on commonly reported adverse events as experience with the investigational

---

[vii] Please refer to Gardener *et al.*, Issues in designing and conducting clinical trials for reward disorders: a clinical view in Volume 3, *Reward Deficit Disorders*, for further discussion of end point selection and statistical analyses in clinical trials.

compound grows. Open-ended questions about "any other problems" should be asked at the beginning and end of tolerability assessments with the intent of identifying unanticipated adverse events. Vital signs and laboratory measures of systemic health should be extensively recorded throughout development.

It can be informative to collect patients' subjective experiences of the benefit and tolerability of their assigned treatments. These experiences are often embedded in very different conceptual frameworks from those of research staff and they may be idiosyncratic from patient to patient. Simple global measures that integrate patients' perceptions of the worth of the drug and its burden of side effects can be informative.

IMPROVEMENTS ARE NEEDED AND TRANSLATIONAL MODELS WILL HELP

Patient Population

Diagnosis is syndrome-based in psychiatry, made on the basis of clusters of signs and symptoms and their course of appearance.[viii] No external validating measures exist that consistently discriminate those who truly have a circumscribed disorder from those who have overlapping features from some other cause. We believe that the most common cause of failed efficacy trials is the inclusion of patients who do not suffer from the target illness, who have the target illness but in a quiescent state, or whose illness is minimally responsive or unresponsive to any treatment. In any of these latter cases, the width of a placebo-active comparator difference will be reduced. Our understanding of the pathophysiology of psychiatric disorders evolved through iterative interactions between clinical observations and translational models. Some drugs that affect dopamine and glutamate neurotransmission were noted to reduce psychotic features in people with psychotic disorders. Other drugs that affect these neurotransmitter systems in other ways were found to produce psychosis in people not previously psychotic; these latter drugs also induce observable features of psychosis (disorganized behaviors, stereotypical movements) in laboratory animals.

Psychotic features are seen across many of our current diagnostic entities and respond consistently to antipsychotic drugs, irrespective of diagnosis. In no case do we understand the fundamental abnormalities that lead to malfunctions in the neurotransmitter systems antipsychotic drugs affect, or whether these fundamental abnormalities cluster as our current diagnostic syndromes do.[ix]

We have promising, *albeit* cumbersome, models of the dynamic activity levels of some psychiatric disorders. For example, antipsychotic-treated patients with schizophrenia

---

[viii] Please refer to the *Diagnostic and Statistical Manual of Mental Disorders, Fourth Edition – Text Revision* (DSM-IV-TR), or *The International Statistical Classification of Diseases and Related Health Problems 10th Revision*, published by the American Psychiatric Association and the World Health Organization, respectively, for current diagnostic criteria manuals in use.

[ix] For a comprehensive discussion of diversity within patient populations with ostensibly similar diagnosis, and the difficulties of matching abnormal animal behavior to syndrome-based diagnoses. Please refer to Steckler *et al.*, Developing novel anxiolytics: Improving preclinical detection and clinical assessment, in this volume.

who demonstrate large increases in psychosis and high levels of brain dopamine release (evident on PET) when challenged with stimulant drugs are at high risk for rapid relapse if the antipsychotic drug is discontinued. Patients who do not show such responses to stimulant challenge may remain stable without treatment for many months without relapse.

Better understanding of the fundamental causes (genetic, environmental, etc.) of psychiatric disorders will permit "foundation-up" construction of models that can be more effective in clustering patients into diagnostic and treatment-response subgroups. Such models will allow more objective evaluation of the appropriateness of candidate drugs and appropriate patients for clinical trials, provide indicators of effective dose ranges, serve as measures of change with treatment, and ultimately lead to individual tailoring of treatments for patients in clinical settings.[x]

Patients who show minimal or no response to available treatments should only be included in trials of investigational compounds believed to have novel mechanisms of action that have the potential to offer these patients added benefit. Animal and translational models of what is different about the pathophysiology of treatment-non-responsive patients can help to screen for compounds with expanded therapeutic benefit.

Pharmacological Treatments

Dosing that is too low will be inadequate to produce the desired therapeutic benefit. When dosing is too high, therapeutic benefit will be attenuated by unnecessary side effects. A translational model of pharmacological actions linked to therapeutic benefit can offer evidence of when adequate doses have been achieved. Translational models of side effects can help to demarcate the upper bound or maximum tolerated doses of drugs. For example, coarse rigidity and bradykinesia during treatment with dopamine-blocking antipsychotic drugs document that excessive levels of receptor blockade have been reached in brain, higher than necessary for the therapeutic action of these agents.[30] Although the coarse rigidity and bradykinesia can be partially relieved by adding anticholinergic anti-Parkinson drugs, this does not reverse the fundamental alterations in motor systems caused by the excessive dosages and leaves patients at increased risk for later, irreversible tardive dyskinesias. The maximum-tolerated doses of these agents are signaled by sub-clinical rigidity and bradykinesia, detectable only on careful examination (the neuroleptic threshold).

Excluding numerous adjunctive and concomitant medications without good cause makes clinical trial implementation unnecessarily difficult. Determining the effects, or lack thereof, of adjunctive and concomitant medications in translational models may allow their use with the reassuring knowledge that they do not compromise key outcome.

Duration of Trials

We believe that efficacy trials should only last long enough to permit the unfolding of the therapeutic mechanisms of action of assigned medications. Highly efficacious

---

[x] For an example of patient selection in psychiatric clinical trials, please refer to Large *et al.*, Developing therapeutics for bipolar disorder: from animal models to the clinic in this Volume.

treatments may demonstrate the bulk of their benefit early (e.g., within 2 weeks). To run a trial for such agents for more than 4 weeks invites confounds (e.g., change from inpatient to outpatient status) and incomplete data sets. Translational models of mechanism of pharmacological action can help to determine trial duration. Changes in markers associated with therapeutic response may be demonstrable early and serve as trial endpoints. Dopamine-blocking antipsychotic drugs block D_2 receptors within minutes of administration. However, it is the gradual development of depolarization block in dopamine-releasing neurons that corresponds in time with therapeutic efficacy.

Efficacy trials addressing patients unresponsive to standard treatments should err in the direction of longer durations, for example, 8–12 weeks. The processes involved in resistance to treatment may be slower to change than the processes underlying acute treatment response. Patients eligible for such trials often reside in supervised locations where attrition is unlikely, and little is to be lost with the longer duration.

Longer periods of follow-up are usually desirable in maintenance treatment trials. If time to relapse is a primary outcome measure, it may take two or more years for a sufficient number of relapses to occur to demonstrate small relapse rate differences. Other complex outcomes such as social or occupational functioning may take years to develop and mature. Long periods of follow-up are necessary for safety monitoring.[16,17]

Outcome Measures

Determining whether participating patients received their assigned medications and no confounding medications is the first step in evaluating the outcomes of clinical trials. Mistakes can be made in the assignment, dispensing, and administration of medication. Patients may not take the medications they are sent home with, and/or take other medications prohibited by the protocol and fail to inform the investigators. Monitoring blood samples for the presence of the assigned medication and the absence of excluded medications is the best way to ascertain if treatment was ingested as assigned.

Persistence on an assigned medication is indicative that the medication relieves unwanted features of the target illness and does not produce intolerable side effects. Time to treatment discontinuation provides a summary measure for comparing the overall effectiveness and tolerability of medications. Rates of study completion can be highly informative about the integrity of a trial; if 90% of patients assigned to placebo complete a trial, questions should be raised as to who the patients were who participated. If the percentage of patients completing the trial on the investigational compound is similar to the percentage of patients completing on placebo, the overall benefit of the investigational compound is not impressive.

Correct assessment of psychopathology depends upon the experience of the rater and his or her familiarity with the dynamics of the disease, the integrity of the rater in striving for objectivity, the exposure of the rater to the patient and additional informant reports regarding the patient, and the success of the rater's training on the proper use of the rating instrument. Central rating systems accomplished via improving videoconferencing technologies will provide consistency and quality in many situations. However, studies of agitated or suspicious patients may have difficulty recruiting patients for studies in which videoconferencing is mandatory.[31]

Given the subjective nature of clinical ratings, it is obvious that objective translational models of the pathophysiology that contributes to psychopathology are highly desirable. Readily accessible indicators developed from such models will be less subject to bias than clinical ratings and may permit separations or documentation of change that are not evident clinically.

THE BUSINESS OF RESEARCH

Over the past two decades, the relationships between pharmaceutical companies and clinical investigators have changed. Twenty years ago, pharmaceutical company professionals experienced with the investigational compound and with the target illness would meet clinical investigators face-to-face in individual visits or at an investigators' meeting. They would discuss a draft protocol with the investigators and together make pragmatic changes to improve the protocol design and simplify implementation. Most clinical research sites were academic, led by investigators with established independent research records and documented scholarship on the target illness. Payment rates were adequate.

Rapid expansion of new drug development for psychiatric disorders overwhelmed this system. There were too few sites to handle the workload. In keeping with the law of supply and demand, payment rates increased, and then large numbers of independent clinical research centers sprang up. These centers require initial capital expenditures for office space and equipment, and have substantial ongoing budgets for personnel, utilities, supplies, etc. Pharmaceutical pipelines are capricious and unreliable; sensible businessmen/investigators diversified across multiple disease areas to maintain income, and developed marketing strategies (such as advertising for patients) for attracting a continuous stream of potential study candidates.

Monitoring multiple large clinical trials became too much for pharmaceutical companies to do in house and they began to outsource the oversight of trials to contract research organizations (CROs) that initially helped to manage and analyze data and prepare NDA submissions.[32-35] The CROs later expanded their portfolios to offer site selection, rater training, and project medical officers (physicians who might serve across specialties and disease areas).

Now pharmaceutical companies finalize protocols with CRO staff and consultant experts, many of whom have not recently treated patients or implemented trials. Site investigators are contacted by junior CRO staff, with an immutable and sometimes impractical protocol, and offered the opportunity to apply to serve as a contract worker doing piecework for the trial. The atmosphere of collegial, shared exploration has been replaced by the atmosphere of the factory floor. Investigators with sensible questions speak with CRO project medical officers who dutifully read the protocol over the phone to the investigators. This atmosphere is not conducive to investigators erring on the side of scientific integrity. Faced with a marginal patient who may be sub-optimal for addressing the central question of the trial, but who, if included, will generate many thousands of dollars for the site, businessmen/investigators are sorely tempted.

In such an atmosphere, one can see advertisements on local television seeking patients with schizophrenia to participate in clinical trials (for substantial compensation). Those familiar with patients with schizophrenia would immediately rule out from participation in a schizophrenia trial anyone who would answer such an advertisement; a lack of acknowledgment of illness and need for treatment is the most common psychopathological feature of the disease. We and several of our colleagues in the area recently received the email below:

> *My name is _____, and I was inquiring as to whether you have any upcoming inpatient clinical trials. I have been diagnosed with schizophrenia, chronic, undifferentiated, and I live in the _____ area. I am 39 years old and currently taking risperidone for my schizophrenia. I have no other medical problems, other than astigmatism in my eyes. Please do let me know if there are any compensated inpatient clinical trials upcoming in your hospital.*

The likelihood that the writer of this email has schizophrenia is low; the likelihood that he will evidence a difference in his condition after 4 weeks of treatment with placebo versus active comparator is very low.

There is little understanding of how business practices like projected timelines impact upon the quality of trials. These timelines are usually unrealistic, and lead to a frenzied, badgering atmosphere that corrodes attention to quality. Investigators are always tempted to push into trials patients who are on the border of eligibility; they are paid for patients that enter trials, and they are not paid for patients who do not enter trials. Pressure to hurry will only increase the temptation to include sub-optimal patients. If investigators realize that a multi-site study's recruitment is drawing to a close, marginal patients look especially eligible.

Inpatient trials may offer payment for "bed costs," for example, for up to 14 days, with additional days paid for only inpatients who are not doing well. Patients with a good response at day 14 may then be released from hospital, not take their medications reliably, abuse substances, or experience stressful events, and have a last observation reflecting substantially less benefit than the assigned treatment could have really offered. Alternatively, investigators may inflate psychopathology ratings to justify continued financial support for patients who need to remain in hospital.

Maintenance trials that only pay investigators for the duration of time patients stay in study may lead investigators to continue patients on assigned treatments longer than they would otherwise, covering differences in survival that would otherwise be apparent.

Creative budgeting solutions that reward unbiased, best practices are needed. Translational models that provide objective measures of the appropriateness of patients for inclusion, and of their clinical condition as they proceed through trials will make clinical trials more scientifically rigorous. However, improved contact between scientists in the pharmaceutical industry and investigators in the field is needed to re-instate the collegial and exciting atmosphere of drug discovery.

CONCLUSIONS

The implementation of clinical trials is fraught with hazard. Present methods are incapable of assuring that the best patients are included in trials, and that the true effects of assigned treatments are consistently captured. Inference making should be cautious and restrained. Only after multiple trials are completed by several groups of investigators using differing methodologies produce concordant results should we believe that findings are well supported and are to be used in our practice. As the back and forth process of developing translational models of pathophysiology and pharmacological actions in laboratory and clinical settings proceeds, we will become more objective in clinical trials, and this will hasten the development of clinically useful medicines. Re-engaging dedicated clinical investigators will enhance the quality of this process.

REFERENCES

1. Kola, I. and Landis, J. (2004). Can the pharmaceutical industry reduce attrition rates?. *Nat Rev Drug Discov*, 3:711–715.
2. Lappin, G. and Garner, R.C. (2005). The use of accelerator mass spectrometry to obtain early human ADME/PK data. *Expert Opin Drug Metab Toxicol*, 10:890–894.
3. Littman, B.H. and Williams, S.A. (2005). The ultimate model organism: Progress in experimental medicine. *Nat Rev Drug Discov*, 4:631–638.
4. European Medicines Agency. (2004). *Position paper on non-clinical safety studies to support clinical trials with a single microdose CPMP/SWP/2599/02/Rev1*, . http://www.emea.eu.int/pdfs/human/swp/259902en.pdf
5. Center for Drug Evaluation and Research. (2005). Guidance for industry, investigators and reievers: Exploratory IND studies. Draft guidance. US Department of Health and Human Services, Food and Drug Administration. Center for Drug Evaluation and Research, www.fda.gov/cder/guidance/6284dft.htm
6. Laska, E.M., Klein, D.F., Lavori, P.W., Levine, J., and Robinson, D.S. (1994). Design issues for the clinical evaluation of psychotropic drugs. In Prein, R.F. and Robinson, D.S. (eds.), *Clinical Evaluation of Psychotropic Drugs*. Raven Press, New York, pp. 29–68.
7. Posner, J. (2000). The first administration of a new active substance to humans. In Cohen, A. and Posner, J. (eds.), *A Guide to Clinical Drug Research*. Kluver Academic Publishers, Norwell, MA, pp. 47–63.
8. Kartizinel, R., Lisook, A.B., Rullo, B., Severe, J.B., and Spilker, G. (1994). Clinical trial implementation. In Prein, R.F. and Robinson, D.S. (eds.), *Clinical Evaluation of Psychotropic Drugs*. Raven Press, New York, pp. 161–184.
9. Guarino, R.A. (2000). Clinical research protocols. In Guarino, R.A. (ed.), *New Drug Approval Process*. Marcel Dekker, New York, pp. 219–246.
10. Wooding, W.M. (1994). *Planning Pharmaceutical Clinical Trials*. John Wiley and Sons, New York.
11. Reele, S.B. (1997). Decision points in human drug development. In O'Grady, J. and Joubert, P. H. (eds.), *Phase I/II Clinical Drug Trials*. CRC Press, Boca Raton, FL, pp. 67–80.
12. Chang, M., Chow, S.C., Pong, C. (2006 May). Adaptive design in clinical research: Issues, opportunities, and recommendations, *J Biopharm Stat*, 16(3)299–309, discussion 311-2.
13. Gottlieb, S. (2006). Remarks, Conference on Adaptive Trial Design, http://www.fda.gov/oc/speeches/2006/trialdesign0710.html
14. Baber, N. (2000). What does the investigator need to know about the drug? – The clinical investigators' brochure. In Cohen, A. and Posner, J. (eds.), *A Guide to Clinical Drug Research*. Kluver Academic Publishers, Norwell, MA, pp. 19–45.
15. Laughren, T.P., Levine, J., Levine, J.G., and Thompson, W.L. (1994). Pre-marketing safety evaluation of psychotropic drugs. In Prein, R.F. and Robinson, D.S. (eds.), *Clinical Evaluation of Psychotropic Drugs*. Raven Press, New York, pp. 185–216.

16. Thomas, M. (1997). Study design and assessment of wanted and unwanted drug effects in phase I/II trials. In O'Grady, J. and Joubert, P.H. (eds.), *Phase I/II Clinical Drug Trials*. CRC Press, Boca Raton, FL, pp. 157–169.

17. Heres, S., Davis, J., Maino, K., Jetzinger, E., Kissling, W., and Leucht, S. (2006). Why olanzapine beats risperidone, risperidone beats quetiapine, and quetiapine beats olanzapine: An exploratory analysis of head-to-head comparison studies of second-generation antipsychotics. *Am J Psychiatry*, 163:185–194.

18. Perlis, R.H., Perlis, C.S., Wu, Y., Hwang, C., Joseph, M., and Nierenberg, A.A. (2005). Industry sponsorship and financial conflict of interest in the reporting of clinical trials in psychiatry. *Am J Psychiatry*, 162:1957–1960.

19. Lieberman, J.A., Stroup, S., McEvoy, J., Swartz, M.S., Rosenheck, R.A., Perkins, D.O. *et al.* (2005). Effectiveness of antipsychotic drugs in patients with chronic schizophrenia. *New Engl J Med*, 353:1209–1223.

20. March, J.S., Silva, S.G., Compton, S., Shapiro, M., Califf, R., and Krishnan, R. (2005). The case for practical clinical trials in psychiatry. *Am J Psychiatry*, 162:836–846.

21. Kemmler, G., Hummer, M., Widschwendter, C., and Fleischhacker, W.W. (2005). Dropout rates in placebo-controlled active-control clinical trials of antipsychotic drugs. *Arch Gen Psychiatry*, 62:1305–1312.

22. Kassalow, L.M. (2000). Statistical and data management. In Guarino, R.A. (ed.), *New Drug Approval Process*. Marcel Dekker, New York, pp. 289–310.

23. Csernansky, J.G., Mahmoud, R., and Brenner, R. (2002). A comparison of risperdone and haloperidol for the prevention of relapse in patients with schizophrenia. *N Engl J Med*, 346:16–22.

24. Schooler, N., Rabinowitz, J., Davidson, M., Emsley, R., Harvey, P.D., Kopala, L. *et al.* (2005). Risperdone and haloperidol in first-episode psychosis: A long-term randomized trial. *Am J Psychiatry*, 162(5):947–953.

25. Kraemer, H.C., Mintz, J., Noda, A., Tinklenberg, J., and Yesavage, J.A. (2006). Caution regarding the use of pilot studies to guide power calculations for study proposals. *Arch Gen Psychiatry*, 63:484–489.

26. Halpern, S.D., Karlawish, J.H.T., and Berlin, J.A. (2002). The continuing unethical conduct of underpowered clinical trials. *JAMA*, 288:358–362.

27. McEvoy, J.P. and Barnes, T. (2003). *Guide to Assessment Scales in Schizophrenia*, 2nd edition. Science Press, London.

28. Kay, S.R. (1991). *Positive and Negative Syndromes in Schizophrenia*. Brunner/Mazel, New York.

29. Young, R.C., Biggs, J.T., Ziegler, V.E. *et al.* (1978). A rating scale for mania: Reliability, validity and sensitivity. *Br J Psychiatry*, 133:429–435.

30. McEvoy, J.P., Hogarty, G.E., and Steingard, S. (1991). Optimal dose of neuroleptic in acute schizophrenia. *Archives of General Psychiatry*, 48:739–745.

31. Koback, K.A., Kane, J.M., Thase, M.E., and Nierenberg, A.A. (2007). Why do clinical trials fail? The problem of measurement error in clinical trials: Time to test new paradigms?. *J Clin Psychopharmacol*, 27:1–4.

32. Rowland, C. (2004). Clinical trials seen shifting overseas. *Int J Health Serv*, 34:555–556.

33. Rettig, R.A. (2000). The industrialization of clinical research. *Health Affairs*, 19:129–146.

34. Mirowski, P. and Van Horn, R. (2005). The contract research organization and the commercialization of scientific research. *Soc Stud Sci*, 35:503–548.

35. Schuchmann, M. (2007). Commercializing clinical trials – risks and benefits of the CRO boom. *NEJM*, 357:1365–1368.

CHAPTER 4

Challenges for Translational Psychopharmacology Research: The Need for Conceptual Principles

Klaus A. Miczek

Department of Psychology, Tufts University, Bacon Hall 530 Boston Avenue, Medford, MA 02155 USA

INTRODUCTION

After the first decade of modern psychopharmacology, Kelleher and Morse[1] organized the conceptual and methodological approaches by identifying two types of experiments in this emerging field: type 1 experiments use behavioral and physiological procedures as tools to characterize the effects of drugs, and type 2 experiments use a drug as a tool to analyze behavior and its underlying neural mechanisms. Already in this nascent phase of psychopharmacology, one of the research goals was to construct behavioral profiles of prototypic drugs mainly in laboratory animals and to identify in these profiles features that can be translated to clinical applications. These concerns range from drug responses that characterize individuals as being particularly vulnerable or resilient for disorders of varying psychiatric diagnoses to identifying compounds that are promising as pharmacotherapies. For example, in the very first issues

Similar material has been presented in Miczek, K.A and Wit, H. de (2008). Challenges for translational psychopharmacology research—some basic principles. *Psychopharmacology*, (in press), DOI: 10.1007/s00213-008-1198-4.

Animal and Translational Models for CNS Drug Discovery,
Vol. 1 of 3: Psychiatric Disorders
Robert McArthur and Franco Borsini (eds), Academic Press, 2008

of the journal *Psychopharmacology*, which was founded by researchers in academic institutions, several articles became citation classics on account of reporting type 1 experiments that translated preclinical findings (1) to characterize potentially useful anxiolytic pharmacotherapies,[2] (2) to identify the abuse liability of drugs,[3] or (3) to induce behavioral features such as stereotyped motor routines that could serve as models of psychotic disorders.[4]

The 2006 NIH roadmap for medical research demands more rapid and efficient translation of research findings from the bench to the bedside, and vice versa, better clinical diagnoses that enable the development of more appropriate experimental model systems. To apply this principle to psychiatric disorders is particularly challenging on account of the ever-evolving diagnostic criteria of complex disorders that rely on symptom clusters and are multi-factorially determined.[5] Moreover, some of the cardinal symptoms of psychiatric disorders such as intense craving for drugs, feelings of sadness, or unworthiness rely on the patient's verbal reports that are more or less reliable and that have no counterpart in speechless animals. The current discourse introduces several principles that recur in the discussion of translating preclinical findings to clinical applications, and vice versa.

WHAT EXACTLY IS MODELED IN PRECLINICAL PROCEDURES? ARE EXPERIMENTAL PROCEDURES SCREENS, ASSAYS, MODELS, OR PARADIGMS?

To answer these questions, one can resort to the maxim by Rosenblueth and Wiener some 60 years ago,[6] "… the best material model for a cat is another, or preferably the same cat?" Lexical definitions of a scientific "model" refer to a simplified and systematic description of a phenomenon with which it shares essential characteristics. The development of a productive and theoretically satisfactory model in psychopharmacology is hindered by the imprecise and incomplete specification of the factors that engender the symptoms being modeled or signs of the disorder. Definitions of the disorders are revised and updated continuously, with the fifth edition scheduled to appear in 2011 (see[5]). Current usage refrains from proposing and implementing a model at the *homologous* level and restricts the approach to certain *isomorphic* signs and symptoms.[7] One can argue that a preclinical model becomes superfluous, once the etiology, phenotypic expression, and therapeutic response are homologous between the clinical case and the preclinical experimental preparation. Preclinical models capture some, but not necessarily all features of the disorder. As early efforts with stereotyped motor routines have shown, a secondary symptom of schizophrenia is much more readily modeled than the primary symptoms, namely disturbances in thought. Consider the hyperactive and stereotyped movement patterns in rodents or primates as generated by high amphetamine doses that are effectively blocked by drugs with antipsychotic potential.[8] Yet, the primary or cardinal symptoms of attentional filtering and higher-level cognitive processes remain challenging for modeling in rodents, although the evolution of more adequate models for these symptoms is most promising.[9,10]

Principle 1: *The translation of preclinical data to clinical concerns is more successful when the development of experimental models is restricted in their scope* *to a cardinal or core symptom of a psychiatric disorder. The earlier approach to mimic the entire disorder with a preclinical model has been less productive.*

For several decades, the preclinical conflict procedures that engender a suppression of a positively reinforced licking or lever pressing or key pecking response by a punishment contingency, served as standard to evaluate the punishment-attenuating effects of compounds with anxiolytic potential.[2,11,12] These objective and automated procedures continue to generate systematic dose-dependent data in various animal species that translate to corresponding measurements in human subjects. Moreover, the effects of compounds that act as positive allosteric modulators of GABA$_A$ receptors translate from preclinical to clinical versions of this research procedure. Is the reversal of behavioral suppression due to a punishment contingency a critical characteristic of clinically effective anxiolytic compounds? The benzodiazepine anxiolytics provided validation for this question (Figure 4.1,[13]), whereas studies with compounds targeting serotonergic or glutamatergic receptor subtypes and transporter molecules required intricate experimental protocols and animal species, in order to confirm validly a punishment-attenuating effect.[14-19] This research strategy focuses on two objectively assessed behavioral changes, one of which (punishment-attenuating) is predictive of potentially anxiolytic effects, and the second detects sedative and other behaviorally disruptive effects. A similar strategy guides the fear-potentiated startle procedure, where treatments with anxiolytic potential attenuate the classically conditioned potentiation effect, but leave the non-potentiated startle reflex intact.[17,20,21] The same logic is also the basis for comparing potentially anxiolytic treatments in rodents that promote exploration of open and brightly lit spaces relative to dark and safe spaces (e.g., elevated plus- or zero-maze, light/dark transitions, open-field tests).

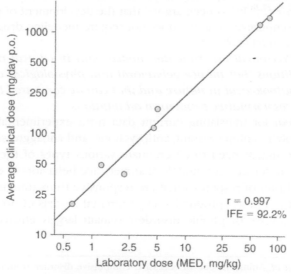

Figure 4.1   Relationship of laboratory dose to clinical dose for seven different anxiolytics: (left to right) diazepam (Valium®), chlordiazepoxide (Librium®), oxazepam (Serax®), phenobarbital (Pb®), amobarbital (Amytal®), tybamate (Solacen®), and meprobamate (Miltown®). Data are from Cook and Davidson (1973) and Shader (1975); figure from Carlton.[13]

These latter procedures are rapidly implemented, since they require no conditioning, but limit each research subject to a single trial.[22]

From a translational perspective, the preceding discussion of the experimental procedures or models used most frequently for developing anxiolytic treatments highlights the problem of shared pathogenesis. In the current phase of model development, the critical measurements focus on adaptive responses to aversive events either distress calls due to maternal separation or behavioral inhibition due to punishment contingencies or suppressed exploratory behavior or fear-potentiated startle reflexes represent behavioral adaptations that are important in the survival of the individual and the species. Similarly, the experimental models for the discovery of antidepressant treatments rely on behavioral adaptations to inescapable, highly aversive situations. When an experimental rat or mouse assumes a floating posture after its attempt to escape from a water tank was unsuccessful, this immobility response was initially labeled "behavioral despair."[23] In fact, a more parsimonious interpretation of the functionality of an energy-conserving passive immobile floating response in an inescapable situation emphasizes the survival value of this behavior and portrays the immobility as a passive coping response.[24,25] As a further example, it may be instructive to examine species-typical aggressive and defensive behavior in confrontations between territorial resident and intruder animals as model systems for investigating potentially therapeutic interventions of violent patients. In contrast to the species-typical behavioral adaptations to situations of conflict, it is useful to focus on escalated forms of aggressive behavior in an attempt to model violent outbursts.[26] Treatments that interfere with or suppress adaptive responses appear problematic and may not offer themselves for direct translation to solving a clinical problem. This point remains controversial in models of drug abuse which focus mostly on stable patterns of drug intake and only rarely model the transition to escalated, compulsive-like drug use and relapse.[27,28] It has been argued that the development of potential medications that target compulsive drug use, does not require modeling drug taking behavior as it occurs in the natural ecology.[29]

Principle 2: *Preclinical experimental models gain in clinical relevance, if they incorporate conditions that induce behavioral and physiological changes that are maladaptive or pathological in nature and that can be compared to the conditions engendering species-normative behavioral adaptations.*

A further *caveat* for translating current data from experimental models for the detection of anxiolytic, antidepressant, antipsychotic, and antiaggressive treatments to the bedside is the urgent need to differentiate various types of these disorders. For example, nearly all of the current models of anxiety-like behaviors in experimental animals focus on a cluster of responses that are responsive to treatments for generalized anxiety disorder. By contrast, productive experimental models of posttraumatic stress or obsessive–compulsive or phobic disorders remain largely elusive.[i] An instructive

---

[i] Please refer to Joel *et al.*, Animal models of obsessive–compulsive disorder: from bench to bedside via endophenotypes and biomarkers, in this volume for further discussion of Obsessive–compulsive disorders, or to Williams *et al.*, Current concepts in the classification, treatment and modeling of pathological gambling and other impulse control disorders, in Volume 3, *Reward Deficit Disorders*, for further discussion regarding modeling aspects of these disorders.

approach comprises the study of startle responses that are exaggerated by either discrete, sudden fear-provoking stimuli, or uncertain distal anxiety-inducing contexts.[17,21] It may be possible to capture a core symptom of phobias, posttraumatic stress or panic disorders with the phasic startle potentiation, whereas an essential feature of generalized anxiety is more adequately contained in the sustained form of aversive conditioning.

Similarly, the spectrum of affective disorders would benefit from developing models that go beyond the current screens for treatments that are validated by their limited effects in unipolar depression. A promising model focuses on depression-like impairments of reward processes during withdrawal from chronic administration of psychomotor stimulant drugs as quantified by the rise in threshold for intracranial electrical self-stimulation (ICSS).[30][ii] Still, it is difficult to translate the ICSS model directly to human subjects, and this methodological approach appears more suited for neurobiological inquiries. A further example shows that both clinical and preclinical studies of aggressive behavior differentiate various types of aggression, the most fundamental of which is the distinction of hostile – impulsive –antisocial – intensely violent outbursts from the calculating, instrumental aggressive acts.[26,31-33]

At present, a common strategy to enhance the value of preclinical contributions to the development of promising pharmacotherapies is to employ a battery of tests. What is the added value of measuring a laboratory rat's locomotion from a dark, safe place to a brightly lit, open area in the elevated plus- or zero-maze, light/dark box and open-field test in an effort to characterize a potentially anxiolytic treatment? In fact, it is sometimes quite challenging to define operationally the hypothetical construct "anxiety" in a single experimental protocol. Consider the popular elevated plus-maze procedure, where the animal's exploratory behavior of an unprotected open arm has been proposed as such an operational definition.[34] At the same time, a rodent's quick approach and exploration of an open area in an elevated plus-maze may reflect an impulsively sensation-seeking behavior. Are the risk-assessment and avoidance of an open space or the approach to novel environs the primary driving forces for these behavioral measures, or do the preclinical tests reflect the resolution of these conflicting forces? A single test at one time point may be insufficient to answer these questions. In order to characterize the hypothetical construct "anxiety" more adequately, several converging behavioral measurements in a range of conditions are advisable. Quantitative trait analysis has identified a locus (QTL) on the first chromosome that may influence exploration, whereas the level of activity may be influenced by a QTL on the fourth chromosome and avoidance by a QTL on chromosome 15.[35] To unravel the behavioral features that are specific to the hypothetical construct "anxiety" in these common procedures remains unresolved. So far, pharmacological validation via medications that are clinically effective in the treatment of generalized anxiety disorders constitutes the major support for these frequently used procedures. As discussed

---

[ii] See also, Koob, The role of animal models in reward deficit disorders: views from academia, or Markou *et al.*, Contribution of animal models and preclinical human studies to medication development for nicotine dependence, in Volume 3, *Reward Deficits Disorders*, for further discussion on ICSS.

below, this type of validation is built on circular reasoning and curtails innovative research efforts.[iii]

Many experimental procedures for detecting pharmacotherapies that are potentially useful in the treatment of anxiety rely on behavioral inhibition in animal and human subjects. As a matter of fact, a behavioral inhibition system has been postulated as the common neural target for the action of anxiolytic drugs,[36] although the suppression of behavior due to non-reinforcement (i.e., extinction) and due to punishment contingencies are readily dissociated pharmacologically.[37,38] It should be noted that an exacting analysis of behavior in tasks that differentiate between the inhibition of ongoing behavior from inhibiting the initiation of a behavioral response clearly dissociates the underlying neurobiological mechanisms.[39] An alternative strategy in developing experimental models for characterizing anxiolytic treatments is the focus on exaggerated responses to innocuous stimuli such as the fear-potentiated startle. In fact, the potentiation of the startle response by prior presentation of a stimulus that was associated with electric shock is particularly sensitive to the effects of compounds that act either as positive modulators at $GABA_A$ receptors or as agonists at serotonergic 5-HT_{1A} or as glutamatergic $mGlu_{2/3}$ receptors.[40,41]

Principle 3: *Preclinical data are more readily translated to the clinical situation when they are based on converging evidence from at least two, and preferably more, experimental procedures, each capturing cardinal features of the modeled disorder*.

The demand for preclinical results that are readily and efficiently translated into clinical practice can be viewed as advocacy for more pragmatic research strategies and tactics. In fact, psychopharmacological research often incorporates experimental screens at an initial stage. An early example is the popular and highly cited Irwin screen[42] that identified basic and simple drug-induced changes in a broad range of behavioral categories in mice. This type of observational screen has evolved into the current high throughput computerized systems for behavioral phenotyping,[43] but the rationale and expected outcome remain limited to relatively large, basic, and coarsely measured functions of CNS activity. The theoretical basis to screen for compounds with a more specific pharmacotherapeutic potential was most often quite removed from the pathogenesis or symptomatology of the targeted disorder. For example, considerable discussion revolves around the rationale for the olfactory bulbectomized rat preparation or the tail suspension test as rapid and efficient screens for compounds with antidepressant potential, primarily due to the limited conceptual rationale.[44,45] Furthermore, experimental preparations such as the antimuricidal

---

[iii] Pharmacological isomorphism, or the amelioration of abnormal behaviors present in the animal model by clinically effective drugs, is an important, but not necessarily sufficient criterion for the establishment of the predictive validity of that behavioral model of a disorder. Please refer to Steckler *et al.*, Developing novel anxiolytics: improving preclinical detection and clinical assessment, Joel *et al.*, Animal models of obsessive–compulsive disorder: From bench to bedside via endophenotypes and biomarkers, in this volume; Lindner *et al.*, Development, optimization and use of preclinical behavioral models to maximize the productivity of drug discovery for Alzheimer's Disease, Merchant *et al.*, Animal models of Parkinson's Disease to aid drug discovery and development, in Volume 2, *Neurological Disorders*, among other chapters, for further discussion of the strengths and limitations of pharmacological isomorphism in establishing model validity.

test for antidepressant-like drugs have not withstood critical and ethical analysis, and disappeared from the preclinical laboratory.[46,47]

Which are the criteria that allow a screen to be considered as model, given the often interchangeable and indiscriminate usage of both terms for experimental preparations that are used in the study of compounds with pharmacotherapeutic potential?[iv] Among the important considerations is the theoretical principle on which even a very simple experimental preparation is based. So far, no model has captured the essence of the multi-factorially determined, polygenic, developmentally organized disorders in a truly homologous manner, and homology maybe an unrealistic criterion for a preclinical model. A screen is usually characterized by practical considerations of being a rapid, high throughput, preferably automated procedure. Most often, the term model is applied to an experimental preparation that has more theoretical aspirations; ideally, a model consists of an experimental preparation that engenders a cardinal symptom of a psychiatric disorder. Consider the escalation in cocaine taking over time when the individual has prolonged access to the drug[28] or persistent cocaine taking that is resistant to aversive consequences.[48,49] These procedures begin to capture essential features of the compulsive nature of cocaine addiction. In recent years, the most pretentious term "paradigm" is used interchangeably with the terms "model" or "screen" in emulation of Isaac Newton's introduction of the experimental paradigm in physics.

Principle 4: *The progression from a simple screen to a theoretically adequate model depends on the incorporation of a cardinal symptom characterizing the disorder under investigation. The closer the model approximates a symptom of clinical significance, the more likely will its use generate data that can be translated to clinical benefits.*

THE THEORETICAL ASSUMPTIONS FOR SELECTING ENVIRONMENTAL, NEUROCHEMICAL AND GENETIC MANIPULATIONS IN ORDER TO MODEL CORE SYMPTOMS

Historically, the independent variables for generating psychiatric symptoms in experimental models can be classified as environmental, neurochemical, and genetic insults or combination of these manipulations, each of these conveying the theoretical framework of the model's origin. For example, separation from the maternal attachment or deprivation of social contact during a critical developmental period are potent determinants of behavioral disturbances that persist throughout the lifetime.[50,51] These

---

[iv] As Miczek points out, historically, there has been a good deal of confusion regarding the terms "models" and "tests or procedures" used in psychopharmacological research. The interested reader is invited to consult Steckler *et al.*, Developing novel anxiolytics: Improving preclinical detection and clinical assessment, Cryan *et al.*, Developing more efficacious antidepressant medications: Improving and aligning preclinical detection and clinical assessment tools, in this volume; Lindner *et al.*, Development, optimization and use of preclinical behavioral models to maximize the productivity of drug discovery for Alzheimer's Disease, Wagner *et al.*, Huntington Disease, in Volume 2, *Neurological Disorders*; or Koob, The role of animal models in reward deficit disorders: views from academia, Markou *et al.*, Contribution of animal models and preclinical human studies to medication development for nicotine dependence, in Volume 3, *Reward Deficits Disorders*, for further discussion regarding "models" or "procedures."

disturbances appear not only relevant to affective disorders, but also to alcohol drinking in adulthood.[52,53] A most striking example of salient experiences during a critical developmental period was the high rates of antisocial violent behavior in men who were maltreated as boys and were characterized with an allelic variant of the MAO-A gene.[54] The example of stressful experiences during an early critical developmental period in conjunction with a specific polymorphism demonstrates a powerful approach to induce symptoms that are relevant to affective disorders, violence, drug, and alcohol abuse and that are readily translated from the preclinical to the clinical realm.

One of the most complex set of environmental manipulations has been developed for the chronic mild stress model that has been proposed for the study of depressive-like symptoms.[55,56] Several weeks of continuous exposure to unpredictable and varied stressors can produce deficits in the preference for sweets that are reversed by chronic treatment with antidepressants. So far, it remains challenging and often elusive to identify the necessary and sufficient environmental manipulations in the chronic mild stress protocol that are responsible for the emergence of deficient reward processes. Given the difficulties with replicating the anhedonia-like outcome after chronic mild stress,[57,58] it is not surprising that many variations of this complex procedure have been reported in order to overcome these problems.

A more successful implementation of stressful environmental manipulations has led to a productive model of activity-based anorexia in rodents.[59] When rodents are given access to a running wheel and limited access to food, they eventually fail to compensate with increased food intake, decline in body weight, but increase in activity, develop immunodeficiency, atrophy of the spleen and thymus, stress ulcers, and are on a morbid course, if not rescued.[60] This behavioral and physiological profile incorporates essential features of anorexia nervosa such as lower food intake while hungry, weight loss, escalated activity, and associated endocrine changes.[61] Manipulations with other stressors such as food restriction, restraint, or social isolation have been explored for modeling appetite loss, but do not capture essential features of anorexia nervosa. It is evident that not all stressors engender a common behavioral and neurobiological response pattern. Contrary to earlier conceptualizations, physiological and neuroanatomical data point to considerable stressor specificity.[62]

One of the most venerable environmental stressful manipulations for engendering behavioral abnormalities with relevance to psychiatric symptoms is isolated housing, as studied in captive feral and laboratory-bred animals. A hallmark characteristic of the "isolation syndrome," as originally termed,[63] was the gradual induction of aggressive behavior, which was viewed as a psychopathology in otherwise placid laboratory mice. In fact, adult male members of the genus *Mus* are quite intolerant of rival males and expel them from their territories, and the isolated male mouse resembles in many respects a territorial male.[64] Social isolation in a territorial species like mice differs considerably in behavioral outcome from a similar manipulation in colonial species such as rats or most primates. For example, when rats are isolated early in life, profound behavioral deficits emerge that are relevant to sensorimotor gating in the prepulse inhibition procedure.

A classic manipulation to induce symptoms in psychiatric disorders relies on pharmacological or neurotoxic treatments. Here, the conceptual framework is determined by the presumed mechanism that is targeted by the chemical substance that is employed as the inducing agent.[65] If the inducing drug treatment is an agent with a glutamatergic mechanism of action such as phencyclidine, dizocilpine, or ketamine in order to impair a sensory gating function as detected by the prepulse inhibition model, then the potentially therapeutic intervention will be in all likelihood related to glutamate. The best-known example is the identification of potentially antipsychotic drugs that act as antagonists at dopamine (DA) D_2 receptors when, in fact, the inducing agent is a dopamine agonist. This is readily illustrated in the attempts to reverse the apomorphine-induced disruption of prepulse inhibition or the reversal of apomorphine-induced stereotypies. Such an approach is aptly labeled as "receptor" or "neurotransmitter tautology," clearly not conducive to innovative efforts.[7]

A similar approach to induce symptoms that are related to major psychiatric disorders relies on neural insults. A particularly productive model involves the lesioning of hippocampal tissue in 1-week old rat pups that later show hyperresponsivity to stimulant and stress challenges and deficits in sensory gating and social interactions in adulthood.[66-68] These and other characteristics of neonatally, hippocampally lesioned rats led to their proposed usefulness for the study of schizophrenia-like symptoms. Of course, the insult to a specific brain region or a specific receptor population should be viewed as a localized interruption of a neural circuit that is much more distributed.

During the past two decades, the most intensively studied experimental manipulations to induce one or more core symptoms relies on molecular genetic methods.[7,60,69] By now, it is evident that the bottom-up genetic approach that focuses on the overexpression or deletion of single genes becomes only relevant when it is developmentally time-limited, specific to brain regions and independent from the genetic background. So far, the gene knockout methodology has been of limited value to focus the mechanistic inquiry into the neurobiological mechanisms of aggressive behavior, with gene manipulations on every chromosome having some influence (Figure 4.2,[70]). Studies of the melanocortin system in obesity reveal a most productive use of manipulating the expression of a particular gene.[60] The deletion of the gene for the melanocortin-4 receptor produced a mouse that showed early onset obesity, hyperphagia, hyperinsulinemia, and increased linear growth.[71] The role of this receptor in obesity was further established by pharmacological agonist and antagonist effects, and eventually led to the identification of mutations in the melanocortin system in obese humans.[72] This sequence of preclinical and clinical studies illustrates the value of translational research that is facilitated by the fact that 4–6% of morbidly obese individuals commonly show mutations of the gene encoding the melanocortin-4 receptor. In contrast to monogenic obesity, polygenic, developmentally and multi-factorially determined disorders are more common and require alternative strategies for translational research.

Principle 5: *The inducing conditions for modeling a cardinal symptom or cluster of symptoms may be environmental, genetic, physiological, or a combination of these factors. The choice of the type of manipulation that induces the behavioral and physiological symptoms reveals the theoretical approach to the model construction.*

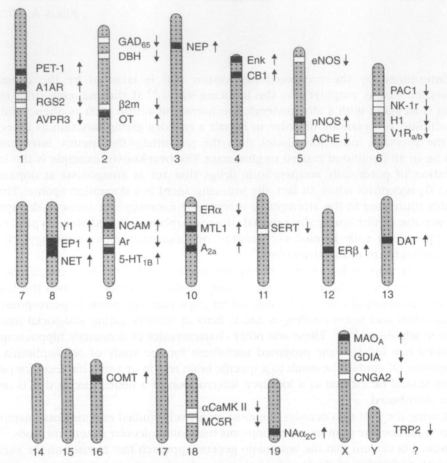

Figure 4.2 Gene deletions affecting aggressive phenotypes in mice. This figure portrays representations of 21 chromosomes (vertical bars) and the approximate location of genes (filled and open horizontal bars) that have been knocked out in mice and engendered heightened- (filled bars, upward arrow) or suppressed-(open bars, downward arrow) levels of aggression. The proteins targeted by the gene deletion are indicated in abbreviated text. Deletions that have not affected aggressive behavior are not shown. Abbreviations and references: 5-HT1B, serotonin receptor 1B; A1AR, adenosine receptor A1; A2a, adenosine receptor 2A; AchE, acetylcholinesterase; αCaMK II, alpha-calcium-calmodulin kinase II; Ar, aromatase; AVPR3, arginine vasopressin 1B receptor; β2m, beta2-microglobulin; CB1, cannabinoid receptor 1; CNGA2, cyclic nucleotide gated channel alpha 2;COMT, catechol-O-methyltransferase; DAT, dopamine transporter; DBH, dopamine beta hydroxylase; eNOS, endothelial nitric oxide synthase; ENK, enkephalin; EP1, prostaglandin E receptor 1; ERα, estrogen receptor alpha; ERβ, estrogen receptor beta; GAD65, glutamic acid decarboxylase (65 amino acids); GDIA, guanosine diphosphate (GDP) dissociation inhibitor 1; H1, histamine receptor 1; MAOA, monoamine oxidase A; MC5R, melanocortin-5 receptor; MTL1, nuclear receptor subfamily 2, group E, member 1 (aka "FIERCE"); Naα2C, adrenergic alpha receptor 2C; NCAM, neural cell adhesion molecule; NEP, neutral endopeptidase; NET, norepinephrine transporter; NK-1r, neurokinin receptor 1; nNOS, neuronal nitric oxide synthase; OT, oxytocin; PAC1, adenylate cyclase activating polypeptide 1 receptor 1; PET-1, ETS (E26 transformation specific) domain transcription factor; RGS2, regulator of G protein signaling; SERT, serotonin transporter; Trp2, transient receptor potential family 2; V1Ra/b, a cluster of vomeronasal receptor genes located on chromosome six, V1ra1-9 and V1rb1-4,7-9;Y1, neuropeptide Y receptor 1. Figure from Miczek et al.[32]

WHICH KIND OF VALIDITY IS NECESSARY FOR A PRECLINICAL MODEL TO RENDER IT TRANSLATABLE TO CLINICAL CONCERNS?

Issues of validity have been discussed elaborately and repeatedly ever since the initial preclinical studies of prototypic compounds with antipsychotic, anxiolytic, antidepressant potential, or abuse liability.[7,73-76] All discussants find it useful to distinguish between different types of validity, ranging from construct, predictive to face validity. Does the amphetamine-induced hyperactivity represent a valid model of amphetamine – or even endogenous psychosis? In terms of face validity, this experimental preparation is severely lacking, but in terms of predictive validity for the reversal by so-called typical and atypical compounds with antipsychotic activity, it represents a simple initial screen for compounds with dopamine D2 receptor antagonism. Similarly, the forced-swim test,[23] particularly in its modified form,[77] achieves very good predictive validity in identifying a large number of currently used antidepressant treatments and rejecting ineffective therapeutic approaches.[78] By contrast, the construct and face validity of this and the related tail-suspension test remain problematic due to their limited relationship to the etiology and symptomatology of the modeled disorder.

Principle 6: *Preclinical experimental preparations can be useful screens that are often validated by predicting reliably treatment success with a prototypic agent. These screens detect "me-too" treatments that are based on the same principle as an existing treatment that has been used to validate the screen.*

From the viewpoint of translational medicine, simple screens, although reliable and efficient, fail to foster innovation in characterizing core features of a psychiatric disorder. It is essential to break the circularity of identifying treatments that work principally on a target and mechanism of a known, but problematic treatment. Behavioral and physiological functions, preferably approximations of cardinal symptoms of a disorder, appear to be more productive and theoretically satisfactory targets for model development. This constraint is apparent in a pharmacologically most useful experimental procedure that relies on the stimulus properties of compounds with CNS activity. The drug discrimination method translates well from implementations in a range of laboratory animals to human subjects, but its innovation is limited by being validated with a well-characterized prototypic drug.

Another model that relies primarily on pharmacological validation is the neurotoxin-induced selective nigrostriatal cell death and motor dysfunctions for capturing essential symptoms of the neurodegenerative Parkinsonian movement disorder (PD).[65] The intra-nigral microinjections of 6-hydroxydopamine (6-OHDA) in rodents or the 1-methyl 4-phenyl 1,2,3,6-tetrahydropyridine (MPTP)-treated monkeys exhibit the long-lasting dopaminergic depletion and many of the cardinal features of motor dysfunctions.[79-81] The primary attraction of these pharmacological models is their validation by the L-dopa therapy. This feature constitutes their translational value, since this compound still continues to be the primary means to provide symptomatic relief for PD patients. At the same time, the lack of effect on non-dopaminergic cells and the lack of neuronal Lewy body aggregations constitute major shortcomings of the toxin-based models. These latter features may be one of the reasons why novel pharmacotherapies have not translated well into the clinic.[v]

Pharmacological validation is the major criterion by which experimental models for assessing liability for drug abuse and for developing pharmacotherapy are evaluated.[29] One of the most noteworthy features of the efforts to predict therapeutic success with novel medications to reduce cocaine use is the dissociation between treatments that decrease the subjective effects of craving for cocaine and the actual cocaine intake. A long list of compounds [e.g., gabapentin (Neurontin®), desipramine (Norpramin®), pergolide (Permax®), risperidone (Risperdal®), ecopipam (SCH 39166), selegeline (Eldepryl®), venlafaxine (Effexor®), and naltrexone (Revia®)] decrease ratings for cocaine craving, but do not change cocaine use under controlled conditions (e.g.,[82,83]). This dissociation of potential medication effects between subjective ratings and actual cocaine use has been difficult to predict on the basis of the current preclinical models.[vi] The intravenous and oral self-administration models reliably predict medication effects that treat opioid dependence. The most promising results in the human self-administration laboratory were obtained with modafinil (Provigil®), an alpha-adrenergic agonist with significant glutamatergic and dopaminergic actions, which reduced both cocaine's subjective and self-administration effects.[84] These observations should prompt preclinical studies to characterize modafinil's profile more adequately.

Given the continuous revisions of the definition of psychiatric disorders, it is unreasonable to expect complete homology between a disorder and an experimental model in the laboratory, and as such, face validity can be achieved only partially. Moreover, some of the cardinal symptoms of psychiatric disorders such as, for example, sadness or feelings of guilt or cravings are difficult to define operationally.

Principle 7: *The degree to which an experimental model fulfills the criteria of high internal or constructs validity relative to face validity or predictive validity depends on the purpose of the model. It is more difficult to develop a model that provides insight into the etiology of a disorder than to predict therapeutic potential relative to a prototypic treatment.*

HOW TO STUDY AFFECTIVE PROCESSES IN PRECLINICAL MODELS AND TRANSLATE THEM TO THE CLINIC?

Ever since Darwin,[85] the evolutionary history of emotional expressions have been traced to non-human organisms. There are several indications that point to the evolutionary roots of affective and cognitive disorders, and it appears to be a reasonable supposition to model the precursors of affective expressions and cognitive processes

---

[v] For further discussion on animal and translational models of Parkinson's Disease, including the 6-OHDA and MPTP models, please refer to Merchant *et al.*, Animal models of Parkinson's Disease to aid drug discovery and development, in Volume 2, *Neurological Disorders*.

[vi] Please refer to Rocha *et al.*, Development of medications for heroin and cocaine addiction and regulatory aspects of abuse liability testing, in Volume 3, *Reward Deficit Disorders*, for further discussion models for assessing liability for drug abuse.

validly in non-human species.[86,87] For example, the distress of infants that are separated from maternal care, can be quantified in myomorph rodent species by the rate of emitting ultrasonic vocalizations in precisely defined frequency ranges.[22,88,89] A most intriguing analysis of different kinds of vocalizations proposes differentiating calls that represent distinctive affective expressions in specific behavioral contexts; these vocalizations may communicate affect during sexual intercourse, agonistic confrontations, maternal care, nociceptive reactions, withdrawal from intense drug taking and during drug seeking.[22,90-93] These species-typical vocal responses during situations of marked salience for the individual may represent the precursors to expressions of affect in humans, although the latter have not received rigorous examination and might be a worthwhile target for model development in humans.

Classically, one of the earliest preclinical models of emotional behavior in rodents and non-human primates is the conditioned emotional response (CER) consisting of the suppression of ongoing instrumental behavior during the presentation of a stimulus that predicted the delivery of an aversive electric shock.[94] The first-generation antipsychotic drugs demonstrated effective attenuation of the behavioral suppression by the conditioned stimulus; the subsequently introduced benzodiazepine anxiolytic drugs showed less consistent effects, and this experimental model fell into disuse, being replaced by punishment procedures.[16,95] By inference, the suppression of ongoing behavior is attributed to the disruptive effects of emotions that are conditioned by their association with the application of an electric shock. Similarly, the pairing of an innocuous light stimulus with the subsequent delivery of an electric shock leads to a potentiated startle response, when this light stimulus is presented prior to a startling loud tone. By inference, this potentiation effect is attributed to a discrete fear state that is induced by the classically conditioning procedure.[20,21]

Principle 8: *It is more productive to focus on behaviorally defined symptoms when translating clinical to preclinical measures, and vice versa. Psychological processes pertinent to affect and cognition are hypothetical constructs that need to be defined in behavioral and neural terms.*

The study of pleasure and its neural basis is of particular significance to disorders in which severe disturbances in these processes are symptomatic such as anhedonia in depressives or in schizophrenics or in drug abusers.[28,30,55,86] Newborn human infants exhibit distinctive tongue protrusions when encountering sweet tastes, which contrast with the gaping response to bitter tastes. These behavioral expressions of affect have their homologues in great apes, monkeys, and rodents.[96,97] The early hypothesis for mesolimbic DA as a critical neurotransmitter system in the mediation of the hedonic features of reward in the context of social, sexual, and alimentary behavior and in drug taking[98] has yielded to a range of alternative interpretations.[99-101] Evidence from preclinical recording and microinjection studies in rodents and monkeys point to a role of mesolimbic DA in reward prediction, motivation, attention, learning about reward and incentive salience.[86,102,103] In fact, phasic and tonic DA activity in mesocorticolimbic projections may characterize the anticipation as well as the consequence of highly salient events, both intensely rewarding and ostensibly aversive.[104-106] The efforts to decompose the reinforcement and reward processes in terms of behavior and neural coding offer opportunities for translation to studies in humans where imaging studies have begun to focus on generator mechanisms for basic and higher-order pleasures in subcortical structures and orbitofrontal cortex.[87,107]

While the taste for sweet appears as a readily implemented index of pleasure, the confounding influences of calories and fluid balance require careful analysis, particular in experimental models that incorporate environmental stressors. Decreased intake of sweet fluids as well as increased current thresholds for ICSS constitute the most prominent measures of anhedonia.[30,96] Obviously, the latter measure is limited to preclinical studies, and it has been proven informative in studies characterizing drugs of abuse, antidepressants, and antipsychotic treatments.[108,109] Nonetheless, the limited success of the antidepressant pharmacotherapies currently available should prompt a concerted effort to develop more insightful and predictive experimental models of disturbances in affect.

CONCLUSIONS

The link between preclinical and clinical studies in psychopharmacology is intensified by continuously emerging methodological innovations that seek to enhance the translational value of experimental models. In the course of the first six decades of psychopharmacological research, experimental models prevailed and were refined that successfully contributed to the study of neurobiological mechanisms and medication development. The current discussion of principles that govern translational research in psychopharmacology emphasizes the importance of a sound conceptual basis for selecting core symptoms of psychiatric disorders when constructing and refining experimental models.

REFERENCES

1. Kelleher, R.T. and Morse, W.H. (1968). Determinants of the specificity of behavioral effects of drugs. *Ergeb Physiol*, 60:1-56.
2. Geller, I. and Seifter, J. (1960). The effects of meprobamate, barbiturates, d-amphetamine and promazine on experimentally induced conflict in the rat. *Psychopharmacologia*, 1:482-492.
3. Deneau, G., Yanigita, T., and Seevers, M.H. (1969). Self-administration of psychoactive substances in the monkey. *Psychopharmacologia*, 16:30-48.
4. Ernst, A.M. (1967). Mode of action of apomorphine and dexamphetamine in gnawing compulsion in rats. *Psychopharmacologia*, 10:316-323.
5. American Psychiatric Association. (2000). *Diagnostic and Statistical Manual of Mental Disorders*. American Psychiatric Association, Washington, DC.
6. Rosenblueth, A. and Wiener, N. (1945). The role of models in science. *Philos Sci*, 12:316-321.
7. Geyer, M.A. and Markou, A. (2002). The role of preclinical models in the development of psychotropic drugs. In Davis, K.L., Charney, D., Coyle, J.T., and Nemeroff, C. (eds.), *Neuropsychopharmacology. The Fifth Generation of Progress*. Lippincott William & Wilkins, Philadelphia, pp. 445-455.
8. Janssen, P.A.J., Niemegee, C.J., and Schellek, K.H. (1965). Is it possible to predict clinical effects of neuroleptic drugs (major tranquillizers) from animal data. I. Neuroleptic activity spectra for rats. *Arzneimittelforschung*, 15:104.
9. Geyer, M.A., Krebs-Thomson, K., Braff, D.L., and Swerdlow, N.R. (2001). Pharmacological studies of prepulse inhibition models of sensorimotor gating deficits in schizophrenia: A decade in review. *Psychopharmacology (Berl)*, 156:117-154.

10. Robbins, T.W. (2002). The 5-choice serial reaction time task: Behavioural pharmacology and functional neurochemistry. *Psychopharmacology*, 163:362–380.

11. Barrett, J.E. and Vanover, K.E. (1993). 5-HT receptors as targets for the development of novel anxiolytic drugs: Models, mechanisms and future directions. *Psychopharmacology*, 112:1–12.

12. Vogel, J.R., Beer, B., and Clody, D.E. (1971). A simple and reliable conflict procedure for testing anti-anxiety agents. *Psychopharmacologia*, 21:1–7.

13. Carlton, P.L. (1983). *A Primer of Behavioral Pharmacology. Concepts and Principles in the Behavioral Analysis of Drug Action*. W.H. Freeman and Company, New York, San Francisco.

14. Barrett, J.E., Witkin, J.M., Mansbach, R.S., Skolnick, P., and Weissman, B.A. (1986). Behavioral studies with anxiolytic drugs. III. Antipunishment actions of buspirone in the pigeon do not involve benzodiazepine receptor mechanisms. *J Pharmacol Exp Ther*, 238:1009–1013.

15. Griebel, G. (1995). 5-Hydroxtryptamine-interacting drugs in animal models of anxiety disorders: More than 30 years of research. *Pharmacol Ther*, 65:319–395.

16. Millan, M.J. (2003). The neurobiology and control of anxious states. *Prog Neurobiol*, 70:83–244.

17. Nordquist, R.E., Steckler, T., Wettstein, J.G., Mackie, C., and Spooren, W. (2008). Metabotropic glutamate receptor modulation, translational methods, and biomarkers: relationship with anxiety. *Psychopharmacology*.

18. Sanger, D.J. (1992). Increased rates of punished responding produced by buspirone-like compounds in rats. *J Pharmacol Exp Ther*, 261:513–517.

19. Spooren, W.P., Gasparini, F., Salt, T.E., and Kuhn, R. (2001). Novel allosteric antagonists shed light on mGlu(5) receptors and CNS disorders. *Trends Pharmacol Sci*, 22:331–337.

20. Davis, M., Falls, W.A., Campeau, S., and Kim, M. (1993). Fear-potentiated startle: A neural and pharmacological analysis. *Behav Brain Res*, 58:175–198.

21. Grillon, C. (2008). Models and mechanisms of anxiety: Evidence from startle studies. *Psychopharmacology*.

22. Miczek, K.A., Weerts, E.M., Vivian, J.A., and Barros, H.M. (1995). Aggression, anxiety and vocalizations in animals: GABA(A) and 5-HT anxiolytics. *Psychopharmacology*, 121:38–56.

23. Porsolt, R.D., Anton, G., Balvet, N., and Jalfre, M. (1978). Behavioural despair in rats: New model sensitive to antidepressant treatments. *Eur J Pharmacol*, 47:379–391.

24. Koolhaas, J.M., Korte, S.M., de Boer, S.F., Van Der Vegt, B.J., Van Reenen, C.G., Hopster, H., De Jong, I.C., Ruis, M.A.W., and Blokhuis, H.J. (1999). Coping styles in animals: Current status in behavior and stress-physiology. *Neurosci Biobehav Rev*, 23:925–935.

25. Weiss, J.M. and Kilts, C.D. (1995). Animal models of depression and schizophrenia. In Schatzberg, A.F. (ed.), *The American Psychiatric Press Textbook of Psychopharmacology*. American Psychiatric Press, Washington, DC, pp. 81–123.

26. Miczek, K.A., Faccidomo, S., de Almeida, R.M.M., Bannai, M., Fish, E.W., and DeBold, J.F. (2004). Escalated aggressive behavior: New pharmacotherapeutic approaches and opportunities. *Ann N Y Acad Sci*, 1036:336–355.

27. Ahmed, S.H. (2005). Imbalance between drug and non-drug reward availability: A major risk factor for addiction. *Eur J Pharmacol*, 526:9–20.

28. Ahmed, S.H. and Koob, G.F. (1998). Transition from moderate to excessive drug intake: Change in hedonic set point. *Science*, 282:298–300.

29. Haney, M. and Spealman, R. (2008). Controversies in translational research: Drug self-administration. *Psychopharmacology*.

30. Markou, A. and Koob, G.F. (1991). Postcocaine anhedonia: An animal model of cocaine withdrawal. *Neuropsychopharmacology*, 4:17–26.

31. Miczek, K.A., Haney, M., Tidey, J., Vivian, J., and Weerts, E. (1994). Neurochemistry and pharmacotherapeutic management of violence and aggression. In Reiss, A.J., Miczek, K.A., and

Roth, J.A. (eds.), *Understanding and Preventing Violence: Biobehavioral Influences on Violence*. National Academy Press, Washington, DC, pp. 244–514.

32. Miczek, K.A., Faccidomo, S.P., Fish, E.W., and De Bold, J.F. (2007). Neurochemistry and molecular neurobiology of aggressive behavior. In Blaustein, J. (ed.), *Behavioral Neurochemistry, Neuroendocrinology and Molecular Neurobiology*. Springer, New York, pp. 285–336.

33. Vitiello, B. and Stoff, D.M. (1997). Subtypes of aggression and their relevance to child psychiatry. *J Am Acad Child Adolesc Psychiatry*, 36:307–315.

34. Montgomery, K.C. (1955). The relation between fear induced by novel stimulation and exploratory behaviour. *J Comp Physiol Psychol*, 48:254–260.

35. Turri, M.G., Datta, S.R., DeFries, J., Henderson, N.D., and Flint, J. (2001). QTL analysis identifies multiple behavioral dimensions in ethological tests of anxiety in laboratory mice. *Curr Biol*, 11:725–734.

36. Gray, J.A., Mellanby, J., and Buckland, C. (1984). Behavioural studies of the role of GABA in anxiolytic drug action. *Neuropharmacology*, 23:827.

37. Miczek, K.A. (1973). Effects of scopolamine, amphetamine and chlordiazepoxide on punishment. *Psychopharmacologia*, 28:373–389.

38. Sanger, D.J. (1985). GABA and the behavioral effects of anxiolytic drugs. *Life Sci*, 36:1503–1513.

39. Eagle, D.M., Bari, A, and Robbins, T.W. (2008). The neuropsychopharmacology of action inhibition: Cross-species translation of the stop-signal and go/no-go tasks. *Psychopharmacology*.

40. Grillon, C., Cordova, J., Levine, L.R., and Morgan, C.A. (2003). Anxiolytic effects of a novel group II metabotropic glutamate receptor agonist (LY354740) in the fear-potentiated startle paradigm in humans. *Psychopharmacology*, 168:446–454.

41. Helton, D.R., Tizzano, J.P., Monn, J.A., Schoepp, D.D., and Kallman, M.J. (1998). Anxiolytic and side-effect profile of LY354740: A potent, highly selective, orally active agonist for group II metabotropic glutamate receptors. *J Pharmacol Exp Ther*, 284:651–660.

42. Irwin, S. (1968). Comprehensive observational assessment: Ia. A systematic, quantitative procedure for assessing the behavioral and physiologic state of the mouse. *Psychopharmacologia*, 13:222–257.

43. Crawley, J.N., Belknap, J.K., Collins, A., Crabbe, J.C., Frankel, W., Henderson, N., Hitzemann, R.J., Maxson, S.C., Miner, L.L., Silva, A.J. *et al.* (1997). Behavioral phenotypes of inbred mouse strains: Implications and recommendations for molecular studies. *Psychopharmacology*, 132:107–124.

44. Kelly, J.P., Wrynn, A.S., and Leonard, B.E. (1997). The olfactory bulbectomized rat as a model of depression: An update. *Pharmacol Ther*, 74:299–316.

45. Steru, L., Chermat, R., Thierry, B., and Simon, P. (1985). The tail suspension test: A new method for screening antidepressants in mice. *Psychopharmacology*, 85:367–370.

46. Fuller, R.W. (1996). Fluoxetine effects on serotonin function and aggressive behavior. In Ferris, C.F. (ed.), *Understanding Aggressive Behavior in Children*. The New York Academy of Sciences, New York, pp. 90–97.

47. Horovitz, Z.P., Ragozzino, P.W., and Leaf, R.C. (1965). Selective block of rat mouse-killing by antidepressants. *Life Sci*, 4:1909–1912.

48. Deroche-Gamonet, V., Belin, D., and Piazza, P.V. (2004). Evidence for addiction-like behavior in the rat. *Science*, 305:1014–1017.

49. Vanderschuren, L.J. and Everitt, B.J. (2004). Drug seeking becomes compulsive after prolonged cocaine self-administration. *Science*, 305:1017–1019.

50. Harlow, H.F. and Suomi, S.J. (1974). Induced depression in monkeys. *Behav Biol*, 12:273–296.

51. Suomi, S.J., Eisele, C.D., Grady, S.A., and Harlow, H.F. (1975). Depressive behavior in adult monkeys following separation from family environment. *J Abnorm Psychol*, 84:576–578.

52. Fahlke, C., Lorenz, J.G., Long, J., Champoux, M., Suomi, S.J., and Higley, J.D. (2000). Rearing experiences and stress-induced plasma cortisol as early risk factors for excessive alcohol consumption in nonhuman primates. *Alcohol Clin Exp Res*, 24:644–650.

53. Huot, R.L., Thrivikraman, K.V., Meaney, M.J., and Plotsky, P.M. (2001). Development of adult ethanol preference and anxiety as a consequence of neonatal maternal separation in Long Evans rats and reversal with antidepressant treatment. *Psychopharmacology (Berl)*, 158:366–373.

54. Caspi, A., McClay, J., Moffitt, T.E., Mill, J., Martin, J., Craig, I.W., Taylor, A., and Poulton, R. (2002). Role of genotype in the cycle of violence in maltreated children. *Science*, 297:851–854.

55. Willner, P., Towell, A., Sampson, D., Sophokleous, S., and Muscat, R. (1987). Reduction of sucrose preference by chronic unpredictable mild stress, and its restoration by a tricyclic antidepressant. *Psychopharmacology*, 93:358–364.

56. Willner, P. (1997). Validity, reliability and utility of the chronic mild stress model of depression: a 10-year review and evaluation. *Psychopharmacology*, 134:319–329.

57. Phillips, A.G. and Barr, A.M. (1997). Effects of chronic mild stress on motivation for sucrose: Mixed messages. *Psychopharmacology*, 134:361–362.

58. Reid, I., Forbes, N., Stewart, C., and Matthews, K. (1997). Chronic mild stress and depressive disorder: A useful new model?. *Psychopharmacology*, 134:365–367.

59. Routtenberg, A. and Kuznesof, A.W. (1967). Self-starvation of rats living in activity wheels on a restricted feeding schedule. *J Comp Physiol Psychol*, 64:414.

60. Casper, R.C., Sullivan, E.L., and Tecott, L. (2008). Relevance of animal models to human eating disorders and obesity. *Psychopharmacology*.

61. Pirke, K. and Ploog, D. (1987). Biology of human starvation. In Beumont, P., Burrows, G., and Casper, R. (eds.), *Eating disorder: Anorexia and bulemia nervosa*. Elsevier, Amsterdam, pp. 80–102.

62. Pacak, K. and Palkovits, M. (2001). Stressor specificity of central neuroendocrine responses: Implications for stress-related disorders. *Endocr Rev*, 22:502–548.

63. Valzelli, L. (1973). The "Isolation syndrome" in mice. *Psychopharmacologia*, 31:305–320.

64. Brain, P.F. (1975). What does individual housing mean to a mouse?. *Life Sci*, 16:187–200.

65. Lane, E. and Dunnett, S. (2008). Animal models of Parkinson's disease and L-dopa induced dyskinesia: How close are we to the clinic? *Psychopharmacology*.

66. Lipska, B.K., Jaskiw, G.E., and Weinberger, D.R. (1993). Postpubertal emergence of hyperresponsiveness to stress and to amphetamine after neonatal excitotoxic hippocampal damage-a potential animal-model of schizophrenia. *Neuropsychopharmacology*, 9:67–75.

67. Lipska, B.K., Swerdlow, N.R., Geyer, M.A., Jaskiw, G.E., Braff, D.L., and Weinberger, D.R. (1995). Neonatal excitotoxic hippocampal damage in rats causes post pubertal changes in prepulse inhibition of startle and its disruption by apomorphine. *Psychopharmacology*, 122:35–43.

68. Sams Dodd, F., Lipska, B.K., and Weinberger, D.R. (1997). Neonatal lesions of the rat ventral hippocampus result in hyperlocomotion and deficits in social behaviour in adulthood. *Psychopharmacology*, 132:303–310.

69. Zhuang, X., Gross, C., Santarelli, L., Compan, V., Trillat, A.C., and Hen, R. (1999). Altered emotional states in knockout mice lacking 5-HT{-1A} or 5-HT{-1B} receptors. *Neuropsychopharmacology*, 21:S52–S60.

70. Miczek, K.A., Maxson, S.C., Fish, E.W., and Faccidomo, S. (2001). Aggressive behavioral phenotypes in mice. *Behav Brain Res*, 125:167–181.

71. Huszar, D., Lynch, C.A., FairchildHuntress, V., Dunmore, J.H., Fang, Q., Berkemeier, L.R., Gu, W., Kesterson, R.A., Boston, B.A., Cone, R.D. *et al.* (1997). Targeted disruption of the melanocortin-4 receptor results in obesity in mice. *Cell*, 88:131–141.

72. Krude, H., Biebermann, H., Luck, W., Horn, R., Brabant, G., and Gruters, A. (1998). Severe early-onset obesity, adrenal insufficiency and red hair pigmentation caused by POMC mutations in humans. *Nat Genet*, 1:155–157.

73. Kornetsky, C. (1989). Animal models: Promises and problems. In Koob, G.F. (ed.), *Animal Models of Depression*. Birkhauser, Boston, pp. 18–29.

74. McKinney, W.T. and Bunney, W.E. (1969). Animal model of depression. I. Review of evidence-implications for research. *Arch Gen Psychiatry*, 21:40.

75. Schuster, C.R. (1975). Drugs as reinforcers in monkey and man. *Pharmacol Rev*, 27:511–521.

76. Willner, P. (1984). The validity of animal models of depression. *Psychopharmacology*, 83:1–16.

77. Detke, M.J., Rickels, M., and Lucki, I. (1995). Active behaviors in the rat forced swimming test differentially produced by serotonergic and noradrenergic antidepressants. *Psychopharmacology*, 121:66–72.

78. Cryan, J.F., Markou, A., and Lucki, I. (2002). Assessing antidepressant activity in rodents: Recent developments and future needs. *Trends Pharmacol Sci*, 23:238–245.

79. Jenner, P., Rupniak, N.M.J., Rose, S., Kelly, E., Kilpatrick, G., Lees, A., and Marsden, C.D. (1984). 1-Methyl-4-phenyl-1,2,3,6-tetrahydropyridine-induced parkinsonism in the common marmoset. *Neurosci Lett*, 50:85–90.

80. Ungerstedt, U. (1971). Adipsia and aphagia after 6-hydroxydopamine induced degeneration of nigro-striatal dopamine system. *Acta Physiol Scand*, 367:95–122.

81. Ungerstedt, U. (1971). Postsynaptic supersensitivity after 6-hydroxydopamine induced degeneration of nigro-striatal dopamine system. *Acta Physiol Scand*, 367:69–93.

82. Fischman, M.W., Foltin, R.W., Nestadt, G., and Pearlson, G.D. (1990). Effects of desipramine maintenance on cocaine self-administration by humans. *J Pharmacol Exp Ther*, 253:760–770.

83. Hart, C.L., Ward, A.S., Collins, E.D., Haney, M., and Foltin, R.W. (2004). Gabapentin maintenance decreases smoked cocaine-related subjective effects, but not self-administration by humans. *Drug and Alcohol Depend*, 73:279–287.

84. Hart, C.L., Haney, M., Vosburg, S.K., Rubin, E., Foltin, R.W. (2008). Human smoked cocaine self-administration is decreased by modafinil. *Neuropsychopharmacology*.

85. Darwin, C. (1872). *The Expression of the Emotions in Man and Animals*. John Murray, London.

86. Berridge, K.C., Kringelbach, M.L. (2008). Affective neuroscience of pleasure: Reward in humans and animals. *Psychopharmacology*.

87. Panksepp, J. (2003). At the interface of the affective, behavioral, and cognitive neurosciences: Decoding the emotional feelings of the brain. *Brain and Cognition*, 52:4–14.

88. Fish, E.W., Sekinda, M., Ferrari, P.F., Dirks, A., and Miczek, K.A. (2000). Distress vocalizations in maternally separated mouse pups: Modulation via 5-HT1A, 5-HT1B and GABAA receptors. *Psychopharmacology*, 149:277–285.

89. Vivian, J.A., Barros, H.M.T., Manitiu, A., and Miczek, K.A. (1997). Ultrasonic vocalizations in rat pups: Modulation at the gamma-aminobutyric acid A receptor complex and the neurosteroid recognition site. *J Pharmacol Exp Ther*, 282:318–325.

90. Burgdorf, J., Knutson, B., Panksepp, J., and Shippenberg, T.S. (2001). Evaluation of rat ultrasonic vocalizations as predictors of the conditioned aversive effects of drugs. *Psychopharmacology (Berl)*, 155:35–42.

91. Mutschler, N.H. and Miczek, K.A. (1998). Withdrawal from a self-administered or non-contingent cocaine binge: Differences in ultrasonic distress vocalizations in rats. *Psychopharmacology*, 136:402–408.

92. Panksepp, J., Meeker, R., and Bean, N.J. (1980). The neurochemical control of crying. *Pharmacol Biochem Behav*, 12:437–443.

93. Winslow, J.T. and Insel, T.R. (1991). Infant rat separation is a sensitive test for novel anxiolytics. *Prog Neuropsychopharmacol Biol Psychiatry*, 15:745–757.

94. Brady, J.V. (1956). Assessment of drug effects on emotional behavior. *Science*, 123:1033–1034.

95. Wuttke, W., Kelleher, R.T. (1970). Effects of Some Benzodiazepines on Punished and Unpunished Behavior in the Pigeon. pp. 397–405.

96. Grill, H.J. and Norgren, R. (1978). Taste reactivity test: I. Mimetic responses to gustatory stimuli in neurological normal rats. *Brain Res*, 143:263–279.

97. Steiner, J.E., Glaser, D., Hawilo, M.E., and Berridge, K.C. (2001). Comparative expression of hedonic impact: Affective reactions to taste by human infants and other primates. *Neurosci Biobehav Rev*, 25:53–74.

98. Wise, R.A. (2006). Role of brain dopamine in food reward and reinforcement. *Philos Trans R Soc B Biol Sci*, 361:1149–1158.

99. Baldo, B.A. and Kelley, A.E. (2007). Discrete neurochemical coding of distinguishable motivational processes: Insights from nucleus accumbens control of feeding. *Psychopharmacology*, 191:439–459.

100. Berridge, K.C. (2007). The debate over dopamine's role in reward: The case for incentive salience. *Psychopharmacology*, 191:391–431.

101. Salamone, J.D., Correa, M., Farrar, A., and Mingote, S.M. (2007). Effort-related functions of nucleus accumbens dopamine and associated forebrain circuits. *Psychopharmacology*, 191:461–482.

102. Barbano, M.F. and Cador, M. (2007). Opioids for hedonic experience and dopamine to get ready for it. *Psychopharmacology*, 191:497–506.

103. Robbins, T.W. and Everitt, B.J. (2007). A role for mesencephalic dopamine in activation: Commentary on Berridge (2006). *Psychopharmacology*, 191:433–437.

104. Ferrari, P.F., Van Erp, A.M.M., Tornatzky, W., and Miczek, K.A. (2003). Accumbal dopamine and serotonin in anticipation of the next aggressive episode in rats. *Eur J Neurosci*, 17:371–378.

105. Horvitz, J.C. (2000). Mesolimbocortical and nigrostriatal dopamine responses to salient non-reward events. *Neuroscience*, 96:651–656.

106. Scott, D.J., Heitzeg, M.M., Koeppe, R.A., Stohler, C.S., and Zubieta, J.K. (2006). Variations in the human pain stress experience mediated by ventral and dorsal basal ganglia dopamine activity. *J Neurosci*, 26:10789–10795.

107. Kringelbach, M.L. (2008). The hedonic brain: A functional neuroanatomy of human pleasure. In Kringelbach, M.L. and Berridge, K.C. (eds.), *Pleasures of the Brain*. Oxford University Press, Oxford.

108. Moreau, J.L., Scherschlicht, R., Jenck, F., and Martin, J.R. (1995). Chronic mild stress-induced anhedonia model of depression-sleep abnormalities and curative effects of electroshock treatment. *Behav Pharmacol*, 6:682–687.

109. Wise, R.A., Bauco, P., Carlezon, W.A., and Trojniar, W. (1992). Self-stimulation and drug reward mechanisms. *Neurobiol Drug Alcohol Addict*, 654:192–198.

ADDITIONAL REFERENCES

Cook, L. and Davidson, A.B. (1973). Effects of behaviorally active drugs in a conflict-punishment procedure in rats. In: Garattini, S., Mussini, E., and Randall, L.O. (Eds.), *The Benzodiazepines*, Raven Press, New York.

Shader, R.I. (1975). *Manual of Psychiatric Therapeutics*. Little, Brown, Boston.

CHAPTER 5

Developing Novel Anxiolytics: Improving Preclinical Detection and Clinical Assessment

Thomas Steckler[1], Murray B. Stein[2] and Andrew Holmes[3]

[1]Department of Psychiatry, RED Europe, Johnson and Johnson Pharmaceutical Research and Development, Beerse, Belgium
[2]Anxiety and Traumatic Stress Disorders Program, Departments of Psychiatry and Family and Preventive Medicine, University of California San Diego; and VA San Diego Healthcare System, La Jolla, CA, USA
[3]Section on Behavioral Science and Genetics, Laboratory for Integrative Neuroscience, National Institute on Alcohol Abuse and Alcoholism, National Institutes of Health, Bethesda, MD, USA

INTRODUCTION

Anxiety disorders are the most prevalent class of psychiatric conditions in the world today.[1,2] While it is impossible to quantify the cost of these highly debilitating conditions to sufferers' lives, the financial burden in healthcare costs and lost productivity is estimated to be in the tens of billions of dollars annually in the United States alone.[3] Unfortunately, existing treatments for anxiety disorders (Table 5.1) do not meet the challenge of this growing health crisis. Various classes of anti-anxiety (anxiolytic) medications are currently available but suffer from significant rates of non-response, a potentially dangerous delay in onset of action and poor tolerability caused by unpleasant side-effects.[4-6]

The most commonly prescribed medication class for anxiety remains the benzodiazepines despite educational efforts over the past decade to increase use of selective serotonin reuptake inhibitors (SSRIs) and reduce use of benzodiazepines.[7] It may be inferred from these data that despite the widespread popularity and use of SSRIs, clinicians and

Animal and Translational Models for CNS Drug Discovery,
Vol. 1 of 3: Psychiatric Disorders
Robert McArthur and Franco Borsini (eds), Academic Press, 2008

Table 5.1 The anxiolytic pharmacopoeia

Class	Putative mechanism of action	Primary indication	Therapeutic limitations
Benzodiazepine (e.g., diazepam)	Allosteric modulator of GABA_A receptor	GAD	Cognitive impairment, sedation, ataxia, dependency, withdrawal
High potency benzodiazepine (e.g., alprazolam)	Allosteric modulator of GABA_A receptor	GAD, PD	Cognitive impairment, sedation, ataxia, dependency, withdrawal
Tricyclic antidepressant (e.g., imipramine)	Increased 5-HT, NE, DA availability	GAD, OCD, PD	Slow therapeutic onset, sleep disturbance, orthostatic hypotension, sexual dysfunction, weight gain
Monoamine oxidase inhibitor (e.g., phenelzine)	Increased 5-HT, NE, DA availability	GAD, OCD, PD	Slow therapeutic onset, orthostatic hypotension, sexual dysfunction, contraindication with tyramine-containing foods
Selective 5-HT reuptake inhibitor (e.g., fluoxetine)	Increased 5-HT (NE, DA) availability	GAD, OCD, PD, PTSD, SAD	Slow therapeutic onset, nausea, sexual dysfunction, weight gain
Dual (5-HT and NE) reuptake inhibitor (e.g., venlafaxine)	Increased NE and 5-HT, (DA) availability	GAD, OCD, PD, PTSD, SAD	Slow therapeutic onset, sexual dysfunction, dizziness, nausea
Azapirone (buspirone)	Partial 5-HT1A receptor agonism	GAD	Slow therapeutic onset, dizziness, headache, hyperprolactinemia

GAD: generalized anxiety disorder; OCD: obsessive-compulsive disorder; PD: panic disorder; PTSD: posttraumatic stress disorder; SAD: social anxiety disorder; 5-HT: serotonin; NE: norepinephrine; DA: dopamine.

consumers are somewhat dissatisfied with their usefulness and continue to rely, at least in part, on benzodiazepines. There is also evidence that consumers rarely take SSRIs for the full recommended duration, usually quitting early due to adverse events.[8] Even when used optimally, pharmacotherapy response rates in anxiety disorders are typically in the range of 50-55%, with remission rates even lower (25-30%).[9] Efforts to improve upon these outcomes with adjunctive therapies (e.g., benzodiazepines or atypical anti-psychotics) are common, with some studies showing benefits of augmentation pharma-cotherapy with these agents.[10,11] But the fact that so few patients achieve compliance or remission with current evidence-based pharmacotherapies signifies a monumental unmet need for better anxiolytics.[6]

The pharmaceutical industry and academia are engaged in enormous investments in developing novel pharmacotherapeutics for anxiety disorders. However, the jury is still out as to how successful these efforts will be, and the field finds itself at a critical juncture. Our aim in this chapter is to provide a frank and critical overview of the field and offer some suggestions on how the process of anxiolytic drug discovery, from the laboratory to the clinic, could be improved.

The identification of novel anxiolytics is still largely based upon the assessment of drug effects in non-humans, chiefly rodents. Therefore, we begin by introducing the concept of "anxiety" in rodents and how rodent models of anxiety help elucidate the neural systems and molecules mediating anxiety and, in so doing, serve to iden-tify anxiolytic targets. We then move on more directly to discuss the place of rodent assays of anxiety-related behaviors in the drug discovery process and note the major *caveats* associated with their use in this context. Finally, we turn to the measurement of anxiety levels in humans and the assessment of anxiolytic efficacy of novel pharma-cotherapeutics in clinical trials. We conclude with a call for closer dialogue between researchers in the preclinical and clinical realms to better bridge the translational gap.

MEASURING "ANXIETY" IN ANIMALS

Anxiety can be defined as the subjective experience of anticipating a future aversive event (or state). Whether pathological anxiety is qualitatively or merely quantitatively different from normal anxiety is a matter of debate.[12] However, by diagnostic defini-tions, clinical forms of anxiety requiring treatment are those in which the perceived level of threat is in excess of that which is actually present (or occurs in the absence of any threat).[13] Yet for most of us a modest level of anxiety and apprehension is a nor-mal and indeed highly adaptive response to the dangers we encounter in everyday life. Anxiety keeps us attuned to future threats, and helps us avoid them guided, in part, on our prior experiences in similar situations. A basic assumption when using animals to study anxiety is that neural and behavioral processes analogous to human anxiety can be evoked in situations that are a real threat to the animal's survival.[14] For nocturnal small prey animals like rats and mice, open and well-lit spaces are putatively danger-ous but, on the other hand, must be explored in order to obtain food, and find a better home or a potential mate. This ethological premise has underpinned the development of the so-called approach–avoidance conflict tests of rodent "anxiety" that have become the most widely used assays for "anxiety-like behavior" and anxiolytic-like activity.[15] For example, in the popular elevated plus-maze test the rat or mouse is faced with a conflict between remaining in protected enclosed arms or venturing out into exposed arms;[16] with relatively high open arm avoidance being the readout of relatively high anxiety-like behavior. Along similar lines, conflict between approach and avoidance in various forms underlies most of the frequently used rodent tests of anxiety-related behavior (e.g., novel open field, light/dark exploration, Vogel conflict, Geller-Seifter, social interaction, hyponeophagia, defensive burying, marble burying); although with exceptions (e.g., stress-induced hyperthermia). For a fuller description of these tests, see.[17]

It should be made clear at this point that a *test* for anxiety in an animal is not necessarily the same as a *model* of anxiety. A test typically assays specific features of behavior, endocrinology or physiology that is symptomatic in anxiety disorders. A model by contrast aims to recapitulate the pathophysiology of an anxiety disorder by experimentally manipulating environment, neurophysiology, neurochemistry or genetics. Models of complex disease states such as anxiety disorders are of course more difficult to devise, and the majority of studies on potential anxiolytics employ tests rather than models.

The utility of both tests and models of anxiety is evaluated in terms of various factors, including practicality, replicability and most importantly, validity. The aforementioned approach–avoidance conflict tests have "*face validity*;" that is, to the human eye they look like reasonable analogues of anxiety. But, as discussed in the next section, they only have a limited degree of "*predictive validity*" (i.e., they respond to) for at least some classes of known anxiolytics. A third main benchmark for animal models of anxiety is "*construct validity*": whether a model recruits the same neurobiological substrates as anxiety in humans, and whether it involves at least some of the pathophysiological mechanisms as the human condition, be they neural, genetic or environmental in nature. This is the most difficult criterion for any animal model of a complex disease state to attain, but particularly so for a disease in which the pathophysiology is itself not fully understood, as with anxiety disorders. The issue of construct validity also raises the question of whether a test that evokes a "normal" adaptive anxiety-like response, as do the ethological tests, can in of itself sufficiently model the type of *abnormal* anxiety seen in anxiety disorders. The argument that it can is based upon the assumption that abnormal anxiety simply represents the extreme end of a continuum, and that normal and abnormal forms recruit the same underlying mechanisms, just to a different degree. As noted above, this is an assumption that may not necessarily hold true and there is growing interest in finding experimental manipulations that generate an anxiety-like response in rodents that is over and above that produced by exposure to a test apparatus *per se*. The idea is that such models might more closely equate to clinical forms of anxiety, thereby improving their construct validity and better serve to elucidate the mechanistic basis of "pathological" or trait anxiety (Figure 5.1).

Rodent Models of "Pathological" Anxiety

Models of abnormal anxiety in rodents can be loosely grouped into those that induce an altered anxiety-like state by either chemical treatment, exposure to stress or genetic variation/modification. Rather than offer an exhaustive review of each approach, we discuss some of the key findings and *caveats* pertinent to each.

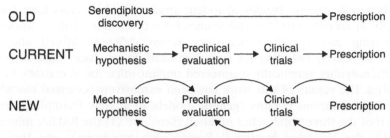

Figure 5.1 Paradigms for anxiolytic drug discovery: old and new. The major classes of drug compounds that are currently prescribed for anxiety disorders are largely based upon the serendipitous discovery of their anti-anxiety properties. A current paradigm advocates a more systematic approach based upon the generation of mechanistic hypotheses regarding the putative role of a target system in the mediation of anxiety, followed by thorough preclinical evaluation using a panel of well-validated animal models and assessment of therapeutic efficacy in double-blind clinical trials. Ideally, the flow of information should be bidirectional, with constant feedback from the clinic to the preclinical researcher and from the market place to the drug developer, which will ensure refinement and innovation in both preclinical models and clinical trial, design, and should lead to the generation of new and testable hypotheses.

Anxiety states analogous to those seen clinically can be induced in normal human subjects by various psychological (e.g., public speaking for social anxiety), chemical (e.g., lactate infusion for panic attacks) and pharmacological (e.g., yohimbine for panic attacks or non-specific anxiety) challenges. Treatment with various pharmacological and chemical agents (e.g., lactate, carbon dioxide, drugs acting at 5-HT2 receptors, adrenoreceptors, or cholecystokinin receptors) can produce increases in anxiety-like behaviors on the aforementioned rodent tests (reviewed in[18,19]). This has led to some elegant research mapping common brain regions activated by anxiety-provoking drugs in rodents as a means to elucidating those neural circuits subserving human anxiety, typically via quantification of immediate early genes such as c-Fos.[20,21] Many of the brain regions (e.g., prefrontal cortex, amygdala, hippocampus, hypothalamus) that are activated by anxiogenic substances are regions implicated in the pathophysiology of anxiety disorders.[22-25] Thus, this approach supports a convergence of evidence identifying key neural circuits subserving pathological forms of anxiety in animals and humans. Establishing such neural correlates of anxiety would have implications not only for understanding the pathophysiology of anxiety, but also for screening novel anxiolytics that effectively normalize the neural effects of chemical agents.

Anxiety disorders are sometimes explicitly associated with a highly stressful event, as in the case of posttraumatic stress disorder (PTSD), or can be provoked and exacerbated by exposure to stress, as in the case of all anxiety (and depressive) disorders. Exposure to stressors such as maternal separation early in life or stressors such restraint or social defeat in adulthood can lead to increases anxiety-like behaviors in rodents.[26-30] Interestingly, recent studies have shown that some of the same brain regions recruited during anxiety are also highly sensitive to stress, and show structural alterations in response to stress.[31-33] Another interesting line of research to emerge from studies of stress effects in rodents is the interaction between stress vulnerability and genetic factors. For example, there are recent examples in humans and rodents, where the effects of stress were only evident in certain "genetically susceptible" populations.[34,35]

More generally, genetic studies of rodent anxiety-like behaviors have burgeoned dramatically in recent years. Genetic studies have taken one of three approaches:[36] (1) comparing anxiety-related behaviors across different inbred and outbred strains, (2) selectively breeding for such behaviors to produce "high anxiety lines" and (3) phenotyping genetically engineered mutant mice for alterations in anxiety-like behavior. The results of this work has been extensively reviewed elsewhere[37–40] and has provided various putative "genetic models" of anxiety. Examples, corresponding to each of the three approaches outlined above, are (1) the BALB/c inbred mouse strain;[40] (2) the Maudsley reactive,[41] Roman high avoidance[42] and High Anxiety Behavior rat lines and the High Anxiety Behavior mouse line;[43] and (3) mice with gene mutations of the serotonin 5-HT_{1A} receptor,[44] serotonin transporter[45] regulator of G protein signaling 2,[46] and overexpression of corticotrophin releasing factor (CRF).[47] As with chemical- and stress-induced anxiety paradigms, these genetically related models have the potential to provide novel ways to study the neurobiology and treatment of anxiety. In addition, these models can be used to identify specific genetic variants contributing to abnormal anxiety (for review see[48]). To date, however, there has not been good integration of these models into the drug discovery process.

Preclinical Tests for Anxiolytic Drug Discovery

Because it is the ultimate goal of pharmaceutical industry to develop novel drugs for the treatment of disorders in man, predictive validity is the primary driver amongst the three types of validity mentioned above for industrial research. Unfortunately, as already noted above predictive validity of the available tests is limited. One reason is that the vast majority of preclinical anxiety tests have been validated with acutely administered GABAergic compounds, especially the benzodiazepines. Hence, it comes as no surprise that these tests are exquisitely sensitive to detect compounds acting through GABAergic mechanisms, but that when it comes to other mechanisms of action, they often fail. SSRIs, for example, are nowadays considered the gold standard in the treatment of many anxiety disorders, yet show up as false negatives after acute administration in many contemporary tests measuring anxiety-related behavior in rodents, such as in tests based on spontaneous exploration (elevated plus-maze, light/dark box), in tests based on suppression of responding (e.g., conditioned freezing, four-plates test, novelty-suppressed feeding), in conflict tests (e.g., Vogel conflict test, Geller-Seifter test), in fear-potentiated startle (FPS), social interaction or stress-induced hyperthermia (reviewed in.[49] Only limited evidence exists for the effects of antidepressant drugs on anxiety-related behavior following chronic administration (e.g., see[50]).

In general, the available tests can be considered "*screening paradigms*," that is, they are relatively fast, reliable and reproducible, with high sensitivity to detect a certain class of true positives; that is the GABAergic anxiolytic drugs. However, because of their lower sensitivity to detect other classes of anxiolytics the worrisome possibility is raised that these paradigms may also lack sensitivity to detect other, novel drugs with anxiolytic properties and novel molecular mechanisms of action. Thus, if used as primary tests to screen broadly for novel anxiolytics there is the danger that we will simply detect more of the same ("me same"), that is, other drugs acting either directly or indirectly via GABAergic mechanisms.[51] This *caveat* has led to increasing concern about the reliance on the available anxiety screening tests in drug development programs.

An alternative approach is to develop *"mechanistic tests."* Here, the focus is simply on any easily measurable physiological outcome that determines whether a compound acts at the desired target (e.g., CRF-induced forepaw treading[52]). Although these tests do not necessarily need to be related to the therapeutic effect (e.g., anxiolytic-like activity), they do provide important information about the *in vivo* activity at the target at the site of action (i.e., the brain), which is highly valuable information for drug development. Mechanistic tests are particularly well suited when assessing the pharmacokinetic–pharmacodynamic (PK/PD) profile of a novel drug and hence allow for allometric scaling, which estimates doses in animals that can be expected to result in comparable drug-induced changes in man.

Another complementary approach in drug discovery uses *"simulation models."* These models attempt to incorporate the neuropathology of anxiety disorders and to measure the same behavioral constructs as seen in the psychiatric disease. Hence, they aim to have high construct validity. The rodent models of pathological anxiety discussed above fall within this category, given that the neurobiology of anxiety disorders is modeled and disease-relevant behavioral measures are taken. As such, these models could be well suited as translational models. However, these models must allow for reproducible results within and across laboratories to be of use in an industrial setting, which is not always the case. The models are also in many cases insufficiently characterized. To take one example, Maudsley reactive and non-reactive rat strains are known to differ in their sensitivity to benzodiazepines,[53] but have not been well characterized for responses to other true positives (e.g., SSRIs) or true negatives (e.g., antipsychotics).

A factor further complicating the generating of good animal models for drug development is the ever changing classification of psychiatric disorders, including anxiety disorders. Many preclinical anxiety tests were developed before anxiety disorders were split into different categories by the third edition of DSM-III, published in 1980. Currently, we need models that adhere to the classification scheme of the next edition, DSM-IV, published in 1994, and in the future DSM-V it can be anticipated that classification schemes will change again. Based on these classification schemes, claims have been made to link certain preclinical anxiety models and tests with specific anxiety disorders, but again full validation is often missing. Take marble-burying behavior in mice as an example. Here, the natural tendency of mice to bury unfamiliar objects in sawdust is quantified and postulated to serve as a model of obsessive-compulsive disorder (OCD).[54] At face value, such burying behavior could be seen as a type of compulsive hoarding behavior.[i] But benzodiazepines are active in this test,[55] whereas they are of limited therapeutic use in OCD. Thus, it could be argued that this class of drugs yields a false positive in the marble-burying test, and that the test is therefore questionable as a screen for novel OCD medications.

Taken together, these *caveats* raise some serious questions regarding the utility of the existing preclinical tests and models of anxiety in drug development. In fact, one could go as far as to argue that basing drug discovery on preclinical animal models is no longer either the most effective or economical way of using increasingly limited resources.

---

[i]Refer to Joel *et al.*, Animal models of obsessive-compulsive disorder: From bench to bedside via endophenotypes and biomarkers, in this volume for further discussion of and description of models of OCD-like behaviors.

TRANSLATIONAL MODELS FOR ANXIOLYTIC DRUG DISCOVERY

There is a growing effort to develop and use *translational models* to improve anxiolytic drug identification. These models aim to identify promising targets early in the process by integrating biology, discovery medicine and PK/PD modeling expertise, and then ensure good rationale for progression (and dose selection) based on the link between target access, target activation and pharmacodynamic response. The aforementioned mechanistic models play an important role here.

Presumptive surrogate markers for anxiety may also be employed to test for novel anxiolytics in animals, such as measures of autonomic arousal (cardiovascular measures such as heart rate and blood pressure, body temperature and defecation), measures of stress reactivity (plasma corticosterone/cortisol and plasma adrenocorticotropic hormone, ACTH) and imaging studies. For example, regional cerebral glucose utilization can be studied in conscious rats in response to potential anxiolytic drugs,[56] which can then be extrapolated to human flourodoxhyglucose-positron emission tomography (FDG-PET) studies. Imaging technologies can also help to understand the time course of receptor occupancy better, indicating that a compound of interest penetrates the brain and occupies the target at sufficient concentration.[57]

As discussed above, there are a number of so-called "challenge tests" that have been used in patients suffering from panic disorder or generalized anxiety disorder (GAD) to provoke panic attacks. These challenge tests involve the administration of substances or drugs such as sodium lactate, carbon dioxide, cholecystokinin, pentagastrin or yohimbine in healthy volunteers with the aim of determining differential dose–response relationships and/or differences in physiological responding between healthy subjects and patients with anxiety disorders. As noted, preclinical studies have also investigated the effects of the various challenges in animals (reviewed in[17]). However, the same criticism regarding the relative paucity of solid validation applies here as it does for the more "classical" tests and models. Moreover, and as will be discussed below, challenge tests in humans themselves face limitations when it comes to predicting clinical efficacy of anxiolytic drugs. Indeed, many of the translational models currently enjoy the benefit of the doubt, and there is no guarantee that they will prove any better than the existing tests. Faith in this approach may reflect desperation in the pharmaceutical industry. At present, we can merely conclude that they offer another alternative to the classical models.

CHALLENGES IN MEASURING HUMAN ANXIETY AND RESPONSE TO TREATMENTS

The neurobiology of anxiety disorders – in fact, of any psychiatric disorder – is incompletely understood. Although structural abnormalities and alterations in functional neural circuits for anxiety disorders are being identified,[58] it is unclear to what extent these abnormalities are central to their pathophysiology and, even more importantly, whether altering function in these regions is necessary or sufficient for successful treatment. Further complicating the situation is the fact that our current psychiatric diagnostic systems (DSM-IV, ICD-10)[ii] are built almost exclusively upon phenomeno-logical (i.e., descriptive) characterization, rather than upon an understanding of patho-physiological bases. This means that our diagnoses cannot be expected to reflect a uniform categorization of biologically distinct entities; rather, they are more likely than not to represent a heterogeneous group of syndromes that may share little more than symptoms. These problems are exceptionally well recognized by clinicians and clinical researchers alike.

Less well understood – or perhaps just less well acknowledged – is the inevitable consequence that because the diagnostic criteria consist of a menu of common symp-toms, the modal patients have *some but not all* of the symptoms, and patients differ considerably in terms of which symptoms they manifest. Thus, it is possible, for exam-ple, to have two patients with PTSD who, other than sharing a pathological response to life-threatening trauma, have virtually no overlapping symptoms: one patient with PTSD may have recurrent nightmares of the trauma, emotional numbing and an exag-gerated startle response, whereas a second patient with PTSD may have daytime flash-backs, extensive behavioral avoidance and insomnia without nightmares. Due to the fact that treatment success is identified as symptom reduction, this variable expression of symptoms across individuals within a diagnostic category means that treatment effects will be inherently variable.

Variability in symptom presentation across individuals within the same diagnostic category (e.g., PTSD) presents serious problems for the successful conduct of large-scale controlled trials for anxiety (and, indeed, all psychiatric) disorders. Regulatory bodies, in the absence of a better alternative, have used DSM-IV or ICD-10 criteria as therapeutic targets and outcome measures have, accordingly, been geared toward mea-suring response on all the symptom dimensions that characterize the syndrome of interest. For example, the most widely accepted measure of clinical outcome in social phobia (also known as social anxiety disorder), the Liebowitz Social Anxiety Scale (LSAS),[59] assesses fear (rated 0–3) and avoidance (0–3) in 24 different situations (e.g., speaking in front of a small group; using a public lavatory; expressing disagreement) in order to survey the intra-individual variability in specific symptoms that can occur across individuals who meet diagnostic criteria for the disorder. Not surprisingly, some symptoms are common to many individuals with the diagnosis (e.g., fear and avoid-ance of speaking in front of a large group of people), whereas others are much rarer (e.g., fear and avoidance of writing in front of other people). As in the aforementioned case of PTSD, it is theoretically possible for two individuals to have absolutely no over-lap in symptoms – indeed, to endorse, for example, scores of "3" for fear and "3" for avoidance on 12 of 24 completely different items on the LSAS – and yet to score well into the clinical range (in this example, scoring a total of "72," which would be consid-ered moderately severe). Although it is possible to imagine that a therapeutic agent might exert an impact across such a heterogeneous group of situations that a clini-cal trial using an instrument such as the LSAS could successfully detect a signal (and,

---

[ii] Please refer to the Diagnostic and Statistical Manual of Mental Disorders, Fourth Edition – Text Revision (DSMIV-TR), or The International Statistical Classification of Diseases and Related Health Problems, 10th Revision, published by the American Psychiatric Association and the World Health Organization, respec-tively, for current diagnostic criteria manuals in use.

indeed, the LSAS has done so in the case of the SSRIs in numerous clinical trials), it seems to be asking too much of an assessment measure to gauge outcome across such a vast expanse of symptomatic possibilities.

It is reasonable to ask the question, then, as to whether some anxiety disorders offer more distinct symptomatic domains than others, and might therefore prove riper as therapeutic targets for preclinical drug discovery research. Panic disorder is characterized by the occurrence of recurrent, sometimes unexpected panic attacks. Early pharmacological clinical trials focused on reducing the number of panic attacks as a means of tracking outcome. But as experience with the treatment of panic disorder has progressed, it has become clear that the measurement of panic attacks is notoriously subjective and subject to recall problems when assessed retrospectively (e.g., "Over the past week, how many panic attacks have you had?"), and that the very act of drawing attention to symptoms by asking patients to write them down in diaries (with the aim of improving accurate recall) results in a change in the reporting of number of attacks.[60] In short, an entity that was previously thought to be easy and reliable to measure – the number of panic attacks experienced in a given timeframe – turns out to be remarkably fluctuant, unstable and unreliable. This realization has led to the development of outcome scales for panic disorder that accommodate the clinical complexity of the disorder better, including not only the symptom dimension of panic attack frequency, but also panic attack severity, associated phobic avoidance, and distress and disability. One such example, the Panic Disorder Severity Scale (PDSS),[61] has been widely used in academic circles and federally funded trials (e.g.,[62]) but hardly at all in industry-sponsored trials, presumably because regulatory drug licensing authorities (Food and Drug Administration) have relied upon a reduction in the frequency of panic attacks as a requisite for granting a panic disorder indication to a new drug.

To what extent are these problems with symptom measurement tractable? In theory, it should be possible to design measures that are reliable and valid indicators of clinical outcome both across and within anxiety disorders. Indeed, efforts are underway to design and validate pan-anxiety disorder scales that would de-emphasize reliance on symptoms alone (though these cannot be altogether abandoned, for obvious reasons) and would simultaneously do a better job of incorporating distress and dysfunction that are associated with those symptoms in a given individual. One such example of a scale-in-progress is the Overall Anxiety Impairment and Severity Scale (OASIS).[63] As noted above, efforts to develop better anxiety disorder-specific scales have progressed (e.g., PDSS for panic disorder), but regulatory agencies have been, somewhat understandably, slow to adopt these newer measures, tending to favor the same outcome measures (e.g., reduction in frequency of panic attacks, in the case of panic disorder studies) they have relied upon in the past when granting indications for a specific disorder. To address this problem of slow uptake of newer measures by regulatory agencies, experts need to speak in a coherent voice about the superiority of these newer measures, when such evidence exists.

Another approach that should be further explored – and discussed with regulatory agencies – is the use of measures that do not necessarily match up one-to-one with DSM disorder-specific symptom measures – but nonetheless do a superb job of measuring the "core" construct of the disorder. One such example is the use of an instrument such as the Anxiety Sensitivity Index (ASI) to measure the core belief among patients with panic disorder that the anxiety symptoms they experience are dangerous or threatening.[64] The ASI is sensitive to change among patients with panic disorder, and in federally funded studies has been successfully used as an indicator of treatment outcome (e.g.,[65]). Another example would be to focus on the core "worry" construct in GAD with an instrument such as the Penn State Worry Questionnaire (PSWQ).[66] A considerable advantage over this type of approach is that whereas DSM-IV or ICD-10 diagnoses may change over time, to the extent that the core symptoms of the disorders remain invariant (e.g., panic disorder, in whatever reincarnation it assumes in DSM-V[67] will still be characterized by heightened anxiety sensitivity), these measures should continue to be applicable and useful for treatment trials.

LOST IN TRANSLATION?

As discussed above, anxiety disorders in humans are characterized by a complex set of cognitive and emotional features. Anxious individuals focus on the likelihood (or, as they sometimes perceive it, inevitability) of a future aversive emotional (or bodily) state in certain contexts.[68] Cognitive behavioral theories recognize the importance of anxious thinking in the maintenance (if not necessarily the genesis) of anxiety disorders.[69] By the very nature of this conceptualization, we have no way to know what rodents are thinking when they engage in approach–avoidance behaviors. We can make inferences about their motivation in such tasks, but we have no way of objectifying their cognitions, and therefore must make assumptions about the comparability of these behaviors to those observed in patients with anxiety disorders. Not surprisingly, these assumptions are difficult to verify, and the anxious anticipation and worry that characterize anxiety disorders are subjective, introspective states that cannot be queried using animal models. Consequently, we rely on the kinds of tests described earlier to assess the anxiolytic potential of novel compounds. Is there a better way?

FUTURE PERSPECTIVES

One approach that is gaining some popularity is the automatic measure of several behavioral variables of mice or rats in their home cage or specially designed set-ups over time, with subsequent multivariate analysis of drug effects to identify patterns of behavior that allow clustering of novel compounds into drug classes, for example, to identify fingerprints of anxiolytic drugs.[70,71] Although this approach offers the advantage of potentially identifying behavioral responses with greater precision, being automated and unbiased, it still suffers from the same limitations as other, more classical approaches, that is, it has to be validated, relying on a database using clinically available drugs acting at a limited number of molecular mechanisms. Hence, it also has the "me same" problem. It is still too early to draw conclusions about the predictive validity of this approach. However, the throughput that can be achieved with such systems clearly has the potential to build the detailed and solid databases required for that discrimination.

Another approach that is being increasingly explored is a process that can best be described as "back-translation," or moving from animal tests to human versions of these tests. One such example would be the use of FPS. FPS is a well-studied process in animals wherein a conditioned stimulus (e.g., shock) is associated with a cue (or unconditioned stimulus, such as a light, or even a contextual cue such as a cage where shock had previously been administered) will augment the naturally occurring startle response to a loud noise. The neural circuitry of the startle response has been well worked out, and the involvement of anxiety-relevant structures such as the amygdala in certain types of conditioned fear is well established.[72] In an example of an effort at back-translation, the reduction in humans of FPS with a presumptive therapeutic agent has been used to make inferences about the drug's anxiolytic potential.[73] Although promising and deserving of further study in this regard, the fact that benzodiazepines – a well-established class of anxiolytic drugs – have no effect on FPS in humans[74] suggests that this particular approach has limitations as a predictive human test for anxiolytic efficacy.

Other approaches, such as the use of functional magnetic resonance imaging in conjunction with pharmacotherapy (sometimes referred to as pharmacofMRI), are currently being investigated.[75] This is another, somewhat different example of back-translation, in that pharmacofMRI uses information from animal lesion and genetic studies of anxiety to focus on critical brain structures or circuits the function of which can be altered in predictable ways by anxiolytic drugs. At present, proof-in-principle of this approach has been shown for a single class of drugs, benzodiazepines, exhibiting dose-related reductions in amygdala and insular cortex activation during an emotional face processing task.[76] Work is ongoing to extend these observations to other known anxiolytic classes (e.g., SSRIs) and, if warranted, to novel classes of anxiolytic drugs. Only time will tell to what extent this type of approach will prove useful in bridging the gap between bench and bedside.

Can the growing neuroimaging literature identifying key neural circuit abnormalities in anxiety (e.g., amygdala hyperfunction, prefrontal cortex hypofunction) be taken back to the preclinic with a view to devising animal models of amygdala/prefrontal dysfunction that would then serve as models for validating compounds? First, encouraging studies are being published using small animal fMRI[77] or other imaging methods. But again, it is too early to come to conclusions about the added value of these approaches. New does not necessarily mean better and added value has still to be shown. Care has to be taken not to just fall for the hype and just to run behind a new concept for the sake of being different.

From the clinical side, the next step forward for translational research on anxiolytic actions will be greatly aided by a better diagnostic definition of psychiatric patient populations. Improved diagnostic systems with better clinical (sub) classification based on neurobiological and neurophysiological endophenotypes will permit clearer translation to measures in animals. Achieving these objectives will depend on the academic researchers, pharmaceutical laboratories and clinicians working together with the common goal of improving the lives of the increasing number of people afflicted with anxiety disorders.

REFERENCES

1. Andrade, L., Caraveo-Anduaga, J.J., Berglund, P., Bijl, R.V., De Graaf, R., Vollebergh, W. et al.. (2003). The epidemiology of major depressive episodes: Results from the International Consortium of Psychiatric Epidemiology (ICPE) Surveys. *Int J Method Psychiat Res*, 12(1):3–21.

2. Demyttenaere, K., Bruffaerts, R., Posada-Villa, J., Gasquet, I., Kovess, V., Lepine, J.P. et al. (2004). Prevalence, severity, and unmet need for treatment of mental disorders in the World Health Organization World Mental Health Surveys. *J Am Med Assoc*, 291(21):2581–2590.

3. Greenberg, P.E., Kessler, R.C., Birnbaum, H.G., Leong, S.A., Lowe, S.W., Berglund, P.A. et al. (2003). The economic burden of depression in the United States: How did it change between 1990 and 2000? *J Clin Psychiat*, 64(12):1465–1475.

4. Insel, T.R. and Charney, D.S. (2003). Research on major depression: Strategies and priorities. *JAMA*, 289(23):3167–3168.

5. Holmes, A., Heilig, M., Rupniak, N.M., Steckler, T., and Griebel, G. (2003). Neuropeptide systems as novel therapeutic targets for depression and anxiety disorders. *Trend Pharmacol Sci*, 24(11):580–588.

6. Stein, D.J. and Seedat, S. (2004). Unresolved questions about treatment-resistant anxiety disorders. *CNS Spectr*, 9(10):715.

7. Bruce, S.E., Vasile, R.G., Goisman, R.M., Salzman, C., Spencer, M., Machan, J.T. et al. (2003). Are benzodiazepines still the medication of choice for patients with panic disorder with or without agoraphobia? *Am J Psychiat*, 160(8):1432–1438.

8. Stein, M.B., Cantrell, C.R., Sokol, M.C., Eaddy, M.T., and Shah, M.B. (2006). Antidepressant adherence and medical resource use among managed care patients with anxiety disorders. *Psychiat Serv*, 57(5):673–680.

9. Stein, M.B. (2005). Anxiety disorders: somatic treatment. In Kaplan, H.I. and Sadock, B.J. (eds.), *Comprehensive Textbook of Psychiatry*. Williams & Wilkins, Baltimore, pp. 1780–1788.

10. Seedat, S. and Stein, M.B. (2004). Double-blind, placebo-controlled assessment of combined clonazepam with paroxetine compared with paroxetine monotherapy for generalized social anxiety disorder. *J Clin Psychiat*, 65(2):244–248.

11. Pollack, M.H., Simon, N.M., Zalta, A.K., Worthington, J.J., Hoge, E.A., Mick, E. et al. (2006). Olanzapine augmentation of fluoxetine for refractory generalized anxiety disorder: a placebo controlled study. *Biol Psychiat*, 59(3):211–215.

12. Belzung, C. and Griebel, G. (2001). Measuring normal and pathological anxiety-like behaviour in mice: A review. *Behav Brain Res*, 125(1–2):141–149.

13. DSM-IV (1994). *Diagnostic and Statistical Manual of Mental Disorders*, 4th edition. American Psychiatric Association.

14. Darwin, C.R. (1867). *The Expression of the Emotions in Man and Animals*. Oxford University Press, Oxford.

15. Rodgers, R.J., Cao, B.J., Dalvi, A., and Holmes, A. (1997). Animal models of anxiety: An ethological perspective. *Braz J Med Biol Res*, 30(3):289–304.

16. Handley, S.L. and Mithani, S. (1984). Effects of alpha-adrenoceptor agonists and antagonists in a maze-exploration model of 'fear'-motivated behaviour. *Naunyn Schmiedebergs Arch Pharmacol*, 327(1):1–5.

17. Cryan, J.F. and Holmes, A. (2005). The ascent of mouse: Advances in modelling human depression and anxiety. *Nat Rev Drug Discov*, 4(9):775–790.

18. Griebel, G. (1995). 5-Hydroxytryptamine-interacting drugs in animal models of anxiety disorders: More than 30 years of research. *Pharmacol Ther*, 65(3):319–395.

19. Millan, M.J. (2003). The neurobiology and control of anxious states. *Prog Neurobiol*, 70(2):83–244.

20. Singewald, N. (2007). Altered brain activity processing in high-anxiety rodents revealed by challenge paradigms and functional mapping. *Neurosci Biobehav Rev*, 31(1):18–40.

21. Blanchard, D.C., Canteras, N.S., Markham, C.M., Pentkowski, N.S., and Blanchard, R.J. (2005). Lesions of structures showing FOS expression to cat presentation: Effects on responsivity to a Cat, cat odor, and nonpredator threat. *Neurosci Biobehav Rev*, 29(8):1243–1253.

22. Phillips, M.L., Drevets, W.C., Rauch, S.L., and Lane, R. (2003). Neurobiology of emotion perception II: Implications for major psychiatric disorders. *Biol Psychiat*, 54(5):515–528.

23. Phelps, E.A., Delgado, M.R., Nearing, K.I., and LeDoux, J.E. (2004). Extinction learning in humans: Role of the amygdala and vmPFC. *Neuron*, 43(6):897–905.

24. Drevets, W.C. (2001). Neuroimaging and neuropathological studies of depression: Implications for the cognitive-emotional features of mood disorders. *Curr Opin Neurobiol*, 11(2):240–249.

25. Stein, M.B., Simmons, A.N., Feinstein, J.S., and Paulus, M.P. (2007). Increased amygdala and insula activation during emotion processing in anxiety-prone subjects. *Am J Psychiat*, 164(2):318–327.

26. Meaney, M.J. (2001). Maternal care, gene expression, and the transmission of individual differences in stress reactivity across generations. *Annu Rev Neurosci*, 24:1161–1192.

27. de Kloet, E.R., Sibug, R.M., Helmerhorst, R.M., and Schmidt, M. (2005). Stress, genes and the mechanism of programming the brain for later life. *Neurosci Biobehav Rev*, 29(2):271–281.

28. Levine, S. (2000). Influence of psychological variables on the activity of the hypothalamic-pituitary–adrenal axis. *Eur J Pharmacol*, 405(1–3):149–160.

29. Pryce, C.R. and Feldon, J. (2003). Long-term neurobehavioural impact of the postnatal environment in rats: Manipulations, effects and mediating mechanisms. *Neurosci Biobehav Rev*, 27(1–2):57–71.

30. Holmes, A., le Guisquet, A.M., Vogel, E., Millstein, R.A., Leman, S., and Belzung, C. (2005). Early life genetic, epigenetic and environmental factors shaping emotionality in rodents. *Neurosci Biobehav Rev*, 29(8):1335–1346.

31. Izquierdo, A., Wellman, C.L., and Holmes, A. (2006). Brief uncontrollable stress causes dendritic retraction in infralimbic cortex and resistance to fear extinction in mice. *J Neurosci*, 26(21):5733–5738.

32. Vyas, A., Mitra, R., Shankaranarayana Rao, B.S., and Chattarji, S. (2002). Chronic stress induces contrasting patterns of dendritic remodeling in hippocampal and amygdaloid neurons. *J Neurosci*, 22(15):6810–6818.

33. McEwen, B.S. (1999). Stress and hippocampal plasticity. *Annu Rev Neurosci*, 22:105–122.

34. Wellman, C.L., Izquierdo, A., Garret, J.E., Martin, K.P., Carroll, J., Millstein, R. et al. (2007). Impaired stress-coping and fear extinction and abnormal corticolimbic morphology in serotonin transporter knock-out mice. *J Neurosci*, 27:684–691.

35. Caspi, A., Sugden, K., Moffitt, T.E., Taylor, A., Craig, I.W., Harrington, H. et al. (2003). Influence of life stress on depression: Moderation by a polymorphism in the 5-HTT gene. *Science*, 301(5631):386–389.

36. Holmes, A. (2007). Strains, SNPs and selected lines: Genetic factors influencing variation in murine anxiety-like behavior. In Crusio, W.E., Sluyter, F., and Gerlai, R. (eds.), *Handbook of Behavioral Genetics of the Mouse*. Cambridge University Press, Cambridge.

37. Holmes, A. (2001). Targeted gene mutation approaches to the study of anxiety-like behavior in mice. *Neurosci Biobehav Rev*, 25(3):261–273.

38. El Yacoubi, M., Vaugeois, J.M. (2007). Genetic rodent models of depression, *Curr Opin Pharmacol*, 7(1): 3–7.

39. Finn, D.A., Rutledge-Gorman, M.T., and Crabbe, J.C. (2003). Genetic animal models of anxiety. *Neurogenetics*, 4(3):109–135.

40. Belzung, C. (2001). The genetic basis of the pharmacological effects of anxiolytics: A review based on rodent models. *Behav Pharmacol*, 12(6–7):451–460.

41. Broadhurst, P.L. (1975). The Maudsley reactive and nonreactive strains of rats: A survey. *Behav Genet*, 5(4):299–319.

42. Bignami, G. (1965). Selection for high rates and low rates of avoidance conditioning in the rat. *Anim Behav*, 13(2):221–227.

43. Kromer, S.A., Kessler, M.S., Milfay, D., Birg, I.N., Bunck, M., Czibere, L. et al. (2005). Identification of glyoxalase-I as a protein marker in a mouse model of extremes in trait anxiety. *J Neurosci*, 25(17):4375–4384.

44. Gross, C. and Hen, R. (2004). The developmental origins of anxiety. *Nat Rev Neurosci*, 5(7):545–552.

45. Hariri, A.R. and Holmes, A. (2006). Genetics of emotional regulation: the role of the serotonin transporter in neural function. *Trend Cogn Sci*, 10(4):182–191.

46. Yalcin, B., Willis-Owen, S.A., Fullerton, J., Meesaq, A., Deacon, R.M., Rawlins, J.N. et al. (2004). Genetic dissection of a behavioral quantitative trait locus shows that Rgs2 modulates anxiety in mice. *Nat Genet*, 36(11):1197–1202.

47. van Gaalen, M.M., Stenzel-Poore, M.P., Holsboer, F., and Steckler, T. (2002). Effects of transgenic overproduction of CRH on anxiety-like behaviour. *Eur J Neurosci*, 15(12):2007–2015.

48. Flint, J. (2003). Amimal models of anxiety. In Plomin, R., DeFries, J., Craig, I.W., and McGuffin, P. (eds.), *Behavioral genetics in the post-genome era*. American Psychological Association, Washington, DC.

49. Borsini, F., Podhorna, J., and Marazziti, D. (2002). Do animal models of anxiety predict anxiolytic-like effects of antidepressants? *Psychopharmacology (Berl)*, 163(2):121–141.

50. Dulawa, S.C. and Hen, R. (2005). Recent advances in animal models of chronic antidepressant effects: The novelty-induced hypophagia test. *Neurosci Biobehav Rev*, 29(4–5):771–783.

51. Rodgers, R.J. (1997). Animal models of 'anxiety': where next? *Behav Pharmacol*, 8(6–7): 477–496. discussion 497–504.

52. Chaki, S., Nakazato, A., Kennis, L., Nakamura, M., Mackie, C., Sugiura, M. et al. (2004). Anxiolytic- and antidepressant-like profile of a new CRF1 receptor antagonist, R278995/CRA0450. *Eur J Pharmacol*, 485(1–3):145–158.

53. Commissaris, R.L., Harrington, G.M., and Altman, H.J. (1990). Benzodiazepine anticonflict effects in Maudsley reactive (MR/Har) and non-reactive (MNRA/Har) rats. *Psychopharmacology (Berl)*, 100(3):287–292.

54. Njung'e, K. and Handley, S.L. (1991). Evaluation of marble-burying behavior as a model of anxiety. *Pharmacol Biochem Behav*, 38(1):63–67.

55. Broekkamp, C.L., Rijk, H.W., Joly-Gelouin, D., and Lloyd, K.L. (1986). Major tranquillizers can be distinguished from minor tranquillizers on the basis of effects on marble burying and swim-induced grooming in mice. *Eur J Pharmacol*, 126(3):223–229.

56. Grasby, P.M., Sharp, T., Allen, T., Kelly, P.A., and Grahame-Smith, D.G. (1992). Effects of the 5-HT1A partial agonists gepirone, ipsapirone and buspirone on local cerebral glucose utilization in the conscious rat. *Psychopharmacology (Berl)*, 106(1):97–101.

57. Patel, S., Ndubizu, O., Hamill, T., Chaudhary, A., Burns, H.D., Hargreaves, R. et al. (2005). Screening cascade and development of potential Positron Emission Tomography radiotracers for mGluR5: In vitro and in vivo characterization. *Mol Imaging Biol*, 7(4):314–323.

58. Deckersbach, T., Dougherty, D.D., and Rauch, S.L. (2006). Functional imaging of mood and anxiety disorders. *J Neuroimag*, 16(1):1–10.

59. Heimberg, R.G., Horner, K.J., Juster, H.R., Safren, S.A., Brown, E.J., Schneier, F.R. et al. (1999). Psychometric properties of the Liebowitz Social Anxiety Scale. *Psychol Med*, 29(1):199–212.

60. Antony, M.M. and Rowa, K. (2005). Evidence-based assessment of anxiety disorders in adults. *Psychol Assess*, 17(3):256–266.

61. Houck, P.R., Spiegel, D.A., Shear, M.K., and Rucci, P. (2002). Reliability of the self-report version of the panic disorder severity scale. *Dep Anxiety*, 15(4):183–185.

62. Barlow, D., Gorman, J.M., Shear, M.K., and Woods, S.W. (2000). Cognitive-behavioral therapy, imipramine, or their combination for panic disorder: A randomized controlled trial. *J Am Med Assoc*, 283(19):2529–2536.

63. Norman, S.B., Cissell, S.H., Means-Christensen, A.J., and Stein, M.B. (2006). Development and validation of an Overall Anxiety Severity and Impairment Scale (OASIS). *Depress Anxiety*, 23(4):245–249.

64. McNally, R.J. (2002). Anxiety sensitivity and panic disorder. *Biol Psychiat*, 52(10):938–946.

65. Roy-Byrne, P.P., Craske, M.G., Stein, M.B., Sullivan, G., Bystritsky, A., Katon, W. et al. (2005). A randomized effectiveness trial of cognitive-behavioral therapy and medication for primary care panic disorder. *Arch Gen Psychiat*, 62(3):290–298.

66. Meyer, T.J., Miller, M.L., Metzger, R.L., and Borkovec, T.D. (1990). Development and validation of the Penn State Worry Questionnaire. *Behav Res Ther*, 28(6):487–495.

67. Stein, M.B. and Bienvenu, O.J. (2004). Diagnostic classification of anxiety disorders: DSM-V and beyond. In Charney, D.S. and Nestler, E.J. (eds.), *The Neurobiology of Mental Illness*, 2nd edition. Oxford University Press, New York.

68. Paulus, M.P., Feinstein, J.S., Simmons, A., and Stein, M.B. (2004). Anterior cingulate activation in high trait anxious subjects is related to altered error processing during decision making. *Biol Psychiat*, 55(12):1179–1187.

69. Barlow, D.H. (2002). *Anxiety and its disorders: The nature and treatment of anxiety and panic*, 2nd edition. Guilford Press, New York.

70. Tecott, L.H. and Nestler, E.J. (2004). Neurobehavioral assessment in the information age. *Nat Neurosci*, 7(5):462–466.

71. Brunner, D., Nestler, E., and Leahy, E. (2002). In need of high-throughput behavioral systems. *Drug Discov Today*, 7(18(Suppl)):S107–S112.

72. Davis, M., Falls, W.A., Campeau, S., and Kim, M. (1993). Fear-potentiated startle: A neural and pharmacological analysis. *Behav Brain Res*, 58(1–2):175–198.

73. Grillon, C. and Baas, J. (2003). A review of the modulation of the startle reflex by affective states and its application in psychiatry. *Clin Neurophysiol*, 114(9):1557–1579.

74. Baas, J.M., Grillon, C., Bocker, K.B., Brack, A.A., Morgan III, C.A., Kenemans, J.L. et al. (2002). Benzodiazepines have no effect on fear-potentiated startle in humans. *Psychopharmacology (Berl)*, 161(3):233–247.

75. Paulus, M.P. and Stein, M.B. (2007). Role of functional magnetic resonance imaging in drug discovery. *Neuropsychol Rev*, 17:179–188.

76. Paulus, M.P. and Stein, M.B. (2006). An insular view of anxiety. *Biol Psychiat*, 60(4):383–387.

77. Hackler, E.A., Turner, G.H., Gresch, P.J., Sengupta, S., Deutch, A.Y., Avison, M.J. et al. (2007). 5-Hydroxytryptamine2C Receptor Contribution to m-Chlorophenylpiperazine and N-Methyl-beta-carboline-3-carboxamide-Induced Anxiety-Like Behavior and Limbic Brain Activation. *J Pharmacol Exp Ther*, 320(3):1023–1029.

CHAPTER 6

Animal Models of Obsessive–Compulsive Disorder: From Bench to Bedside via Endophenotypes and Biomarkers

Daphna Joel[1], Dan J. Stein[2] and Rudy Schreiber[3]

[1]Department of Psychology, Tel Aviv University, Ramat-Aviv, Tel Aviv, Israel
[2]Department of Psychiatry, University of Cape Town, Groote Schuur Hospital, Cape Town, South Africa
[3]Sepracor, Marlborough, MA, USA

Animal and Translational Models for CNS Drug Discovery,
Vol. 1 of 3: Psychiatric Disorders
Robert McArthur and Franco Borsini (eds), Academic Press, 2008

INTRODUCTION

This chapter focuses on animal models of obsessive–compulsive disorder (OCD). We begin by briefly summarizing the clinical phenomenology and psychobiology of OCD, focusing in particular on the question of whether understanding the heterogeneity of OCD or its underlying endophenotypes may be useful for future research on this disorder. We then review existing animal models of OCD, discussing recent work in this area in terms of the face, construct, and predictive validity of models. We also provide a current perspective from the pharmaceutical industry, focusing on selected targets and how the use of neurocognitive testing can perhaps facilitate the development of novel drugs for these targets. We conclude that a better understanding of OCD spectrums and subtypes, their mediating circuitry, and the relevant genes and proteins in these circuits, will help bring about new pharmacotherapies for this disorder.

Before moving to the review of clinical material on OCD, a brief comment on why we chose to focus on the concept of endophenotype may be useful.[1] On the one hand, there is increasing evidence that many psychiatric disorders, including OCD, have high heritability.[2] On the other hand, there is deserved skepticism about whether genes code for OCD, rather than for susceptibility to developing obsessions and compulsions. Endophenotypes (which may emerge from clinical studies of biochemistry, imaging, cognition, etc.) may provide more useful clues for translational work. We also continue to employ the term "biomarker" here (defined by the Food and Drug Administration, FDA, as: *"A characteristic that is objectively measured and evaluated as an indicator of normal biologic or pathogenic processes or pharmacological responses to a therapeutic intervention"*), as some phenotypes may be useful for thinking about translational research, but not yet have evidence of heritability.[i]

CLINICAL ASPECTS

Obsessions and Compulsions

OCD has a lifetime prevalence of approximately 2% in many parts of the world,[3] and is one of the most disabling of all medical disorders.[4] The defining symptoms of OCDs are obsessions and compulsions.[5] Obsessions are defined as recurrent intrusive thoughts or images, and they are frequently accompanied by an increase in anxiety. Compulsions are repetitive driven behaviors, or mental acts, typically in response to obsessions, or according to inflexible rules, and often leading to a temporary decrease in anxiety. Most people with OCD have good insight into their symptoms, realizing that their concerns are excessive and inappropriate. The clinical criterion in DSM-IV[5] specifies that the symptoms are accompanied by clinical distress, are time consuming, or lead to impairment.

---

[i] For further discussion of endophenotypes, please see Tannock *et al.*, Towards a Biological Understanding of ADHD and the Discovery of Novel Therapeutic Approaches, Bartz *et al.*, Preclinical Animal Models of Autistic Spectrum Disorders (ASD), Cryan *et al.*, Developing More Efficacious Antidepressant Medications: Improving and Aligning Preclinical Detection and Clinical Assessment Tools, or Large *et al.*, Developing Therapeutics for Bipolar Disorder: From Animal Models to the Clinic, in this Volume.

Contamination concerns (resulting in washing and cleaning) and concerns about potential harm (resulting in repeated checking) were commonly described in initial reports from OCD clinics. More recently, factor analyses have suggested that there are four main subtypes of OCD symptoms; contamination symptoms, harm-focused symptoms, hoarding/ordering, and concerns about sex, religion, aggression and other matters.[6,7] However, a range of other subtypes have also been discussed in the literature, including early-onset OCD, OCD with lack of insight, and OCD as a result of PANDAS (pediatric auto-immune neuropsychiatric disorders associated with streptococcus). As discussed below, there is increased interest in defining the psychobiology that differentiates such subtypes, and in developing more specific treatment approaches for each subtype.

The clinical literature has also devoted significant attention to the putative construct of obsessive–compulsive spectrum disorders.[8,9] The hypothesis is that there is phenomenological and psychobiological overlap across OCD and a number of potentially related disorders such as body dysmorphic disorder, hypochondriasis, Tourette's syndrome (TS), and trichotillomania.[ii] Certainly, there are a number of disorders other than OCD that have symptoms that are strongly reminiscent of obsessions and compulsions.[iii] Family studies show that there is a genetic relationship between patients with OCD and with Tourette's disorder. Also, a range of work, including brain imaging studies, has indicated cortico-striatal involvement in OCD as well as some related disorders, such as TS. To some extent, then, genetic variation or cortico-striatal abnormalities, which result in vulnerability to develop repetitive non-functional behaviors, may represent an important focus for understanding OCDs, and for developing new medications. Indeed, selective serotonin reuptake inhibitors (SSRIs) appear to be selectively effective in OCD as well as in a number of other conditions, while dopamine D_2 receptor blockers are useful as a primary treatment in TS and as an augmentation treatment in OCD.

In the next section we discuss the phenomenology and psychobiology of OCD subtypes and spectrums, keeping in mind the possibility that there are unique mechanisms that underpin these phenomena (with correlative animal models) as well as unique treatment targets (for novel medications).

Phenomenology and Psychobiology of Subtypes and Spectrums

Subtypes: Differentiating Treatment Targets

The literature on factor and cluster analysis has been useful in providing a way of understanding the symptom dimensions of OCD. There is also some evidence that different symptom dimensions have different neuronal[10,11] and genetic[7,12] underpinnings, and they may therefore respond to different interventions. In particular, there is

---

[ii] Please refer to Heidbreder, Impulse and Reward Deficit Disorders: Drug Discovery and Development, or Williams *et al.*, Current Concepts in the Classification, Treatment and Modeling of Pathological Gambling and Other Impulse Control Disorders, in Volume 3, Reward Deficit Disorders for further discussion of obsessive–compulsive spectrum disorders.

[iii] Though not specifically discussed by Joel and colleagues in this chapter, OCD shares many characteristics with Autistic Spectrum Disorders, including its treatment. For further discussion, please refer to Bartz *et al.*, Preclinical Animal Models of Autistic Spectrum Disorders, in this Volume.

evidence that hoarding and symmetry symptoms may involve more dopaminergic circuits, may have a familial component that accounts for the relevant genes involved in underpinning these symptoms, and may respond more poorly to serotonergic agents.

A second potentially useful way of subtyping OCD on a clinical basis is the differentiation between early-onset and later-onset OCD. Early-onset OCD is more common in males, is more commonly associated with tics, and is less treatment responsive to serotonergic agents. There has been relatively little work on differentiating the neuronal circuitry of early-onset OCD, but it has been demonstrated that patients with more neurological soft signs have more diffuse neuronal damage, and respond more poorly to treatment. There is also some data on the genetic basis of early-onset OCD.[13] Dopaminergic targets may be particularly relevant in this form of OCD.

The discovery that OCD symptoms and tics could develop suddenly, in the acute aftermath of a streptococcal infection, has also been useful in suggesting novel targets for intervention. This work has focused on auto-immune mechanisms in OCD, and has suggested both unique neuronal correlates (e.g., increased volume in cortico-striatal circuits),[14] as well as family history correlates. Fascinating work has suggested that immune interventions can reverse symptoms in this subtype of OCD.[15] The role of antibiotic prophylaxis in preventing OCD exacerbation in such patients deserves further study.[16]

Work on various other OCD subtypes, such as lack of insight, has not clearly demonstrated the existence of unique pathogenetic mechanisms, and consequent treatment targets. Indeed, although there are some useful clues for predicting treatment response in OCD (patients with tics or neurological soft signs may be less responsive to SSRIs), in general, a range of studies on clinical predictors of treatment response in OCD underscore that these are not highly precise,[17,18] and that additional work is therefore needed on the underlying psychobiology of OCD in order to inform prognosis, and to develop new drug targets.

Spectrums: Differentiating OCD, Stereotypy, and Perseveration

The current official psychiatric nosology[5] differentiates between OCD (which is classified as an anxiety disorder), various putative OCD spectrum disorders (body dysmorphic disorder and hypochondriasis are characterized as a somatoform disorder, trichotillomania is characterized as an impulse control disorder not otherwise classified, stereotypic movement disorder is classified as a disorder usually diagnosed in infancy, childhood, or adolescence), and perseverative symptoms (which are noted in the diagnosis of delirium, and defined in a glossary as "Tendency to emit the same verbal or motor response again and again to varied stimuli").

A stereotyped movement is described by DSM-IV[5] as a repetitive, seemingly driven non-functional motor behavior (e.g., head banging, body rocking, self-biting). A tic, on the other hand, is a sudden, rapid, recurrent, non-rhythmic stereotyped motor movement or vocalization (e.g., eye blinking, tongue protrusion, throat clearing). Compared with a compulsion, DSM-IV specifies that tics and stereotyped movements are typically less complex and are not aimed at neutralizing an obsession. It is notable, however, that some individuals have both OCD and tics, and a diagnosis of comorbid OCD and TS is suitable in such cases. Indeed, OCD spectrum disorders are quite common in OCD patients.[19]

Comorbidity of OCD and OC spectrums suggests that it would be useful if phenomenological overlaps and distinctions could be substantiated by psychobiological ones. In TS, for example, it can be extremely difficult to differentiate phenomenologically between complex tics (e.g., facial gestures, grooming behaviors, jumping, touching, stamping, and smelling an object) and compulsions. It is therefore reassuring, in some ways, to know that OCD and TS have a strong genetic relationship,[20] and that there may be close overlap in the brain imaging findings of particular probands in the same family, even if they receive disparate diagnoses.[21]

Is there a unifying psychobiology of OC spectrum disorders, which could potentially yield an underlying phenotype, and a target for new medications? It is notable that the basal ganglia are particularly susceptible to anoxic damage early in life. It is possible therefore that damage to these structures (e.g., observable with brain imaging) would constitute an endophenotype, or that genetic variations, which are accompanied by susceptibility to neuronal damage (e.g., variants in neurotrophic systems) would constitute a useful biomarker, for OCD research. Nevertheless, much further clinical research is needed in order to validate such a hypothesis. Animal models focusing on the relevant mechanisms (e.g., striatal neurons and their susceptibility to damage), may ultimately be useful for understanding OCD and developing new treatments.

While a unifying psychobiology of the OC spectrum disorders remains a future goal, there is probably sufficient data to already state that this psychobiology will differ from that which creates vulnerability to anxiety disorders in general. There is increasing evidence that the anxiety disorders (e.g., post-traumatic stress disorder, panic disorder, social anxiety disorder) are mediated by amygdala–hippocampal circuits and component receptors. Although there may be some overlap in psychobiology with OCD, it is notable that OC spectrum disorders involve disturbances in emotions other than anxiety (e.g., disgust),[22] circuitry other than amygdala–hippocampus (e.g., cortico-striatal-thalamo-cortical circuit, CSTC[8]), and unique genes (e.g., SLITRK1).[23] Animal models should be developed with such considerations in mind.[24]

Pharmacotherapy of OCD

Early anecdotal evidence that clomipramine (Anafranil®), a serotonergic tricyclic antidepressant, was effective in OCD ultimately led to multi-centre placebo-controlled trials of this medication in both adults and children, and to rigorous trials comparing clomipramine with the noradrenergic tricyclic desipramine (Norpramin®), and with psychotherapy.[25] The finding that clomipramine was more effective than desipramine in OCD emphasized the distinction between OCD and depression (which responded to all tricyclics), and led researchers to focus on the potential role of 5-HT in the mediation of OCD.[26]

There is certainly significant evidence of 5-HT mediation in OCD. Several methods have been employed, including study of 5-HT and 5-HIAA levels in cerebrospinal fluid; pharmacological challenges with 5-HT agents such as fenfluramine, m-chlorophenylpiperazine (mCPP), and sumatriptan (Mitrex®/Imigran®); molecular imaging studies with serotonergic ligands, and candidate gene studies.[26,27] Although there is no clear evidence that 5-HT plays a causal role in OCD in the majority of patients, genetics research has demonstrated that rare functional variants of the serotonin transporter gene do appear to be causally associated with OCD in a minority of subjects.[28]

Given the efficacy of clomipramine in OCD, once the SSRIs were introduced for the treatment of depression, they were soon studied in OCD. Multi-centre placebo-controlled trials of each of the SSRIs have demonstrated good efficacy and tolerability. A number of these agents have also been studied in children, in the longer term, and in comparison with other drugs (often clomipramine). On the basis of this evidence, current consensus guidelines invariably recommend SSRIs as the first-line pharmaco-therapy of choice for the treatment of OCD.[29,30]

Many OCD patients do not, however, respond to treatment with available pharmacotherapies or psychotherapies.[31] Interest has grown in conducting randomized-controlled trials in treatment-refractory OCD, often focusing on augmentation treatment strategies. On the basis of animal and clinical data suggesting that dopamine plays a role in OCD,[32] one of the first of augmentation studies focused on the D_2 receptor antagonist, haloperidol (Haldol®), in the augmentation of SSRIs in treatment-refractory OCD,[33] and with the introduction of the new generation of antipsychotic agents, these too have received attention in OCD.[34]

This work has also given impetus to understanding the role of the dopamine system in OCD and OC spectrum disorders.[35] Molecular imaging studies of dopamine transporter (DAT) and dopamine D_2 receptors demonstrate abnormalities in striatal density,[36,37] and several genetic studies of OCD have suggested a role for variants in dopaminergic candidate genes. The dopamine system may be particularly relevant to certain OCD subtypes, such as hoarding. The dopamine system also appears to play an important role in a number of OCD-related disorders, including TS and trichotillomania.

Strengths and Limitations of Past Clinical Research

Although the SSRI trials represented an important step forwards, there remain important limitations. These include: (a) relatively few long-term trials, (b) relatively few trials in real-life settings, (c) relatively limited understanding of the mediators and moderators of response to treatment (although secondary analysis of OCD datasets has provided some data on the demographic, clinical, and psychobiological predictors of response[17,19]).

The 2nd generation (atypical) antipsychotic trials have also been valuable. Nevertheless, there have been very few of these, sample sizes were small, and treatment durations short.[34] Thus the efficacy and tolerability of these agents in OCD, and in OCD subtypes and spectrums, remains to be fully understood. While it appears that these antipsychotics are better tolerated than the first generation of agents, much remains to be learned about their optimal use.

Novel Pharmacological Targets for OCD

In the wake of the successful approval of SSRIs for the treatment of OCD, developing new treatment targets represents a scientific challenge. In addition, there is a perception that OCD is a rare disorder, with a market that is too small to allow for a return on commercial investment. Although the current chapter is focused on the need for, and possibility of, developing new drug targets in OCD, it is not unlikely that in the foreseeable future, we can expect that drugs will be developed primarily for mood and other anxiety disorders, and only then considered for OCD trials. This is by no means unique for OCD, as there is a range of examples from CNS drug discovery efforts in the last 10–15 years that have focused on extending the applicability of drugs registered for another reason.[38] One of the questions we are trying to address in this review is whether translational approaches, including the use of animal models to screen drugs with anti-compulsive activity and the use of endophenotypes or biomarkers in early clinical testing, might help lower the risk by allowing quality go/no-go decisions as early as possible during pre-clinical and clinical development. Below we will first briefly summarize some early and potentially interesting approaches for novel drug treatments; next we provide an overview of translational approaches, and finally we conclude with suggestions how these approaches could be successfully employed to facilitate the development of novel anti-OCD treatments.

Serotonergic approaches: 5-HT$_{1B}$, 5-HT$_{2A}$, and 5-HT$_{2C}$ ligands

Many drug discovery efforts have exploited the success of the SSRIs by focusing on serotonergic receptor subtype selective ligands. A very influential set of studies have been carried out by Blier and colleagues in rodents. This group has attempted to delineate changes in 5-HT release and in pre- and postsynaptic 5-HT receptors that follow chronic administration of SSRIs (for review, see[39]). In this respect, this approach may be described as an animal model of drug action. This approach has been largely based on the congruent time courses between the development of increased 5-HT release and receptor adaptations in rodents and (delayed) onset of therapeutic response for SSRIs in OCD patients.[39] Thus, in rodents, the terminal 5-HT$_{1B}$ receptor desensitizes upon chronic treatment with SSRIs and a drug that would prevent the negative feedback of 5-HT$_{1B}$ receptor activation on the release of 5-HT could have a potential anti-OCD effect in humans. This could be achieved by acute blockade of the terminal receptor by a 5-HT$_{1B}$ antagonist or accelerated downregulation of this receptor by a 5-HT$_{1B}$ agonist. Although an antagonist might have a potential quicker onset of action, simultaneous blockade of pre- and postsynaptic receptors would be expected to decrease the effect of an antagonist on net serotonergic transmission[39] (and references therein). Therefore, the challenge will be to find antagonists that are selective for presynaptic receptors.

The rationale for 5-HT$_{2A}$ agonists is based on the anti-OCD effects of hallucinogens with 5-HT$_{2A}$ agonist properties such as lysergic diethylamide (LSD) and psilocybin in humans.[40] Since their hallucinogenic effects are believed to be mediated by the 5-HT$_{2A}$ receptor, this target seems undesirable for the development of novel anti-OCD treatments. In principle, however, 5-HT$_{2A}$ receptors located in the brain areas involved in the anti-OCD effects could be pharmacologically distinct from those mediating hallucinogenic effects.

Further, some recent and interesting developments in the molecular pharmacology of G-protein-couples receptors (GPCRs) may offer innovative concepts to target the desired subpopulations of 5-HT$_{1B}$ or 5-HT$_{2A}$ receptors selectively with novel drugs. Allosteric modulators interact with binding sites that are distinct from the orthosteric site recognized by the receptor's endogenous agonist. Because of their ability to modulate receptor confirmations in the presence of orthosteric ligand, allosteric modulators can fine-tune pharmacological responses.[41] For example, it could be hypothesized that a positive allosteric modulator for 5-HT$_{2A}$ receptors may preferentially act on binding sites in brain areas involved in OCD pathology – areas presumably under a lower serotonergic tone – and have less (if any) activity in these cortical areas involved in hallucinations – areas presumably under a regular serotonergic tone.

Another emerging concept is that of "pathway-biased" drugs. β-Arrestins are cytosolic proteins that bind to activated GPCRs and uncouple them from G-protein-mediated second messenger signaling pathways and/or lead to new signals.[42] There is an example from the opioid field that illustrates that "pathway-based" drugs can be successfully generated. Compounds that recruit β-arrestin, such as the μ-opioid agonist DAMGO, lead to receptor internalization and tolerance. A novel μ-selective agonist, herkinorin, was found to *not* promote the recruitment of β-Arrestin-2 to the μ-opioid receptor, and as a consequence this compound did *not* lead to receptor internalization.

Although speculative, a similar approach might yield pathway-biased 5-HT$_{2A}$ agonists that target the pathways involved in OCD, but not those involved in hallucinations. As illustrated by the concepts of allosteric modulation and pathway-biased drugs, future progress in drug discovery may not only come from the development of new target ideas but also from novel approaches for finding drugs for known targets.

Activation of 5-HT$_{2C}$ receptors (typically by administration of mCPP) can exacerbate OC symptoms in OCD patients,[43–50] although several studies have failed to obtain this effect.[51–54] In addition, several studies reported that the secretion of stress-related hormones and neuropeptides in response to mCPP administration was greater in patients with anxiety disorders compared to healthy controls, suggesting that 5-HT$_{2C}$ receptors may be hypersensitive in subjects with anxiety disorders.[55] The finding that chronic treatment with SSRIs attenuates mCPP-induced symptoms exacerbation in OCD patients,[45,50] suggests that normalization or desensitization of 5-HT$_{2C}$ receptors may play a role in mediating the therapeutic actions of SSRIs.[55–57] It therefore follows that blockade of these receptors may have a beneficial effect in OCD patients. Indeed, 5-HT$_{2C}$ antagonists have been shown to exert an anti-compulsive effect in the signal attenuation rat model of OCD, following both systemic and intra-orbital administration,[58] but an opposite effect has been obtained in the schedule-induced polydipsia model.[59]

Approaches involving a dopaminergic component: dual SERT/DAT inhibitors and dopamine stabilizers

Adding antipsychotic drugs to SSRIs for the treatment of OCD improves the rate of responders and the most parsimonious explanation is that this involves a dopaminergic mechanism. Although various pre-clinical and clinical lines of evidence suggest a role for dopamine in OCD (reviewed in[35]), the pathophysiological mechanism is not altogether clear and it remains therefore somewhat speculative what the preferred dopaminergic treatment approach would be.

Microdialysis studies suggest synergistic effects of atypical antipsychotics in combination with SSRIs on norepinephrine and dopamine release in the prefrontal cortex (PFC).[35,36,60] It can be speculated that a similar mechanism may underlie the effects of augmentation therapy with antipsychotic drugs in combination with SSRIs in OCD patients. A more direct approach for such an augmentation therapy would be to target directly the molecular mechanism involved in the augmentation effects of atypical antipsychotic drugs. Interestingly, an increase in dopaminergic activity may provide a mechanistic basis for 5-HT$_{2C}$ receptors as a potential target for OCD. These receptors exert an inhibitory control on noradrenaline and dopamine terminals in the PFC[61] and atypical antipsychotics such as clozapine possess antagonist activity at these receptors.[62]

The role of dopamine in OCD is complex as preliminary findings with the dual noradrenaline and dopamine reuptake inhibitor bupropion (Wellbutrin®) in a small, open label study suggest a bimodal distribution with some patients *improving* and others getting *worse* upon treatment.[63] Assuming the bimodal distribution would hold up in a larger, controlled study, the data support a dopamine "stabilizer" approach originally proposed for the treatment of Parkinson's disease and schizophrenia.[64] Indeed, preliminary findings suggest that monotherapy with the non-selective dopamine partial agonist, aripiprazole (Abilify®), improves OCD.[65] Other approaches that may facilitate getting more successful outcomes consist of testing dopaminergic ligands in patient populations that might be expected to be more responsive to dopaminergic treatments, such as treatment-resistant patients, early-onset OCD, and patients with hoarding or symmetry symptoms (see Section Differentiating treatment targets).

Excitatory amino acids: mGluR2 agonists, glutamate release inhibitors and glycine agonists

Evidence from human and animal studies suggests that increased glutamatergic activity is associated with OCD (for a review, see[66]). However, most clinical data have served more to generate hypotheses rather than showing proof of mechanism. Decreasing glutamatergic activity may in principle consist of another approach to pharmacologically treat OCD. An attractive approach to this end is agonism at metabotropic glutamate type 2 receptor (mGluR2) since this is an auto-receptor that controls the release of glutamate.[67] The mGluR2 agonist LY354740 has been tested in generalized anxiety disorder but no data have been published from studies in OCD patients. Riluzole (Rilutek®) is thought to act at least partly by decreasing glutamate release and an open label study supports efficacy in patients with treatment-resistant OCD.[68] Another drug with a glutamatergic mechanism, memantine (Namenda®) is under active study for OCD (www.clinicaltrials.gov).

D-cycloserine acts at the strychnine-insensitive glycine recognition site of the N-methyl-D-aspartate (NMDA) receptor complex to *enhance* NMDA receptor function and it has been extensively studied for cognitive enhancing effects in animal models, healthy humans and in patient populations. In a recent double blind, placebo-controlled trial in OCD patients, D-cycloserine augmentation of psychotherapy increased the efficiency, palatability and overall effectiveness of standard exposure therapy[69] (but see also[70]).

These new data open the possibility for a whole new class of targets that increase activity at the glycine recognition site, such as glycine transporter inhibitors and inhibitors of the di-amino acid oxidase, the enzyme that metabolizes d-serine, as augmentors of psychotherapy.

Other Directions in the Development of New Therapies for OCD

There has been interest in a broad range of innovative treatments of OCD. In the area of pharmacotherapy, in addition to the attempts to find new targets for anti-compulsive pharmacotherapy described above, novel methods of drug delivery or higher dosing have been researched.[71] Psychotherapy researchers have attempted to optimize intervention by using cognitive techniques,[72] self-help approaches,[73] or partial hospitalization.[74] Highly specialized OCD treatment centers have long considered neurosurgical intervention as a treatment of last resort,[75] and are now considering interventions such as deep brain stimulation,[76] and repetitive transcranial magnetic stimulation (rTMS).[77] However, much additional work is still needed.

Ultimately, a better understanding of the psychobiology of OCD is needed in order to develop appropriately targeted treatments. As noted above, various studies, including brain imaging, have made an important advance by clearly identifying the importance of CSTC circuits in OCD.[78] It is notable that both pharmacotherapy and psychotherapy normalize functional cortical-striatal neurocircuitry in OCD, but that each modality has a different set of predictors.[79] Nevertheless, much more work remains to be done to fully delineate the nature of the circuitry, and the relevant genes/proteins. Although imaging studies have provided evidence that CSTC circuitry mediates OCD, and that serotonin, dopamine and glutamatergic systems play a role, it is unclear what the nature of the primary lesion is (there is some evidence that increased orbitofrontal function is merely compensatory). Serotonin, dopamine and glutamate are only three of the multiple genes/protein systems involved in CSTC function, and multiple potential additional treatment targets exist.

Where to Next in Clinical Research?

As noted in the previous section, additional work is needed with currently available agents. Despite the high morbidity and costs associated with OCD, relatively little National Institutes of Health (NIH) funds have gone to treatment trials on this disorder. Work on putative OCD spectrum disorders, such as body dysmorphic disorder and trichotillomania is also underfunded relative to their prevalence and disability.[iv]

Another path forward is to extend current attempts to delineate subtypes of OCD, including attempts to understand moderators and mediators of response to treatment. Recent work, for example, on the brain imaging of patients with hoarding[10] suggests that they may have a unique neurobiology. Given that patients with hoarding may not respond as well to SSRIs, targeted treatment trials are needed for this population.[80] And most importantly, new pharmacotherapies are needed. More than 90% of CNS drugs fail in the development phases and most because of a lack of efficacy. Thus, a critical intermediate step between the identification of potentially interesting molecular targets and the investment in expensive, long clinical studies in patients is the assessment of the novel drugs in predictive animal models and/or attempt to provide proof of mechanism or proof of concept in (small) human studies. This explains the high level of interest in translational studies, to which we turn next. We begin by describing animal models of OCD. Next, we turn to attempts to delineate specific endophenotypes or biomarkers of OCD, and when possible, describe animal models of such endophenotypes or biomarkers.

[iv] Please refer to Winsky *et al*. Drug Discovery and Development Initiatives at the National Institute of Mental Health: From Cell-Based System to Proof of Concept, in this Volume for further discussion and description of NIH initiatives for psychiatric disorders.

ANIMAL MODELS OF OCD

During the last 30 years there have been many attempts to develop animal models of OCD, in the hope that they may provide a route for furthering our understanding and treatment of this disorder. Before discussing specific animal models, we shortly discuss the criteria for the validation and evaluation of animal models, with special emphasis on predictive validity.

Face, Predictive and Construct Validity of Animal Models

Although there has been an expansion in the development and use of animal models in psychiatry, and several papers aiming at providing a conceptual framework for guiding the development of this field have been published,[81-88] there is still a lack of clarity regarding the terminology and classification of animal models and their validation criteria (see[89] for a review of the various terminologies and classifications). In the following discussion we will treat phenomenological similarity between the behavior in the animal model and the specific symptoms of the human condition as contributing to face validity; similarity in response to treatment as contributing to the predictive validity; and similarity in the inducing mechanism (physiological or psychological) and in the neural systems involved as contributing to the construct validity of a model. It should be noted that a critical component in the demonstration of a common physiological basis is the demonstration of a similar response to pharmacological treatments, because the latter suggests similarity in the neurotransmitter systems involved. This makes pharmacological isomorphism an important factor in assessing the validity of an animal model, and indeed, the validation process of most animal models of psychopathology involves testing the effects of relevant pharmacological treatments.[v]

Several points should be raised with respect to the assessment of predictive validity in animal models of OCD through the process of pharmacological isomorphism. First, although SSRIs are, to date, the only effective pharmacological treatment of OCD, they are effective in several other psychiatric disorders, including depression, generalized anxiety disorder, panic disorder and social phobia (for recent reviews see[90,91]). Animal models of OCD should therefore demonstrate both sensitivity to SSRIs and insensitivity to other classes of drugs, which are not effective in OCD but are effective in these other conditions (e.g., non-serotonergic antidepressants such as desipramine, anxiolytic agents such as diazepam, Valium®).

Second, SSRIs are not effective in all OCD patients (see also Insel *et al.*'s[92] emphasis of this point). Therefore, a lack of effect of SSRIs in a model may suggest that it is a model of compulsive behavior in the subgroup of OCD patients that do not respond to SSRI treatment, rather than demonstrate that it is not a model of OCD. Importantly, such a model should still demonstrate insensitivity to other types of pharmacological

---

[v] Please refer to Steckler *et al.*, Developing Novel Anxiolytics: Improving Preclinical Detection and Clinical Assessment, Large *et al.*, Developing Therapeutics for Bipolar Disorder: From Animal Models to the Clinic, in this Volume, or to Lindner *et al.*, Development, Optimization and Use of Preclinical Behavioral Models to Maximize the Productivity of Drug Discovery for Alzheimer's Disease, in Volume 2, Neurological Disorders for further discussion of the strengths and limitations of pharmacological isomorphism in establishing model validity.

treatment, because there is currently no other effective monotherapy for this sub-group of OCD patients.

Third, SSRIs are effective in patients only after several weeks of repeated administration. There is currently disagreement on the importance of demonstrating similarity in treatment regime (acute versus chronic) in the animal model and the disease being modeled. Bourin *et al.*[93] stated that a demonstration of a "therapeutic" effect in a model after acute treatment undermines the model's predictive validity. Matthysse[83] included a demonstration that the pharmacological effect grows stronger with time among the requirements for establishing pharmacological isomorphism. Willner[88] argued that the demonstration of drug effects in a model after a period of chronic administration is important for establishing its face validity, but is not relevant to the model's predictive validity and therefore to its ability to serve as a screening test for treatments for the modeled disease. Similarly, Geyer and Markou[82] concluded that a demonstration of therapeutic effects following acute administration does not undermine the screening abilities of a specific paradigm although it may detract from the validity of the model. Furthermore, Matthysse[83] and Geyer and Markou[82] pointed out to some difficulties with the notion of delayed drug effects in psychiatric disorders, such as the fact that in most animal studies acute effects are obtained with much higher doses than would be tolerated by humans, and the possibility that drugs may also have acute effects in humans, but that this effect may be hard to detect statistically (for a recent criticism of the notion of delayed-onset action, see[94]). These difficulties may also be relevant to OCD, especially because in order to prevent side effects, SSRI treatment is typically started with low doses that are gradually increased, and the difference between the initial dose and the therapeutic dose may be very large (e.g., 50 mg/day versus 200–300 mg/day, respectively, for fluvoxamine, Luvox®[95]).

Animal Models of OCD

Animal models of OCD can be divided into three classes, behavioral, pharmacological, and genetic, according to the method used to induce compulsive behavior in the model. Most of these models have been reviewed extensively.[89,92,96,97] In the present chapter we have chosen to focus only on animal models that seem most relevant to the development of new approaches for the treatment of OCD. We therefore discuss only laboratory models (and not veterinarian models – that is models of OCD drawn from animals presenting for treatment in veterinary or animal behavior settings) whose predictive validity has been assessed and that have some construct validity. When there are several models from the same class which fulfill these criteria, we have chosen one example from a class, according to whether it is currently being used.

Behavioral Models

Most animal models of OCD fall under this category. This category can be further divided into naturally occurring repetitive or stereotypic behaviors, such as tail chasing, fur chewing and weaving (for review see[92,97,98]; innate motor behaviors that occur during periods of conflict, frustration, or stress (displacement behaviors), such as grooming, cleaning, and pecking (for review see[92,97,99,100]), or following some behavioral manipulation (adjunctive behaviors), such as schedule-induced polydipsia[101] and food restriction-induced hyperactivity;[102] and learned behaviors that become compulsive-like following a behavioral manipulation, such as signal attenuation-induced compulsive lever-pressing (for review see[103]).

Naturally occurring repetitive or stereotypic behaviors   Although there are differences between stereotypic and compulsive behavior, stereotypies, tics and compulsions may all represent different forms of a similar deficit (e.g., in inhibitory control).[104]

Spontaneous stereotypy in deer mice   Deer mice (*P. maniculatus bairdii*) have been shown to develop stereotypic behaviors consisting of vertical jumping, backward somersaulting, and patterned running. These stereotypies are expressed spontaneously, appear early in development and persist throughout the lifetime of the animals.[105] These features are shared with some human pathologies that involve stereotypic behaviors (e.g., stereotypic movement disorder) as well as with OCD. By comparing high- and low-stereotypy mice, Presti and Lewis[106] have been able to show that high stereotypy is paralleled by a decrease in enkephalin content and an increase in the dynorphin/enkephalin ratio in the striatum, suggesting that high stereotypy may be mediated by decreased functioning of the indirect basal ganglia–thalamo–cortical pathway and an increased functioning of the direct basal ganglia–thalamo–cortical pathway. In line with this hypothesis, blockade of striatal D_1 and NMDA receptors has been shown to reduce spontaneously occurring stereotypies in these mice, without affecting motor activity in general.[107] As CSTC circuits have been implicated in the pathophysiology of OCD (see above), the findings suggesting that imbalance in the direct and indirect pathways of these circuits may mediate spontaneous stereotypy in deer mice lend the model construct validity. Moreover, imbalance between the direct and indirect pathways has been suggested to underlie the emergence of compulsions in OCD patients, and D_1 antagonists have therefore been suggested to ameliorate compulsions.[108] Korff and colleagues[109] have found that clomipramine is more robust than desipramine in decrease stereotypies in deer mice.

In summary, spontaneous stereotypy in deer mice may be an example of an animal model of an endophenotype (e.g., vulnerability to developing repetitive behavior) or, alternatively, as a model of a behavior that is analogous to a human compulsion, and may advance our understanding of neural circuits relevant to OCD. In addition, this model has an important advantage, in that it develops spontaneously, and thus may provide insight into a range of genetic and environmental etiologic factors in OCD. Attempts to establish the model's predictive validity have now been initiated.[vi]

Innate motor behaviors that occur following some behavioral manipulation   Three animal models can be found in this class, namely, schedule-induced polydipsia,[101] food restriction-induced hyperactivity,[102] and marble burying.[110-112] Although the first two models have good predictive validity, in that SSRIs have been shown to reduce "compulsive" behavior in the model, whereas drugs known not to be effective in OCD have not (fluoxetine versus imipramine;[102] fluvoxamine, fluoxetine and clomipramine versus desipramine, haloperidol and diazepam[101]), they have not been used since the original publications. Below

---

[vi] For further discussion of the deer mouse as a model of repetitive behaviors, please refer to Bartz *et al.*, Preclinical Animal Models of Autistic Spectrum Disorders (ASD), in this Volume.

we review the marble burying model, which seems to be an active model, and which highlights the role of anxiety in OCD and in animal models of this disorder.

Marble burying in mice   Rodents use bedding material to bury noxious as well as harmless objects. Inhibition of object burying was originally suggested as a screening test for anxiolytic activity, because the duration and extent of burying of both noxious and harmless objects were reduced by a variety of anxiolytic drugs, at doses that did not reduce behavioral output in general.[113-115] Although later studies have provided further support for the sensitivity of marble burying to anxiolytic drugs, the finding that burying was reduced by SSRIs raised the possibility that this behavior may be related to OCD.[113,116] Indeed, careful analysis of marble burying behavior has later led to the conclusion that it does not model anxiety, but may rather be related to compulsive behaviors.[110-112] Thus, mice do not avoid the marbles when given the opportunity to do so nor will repeated exposure to the marbles lead to habituation of the burying response, suggesting that the marbles have no aversive or fear-provoking properties and that this behavior is not related to novelty or fear.[111,112] Londei *et al.*[111] suggested that marble burying may begin as an appropriate, investigative, activity. However, because the marbles are non-reactive, they cannot provide the animal with the necessary stop signal, thus leading to compulsive burying. This suggestion is in line with the view that compulsive behaviors result from an inability to achieve a sense of task completion (for a recent review see Szechtman and Woody[117]). It is possible that certain behaviors, such as animal hoarding are evolutionary conserved and underpinned by a specific mechanism, and so have more ecological validity.

There are several reports that marble burying is decreased by SSRIs at doses that do not affect locomotor activity,[112,118,119] and this suppressive effect is not shared by desipramine.[120] However, marble burying is also reduced by drugs such as diazepam that do not have anti-compulsive ability.[112,113,116,120] These findings would tend to question the predictive validity of the marble burying model. The report of Ichimaru *et al.*[120] that the effects of diazepam completely disappear with repeated administration, whereas this is not the case with the SSRI fluvoxamine, raises the promising possibility that marble burying may show selective response to SSRIs if repeated rather than acute administration is used. This possibility, however, requires further investigation.

Although the finding that acute administration of anxiolytics reduces marble burying detracts from the model's predictive validity, it may be useful in studying the role of anxiety in OCD. Indeed, as noted earlier, there is ongoing debate about whether OCD is an anxiety disorder or not. There seem to be differences in comorbidity patterns (e.g., OCD is the only anxiety disorder with increased tic disorders) and their underlying neurobiology (e.g., OCD is mediated by CSTC circuits, while amygdala–hippocampal circuitry may be more important in anxiety). Nevertheless, OCD patients certainly suffer from anxiety disorders, and although anxiolytics are not a treatment of choice in OCD, they are sometimes used in the clinical setting to decrease anxiety symptoms.

Learned behaviors that become compulsive-like following a behavioral manipulation
Under this title there is currently only one animal model, namely, the signal attenuation model.

The signal attenuation model   The signal attenuation model[121-126] (for a recent review see[103]) has been developed on the basis of the theoretical proposition that compulsive behaviors result from a failure to cease responding following the successful completion of an action due to a deficient response feedback mechanism[100,117,127,128] (for review see[129]). The model simulates the deficiency in response feedback hypothesized to underlie obsessions and compulsions. The deficiency is induced using the paradigm of post-training signal attenuation, and leads to a pattern of lever-press responding that may be analogous to compulsive behavior. The procedure includes four stages. In Stage 1, a compound stimulus is established as a signal for the delivery of food by classically conditioning it with food. In Stage 2, rats are trained to lever-press for food whose delivery is accompanied by the compound stimulus. Thus, the stimulus is established as a feedback signaling that the lever-press response was effective in producing food. In Stage 3, signal attenuation, the capacity of the signal to serve as a feedback for the effectiveness of the lever-press response is attenuated by extinguishing the classical contingency between the stimulus and food. In the last, test, stage, the effects of *Signal Attenuation* on lever-press responding are assessed under extinction conditions (i.e., pressing the lever results in the presentation of the stimulus but no food is delivered).

Two types of excessive lever-presses appear on this Test stage – excessive lever-presses that are followed by magazine entry, and excessive lever-presses that are *not* followed by magazine entry. Joel and colleagues have suggested that the former type of excessive lever-presses reflects rats' response to the encounter of non-reward in the Test stage, whereas the latter type reflects rats' response to the encounter of an attenuated signal, and is therefore the measure of "compulsive" behavior in this model (for a recent review and discussion see[103]). Excessive lever-presses that are *not* followed by magazine entry bear some face similarity to compulsive behaviors in OCD, because the cessation of the attempts to collect a reward, which indicates that the rat detected the change in response consequences, combined with the increased emission of the lever-press response, makes the operant behavior both excessive and "inappropriate" or "unreasonable", thus fulfilling two important criteria of compulsive behavior.[5]

The signal attenuation model has good predictive validity, as acute administration of SSRIs (paroxetine and fluvoxamine), but not of drugs known not to be effective in OCD (desipramine, diazepam and haloperidol), has been shown to exert an "anti-compulsive" effect in the model.[123,124] Acute administration of two drugs, not currently in use as pharmacotherapies, has been shown to exert an anti-compulsive effect in the model – the D_1 receptor antagonist SCH 23390,[124] and the 5-HT_{2C} receptor antagonist RS 102221.[58] The suggestion that blockade of D_1 receptors may provide a new approach to the treatment of OCD is in line with Saxena *et al.*'s hypothesis[108] made on the basis of a theoretical model of OCD (see above). The suggestion that 5-HT_{2C} receptor antagonists may alleviate symptoms in patients is consistent with the finding that in OCD patients activation of 5-HT_{2C} receptors exacerbates symptoms[43-50] (although others have failed to obtained this effect[51-54]), and with the hypotheses, derived from challenge studies in OCD patients, that 5-HT_{2C} receptors are hypersensitive in OCD patients[55,130] and that SSRI-induced desensitization of these receptors may contribute to the therapeutic effects of SSRIs.[55-57]

In addition to involvement of the serotonergic and dopaminergic systems in compulsive lever-pressing (for the latter, see also[122]), there is evidence for involvement of the orbitofrontal cortex in this behavior,[125,126] in line with data implicating this cortical region in the pathophysiology of OCD (for review see[131]). These findings lend the signal attenuation model construct validity.

In summary, signal attenuation may provide an animal model of OCD with: construct validity, which derives from similarities in the compulsivity-inducing mechanism (i.e., attenuation of an external feedback and a deficient response feedback mechanism, respectively) and in the neural systems involved (the orbital cortex and the serotonergic and dopaminergic systems); face validity, that is, "compulsive" lever-pressing is both excessive and unreasonable, as are compulsions; and predictive validity, that is, selectivity for anti-obsessional/anti-compulsive drugs. The main disadvantage of the signal attenuation model is that it is not well suited for chronic drug administration studies, because repeated drug administration may affect behavior in the early stages of the procedure (e.g., lever-press training, signal attenuation).

Pharmacological Models

Pharmacological models of OCD are based on drug-induced behavioral alterations that bear similarity to some specific characteristics of the behavior of humans diagnosed with OCD, such as perseveration and indecision,[132] or compulsive checking.[133-135] In addition to behavioral similarity, in both models the relevant behavior is induced by manipulations of a neurotransmitter system whose dysfunction has been implicated in OCD. Thus, in Yadin *et al.*'s[132] model, perseveration is induced by manipulations of the serotonergic system, and in Szechtman and colleagues' model,[133-135] compulsive checking is induced by manipulations of the dopaminergic system. Finally, in both models the effects of an SSRI (fluoxetine and clomipramine in Yadin *et al.*'s model,[132,136] and clomipramine in Szechtman and colleagues' model[134]) have been tested. In the present chapter we have chosen to discuss in more detail the quinpirole model because of its strong face validity and evidence supporting its construct validity.

Quinpirole-induced compulsive checking   In this model, developed by Szechtman and colleagues,[134] rats are treated chronically with the D_2/D_3 receptor agonist quinpirole (0.5 mg/kg twice weekly for 5 weeks), and as a result "compulsive" checking emerges in specific locations (typically 1–2) in a large open field. Compulsive checking is characterized by excessive visits to these locations (up to 20-fold more compared to saline-treated rats), much shorter return times to these places and less stops at other locations between returns, compared to control rats. In addition, quinpirole-treated rats perform a characteristic "ritual-like" set of motor acts at these places.[134,135,137] On the basis of published descriptions of compulsive behavior in OCD patients as well as their own observations,[138,139] Szechtman and colleagues[134,135] argued that the behavior of quinpirole-treated rats is similar in several respects to compulsive checking in OCD patients, including a preoccupation with and an exaggerated hesitancy to leave the item(s) of interest; a ritual-like motor activity pattern; dependence of checking behavior on environmental context; and the ability to suspend the compulsive behavior for a period of time. Thus, the quinpirole model has strong face validity established convincingly using formal ethological criteria.

Two lines of evidence seem to support the construct validity of the quinpirole model. First, compulsive checking is induced by a dopaminergic manipulation. Given the evidence for dopamine involvement in OCD and in some OC spectrum disorders (see above) quinpirole-induced compulsive checking may be particularly relevant for modeling the subgroup of patients with a more pronounced DA involvement. Second, high frequency stimulation of the subthalamic nucleus[140] and of the nucleus accumbens shell[141] has been recently shown to selectively reduce compulsive checking in the quinpirole model, in line with recent reports of alleviation of compulsions following bilateral high frequency stimulation of the subthalamic nucleus in three pharmacodynamic patients with severe comorbid OCD,[142,143] and bilateral high frequency stimulation of the nucleus accumbens in OCD patients.[144-146]

An important advantage of the quinpirole model is that once compulsive checking is established (usually by the 8th to 10th quinpirole injection) it remains rather stable on subsequent quinpirole injections.[134] This allows the use of chronic administration of drugs and enables the assessment of the long-term effects of acute manipulations (such as deep brain stimulation) and the use of a within-subject design, which can greatly reduce the number of animals needed for a given experiment.

The major disadvantages of the quinpirole model are that (1) although it has been shown that quinpirole-induced compulsive checking is partially attenuated by clomipramine,[134] the effects of SSRIs and, even more critically, of drugs which are known not to be effective in OCD have not been assessed in the model, detracting from the model's predictive validity, and (2) 5 weeks of repeated quinpirole injections and behavioral testing are needed before compulsive behavior stabilizes, and the assessment of compulsive checking is very time consuming.

Genetic Models

Under this heading there are currently five mice models of OCD, namely, the D1CT-7 transgenic mouse model of comorbid OCD and TS,[147-149] the Hoxb8 mutant mouse model of trichotillomania,[24] the SAP90/PSD95-associated protein 3 (SAPAP3),[150] the $5\text{-}HT_{2c}$ receptor knockout mouse model of OCD[151] and the DAT knockdown mouse model of OCD and TS.[152] It is important to note that the five models are not genetic models in the sense alluded to by Matthysse,[83] that is, they were not created on the basis of a known mutation in humans that was found to be related to OCD. Rather, these models are based on behavioral similarity, that is, the behavior of genetically modified mice was found to be similar in specific respects to that of OCD patients, and this is the main basis for the claim that they may serve as animal models of this disorder. Regretfully, there are few reports on the effects of different pharmacological treatments in these models (the SAPAP3 model is an exception), which could have strengthened their relevance to OCD. An additional problem relevant to at least some of these genetic models is that the mutant mice typically show additional behavioral and neural abnormalities which are not related to OCD. For example, $5\text{-}HT_{2c}$ knockout mice are obese and hyperphagic with impaired satiety mechanisms,[153-155] and exhibit behavioral and neural abnormalities that may be related to cocaine dependence (e.g., increased sensitivity to the psychostimulant and reinforcing effects of cocaine and enhanced cocaine-induced increase in nucleus accumbens dopamine levels[156]) and Alzheimer's disease (e.g., impaired use of a spatial strategy in the Morris water maze and a dentate gyrus-specific deficit in hippocampal long-term potentiation[157]). Similarly, a number of these models involve self-injury, which is not typical of human OCD. It seems therefore unlikely that such genetic models are models of OCD, although clearly, such models may contribute to our understanding of the role of specific genes and proteins in compulsive behaviors.

ENDOPHENOTYPES AND BIOMARKERS

As suggested earlier, the concepts of endophenotypes and biomarkers may be particularly useful in future attempts to understand the pathogenesis of OCD, and to do translational research between bench and bedside. Rather than attempting to establish the psychobiology of OCD by studying OCD patients and animal models of this disorder, it may be useful to determine, in normal humans and animals, the neurocircuitry and molecular basis of intermediate phenotypes which may in turn be important in susceptibility to OCD.

Stereotypy as a Possible Endophenotype

Work on the neurobiology of stereotypies and habits may provide one route to exploring relevant endophenotypes for OCD. Some animals and some humans seem particularly susceptible to developing stereotypic behavior (e.g., in response to environmental poverty, or in response to pharmacological challenge), and it is possible that such mechanisms are similar to those which underpin OCD. For example, dopaminergic agonists lead to stereotypic behavior in both animals and humans, and dopamine appears important in OCD. As noted earlier, although there are differences between stereotypic and compulsive behavior, stereotypics, tics and compulsions may all represent different forms of a similar deficit (e.g., of inhibitors mechanisms). Indeed, it has been suggested that OCD involves disruption in inhibitory control, and that tasks addressing such control may serve as an endophenotype.[158] Animal models of stereotypic behavior may therefore provide important information on the neural systems that also mediate compulsive behavior (e.g., spontaneous stereotypy in deer mice, *P. maniculatus bairdii*).

Emotional Biomarkers

Many anxiety disorders involve maladaptive emotional learning where fear of a specific object, activity, place, or circumstance evokes extensive fear and may lead to inappropriate avoidance. Accordingly, behavioral therapies are modeled on extinction training as a means for reducing pathological anxiety;[159] an approach that is also used for OCD. It is therefore possible that studying the neural mechanisms of extinction, and particularly of extinction of emotions, may reveal neural mechanisms that are dysfunctioning in OCD. Furthermore, it is possible that drugs which facilitate extinction will have a beneficial effect in OCD and other anxiety disorders. The case of D-cycloserine, which enhances NMDA receptor function, is an example of the potential power of this approach.[160] This drug was found to facilitate extinction of conditioned fear in rodents,[161] and these results informed a human study which found that D-cycloserine significantly facilitated extinction of fear in patients with acrophobia undergoing behavioral exposure therapy.[162] Similarly, in a double blind, placebo-controlled trial in OCD patients, D-cycloserine augmentation increased the efficiency, palatability and overall effectiveness of standard exposure therapy.[69]

Neuropsychological studies of particular emotions may be useful in establishing an endophenotype of OCD. Whereas anxiety disorders may involve behavioral inhibition, with increased amygdala response to novelty, other emotions may be more relevant to OCD. It has been suggested, for example, that OCD involves a relative inability to recognize facial expressions of disgust, but also increased response of the insula during disgust-evoking tasks.[163,164] Thus, studies of the neural circuitry of disgust may contribute to the understanding of the neural mechanisms of OCD, and may pave the way for the development of new pharmacotherapies.

Neurocognitive Biomarkers

Animal models of cognitive deficits have been of interest as these involve domains that are often conserved between rodents, primates and humans, and that involve similar neural circuits. Recently, such studies have been combined with genetics and imaging ("genetics imaging"). For example, Weinberger and colleagues[165] reported that carriers of the short allele of the serotonin transporter gene have increased amygdala reactivity,[166] and they may also be at elevated risk of depression. The short allele carriers showed partial uncoupling of the amygdala–cingulate feedback circuit critical for emotional regulation. This raises several interesting questions and opportunities of a general nature that may apply to OCD as well. Can such alterations be reversed by drugs (state marker)? Are there rodent models showing a similar relative uncoupling? And can this be reversed by drugs? And will the phenotype also be reversed? Most importantly, can imaging techniques in rodents and healthy humans with the short SERT allele be used as surrogates for predicting drug efficacy in patients? In this respect it is noteworthy that in OCD, functional variants of the serotonin transporter gene have been identified and they appear to be causally associated with OCD in at least a minority of subjects.[28] Perhaps there are gene variants associated with the striatal dysfunction that appears characteristic of OCD.

Sensorimotor Gating

Because the intrusive, undesired thoughts that patients with OCD experience may involve impaired "cognitive gating", and the pathophysiology of OCD includes impairments in frontostriatal brain areas that control pre-pulse inhibition (PPI) (a procedure to measure sensorimotor gating), it has been hypothesized that OCD patients might have deficient sensorimotor gating.[vii] Indeed, this is what has been found,[167] with preliminary findings suggesting that PPI in a subgroup treated with antidepressants and antipsychotics was similar to healthy controls.[168] Sensorimotor gating studies also start shedding some light on the underlying pathophysiology. PPI is disrupted in DAT knockout mice and this effect is reversed by inhibitors at the serotonin–noradrenalin–DAT (either by one or by all three).[169] Consistent with this, an increase in frequency of the DAT

[vii] Please refer to Jones *et al.*, Developing New Drugs for Schizophrenia: From Animals to the Clinic, in this Volume, or Wagner *et al.*, Huntington Disease, in Volume 2, Neurologic Disorders for further discussion of sensorimotor gating and PPI.

A9-allele containing genotypes has been observed in OCD patients in 2 out of 3 studies and it has been proposed that this allele could alter the function of the transporter, resulting in an impairment of dopamine reuptake[170] (and references therein). It is tempting to speculate that PPI may provide a translational measure for testing dopaminergic OCD treatments. Vulink and colleagues[63] have recently found a bimodal distribution in the response to treatment with the dopaminergic agent bupropion in patients with OCD. It would be of interest to know whether the patients that improved possess the DAT A9-allele, whether they show impaired baseline PPI, and whether such impairment could be reversed by bupropion. Furthermore, PPI may also offer a potential marker of the effects of mGlu2 receptor agonists or positive modulators as these ligands reversed amphetamine – or phencyclidine-induced PPI deficits in mice (but not rats,[171] and references therein). In a next step, these ligands could be tested in a PPI model for sensorimotor gating deficits in OCD – such as the DAT knockdown mouse. In conclusion: PPI data are interesting and "hypothesis generating". An important question that remains to be addressed is if PPI normalizes with successful treatment or whether it is a stable trait that may qualify as an endophenotype or biomarker of OCD.

Executive Function

Functional neuroimaging studies found that OCD symptoms are associated with increased activity in orbitofrontal cortex, caudate nucleus, thalamus and anterior cingulate gyrus.[108,158,172] There is evidence that treatment with SSRIs can normalize activity in these brain areas and result in improved neurocognitive performance (e.g.,[173]), raising the possibility that neurocognitive tasks may be useful for testing novel OCD treatments. Compared with PPI, many more studies are available on the performance of OCD patients on neurocognitive tasks, although problems with small sample sizes, comorbidity, and phenotypic heterogeneity have been confounding.

Recently, it has been suggested to conceptualize OCD in terms of lateral orbitofrontal loop dysfunction, which may result in failures in cognitive and behavioral inhibition processes that may underlie the symptoms and many of the neurocognitive deficits of OCD patients.[158] Cognitive inhibition represents control over internal cognitions and behavioral inhibition represents control over externally manifested motor activities. Neurocognitive indices of these inhibitory failures may be useful in subgrouping patients and for drug testing. Several tasks from the Cambridge Neuropsychological Test Automated Battery (CANTAB) have been used, such as the intradimensional/extradimensional (ID/ED) shift task for the inability to set shift, and spatial recognition and working memory tasks for the memory deficits on tasks assisted by strategy use.[62] Although most of these tasks can be used in animals,[viii] few studies looked at the effects of SSRIs or augmentation with antipsychotics in these neurocognitive tasks in rodents or humans. Indirect support for a beneficial effect of SSRIs derives from studies showing that the functioning of the orbitofrontal cortex, as measured by a probabilistic learning and reversal task, was intact in OCD patients on SSRIs but impaired in drug-free patients.[158,174] In

---

[viii] Please refer to Lindner *et al.*, Development, Optimization and Use of Preclinical Behavioral Models to Maximize the Productivity of Drug Discovery for Alzheimer's Disease, in Volume 2, Neurological Disorders for further discussion and description of CANTAB and assessment of cognitive ability.

a study with OCD patients treated for 12 weeks with the SSRI paroxetine or the noradrenergic and serotonergic reuptake inhibitor venlafaxine, responders showed less spatial working memory deficits in an n-back task and a greater change in brain activity (medial frontal lobe, anterior cingulate, dorsolateral PFC, parietal cortex) during increasing task difficulty.[175] In contrast, spatial memory and planning impairments, which are thought to depend more on the dorsolateral PFC, showed no meaningful improvement in patients treated with fluoxetine.[176] In conclusion: evidence for both state and trait-dependent neurocognitive deficits has been obtained and this may depend on the involvement of orbitofrontal (state) versus dorsolateral prefrontal (trait) cortical regions. Neurocognitive tasks involving the orbitofrontal cortex may therefore be the tasks of choice for drug testing.

One such a task is reversal learning, as lesion studies found that the orbital PFC, but not the dorsolateral PFC in primates or the medial PFC in rats, mediates this type of learning.[177] This task involves serotonergic activity[178] and may offer a potentially sensitive test in rats and humans for novel anti-OCD drugs with a serotonergic mechanism such as 5-HT$_{2A}$ receptor agonists.

Application of Neurocognitive Biomarkers in OCD

Neurocognitive biomarkers can be helpful in establishing a proof of mechanism. But there can be uncertainties whether the cognitive deficit is related to the symptoms, and if drugs that alleviate the cognitive deficits would also alleviate symptoms. For example, PPI is disrupted in schizophrenia, Huntington's disease and other disorders and it could be argued that DAT knockout mice may consist of a model of schizophrenia, Huntington's disease or OCD, and that a drug that alleviates disrupted PPI in these mice may have antipsychotic, anti-Huntington or anti-compulsive, effects. OCD, Huntington's disease and schizophrenia share much in common – they are all basal ganglia-related disorders – and it is possible that disruption of PPI is pathognemonic to basal ganglia-related disorders, rather than pathognemonic to OCD. However, disease specificity may be an advantage rather than a "must" for a biomarker. Indeed, in view of overlapping neuropathology, the high level of comorbidity, and the frequent use of the same drugs for different psychiatric disorders, it would be surprising to find many disease-specific biomarkers. That a biomarker needs not to be disease specific in order to be valuable in drug discovery is illustrated by sleep electroencephalogram (EEG) findings. Sleep EEG is disrupted in several psychiatric disorders but the probabilities of antidepressants, antipsychotics, sedative hypnotics and stimulants to be correctly identified were high (73–87%[179]). Nevertheless, such a strategy has important limitations, given that a molecule that acts at a particular biomarker may be effective for a broad range of disorders.

CONCLUSION

Although there has been considerable progress in understanding the psychobiology of OCD and in developing medications for this disorder, much remains to be done. At a clinical level, although we know that CSTC circuits and 5-HT/dopamine/glutamate are involved in mediating OCD, the precise nature of the dysfunction is unknown. Similarly, it is not clear what the most relevant endophenotypes are. At a pre-clinical level, we have described a number of useful models, with varying degrees of face, construct, and predictive validity. But again, there model can yet be described as definitive.

What, Then, are the Next Steps Going Forwards?

Clinical research on large numbers of probands and unaffected family members would be useful in furthering our study of endophenotypes. These could include detailed phenomenology data, neuropsychological assessment, genetics, imaging, and challenge studies. Advances in large-scale gene and protein expression methods may be relevant to defining biological markers of OCD, or underlying endophenotypes, and may ultimately lead to new drug targets. Gene and protein work should not be a "fishing expedition", but could focus on particular genes/proteins thought to be involved in OCD (e.g., those particularly involved in CSTC function).

Animal research needs to explore different models in greater depth, keeping an eye on developments in the clinical literature which provide relevant endophenotypes and biomarkers. At the same time, basic research needs to occur on several mechanisms which may be relevant to OCD (e.g., PPI, working memory, implicit memory). Ultimately, advances in basic work should provide a platform from which new drug development can occur in the clinical context. Although the pharmaceutical industry is focused primarily on depression and generalized anxiety disorder, we are hopeful that future advances in basic neuroscience will ultimately lead to new therapies for OCD.

REFERENCES

1. Gottesman, I.I. and Gould, T.D. (2003). The endophenotype concept in psychiatry: Etymology and strategic intentions. *Am J Psychiat*, 160:636–645.
2. Hettema, J.M., Neale, M.C., and Kendler, K.S. (2001). A review and meta-analysis of the genetic epidemiology of anxiety disorders. *Am J Psychiat*, 158:1568–1578.
3. Weissman, M.M., Bland, R.C., Canino, G.J., Greenwald, S., Hwu, H.-G., Lee, C.K. *et al.* (1994). The cross national epidemiology of obsessive compulsive disorder. *J Clin Psychiat*, 55S:5–10.
4. Murray, C.J.L. and Lopez, A.D. (1996). *Global Burden of Disease: A Comprehensive Assessment of Mortality and Morbidity from Diseases, Injuries and Risk Factors in 1990 and Projected to 2020.* World Health Organisation, Havard.
5. American Psychiatric Association. (1994). *Diagnostic and Statistical Manual of Mental Disorders*, 4th edition. American Psychiatric Press, Washington, DC.
6. Lochner, C. and Stein, D.J. (2003). Heterogeneity of obsessive–compulsive disorder: A literature review. *Harv Rev Psychiat*, 11:113–132.
7. Mataix-Cols, D., Rosario-Campos, M.C.d., and Leckman, J.F. (2005). A multidimensional model of obsessive–compulsive disorder. *Am J Psychiat*, 162:228–238.
8. Stein, D.J. (2000). Neurobiology of the obsessive-compulsive spectrum disorders. *Biologic Psychiat*, 47:296–304.
9. Stein, D.J. (2002). Seminar on obsessive-compulsive disorder. *Lancet*, 360:397–405.
10. Saxena, S., Brody, A.L., Maidment, K.M., Smith, E.C., Zohrabi, N., Katz, E. *et al.* (2004). Cerebral glucose metabolism in obsessive-compulsive hoarding. *Am J Psychiat*, 161:1038–1048.
11. Phillips, M.L. and Mataix-Cols, D. (2004). Patterns of neural response to emotive stimuli distinguish the different symptom dimensions of obsessive–compulsive disorder. *CNS Spectr*, 9:275–283.

12. Lochner, C., Hemmings, S.M.J., Kinnear, C.J., Niehaus, D.J.H., Nel, D.G., Corfield, V.A. *et al.* (2005). Cluster analysis of obsessive–compulsive spectrum disorders in patients with obsessive–compulsive disorder: Clinical and genetic correlates. *Compr Psychiat*, 46:14–19.

13. Hemmings, S.M.J., Kinnear, C.J., Lochner, C., Niehaus, D.J.H., Knowles, J.A., Moolman-Smook, J.C. *et al.* (2004). Early- versus late-onset obsessive–compulsive disorder: Investigating genetic and clinical correlates. *Psychiat Res*, 128:175–182.

14. Giedd, J.N., Rapoport, J.L., Garvey, M.A., Perlmutter, S., and Swedo, S.E. (2000). MRI assessment of children with obsessive–compulsive disorder or tics associated with streptococcal infection. *Am J Psychiat*, 157:281–283.

15. Leonard, H.L. and Swedo, S.E. (2001). Paediatric autoimmune neuropsychiatric disorders associated with streptococcal infection (PANDAS). *Int J Neuropsychopharmacol*, 4:191–198.

16. Snider, L.A., Lougee, L., Slattery, M., Grant, P., and Swedo, S.E. (2005). Antibiotic prophylaxis with azithromycin or penicillin for childhood-onset neuropsychiatric disorders. *Biologic Psychiat*, 57:788–792.

17. Stein, D.J., Montgomery, S.A., Kasper, S., and Tanghoj, P. (2001). Predictors of response to pharmacotherapy with citalopram in obsessive–compulsive disorder. *Int Clin Psychopharmacol*, 16:357–361.

18. Denys, D. and de Geus, F. (2005). Predictors of pharmacotherapy response in anxiety disorders. *Curr Psychiat Rep*, 7:252–257.

19. Stein, D.J. and Lochner, C. (2006). Obsessive–compulsive spectrum disorders: A multidimensional approach. *Psychiatr Clin North Am*, 29:343–351.

20. Pauls, D.L., Towbin, K.E., Leckman, J.F. *et al.* (1986). Gilles de la Tourette's syndrome and obsessive compulsive disorder: Evidence supporting a genetic relationship. *Arch Gen Psychiat*, 43:1180–1182.

21. Moriarty, J., Eapen, V., Costa, D.C., Gacinovic, S., Trimble, M., Ell, P.J. *et al.* (1997). HMPAO SPET does not distinguish obsessive–compulsive and tic syndromes in families multiply affected with Gilles de la Tourette's syndrome. *Psychol Med*, 27:737–740.

22. Stein, D.J., Liu, Y., Shapira, N.A., and Goodman, W.K. (2001). The psychobiology of obsessive–compulsive disorder: how important is the role of disgust? *Curr Psychiat Rep*, 3:281–287.

23. Abelson, J.F., Kwan, K.Y., O'Roak, B.J., Baek, D.Y., Stillman, A.A., Morgan, T.M. *et al.* (2005). Sequence variants in SLITRK1 are associated with Tourette's syndrome. *Science*, 310:317–320.

24. Greer, J.M. and Capecchi, M.R. (2002). Hoxb8 is required for normal grooming behavior in mice. *Neuron*, 33:23–34.

25. Abramowitz, J.S. (1997). Effectiveness of psychological and pharmacological treatments for obsessive–compulsive disorder: A quantitative review. *J Consult Clin Psychol*, 65:44–52.

26. Barr, C.L., Goodman, W.K., Price, L.H., McDougle, C.J., and Charney, D.S. (1992). The serotonin hypothesis of obsessive compulsive disorder: implications of pharmacologic challenge studies. *J Clin Psychiat*, 53S:17–28.

27. Stein, D.J., Goodman, W.K., and Rauch, S.L. (2000). The cognitive-affective neuroscience of obsessive–compulsive disorder. *Curr Psychiat Rep*, 2:341–346.

28. Ozaki, N., Goldman, D., Kaye, W.H., Plotnicov, K., Greenberg, B.D., Lappalainen, J. *et al.* (2003). Serotonin transporter missense mutation associated with a complex neuropsychiatric phenotype. *Mol Psychiat*, 8:933–936.

29. March, J.S., Frances, A., Carpenter, D., and Kahn, D. (1997). Treatment of obsessive–compulsive disorder. The Expert Consensus Panel for obsessive–compulsive disorder. *J Clin Psychiat*, 58S4:1–72.

30. Bandelow, B., Zohar, J., Hollander, E., Kasper, S., and Moller, H.-J. AWFSBP Task Force on Treatment Guidelines for Anxiety. (2002). World Federation of Societies of Biological

Psychiatry (WFSBP) guidelines for the pharmacological treatment of anxiety, obsessive-compulsive and posttraumatic stress disorders. *World J Biol Psychiat*, 3:171-199.

31. Pallanti, S., Hollander, E., Bienstock, C., Koran, L., Leckman, J., Marazziti, D. *et al.* (2002). Treatment non-response in OCD: methodological issues and operational definitions. *Int Clin Psychopharmacol*, 5:181-191.

32. Goodman, W.K., McDougle, C.J., and Lawrence, L.P. (1990). Beyond the serotonin hypothesis: A role for dopamine in some forms of obsessive–compulsive disorder. *J Clin Psychiat*, 51S:36-43.

33. McDougle, C.J., Goodman, W.K., and Leckman, J.F. (1994). Haloperidol addition in fluvoxamine-refractory obsessive–compulsive disorder: A double-blind placebo-controlled study in patients with and without tics. *Arch Gen Psychiat*, 51:302-308.

34. Ipser, J.C., Carey, P., Dhansay, Y., Fakier, N., Seedat, S., and Stein, D.J. (2006). Pharmacotherapy augmentation strategies in treatment-resistant anxiety disorders, Cochrane Database Syst Rev CD005473.

35. Denys, D., Zohar, J., and Westenberg, H.G.M. (2004). The role of dopamine in obsessive-compulsive disorder: preclinical and clinical evidence. *J Clin Psychiat*, 65:11-17.

36. Denys, D., van der Wee, N., Janssen, J., de Geus, F., and Westenberg, H.G.M. (2004). Low level of dopaminergic D2 receptor binding in obsessive–compulsive disorder. *Biologic Psychiat*, 55:1041-1045.

37. van der Wee, N.J., Stevens, H., Hardeman, J.A., Mandl, R.C., Denys, D.A., van Megen, H.J. *et al.* (2004). Enhanced dopamine transporter density in psychotropic-naive patients with obsessive–compulsive disorder shown by [123I] beta-CIT SPECT. *Am J Psychiat*, 161:2201-2206.

38. Stahl, S.M. (2006). Finding what you are not looking for: strategies for developing novel treatments in psychiatry. *NeuroRx*, 3:3-9.

39. El Mansari, M. and Blier, P. (2006). Mechanisms of action of current and potential pharmacotherapies of obsessive–compulsive disorder. *Prog Neuropsychopharmacol Biol Psychiat*, 30:362-373.

40. Delgado, P.L. and Moreno, F.A. (1998). Hallucinogens, serotonin and obsessive–compulsive disorder. *J Psychoactive Drug*, 30:359-366.

41. May, L.T., Leach, K., Sexton, P.M., and Christopoulos, A. (2007). Allosteric modulation of G protein-coupled receptors. *Annu Rev Pharmacol Toxicol*, 47:1-51.

42. Shenoy, S.K. and Lefkowitz, R.J. (2003). Trafficking patterns of beta-arrestin and G protein-coupled receptors determined by the kinetics of beta-arrestin deubiquitination. *J Biol Chem*, 278:14498-14506.

43. Broocks, A., Pigott, T.A., Hill, J.L., Canter, S., Grady, T.A., L'Heureux, F., and Murphy, D.L. (1998). Acute intravenous administration of ondansetron and m-CPP, alone and in combination, in patients with obsessive–compulsive disorder (OCD): Behavioral and biological results. *Psychiat Res*, 79:11-20.

44. Gross-Isseroff, R., Cohen, R., Sasson, Y., Voet, H., and Zohar, J. (2004). Serotonergic dissection of obsessive compulsive symptoms: A challenge study with m-chlorophenylpiperazine and sumatriptan. *Neuropsychobiology*, 50:200-205.

45. Hollander, E., DeCaria, C., Gully, R., Nitescu, A., Suckow, R.F., Gorman, J.M., Klein, D.F., and Liebowitz, M.R. (1991). Effects of chronic fluoxetine treatment on behavioral and neuro-endocrine responses to meta-chlorophenylpiperazine in obsessive–compulsive disorder. *Psychiat Res*, 36:1-17.

46. Murphy, D.L., Zohar, J., Benkelfat, C., Pato, M.T., Pigott, T.A., and Insel, T.R. (1989). Obsessive-compulsive disorder as a 5-HT subsystem-related behavioural disorder. *Br J Psychiat*, 5(Suppl):15-24.

47. Pigott, T.A., Zohar, J., Hill, J.L., Bernstein, S.E., Grover, G.N., Zohar-Kadouch, R.C., and Murphy, D.L. (1991). Metergoline blocks the behavioral and neuroendocrine effects of orally

administered m-chlorophenylpiperazine in patients with obsessive–compulsive disorder. *Biol Psychiat*, 29:418–426.

48. Pigott, T.A., Hill, J.L., Grady, T.A., L'Heureux, F., Bernstein, S., Rubenstein, C.S., and Murphy, D. L. (1993). A comparison of the behavioral effects of oral versus intravenous mCPP administration in OCD patients and the effect of metergoline prior to i.v. mCPP,. *Biol Psychiatry*, 33:3–14.

49. Stern, L., Zohar, J., Cohen, R., and Sasson, Y. (1998). Treatment of severe, drug resistant obsessive compulsive disorder with the 5HT1D agonist sumatriptan. *Eur Neuropsychopharmacol*, 8:325–328.

50. Zohar, J., Insel, T.R., Zohar-Kadouch, R.C., Hill, J.L., and Murphy, D.L. (1988). Serotonergic responsivity in obsessive–compulsive disorder. Effects of chronic clomipramine treatment,. *Arch Gen Psychiat*, 45:167–172.

51. Charney, D.S., Goodman, W.K., Price, L.H., Woods, S.W., Rasmussen, S.A., and Heninger, G.R. (1988). Serotonin function in obsessive–compulsive disorder. A comparison of the effects of tryptophan and m-chlorophenylpiperazine in patients and healthy subjects,. *Arch Gen Psychiat*, 45:177–185.

52. Goodman, W.K., McDougle, C.J., Price, L.H., Barr, L.C., Hills, O.F., Caplik, J.F., Charney, D.S., and Heninger, G.R. (1995). m-Chlorophenylpiperazine in patients with obsessive–compulsive disorder: absence of symptom exacerbation. *Biol Psychiat*, 38:138–149.

53. Ho Pian, K.L., Westenberg, H.G., den Boer, J.A., de Bruin, W.I., and van Rijk, P.P. (2001). Effects of meta-chlorophenylpiperazine on cerebral blood flow in obsessive–compulsive disorder and controls. *Biol Psychiat*, 44:367–370.

54. Khanna, S., John, J.P., and Reddy, L.P. (2001). Neuroendocrine and behavioral responses to mCPP in Obsessive–Compulsive Disorder. *Psychoneuroendocrinology*, 26:209–223.

55. Yamauchi, M., Tatebayashi, T., Nagase, K., Kojima, M., and Imanishi, T. (2004). Chronic treatment with fluvoxamine desensitizes 5-HT2C receptor-mediated hypolocomotion in rats. *Pharmacol Biochem Behav*, 78:683–689.

56. Kennett, G.A., Lightowler, S., de Biasi, V., Stevens, N.C., Wood, M.D., Tulloch, I.F., and Blackburn, T.P. (1994). Effect of chronic administration of selective 5-hydroxytryptamine and noradrenaline uptake inhibitors on a putative index of 5-HT2C/2B receptor function. *Neuropharmacology*, 33:1581–1588.

57. Quested, D.J., Sargent, P.A., and Cowen, P.J. (1997). SSRI treatment decreases prolactin and hyperthermic responses to mCPP. *Psychopharmacology (Berl)*, 133:305–308.

58. Flaisher-Grinberg, S., Klavir, O., and Joel, D. The role of 5-HT2a and 5-HT2c receptors in the signal attenuation rat model of obsessive compulsive disorder (submitted).

59. Martin, J.R., Ballard, T.M., and Higgins, G.A. (2002). Influence of the 5-HT2C receptor antagonist, SB-242084, in tests of anxiety. *Pharmacol Biochem Behav*, 71:615–625.

60. Zhang, W., Perry, K.W., Wong, D.T., Potts, B.D., Bao, J., Tollefson, G.D., and Bymaster, F.P. (2000). Synergistic effects of olanzapine and other antipsychotic agents in combination with fluoxetine on norepinephrine and dopamine release in rat prefrontal cortex. *Neuropsychopharmacology*, 23:250–262.

61. Gobert, A., Rivet, J.M., Lejeune, F., Newman-Tancredi, A., Adhumeau-Auclair, A., Nicolas, J.P., Cistarelli, L., Melon, C., and Millan, M.J. (2000). Serotonin(2C) receptors tonically suppress the activity of mesocortical dopaminergic and adrenergic. *but not serotonergic, pathways: A combined dialysis and electrophysiological analysis in the rat, Synapse*, 36:205–221.

62. Canton, H., Verriele, L., and Millan, M.J. (1994). Competitive antagonism of serotonin (5-HT)2C and 5-HT2A receptor-mediated phosphoinositide (PI) turnover by clozapine in the rat: A comparison to other antipsychotics. *Neurosci Lett*, 181:65–68.

63. Vulink, N.C., Denys, D., and Westenberg, H.G. (2005). Bupropion for patients with obsessive-compulsive disorder: an open-label, fixed-dose study. *J Clin Psychiat*, 66:228–230.

64. Carlsson, M.L., Carlsson, A., and Nilsson, M. (2004). Schizophrenia: from dopamine to glutamate and back. *Curr Med Chem*, 11:267–277.

65. Connor, K.M., Payne, V.M., Gadde, K.M., Zhang, W., and Davidson, J.R. (2005). The use of aripiprazole in obsessive-compulsive disorder: preliminary observations in 8 patients. *J Clin Psychiat*, 66:49–51.

66. Pittenger, C., Krystal, J.H., and Coric, V. (2006). Glutamate-modulating drugs as novel pharmacotherapeutic agents in the treatment of obsessive-compulsive disorder. *NeuroRx*, 3:69–81.

67. Spooren, W., Ballard, T., Gasparini, F., Amalric, M., Mutel, V., and Schreiber, R. (2003). Insight into the function of Group I and Group II metabotropic glutamate (mGlu) receptors: behavioural characterization and implications for the treatment of CNS disorders. *Behav Pharmacol*, 14:257–277.

68. Coric, V., Milanovic, S., Wasylink, S., Patel, P., Malison, R., and Krystal, J.H. (2003). Beneficial effects of the antiglutamatergic agent riluzole in a patient diagnosed with obsessive-compulsive disorder and major depressive disorder. *Psychopharmacology (Berl)*, 167:219–220.

69. Kushner, M.G., Kim, S.W., Donahue, C., Thuras, P., Adson, D., Kotlyar, M., McCabe, J., Peterson, J., and Foa, E.B. (2007). D-cycloserine augmented exposure therapy for obsessive-compulsive disorder. *Biol Psychiat*, 62:835–838.

70. Storch, E.A., Merlo, L.J., Bengtson, M., Murphy, T.K., Lewis, M.H., Yang, M.C., Jacob, M.L., Larson, M., Hirsh, A., Fernandez, M., Geffken, G.R., and Goodman, W.K. (2007). D-cycloserine does not enhance exposure-response prevention therapy in obsessive-compulsive disorder. *Int Clin Psychopharmacol*, 22:230–237.

71. Fallon, B.A., Liebowitz, M.R., Campeas, R., Schneier, F.R., Marshall, R., Davies, S. *et al.* (1998). Intravenous clomipramine for obsessive-compulsive disorder refractory to oral clomipramine: A placebo-controlled study. *Arch Gen Psychiat*, 55:918–924.

72. Salkovskis, P.M. (1999). Understanding and treating obsessive-compulsive disorder. *Behav Res Ther*, 37S1:29–52.

73. Nakagawa, A., Marks, I.M., Park, J.M., Bachofen, M., Baer, L., Dottl, S.L. *et al.* (2000). Self-treatment of obsessive-compulsive disorder guided by manual and computer-conducted telephone interview. *J Telemed Telecare*, 6:22–26.

74. Bystritsky, A., Munford, P.R., Rosen, R.M. *et al.* (1996). A preliminary study of partial hospital management of severe obsessive-compulsive disorder. *Psychiat Serv*, 47:170–174.

75. Greenberg, B.D., Price, L.H., Rauch, S.L., Friehs, G., Noren, G., Malone, D. *et al.* (2003). Neurosurgery for intractable obsessive-compulsive disorder and depression: critical issues. *Neurosur Clin North Am*, 14:199–212.

76. Abelson, J.L., Curtis, G.C., Sagher, O., Albucher, R.C., Harrigan, M., Taylor, S.F. *et al.* (2005). Deep brain stimulation for refractory obsessive-compulsive disorder. *Biol Psychiatry*, 57:510–516.

77. Alonso, P., Pujol, J., Cardoner, N., Benlloch, L., Deus, J., Menchon, J.M. *et al.* (2001). Right prefrontal repetitive transcranial magnetic stimulation in obsessive-compulsive disorder: a double-blind, placebo-controlled study. *Am J Psychiat*, 158:1143–1145.

78. Whiteside, S.P., Port, J.D., and Abramowitz, J.S. (2004). A meta-analysis of functional neuroimaging in obsessive-compulsive disorder. *Psychiat Res*, 132:69–79.

79. Baxter, L.R., Schwartz, J.M., Bergman, K.S. *et al.* (1992). Caudate glucose metabolic rate changes with both drug and behavior therapy for OCD. *Arch Gen Psychiat*, 49:681–689.

80. Saxena, S. and Maidment, K.M. (2004). Treatment of compulsive hoarding. *J Clin Psychol*, 60:1143–1154.

81. Geyer, M.A. and Markou, A. (1995). Animal models of psychiatric disorders. In Bloom, F.E. and Kupfer, D.J. (eds.), *Psychopharmacology: The Fourth Generation of Progress*. Raven Press Ltd, New York, pp. 787–798.

82. Geyer, M.A. and Markou, A. (2002). The role of preclinical models in the development of psychotropic drugs. In Davis, K.L., Charney, D., Coyle, J.T., and Nemeroff, C. (eds.),

Neuropsychopharmacology: The Fifth Generation of Progress. Philadelphia, Lippincott Williams & Wilkins, pp. 445–455.

83. Matthysse, S. (1986). Animal models in psychiatric research. Prog Brain Res, 65:259–270.

84. McKinney, W.T., Jr. (1988). Models of mental disorders: A new comparative psychiatry. Plenum Medical Book Co., New York.

85. McKinney, W.T., Jr. and Bunney, W.E., Jr. (1969). Animal model of depression. I: Review of evidence: implications for research. Arch Gen Psychiat, 21:240–248.

86. Willner, P. (1984). The validity of animal models of depression. Psychopharmacology (Berl), 83:1–16.

87. Willner, P. (1986). Validation criteria for animal models of human mental disorders: learned helplessness as a paradigm case. Prog Neuropsychopharmacol Biol Psychiat, 10:677–690.

88. Willner, P. (1991). Behavioural models in psychopharmacology. In Willner, P. (ed.), Behavioural Models in Psychopharmacology: Theoretical, Industrial and Clinical Perspectives. Cambridge University Press, Cambridge, pp. 3–18.

89. Joel, D. (2006). Current animal models of obsessive compulsive disorder: a critical review. Prog Neuropsychopharmacol Biol Psychiat, 30:374–388.

90. Argyropoulos, S.V., Sandford, J.J., and Nutt, D.J. (2000). The psychobiology of anxiolytic drug, Part 2: Pharmacological treatments of anxiety. Pharmacol Ther, 88:213–227.

91. Vaswani, M., Linda, F.K., and Ramesh, S. (2003). Role of selective serotonin reuptake inhibitors in psychiatric disorders: a comprehensive review. Prog Neuropsychopharmacol Biol Psychiat, 27:85–102.

92. Insel, T.R., Mos, J., and Olivier, B. (1994). Animal models of obsessive compulsive disorder: A review. In Hollander, E., Zohar, J., Marazzitti, D., and Olivier, B. (eds.), Current Insights in Obsessive Compulsive Disorder. John Wiley & Sons, Chichester, pp. 117–135.

93. Bourin, M., Fiocco, A.J., and Clenet, F. (2001). How valuable are animal models in defining antidepressant activity? Hum Psychopharmacol, 16:9–21.

94. Agid, O., Kapur, S., Arenovich, T., and Zipursky, R.B. (2003). Delayed-onset hypothesis of antipsychotic action: a hypothesis tested and rejected. Arch Gen Psychiat, 60:1228–1235.

95. Masand, P.S. and Gupta, S. (1999). Selective serotonin-reuptake inhibitors: an update. Harv Rev Psychiat, 7:69–84.

96. Korff, S. and Harvey, B.H. (2006). Animal models of obsessive–compulsive disorder: rationale to understanding psychobiology and pharmacology. Psychiat Clin North Am, 29:371–390.

97. Winslow, J.T. and Insel, T.R. (1991). Neuroethological models of obsessive–compulsive disorder. In Zohar, J., Insel, T., and Rasmussen, S. (eds.), The Psychobiology of Obsessive–Compulsive Disorder. Springer Publishing Company, New York, pp. 208–226.

98. Stein, D.J., Dodman, N.H., Borchelt, P., and Hollander, E. (1994). Behavioral disorders in veterinary practice: relevance to psychiatry. *Compr Psychiat*, 35(4):275–285.

99. Ricciardi, J.N. and Hurley, J. (1990). Development of animal models of obsessive–compulsive disorders. In Jenike, M.A., Baer, L., and Minichiello, W.E. (eds.), *Obsessive-Compulsive Disorders: Theory and Management*, 2nd edition. Year Book Medical Publishers, Inc, Chicago, pp. 189–199.

100. Pitman, R.K. (1991). Historical considerations. In Zohar, J., Insel, T., and Rasmussen, S. (eds.), *The Psychobiology of Obsessive-Compulsive Disorder*. Springer Publishing Company, New York, pp. 1–12.

101. Woods, A., Smith, C., Szewczak, M., Dunn, R.W., Cornfeldt, M., and Corbett, R. (1993). Selective serotonin re-uptake inhibitors decrease schedule-induced polydipsia in rats: a potential model for obsessive compulsive disorder. *Psychopharmacology*, 112:195–198.

102. Altemus, M., Glowa, J.R., Galliven, E., Leong, Y.M., and Murphy, D.L. (1996). Effects of serotonergic agents on food-restriction-induced hyperactivity. *Pharmacol Biochem Behav*, 53:123–131.

103. Joel, D. (2006). The signal attenuation rat model of obsessive–compulsive disorder: a review. *Psychopharmacology (Berl)*, 186:487–503.

104. Chamberlain, S.R., Fineberg, N.A., Blackwell, A.D., Robbins, T.W., and Sahakian, B.J. (2006). Motor inhibition and cognitive flexibility in obsessive–compulsive disorder and trichotillomania. *Am J Psychiat*, 163:1282–1284.

105. Powell, S.B., Newman, H.A., Pendergast, J.F., and Lewis, M.H. (1999). A rodent model of spontaneous stereotypy: initial characterization of developmental, environmental, and neurobiological factors. *Physiol Behav*, 66:355–363.

106. Presti, M.F. and Lewis, M.H. (2005). Striatal opioid peptide content in an animal model of spontaneous stereotypic behavior. *Behav Brain Res*, 157:363–368.

107. Presti, M.F., Mikes, H.M., and Lewis, M.H. (2003). Selective blockade of spontaneous motor stereotypy via intrastriatal pharmacological manipulation. *Pharmacol Biochem Behav*, 74:833–839.

108. Saxena, S., Brody, A.L., Schwartz, J.M., and Baxter, L.R. (1998). Neuroimaging and frontal-subcortical circuitry in obsessive–compulsive disorder. *Br J Psychiat Suppl*, 35:26–37.

109. Korff, S., Stein, D.J., and Harvey, B.H. Stereotypic behaviour in the deer mouse: Pharmacological validation, relevance for obsessive compulsive disorder. Neuropsychopharmacology, *Biol Psychiatry* (in press).

110. Gyertyan, I. (1995). Analysis of the marble burying response: marbles serve to measure digging rather than evoke burying. *Behav Pharmacol*, 6:24–31.

111. Londei, T., Valentini, A.M., and Leone, V.G. (1998). Investigative burying by laboratory mice may involve non-functional, compulsive, behaviour. *Behav Brain Res*, 94:249–254.

112. Njung'e, K. and Handley, S.L. (1991). Evaluation of marble-burying behavior as a model of anxiety. *Pharmacol Biochem Behav*, 38:63–67.

113. Broekkamp, C.L., Rijk, H.W., Joly-Gelouin, D., and Lloyd, K.L. (1986). Major tranquillizers can be distinguished from minor tranquillizers on the basis of effects on marble burying and swim-induced grooming in mice. *Eur J Pharmacol*, 126:223–229.

114. Treit, D. (1985). The inhibitory effect of diazepam on defensive burying: anxiolytic vs. analgesic effects. *Pharmacol Biochem Behav*, 22:47–52.

115. Treit, D., Pinel, J.P., and Fibiger, H.C. (1981). Conditioned defensive burying: a new paradigm for the study of anxiolytic agents. *Pharmacol Biochem Behav*, 15:619–626.

116. Broekkamp, C.L. and Jenck, F. (1989). The relationship between various animal models of anxiety, fear-related psychiatric symptoms and response to serotonergic drugs. In Bevan, P., Cools, R., and Archer, T. (eds.), *Behavioural Pharmacology of 5-HT*. Erlbaum, Hillsdale, pp. 321–335.

117. Szechtman, H. and Woody, E. (2004). Obsessive–compulsive disorder as a disturbance of security motivation. *Psychol Rev*, 111:111–127.

118. Hirano, K., Kimura, R., Sugimoto, Y., Yamada, J., Uchida, S., Kato, Y., Hashimoto, H., and Yamada, S. (2005). Relationship between brain serotonin transporter binding, plasma concentration and behavioural effect of selective serotonin reuptake inhibitors. *Br J Pharmacol*, 144:695–702.

119. Takeuchi, H., Yatsugi, S., and Yamaguchi, T. (2002). Effect of YM992, a novel antidepressant with selective serotonin re-uptake inhibitory and 5-HT 2A receptor antagonistic activity, on a marble-burying behavior test as an obsessive–compulsive disorder model. *Jpn J Pharmacol*, 90:197–200.

120. Ichimaru, Y., Egawa, T., and Sawa, A. (1995). 5-HT1A-receptor subtype mediates the effect of fluvoxamine, a selective serotonin reuptake inhibitor, on marble-burying behavior in mice. *Jpn J Pharmacol*, 68:65–70.

121. Joel, D. and Avisar, A. (2001). Excessive lever pressing following post-training signal attenuation in rats: A possible animal model of obsessive compulsive disorder? *Behav Brain Res*, 123:77–87.

122. Joel, D., Avisar, A., and Doljansky, J. (2001). Enhancement of excessive lever-pressing after post-training signal attenuation in rats by repeated administration of the D1 antagonist

SCH 23390 or the D2 agonist quinpirole but not of the D1 agonist SKF 38393 or the D2 antagonist haloperidol. *Behav Neurosci*, 115:1291-1300.

123. Joel, D., Ben-Amir, E., Doljansky, J., and Flaisher, S. (2004). 'Compulsive' lever-pressing in rats is attenuated by the serotonin re-uptake inhibitors paroxetine and fluvoxamine but not by the tricyclic antidepressant desipramine or the anxiolytic diazepam. *Behav Pharmacol*, 15:241-252.

124. Joel, D. and Doljansky, J. (2003). Selective alleviation of 'compulsive' lever-pressing in rats by D1, but not D2, blockade: Possible implications for the involvement of D1 receptors in obsessive compulsive disorder. *Neuropsychopharmacology*, 28:77-85.

125. Joel, D., Doljansky, J., Roz, N., and Rehavi, M. (2005). Role of the orbital cortex and the serotonergic system in a rat model of obsessive compulsive disorder. *Neuroscience*, 130:25-36.

126. Joel, D., Doljansky, J., and Schiller, D. (2005). 'Compulsive' lever pressing in rats is enhanced following lesions to the orbital cortex, but not to the basolateral nucleus of the amygdala or to the dorsal medial prefrontal cortex. *Eur J Neurosci*, 21:2252-2262.

127. Baxter, L.R. (1999). Functional imaging of brain systems mediating obsessive–compulsive disorder. In Nestler W. Bunney, C.E. (ed.), *Neurobiology of Mental Illness*. Oxford University Press, New York, pp. 534-547.

128. Reed, G.F. (1977). Obsessional personality disorder and remembering. *Br J Psychiat*, 130:177-183.

129. Otto, M.W. (1992). Normal and abnormal information processing: A neuropsychological perspective on obsessive–compulsive disorder. In Jenike, M.A. (ed.), *The Psychiatric Clinics of North America. Obsessional Disorders*, Vol. 15. W.B. Saunders Company, Harcourt Brace Jovanovich, Inc, Chicago, pp. 825-848.

130. Graf, M. (2006). 5-HT2c receptor activation induces grooming behaviour in rats: possible correlations with obsessive-compulsive disorder. *Neuropsychopharmacol Hung*, 8:23-28.

131. Rauch, S.L. and Baxter., L.R. (1998). Neuroimaging in obsessive-compulsive and related disorders. In Jenike, M.A., Baer, L., and Minichiello, W.E. (eds.), *Obsessive-Compulsive Disorders: Practical Management*, 3rd Edition. Mosby, St. Louis, MO, pp. 289-316.

132. Yadin, E., Friedman, E., and Bridger, W.H. (1991). Spontaneous alternation behavior: an animal model for obsessive-compulsive disorder? *Pharmacol Biochem Behav*, 40:311-315.

133. Eilam, D. and Szechtman, H. (1995). Towards an animal model of obsessive-compulsive disorder (OCD): Sensitization to dopamine agonist quinpirole. *Soc Neurosci Abstr*, 21:192.

134. Szechtman, H., Sulis, W., and Eilam, D. (1998). Quinpirole induces compulsive checking behavior in rats: a potential animal model of obsessive-compulsive disorder (OCD). *Behav Neurosci*, 112:1475-1485.

135. Szechtman, H., Eckert, M.J., Tse, W.S., Boersma, J.T., Bonura, C.A., McClelland, J.Z., Culver, K.E., and Eilam, D. (2001). Compulsive checking behavior of quinpirole-sensitized rats as an animal model of Obsessive-Compulsive Disorder(OCD): form and control. *BMC Neurosci*, 2:4.

136. Fernandez-Guasti, A., Ulloa, R.E., and Nicolini, H. (2003). Age differences in the sensitivity to clomipramine in an animal model of obsessive–compulsive disorder. *Psychopharmacology (Berl)*, 166:195-201.

137. Ben-Pazi, A., Szechtman, H., and Eilam, D. (2001). The morphogenesis of motor rituals in rats treated chronically with the dopamine agonist quinpirole. *Behav Neurosci*, 115:1301-1317.

138. Eilam, D. and Szechtman, H. (2005). Psychostimulant-induced behavior as an animal model of obsessive-compulsive disorder: An ethological approach to the form of compulsive rituals. *CNS Spectr*, 10:1-12.

139. Szechtman, H. and Eilam, D. (2005). Psychiatric models. In Whishaw, I.Q. and Kolb, B. (eds.), *The Behavior of the Laboratory Rat: A Handbook with Tests*. Oxford University Press, Inc, London, pp. 462–474.

140. Winter, C., Joel, D., Klavir, O., Mundt, A., Jalali, R., Flash, S., Klein, J., Harnack, D., Morgenstern, R., Juckel, G., and Kupsch, A. (2007). Modulation of subthalamic Nucleus activity differentially affects compulsive behavior in rats. *Pharmacopsychiatry*, 40:242.

141. Mundt, A., Klein, J., Heinz, A., Morgenstern, R., Juckel, G., Kupsch, A., and Winter, C. (2007). Deep brain stimulation of the Nucl. accumbens core and shell differentially reduces quinpirole-induced compulsive checking behavior in rats. *Pharmacopsychiatry*, 40:246.

142. Mallet, L., Mesnage, V., Houeto, J.L., Pelissolo, A., Yelnik, J., Behar, C., Gargiulo, M., Welter, M.L., Bonnet, A.M., Pillon, B., Cornu, P., Dormont, D., Pidoux, B., Allilaire, J.F., and Agid, Y. (2002). Compulsions, Parkinson's disease, and stimulation. *Lancet*, 360:1302–1304.

143. Fontaine, D., Mattei, V., Borg, M., von Langsdorff, D., Magnie, M.N., Chanalet, S., Robert, P., and Paquis, P. (2004). Effect of subthalamic nucleus stimulation on obsessive–compulsive disorder in a patient with Parkinson disease. Case report. *J Neurosurg*, 100:1084–1086.

144. Greenberg, B.D., Malone, D.A., Friehs, G.M., Rezai, A.R., Kubu, C.S., Malloy, P.F., Salloway, S.P., Okun, M.S., Goodman, W.K., and Rasmussen, S.A. (2006). Three-year outcomes in deep brain stimulation for highly resistant obsessive–compulsive disorder. *Neuropsychopharmacology*, 31:2384–2393.

145. Rauch, S.L., Dougherty, D.D., Malone, D., Rezai, A., Friehs, G., Fischman, A.J., Alpert, N.M., Haber, S.N., Stypulkowski, P.H., Rise, M.T., Rasmussen, S.A., and Greenberg, B.D. (2006). A functional neuroimaging investigation of deep brain stimulation in patients with obsessive–compulsive disorder. *J Neurosurg*, 104:558–565.

146. Sturm, V., Lenartz, D., Koulousakis, A., Treuer, H., Herholz, K., Klein, J.C., and Klosterkotter, J. (2003). The nucleus accumbens: a target for deep brain stimulation in obsessive–compulsive- and anxiety-disorders. *J Chem Neuroanat*, 26:293–299.

147. Campbell, K.M., de Lecea, L., Severynse, D.M., Caron, M.G., McGrath, M.J., Sparber, S.B., Sun, L.Y., and Burton, F.H. (1999). OCD-Like behaviors caused by a neuropotentiating transgene targeted to cortical and limbic D1+ neurons. *J Neurosci*, 19:5044–5053.

148. Campbell, K.M., McGrath, M.J., and Burton, F.H. (1999). Differential response of cortical-limbic neuropotentiated compulsive mice to dopamine D1 and D2 receptor antagonists. *Eur J Pharmacol*, 371:103–111.

149. McGrath, M.J., Campbell, K.M., Veldman, M.B., and Burton, F.H. (1999). Anxiety in a transgenic mouse model of cortical-limbic neuro-potentiated compulsive behavior. *Behav Pharmacol*, 10:435–443.

150. Welch, J.M., Lu, J., Rodriguiz, R.M., Trotta, N.C., Peca, J., Ding, J.D., Feliciano, C., Chen, M., Adams, J.P., Luo, J., Dudek, S.M., Weinberg, R.J., Calakos, N., Wetsel, W.C., and Feng, G. (2007). Cortico-striatal synaptic defects and OCD-like behaviours in Sapap3-mutant mice. *Nature*, 448:894–900.

151. Chou-Green, J.M., Holscher, T.D., Dallman, M.F., and Akana, S.F. (2003). Compulsive behavior in the 5-HT2C receptor knockout mouse. *Physiol Behav*, 78:641–649.

152. Berridge, K.C., Aldridge, J.W., Houchard, K.R., and Zhuang, X. (2004). Sequential super-stereotypy of an instinctive fixed action pattern in hyper-dopaminergic mutant mice: a model of obsessive compulsive disorder and Tourette's. *BMC Biology*, 3:1–16.

153. Nonogaki, K., Strack, A.M., Dallman, M.F., and Tecott, L.H. (1998). Leptin-independent hyperphagia and type 2 diabetes in mice with a mutated serotonin 5-HT2C receptor gene. *Nat Med*, 4:1152–1156.

154. Tecott, L.H., Sun, L.M., Akana, S.F., Strack, A.M., Lowenstein, D.H., Dallman, M.F., and Julius, D. (1995). Eating disorder and epilepsy in mice lacking 5-HT2c serotonin receptors. *Nature*, 374:542–546.

155. Vickers, S.P., Clifton, P.G., Dourish, C.T., and Tecott, L.H. (1999). Reduced satiating effect of d-fenfluramine in serotonin 5-HT(2C) receptor mutant mice. *Psychopharmacology (Berl)*, 143:309–314.

156. Rocha, B.A., Goulding, E.H., O'Dell, L.E., Mead, A.N., Coufal, N.G., and Parsons, L.H. (2002). L.H. Tecott, Enhanced locomotor, reinforcing, and neurochemical effects of cocaine in serotonin 5-hydroxytryptamine 2C receptor mutant mice. *J Neurosci*, 22:10039–10045.

157. Tecott, L.H., Logue, S.F., Wehner, J.M., and Kauer, J.A. (1998). Perturbed dentate gyrus function in serotonin 5-HT2C receptor mutant mice. *Proc Natl Acad Sci USA*, 95:15026–15031.

158. Chamberlain, S.R., Blackwell, A.D., Fineberg, N.A., Robbins, T.W., and Sahakian, B.J. (2005). The neuropsychology of obsessive compulsive disorder: the importance of failures in cognitive and behavioural inhibition as candidate endophenotypic markers. *Neurosci Biobehav Rev*, 29:399–419.

159. Gillespie, C.F. and Ressler, K.J. (2005). Emotional learning and glutamate: translational perspectives. *CNS Spectr*, 10:831–839.

160. Davis, M., Ressler, K., Rothbaum, B.O., and Richardson, R. (2006). Effects of D-cycloserine on extinction: translation from preclinical to clinical work. *Biol Psychiat*, 60:369–375.

161. Davis, M. (2002). Role of NMDA receptors and MAP kinase in the amygdala in extinction of fear: clinical implications for exposure therapy. *Eur J Neurosci*, 16:395–398.

162. Ressler, K.J., Rothbaum, B.O., Tannenbaum, L., Anderson, P., Graap, K., Zimand, E., Hodges, L., and Davis, M. (2004). Cognitive enhancers as adjuncts to psychotherapy: use of D-cycloserine in phobic individuals to facilitate extinction of fear. *Arch Gen Psychiat*, 61:1136–1144.

163. Aigner, M., Sachs, G., Bruckmuller, E., Winklbaur, B., Zitterl, W., Kryspin-Exner, I., Gur, R., and Katschnig, H. (2007). Cognitive and emotion recognition deficits in obsessive–compulsive disorder. *Psychiat Res*, 149:121–128.

164. Shapira, N.A., Liu, Y., He, A.G., Bradley, M.M., Lessig, M.C., James, G.A., Stein, D.J., Lang, P.J., and Goodman, W.K. (2003). Brain activation by disgust-inducing pictures in obsessive–compulsive disorder. *Biol Psychiat*, 54:751–756.

165. Bertolino, A., Arciero, G., Rubino, V., Latorre, V., De Candia, M., Mazzola, V., Blasi, G., Caforio, G., Hariri, A., Kolachana, B., Nardini, M., Weinberger, D.R., and Scarabino, T. (2005). Variation of human amygdala response during threatening stimuli as a function of 5'HTTLPR genotype and personality style. *Biol Psychiat*, 57:1517–1525.

166. Hariri, A.R., Mattay, V.S., Tessitore, A. *et al.* (2002). Serotonin transporter genetic variation and the response of the human amygdala. *Science*, 297:400–403.

167. Swerdlow, N.R., Benbow, C.H., Zisook, S., Geyer, M.A., and Braff, D.L. (1993). A preliminary assessment of sensorimotor gating in patients with obsessive compulsive disorder. *Biol Psychiat*, 33:298–301.

168. Hoenig, K., Hochrein, A., Quednow, B.B., Maier, W., and Wagner, M. (2005). Impaired prepulse inhibition of acoustic startle in obsessive–compulsive disorder. *Biol Psychiat*, 57:1153–1158.

169. Yamashita, M., Fukushima, S., Shen, H.W., Hall, F.S., Uhl, G.R., Numachi, Y., Kobayashi, H., and Sora, I. (2006). Norepinephrine transporter blockade can normalize the prepulse inhibition deficits found in dopamine transporter knockout mice. *Neuropsychopharmacology*, 31:2132–2139.

170. Hemmings, S.M., Kinnear, C.J., Niehaus, D.J., Moolman-Smook, J.C., Lochner, C., Knowles, J.A., Corfield, V.A., and Stein, D.J. (2003). Investigating the role of dopaminergic and serotonergic candidate genes in obsessive–compulsive disorder. *Eur Neuropsychopharmacol*, 13:93–98.

171. Linden, A.M. and Schoepp, D.D. (2006). MGLUR targets for neuropsychiatric disorders. *Drug Discov Today Therap Strategies*, 3:507–517.

172. Friedlander, L. and Desrocher, M. (2006). Neuroimaging studies of obsessive–compulsive disorder in adults and children. *Clin Psychol Rev*, 26:32–49.

173. Nakao, T., Nakagawa, A., Yoshiura, T., Nakatani, E., Nabeyama, M., Yoshizato, C., Kudoh, A., Tada, K., Yoshioka, K., Kawamoto, M., Togao, O., and Kanba, S. (2005). Brain activation of patients with obsessive-compulsive disorder during neuropsychological and symptom provocation tasks before and after symptom improvement: a functional magnetic resonance imaging study. *Biol Psychiat*, 57:901–910.

174. Remijnse, P.L., Nielen, M.M., van Balkom, A.J., Cath, D.C., van Oppen, P., Uylings, H.B., and Veltman, D.J. (2006). Reduced orbitofrontal-striatal activity on a reversal learning task in obsessive–compulsive disorder. *Arch Gen Psychiat*, 63:1225–1236.

175. van der Wee, N.J., Ramsey, N.F., van Megen, H.J., Denys, D., Westenberg, H.G., and Kahn, R.S. (2007). Spatial working memory in obsessive-compulsive disorder improves with clinical response: A functional MRI study. *Eur Neuropsychopharmacol*, 17:16–23.

176. Nielen, M.M. and Den Boer, J.A. (2003). Neuropsychological performance of OCD patients before and after treatment with fluoxetine: evidence for persistent cognitive deficits. *Psychol Med*, 33:917–925.

177. McAlonan, K. and Brown, V.J. (2003). Orbital prefrontal cortex mediates reversal learning and not attentional set shifting in the rat. *Behav Brain Res*, 146:97–103.

178. Clarke, H.F., Walker, S.C., Dalley, J.W., Robbins, T.W., and Roberts, A.C. (2007). Cognitive inflexibility after prefrontal serotonin depletion is behaviorally and neurochemically specific. *Cereb Cortex*, 17:18–27.

179. Steckler, T. (2007). Preclinical biomarkers and surrogate markers in depression and anxiety. *Proceedings of Translating Depression and Anxiety Therapeutics, MarcusEvans Conferences*, 11 and 12 January 2007, London, UK.

180. Man, J., Hudson, A.L., Ashton, D., and Nutt, D.J. (2004). Animal models of obsessive compulsive disorder. *Curr Neuropharmacol*, 2:1–7.

181. Pitman, R.K. (1989). Animal models of compulsive behavior. *Biol Psychiat*, 26(2):189–198.

182. Gray, J.A. (1982). *The neuropsychology of anxiety: An enquiry into the functions of the septo-hippocampal system*. Oxford University Press, New York.

183. Malloy, P. (1987). Frontal lobe dysfunction in obsessive compulsive disorder. In Perecman, E. (ed.), *The Frontal Lobes Revisited*. IRBN Press, New York.

184. Pitman, R.K. (1987). A cybernetic model of obsessive–compulsive psychopathology. *Compr Psychiat*, 28:334–343.

CHAPTER 7

Developing More Efficacious Antidepressant Medications: Improving and Aligning Preclinical and Clinical Assessment Tools

John F. Cryan[1], Connie Sánchez[2], Timothy G. Dinan[3] and Franco Borsini[4]

[1]Department of Pharmacology and Therapeutics, School of Pharmacy, University College Cork, Cork, Ireland
[2]Lundbeck Research USA, Inc., Neuroscience, 215 College Road, Paramus, NJ 07652, USA
[3]Department of Psychiatry, Cork University Hospital, University College Cork, Cork, Ireland
[4]Sigma-tau S.p.A., Via Pontina Km 30,400, I-00044 Pomezia, Roma, Italy

Animal and Translational Models for CNS Drug Discovery,
Vol. 1 of 3: Psychiatric Disorders
Robert McArthur and Franco Borsini (eds), Academic Press, 2008

INTRODUCTION

Depression is, according to the World Health Organization, among the top five causes of disability and is a major healthcare problem and thus a serious economic burden for society.[1,2] Current treatments for depression and anxiety disorders are of limited efficacy in many patients and are associated with side effects that reduce compliance in others.[3,4] As all antidepressants currently used exert their primary pharmacological action by altering serotonergic and/or noradrenergic pathways in the brain, substantial research efforts have been directed toward the potential to develop novel, more effective, non-monoamine-based antidepressant medications.[5,6] To date this has proved very difficult and along the way there have been a number of high-profile casualties, most notably the neurokinin (NK)-1 receptor antagonists,[7] which demonstrated an excellent preclinical portfolio but failed in clinical trials.[8,9]

All of the present preclinical tests available in depression research were developed after the clinical introduction of the first generation of antidepressants, the tricyclic antidepressants (TCAs) and monoamine oxidase inhibitors, and are more appropriately viewed as tests predictive of antidepressant-activity, or even more reductionistically, as tests of enhanced monoamine function. There is currently a shift away from these traditional animal models to more focused research dealing with an endophenotype-style approach, selective breeding programs and incorporation of new findings from human neuroimaging and genetic studies.[3,10] Moreover, advances in neuroimaging and in biomarker development are also informing the clinical testing of novel drugs. In this review we assess these new directions and the potential impact that they could have in developing novel therapeutics for depression where there is a huge unmet medical need.

THE CHALLENGES OF DEVELOPING THE NEXT GENERATION OF ANTIDEPRESSANTS

Given the high morbidity of depression in the population[11] coupled with its chronic nature and marked socioeconomic implications, there is a huge impetus from the pharmaceutical industry's perspective to view depression as a lucrative therapeutic area to exploit. However, it is also a highly challenging field in modern drug discovery.[12,13] This is compounded by the fact that unlike other medical disorders where pathology is well characterized (although perhaps not understood) such as diabetes or Parkinson's disease, the underlying pathophysiology of depression is still unresolved.

Depressive disorder is a heterogeneous diagnostic entity that is subdivided into diagnostic subclasses, for example, according to the commonly used diagnostic classification system, diagnostic and statistical manual (DSM-IV[14]) of the American Psychiatric Association, among others, major depressive disorder (MDD), dysthymic disorder, premenstrual dysphoric disorder, minor depressive disorder, recurrent brief depressive disorder, bipolar depression, mood disorder due to a medical condition.[14] The diagnostic system ICD-10 (*International Statistical Classification of Diseases and Related Health Problems*, 10th Edition) provided by the World Health Organization (http://www.who.int/classifications/apps/icd/icd10online/) conveys a similar heterogeneity.

MDD, as defined by DSM-IV, is a common, disabling and potentially life-threatening disease associated with substantial costs to society and the affected patients. According to a recent study the lifetime prevalence of MDD is about 16% and the 1-year prevalence about 6.6%.[15] Depression is often chronic, episodic and with high risk of recurrences. It is therefore often a lifelong disease with the need for long-term treatment. Comorbidity with anxiety disorders is frequent. It is also important to note that depressed patients are at significantly greater risk for a variety of somatic conditions such as heart disease, gastrointestinal disorders and obesity.[16-19] Alarmingly, suicide, invariably associated with emotional disturbance, is now the third largest cause of death among young adults in Western countries.[20] Abnormal emotion is also frequently seen in other neuropsychiatric and neurological diagnoses, ranging from Alzheimer's disease to substance abuse, and can oftentimes precipitate symptoms in these conditions.[14] It is important to appreciate that depression is a syndrome diagnosed by the presence of a cluster of symptoms and not by laboratory investigation. Whilst several biological markers have been described,[21] no marker has sufficient sensitivity and specificity to be of use in the diagnosis of the condition. The diagnosis therefore is essentially based on clinical grounds.[14]

The core feature of depression is a sustained lowering of mood or an anhedonia.[14] The latter refers to an inability to gain enjoyment from aspects of one's life.[22] Other symptoms can be of a psychological or biological nature. The psychological symptoms include low self-esteem, pessimistic thoughts about the future, heightened anxiety, poor concentration and suicidal thoughts. Biological symptoms include insomnia which can take the form of early insomnia where the individual has difficulty falling asleep, middle insomnia where the individual wakes in the middle of the night and delayed insomnia where there is early morning wakening.[23] [i] Anorexia is also a frequent component of the syndrome and may be associated with weight loss.[24] Some atypical forms of depression are accompanied by over sleeping and over eating with carbohydrate craving. This is particularly true with milder forms of depression seen in the community, especially in females. Other biological symptoms include a diurnal variation in mood,[25] which is usually worse in the morning, and significantly decreased libido.[26]

All social classes are vulnerable to depression, though certain studies suggest an increased prevalence in lower socio-economic groups and especially in women living in urban areas with large families and unsupportive spouses.[27] While both males and females suffer from depression, almost all epidemiological studies support the view that the disorder is more common in females.[28] This is in contrast to schizophrenia, which is more common in males.[29] The reason, for the increased risk of the disorder in women has been attributed to both biological and social factors.[30] Women may experience more psychosocial stress than men and there are differences in the neuro-endocrine response to stress in both genders.

The basis of all pharmacological treatments currently used for depression is modulation of the monoaminergic neurotransmitter systems, in particular the serotonergic and noradrenergic systems. The selective serotonin reuptake inhibitors (SSRIs), and the serotonin and noradrenaline reuptake inhibitors (SNRIs) are by far the most commonly used antidepressants. These treatments are used across a variety of diagnostic subcategories within depression and a number of the SSRIs and SNRIs are also

---

[i] Refer to Doran *et al.*, Translational models of sleep and sleep disorders, in this volume for further discussion of sleep and sleep-related disorders.

approved for treatment of anxiety disorders.[31] The introduction of SSRIs in the 1980s resulted in a marked increase of the awareness of depression and treatment of depression mainly because these drugs are much safer and better tolerated than the older TCAs.[4,31] In particular the cardio-toxicity, anticholinergic side effect and weight gain of TCAs are major drawbacks that restrict their use.[32] However, because of the overall somewhat better efficacy, TCAs are still being used in more difficult to treat patient groups after response failure to SSRIs.[32,33]

Limitations of Clinical Assessment

Most clinical trials conducted focus entirely on changes in rating scale measures rather than biomarkers. The most widely used scales for assessing severity of depression are the Hamilton rating scale (HAMD)[34] and the Montgomery–Asberg scale.[35] A score of 17 or above on the HAMD is usually the entry requirement in a study of major depression. The scale has the advantage of being sensitive to change but heavily focusing on somatic symptoms. The Montgomery–Asberg scale is also sensitive to change but more focused on psychological aspects of depression. Response is conventionally defined as a 50% drop in HAMD score, while remission is defined as a score of less than seven. Many pivotal studies of SSRIs have found considerable efficacy in terms of producing response but a large percentage of patients in such studies do not achieve remission.

Is the failure to produce more effective antidepressants due to the insensitivity of current rating measures or the failure to produce genuinely more effectively compounds? While the current rating measures are less than perfect it is unlikely that their lack of sensitivity is the reason for the failure to develop more effective antidepressants. Far more important from a clinical perspective is the relatively broad definition of major depression provided in both DSM-IV and ICD-10. These syndromes are highly heterogeneous and this lack of homogeneity presents a problem in the development of new antidepressants. Furthermore, whilst comorbid personality disorder is usually an exclusion criterion in clinical trials, it is not always easy to firmly diagnose this and undoubtedly such patients end up in trials, presenting an important confounding factor.[ii]

Optimal studies should provide tight inclusion criteria paying special attention to the exclusion of patients with comorbid personality disorder and only allowing patients entry after an adequate period of time and not just 2 weeks as required by the DSM-IV criteria. Whilst regulatory authorities do not require the use of biomarkers, it can be of immense help to include biomarkers, especially those involving the hypothalamic–pituitary–adrenal (HPA) axis, at least in Phase II trials. No amount of alteration to ratings scales will produce dramatic improvements in drug discovery. The main challenges at present are the discovery and validation of more

---

[ii] Refer to McEvoy and Freudenreich, Issues in the design and conductance of clinical trials, in this volume for further discussion of patient selection in clinical trials and the consequences of heterogeneous populations.

sensitive biomarkers and in close connection with more innovative drug development approaches.[36,37 iii]

The Need for Better Antidepressant Therapies

All currently available antidepressants have a relatively long onset of action of about 2–4 weeks, a response rate of 60–70% and, even more importantly, a remission rate of only 40–50% after acute treatment of 6–8 weeks resulting in a substantial number of patients not responding to treatment and becoming therapy resistant.[38] No standard predictors exist in clinical practice to help with the choice of the optimal drug for a particular patient.[38] Furthermore, despite achieving a remission, which is defined by standard depression rating scale scores, residual symptoms may still persist in some patients and affect daily functioning of the patients. Current treatments have shown efficacy in relapse prevention and prophylaxis (prevention of recurrent episodes), but no evidence is seen that antidepressants might significantly alter the chronic course of the disease. Although the SSRIs and SNRIs and other monoaminergic antidepressants have proven to be effective in treatment of depression, there are still significant unmet needs in relation to increasing response and remission rates, relapse prevention, increasing recovery rates, reducing sub-syndromal symptoms, improving tolerability and preventing long-term deterioration and disability. Thus, the most significant unmet need remains increased therapeutic effect and an earlier relief of symptoms.

Challenges in the Discovery of New Antidepressants

Coupled with a clear medical need for new more efficacious antidepressant treatment strategies, there is a growing awareness within the pharmaceutical sector that drug discovery for affective disorders must be accelerated. This need is expedited by the fact that the currently used SSRIs and SNRI will all go off patent within the next few years, resulting in dramatic pricing decreases and at the same time the budgets of national healthcare authorities are being increasingly scrutinized, leading to cost containment measures. Thus, new compounds must be clearly differentiated and superior to current treatments and a direct link must be made between the value of the innovation and the additional cost to payers. Several approaches may be followed to achieve this objective. One approach is to identify biologically better defined patients cohorts that may allow for a more rational drug discovery strategy to demonstrate superiority, for example develop new treatments that target-specific patient populations (e.g., bipolar

---

[iii] For further discussion of biomarkers, refer to Tannock *et al.*, Towards a biological understanding of ADHD and the discovery of novel therapeutic approaches; Bartz *et al.*, Preclinical animal models of Autistic Spectrum Disorders (ASD); Joel *et al.*, Animal models of obsessive-compulsive disorder: From bench to bedside via endophenotypes and biomarkers; Large *et al.*, Developing therapeutics for bipolar disorder: From animal models to the clinic; Winsky *et al.*, Drug discovery and development initiatives at the National Institute of Mental Health: from cell-based systems to proof of concept, in Volume 2, Neurologic Disorders; Lindner *et al.*, Development, optimization and use of preclinical behavioral models to maximize the productivity of drug discovery for Alzheimer's Disease; Montes *et al.*, Translational Research in ALS; Wagner *et al.*, Huntington Disease; or Wilding *et al.*, Anti-obesity drugs: From animal models to clinical efficacy in Volume 3, Reward Deficit Disorders.

disorder, non-responders, melancholic depression), residual depressive symptoms (e.g., cognitive symptoms and sleep disturbances), target disease areas with a high incidence of depression (e.g., stress, impulsivity, chronic pain) or in a more long-term perspective develop drugs that target-specific endophenotypes independent of the current diagnostic system. Target identification and validation represents some of the main barriers for central nervous system (CNS) drug discovery and development in general, and psychiatric disorders in particular.[12,13] The absence of adequate animal models has forced the field to focus on available paradigms, most of which involve exposure of normal animals to various forms of acute or chronic stress. Hence, the development and characterization of better preclinical animal models and clinical biomarkers of the disease will pave the way for the development of novel therapeutics.[3,12,13]

BIOMARKERS AND DEPRESSION

As is the case with most other psychiatric disorders major depression is syndromally diagnosed and lacks biomarkers with high sensitivity and specificity. This lack of biomarkers may be due to the heterogeneous nature of the disorder. The dexamethasone (DEX) suppression test is to date the most widely studied biomarker in psychiatry.[39,40] It is a test of negative feedback in the HPA-axis and, while it has less than optimal sensitivity and specificity, it is generally accepted that it is most reliable when applied to more severe forms of depression.[41] Overall, biomarkers relating to HPA-axis function in major depression have helped identify a series of potentially "druggable" target sites. Thus, it is appropriate to discuss in greater depth the relation between unipolar depression and stress.

Stress and Depression

The underlying brain pathophysiology in depressive disorders remains in essence unknown. Furthermore, given the diagnostic heterogeneity of the condition the underlying biological processes are expected to be multiple with depression associated with profound changes in neurochemical, endocrine, metabolic and inflammatory mechanisms. Stressful life events have a substantial causal association with depression, and there is compelling evidence that even early life stress may constitute a major risk factor.[42-46] Emerging evidence suggests that the combination of genetics, early life stress and ongoing stress may ultimately determine individual responsiveness to stress and the vulnerability.[44] The genetic factors and life stressors may contribute not only to neurochemical alterations, but also to the impairments of cellular plasticity and resilience that occurs in depression.[47,48] Moreover, understanding the alterations in stress sensitivity in depression is at the interface of both clinical biomarker development and in novel animal model characterization.[iv]

[iv] For further discussion of effects of stress and changes in the HPA in other behavioral disorders, refer to Large *et al.*, Developing therapeutics for bipolar disorder: From animal models to the clinic; Steckler *et al.*, Developing novel anxiolytics: Improving preclinical detection and clinical assessment; Tannock *et al.*, Towards a biological understanding of ADHD and the discovery of novel therapeutic approaches, in this volume.

HPA Axis Markers

Over-activity of the HPA axis characterized by hypercortisolism, adrenal hyper-plasia and abnormalities in negative feedback is the most consistently described biological abnormality in melancholic depression.[43,46,49-51] Corticotropin-releas-ing hormone (CRH) and arginine vasopressin (AVP) are the main secretagogues of the HPA/stress system. CRH is a 41 amino acid peptide, originally discovered and sequenced by Vale and colleagues in 1981,[52] is produced in the medial parvicellu-lar neurones of the paraventricular nucleus (PVN) of the hypothalamus. These neu-rones project to the external zone of the median eminence, where CRH is released into the portal vasculature to act on CRH1 receptors at the anterior pituitary. CRH and AVP act synergistically in bringing about adrenocorticotropin (ACTH) release from the corticotropes of the anterior pituitary which in turn stimulates cortisol out-put from the adrenal cortex. Following its identification in 1954, vasopressin, a non-apeptide, was considered the principal factor in the regulation of ACTH release,[53] but the subsequent elucidation of the structure of CRH and the domination of the one neurone/one transmitter principle, the role of CRH came to overshadow that of AVP.[54] This dominance has been reflected in neuroendocrine studies conducted in depression.

AVP is released following a variety of stimuli including increasing plasma osmo-lality, hypovolemia, hypotension and hypoglycemia. It has powerful antidiuretic and vasoconstrictor effects.[55-57] AVP has also been implicated in learning and memory processes.[58] Our knowledge of the functional activity and pharmacology of AVP and its receptors in the regulation of HPA activity rests largely on studies conducted in rodents. AVP is released from the magnocellular system and from the parvicellular neurones of the PVN. AVP-containing cell bodies in the PVN are co-localized with CRH-containing neurones. In control non-stressed rats, within the pool of CRH neu-rosecretory cells, 50% co-express AVP.[59] The PVN serves as an important relay site. It receives projections from ascending catecholaminergic pathways including nor-adrenergic projections from the nucleus of the solitary tract and from the locus coeruleus. The PVN also receives input from areas of the limbic system. Whilst it is evident that almost all of the CRH in the hypophyseal portal blood originates from the hypothalamic PVN, the precise origin of AVP is more controversial. It is thought that the bulk of AVP derives from the PVN. However, morphological and neurochemi-cal studies suggest that AVP from supraoptic magnocellular AVP-secreting cells also access the hypophyseal portal blood[60] though this has not been definitively shown in humans. As with other peptide hormones AVP exerts its effects through interac-tion with specific plasma membrane receptors of which three major subtypes have been identified. V1a receptors are widely distributed on blood vessels, and have also been found in the CNS, including the PVN. V2 receptors are predominantly located in the principal cells of the renal collecting system, although there is some evi-dence for central V2 receptors also. The ACTH releasing properties occur via the V3 (V1b) receptor subtype. *In situ* hybridization studies reveal that V3 receptor mRNA is expressed in the majority of pituitary corticotropes, in multiple brain regions and a number of peripheral tissues including kidney, heart, lung and breast and adrenal medulla.[6]

Synergism of CRH and AVP

Vasopressin has ACTH releasing properties when administered alone in humans, a response that may be dependent on the ambient endogenous CRH level. Following the combination of AVP and CRH, a much greater ACTH response is seen and both peptides are required for maximal pituitary–adrenal stimulation.[60] The precise nature of this synergism is incompletely understood. There may also be distinct corticotrope populations in the anterior pituitary some of which require both AVP and CRH for ACTH release.[60]

Glucocorticoids

Glucocorticoids play a pivotal feedback role in the regulation of the HPA axis. Two types of cortisol binding sites have been described in the brain.[61] The type 1 receptor, which is indistinguishable from the peripheral mineralocorticoid receptor, is distributed principally in the septo-hippocampal region. The type 2 or glucocorticoid receptor has a wider distribution.[61] These receptor systems provide negative feedback loops at a limbic, hypothalamic and pituitary level. Overall the type 1 receptor is thought to mediate tonic influences of cortisol or corticosterone, whilst the type 2 receptor mediates stress-related changes in cortisol levels. Under normal conditions the responsiveness of parvicellular neurones to stress is under marked inhibition by the low resting levels of glucocorticoids.[45]

The sensitivity of CRH and AVP transcription to glucocorticoid feedback is markedly different.[62] CRH mRNA and CRH1 receptor mRNA levels are reduced by elevated glucocorticoids, whereas V3 receptor mRNA levels and coupling of the receptor to phospholipase C are stimulated by glucocorticoids, effects which may contribute to the refractoriness of AVP-stimulated ACTH secretion to glucocorticoid feedback.[60]

Vasopressin in Major Depression

Studies of HPA axis function in depression reveal numerous abnormalities. These abnormalities are most pronounced in depressives with melancholic features.[46] A potential role for AVP in affective illness was forwarded in 1978 by Gold and Goodwin.[63] They postulated from animal studies showing that[1] AVP deficiency produces deficits of behavior, which are reversed when the peptide is replaced and[2] that well-developed systems existed for its distribution throughout the CNS, rendered AVP a suitable candidate for involvement in complex behavioral systems. They also describe the symptom complexes in affective illness that AVP is known to influence, notably memory processes, pain sensitivity, synchronization of biological rhythms and the timing and quality of rapid eye-movement (REM) sleep.

A role for AVP was supported not only by the above spectrum of symptoms but also by dynamic tests of HPA axis activity, and in particular, the "DEX/CRH" test. DEX, a potent synthetic glucocorticoid, binds primarily to glucocorticoid receptor on anterior pituitary corticotropes and, by feedback inhibition, suppresses ACTH and cortisol secretion.[64] In the DEX/CRH test, when healthy subjects are treated with DEX prior to CRH infusion, the release of ACTH is blunted and the extent of blunting is proportional to the dose of DEX.[65] Paradoxically, when depressives are pretreated with DEX they show enhanced ACTH response to CRH. It was postulated that VP-mediated ACTH release was responsible for this finding. The combined DEX/CRH test is estimated to have a sensitivity of 80% in differentiating healthy subjects from depressives.[66]

Surprisingly, there are relatively few data on plasma AVP levels in depression. An early report found no change in plasma AVP levels in depression.[67] In contrast, van London *et al.*[68] reported basal plasma levels of AVP to be elevated. In the later study AVP concentrations were found to be higher in the depressed cohort, with greater elevation in in-patient compared to out-patient depressives and in those with melancholic features. A number of studies have shown a significant positive correlation between peripheral plasma levels of AVP and hypercortisolemia in patients with unipolar depression.[69] A postmortem study of depressed subjects reported an increased number of vasopressin-expressing neurones in paraventricular hypothalamic neurones.[70] Radsheer *et al.*[71] has also shown an increase in the number of CRH-neurones in depressives.

Dynamic Tests of HPA Function and the VP-ergic System

Dinan *et al.*[72] examined a cohort of depressed subjects on two separate occasions, with CRH alone, and with the combination of CRH and the synthetic analog of vasopressin desmopressin (ddAVP). A significant blunting of ACTH output to CRH alone was noted. Following the combination of CRH and ddAVP, the release of ACTH in depressives and healthy volunteers was indistinguishable. It was concluded that whilst the CRH1 receptor is downregulated in depression, that a concomitant upregulation of the V3 receptor takes place. This is consistent with the animal models of chronic stress, described below, in which a switching from CRH to AVP regulation is observed. It is interesting that in CRH1 receptor-deficient mice, basal plasma AVP levels are significantly elevated, AVP mRNA is increased in the PVN and there is increased AVP-like immunoreactivity in the median eminence.[73]

In a recent study further evidence has been provided for the upregulation of the anterior pituitary V3 receptor function, assessed as an augmented ACTH and cortisol response to ddAVP in depressed patients.[18] Treatment with fluoxetine (Prozac®) decreases CSF levels of CRH and AVP[74] but [see[75]]. Larger studies are required before any formal conclusions can be drawn about antidepressant effect on central AVP activity. More recently, genetic haplotype studies have implicated the vasopressin system in depression with the identification of five single nucleotide polymorphisms in the V1b receptor gene in patients with major depression thus they describe as a protective haplotype.[76] In a recent study Dempster *et al.*[77] also implicate the V1b gene in early onset depression especially in females.

HPA axis as Antidepressant Target

Clinical studies to date indicate several potential antidepressant target sites within the HPA axis.[46,49] Given the earlier analysis it is clear that the V1b receptor is a potential target site and studies of compounds targeting the receptor in animal models support the clinical observations[78]; however, the clinical value of a V1b receptor antagonist remains to be shown. Many pharmaceutical companies continue to pursue the CRH1 receptor site as a potential therapeutic target.[79][v] However, from a purely endocrine perspective this strategy is problematic as the receptor is downregulated in major depression. It is therefore unlikely an antagonist will remedy the hypercortisolism characteristic of severe depression. An alternative strategy involves the antagonism of the glucocorticoid receptor and RU 486 and analogs have been used in this regards. It has been suggested that this strategy is most likely to be effective in psychotic depression.[80] A related approach involves the inhibition of cortisol synthesis and a variety of drugs have been employed including metyrapone (Metopirone®) and ketoconazole (Nizoral®.[81,82]) While numerous studies have been conducted using the approach and most report positive findings they can generally be criticized because of small sample size and tolerability appears to be an issue. Enhancing negative feedback using steroids such as DEX has been advocated. In the best study of its kind, Arana et al.[83] administered DEX 4 mg/kg/day for 4 days or placebo. All patients then received placebo for 21 days. On study completion those receiving DEX at baseline were significantly improved relative to those receiving placebo throughout the study. Thus further bolstering the link between HPA axis and depression.

Lessons from Clinical Studies of HPA-Axis Modulating Drug Candidates

Clinical trials in the USA are reported in www.clinicaltrial.com but there is no systematic information on clinical trials in other countries of the world. The trend is also that pharmaceutical companies report their clinical trials on their web site and commit to publish the results of all clinical studies; however, this is not being adhered to by all companies yet. Earlier but less detailed sources of information about clinical studies may be company press releases. Based on these various sources of information it appears that among stress axis modulating compounds, mifepristone (Mifeprex®), a GR antagonist, has been in clinical Phase II since 1985 and it seems that it has entered Phase III in 2007. Another GR antagonist, ORG34517, has been in Phase II since 2002. R121919, a CRH1 receptor antagonist, appears to have been in clinical Phase I/II since 2001. Two other CRH1 receptor antagonists, NBI34041 and SB723620, were in Phase I in 2002 but no more information is available. Thus, it seems that clinical trials with these compounds are difficult to run. If the reasons of such difficulty are due to safety issues, lack of efficacy or "druggability" issues or a combination is unknown. The V1b receptor antagonist, SSR149415, entered Phase II in 2007. In spite of these apparently disappointing results, companies still seem to believe in the concept and four CRH1 receptor antagonists are in the preclinical stage (i.e., DPC-368 (Bristol-Myers Squibb), NB-876008 (Neurocrine Biosciences), ONO-2333Ms (Ono) and CP-154,526 (Pfizer)). However, the latter has not moved phase since 1996. The GR antagonist, ORG-34850 (Organon) is also reported to be at the preclinical stage. Thus, so far there are no drugs acting on the stress system that has confirmed antidepressant activity in clinical Phase III, despite the many years that scientists have been working in this area.

---

[v] See also Steckler et al., Developing novel anxiolytics: Improving preclinical detection and clinical assessment, in this volume.

PRECLINICAL MODELS OF DEPRESSION IN DRUG DISCOVERY

The lack of understanding of the underlying pathophysiology of the state(s) of depression has always been a major challenge for the validity of preclinical models used to discover antidepressants. Clearly, a better understanding of the pathophysiology of these disorders and the development of novel, improved therapeutic treatments would fill a major unmet medical need. However, the cost of Phase II and Phase III clinical trials in pharmaceutical drug development is enormous and growing annually[84] with the cost of CNS drug development higher than that of any other major therapeutic area.[85] Further, clinical research in psychiatry is burdened, as in many medical disease trials, with a very high placebo response.[86] As a result, before embarking on costly trials, pharmaceutical companies and research funding agencies increasingly seek assurance that any specific biological target is indeed relevant to the disease. Thus, there is a growing emphasis on first obtaining proof that a new chemical entity designed to alter the function of a specific target will do so predictably and safely. Of central importance to this approach is the availability of valid preclinical animal models for evaluating the potential utility of novel pharmacotherapeutics.[3] Moreover, blame for clinical trial failures involves criticism directed toward preclinical models, which attempt to model depression.[87] However, it is becoming clear that increased interaction between clinical and basic sciences is allowing new insights into the generation of tractable, valid and translational animal models. There have been a number of recent reviews focusing on animal models of depression.[3,88,89]

The classical requirements of preclinical models for drug discovery have been that they should be cost effective and easy to use with a relatively high throughput so that results are provided within a short time frame and fed back to allow for further refinement of the molecule.[90] Traditional approaches have therefore been to use mechanistic *in vitro* assays and simple high throughput *in vivo* models closely related to particular mechanisms of action (i.e., inhibition of 5-HT or NA reuptake or monoamine oxidase inhibition), for example antagonism of reserpine-, tetrabenazine- or clonidine-induced behavioral effects; and potentiation of tryptophan-, 5-hydroxytryptophan, apomorphine- or yohimbine-induced behavioral effects in combination with high-throughput models with a high level of predictive validity but low level of face and construct validity such as the forced swim test.[87] More complex preclinical models (e.g., stress based or genetically selected) that show some level of face and construct validity to symptoms associated with depression but often with a limited exploration of predictive validity have typically been investigated more in academic settings and to a less extent played a role for discovery of drugs.[vi]

[vi] For further discussion of screening assays in drug discovery, refer to Bartz *et al.*, Preclinical animal models of Autistic Spectrum Disorders (ASD); Large *et al.*, Developing therapeutics for bipolar disorder (BPD): from animal models to the clinic; Steckler *et al.*, Developing novel anxiolytics: Improving preclinical detection and clinical assessment; McCann *et al.*, Drug discovery and development for reward disorders: Views from government, in this volume; Klitgaard *et al.*, Animal and translational models of the epilepsies; Lindner *et al.*, Development, optimization and use of preclinical behavioral models to maximize the productivity of drug discovery for Alzheimer's Disease; Montes *et al.*, Translational Research in ALS, in Volume 2, Neurologic Disorders; Heidbreder, Impulse and reward deficit disorders: Drug discovery

Future Challenges for Preclinical Models in Drug Discovery

An inherent bias and obvious weakness in the use of classical tests is that they have been pharmacologically validated with agents, *albeit* clinically active, that modulate the monoamine neurotransmitter systems. This reliance on pharmacological isomorphism can limit their predictive validity for novel drugs working through a monoaminergic mechanism of action, while the predictive validity for compounds with novel therapeutically relevant mechanisms such as peptide receptor mechanisms, or interactions with glutamate receptors is largely unknown.[5,6,9,88,90-94][vii] With the increasing demand for novelty and significant clinical advantages of antidepressants in the future, there is an associated increased need for novelty in preclinical models and for a strengthening of the interface between clinical and preclinical research to enable forward as well as backward translational between the two disciplines.

This strengthening of the link between preclinical and clinical research will be essential for future success at all levels of the drug discovery and drug development process, in particular for the early stages of target identification and target validation and for the transition of a drug candidate into the clinical programs. The lead identification and lead optimization stages in drug discovery will still rely on simple mechanism defined *in vitro* and *in vivo* readouts with reasonable throughput addressing key efficacy, Drug Metabolism/PharmacoKinetic (DMPK) studies and tolerability criteria. For example at the level of target identification and target validation, information from clinical biomarker studies, pharmacogenomics/genetics, imaging studies, etc., may provide insight into the underlying pathophysiology and thereby provide ideas for novel treatment approaches and preclinical models. When novel mechanisms are being evaluated as therapeutic principles the risk of failure increases. Given the huge investment that development of a new drug requires there is a strong need to reduce the risk of clinical failure as much as possible and as early as possible in the drug development process. Optimization of the translation between preclinical and clinical models will play an important role in reducing this risk. Thus a paradigm shift in how new antidepressants are going to be discovered seems unavoidable. This is an onerous task that requires new forms of collaboration between industry and academia in order to be successful.

and development; McCann *et al.*, Drug discovery and development for reward disorders: Views from government; Markou *et al.*, Contribution of animal models and preclinical human studies to medication development for nicotine dependence in Volume 3, Reward Deficit Disorders.

[vii] For further discussion regarding the pharmacological isomorphism validation of animal models of behavioral disorders, refer to Joel *et al.*, Animal models of obsessive-compulsive disorder: From bench to bedside via endophenotypes and biomarkers; Large *et al.*, Developing therapeutics for bipolar disorder (BPD): From animal models to the clinic; Steckler *et al.*, Developing novel anxiolytics: Improving preclinical detection and clinical assessment in this volume; Lindner *et al.*, Development, optimization and use of preclinical behavioral models to maximize the productivity of drug discovery for Alzheimer's disease, in Volume 3, Neurologic Disorders.

Traditional Animal Models of Depression

An ideal animal model of depression would be to have identical causative factors, symptomatology and treatment modalities (see[95]).[viii] However, a number of symptoms of depression are clearly not measurable in preclinical paradigms, such as recurrent thoughts of death or suicide, or excessive thoughts of guilt. It is clear that evolutionary progression has provided humans with a much more elaborated cerebral cortex, that facilitates integration of complex psychological concepts also relevant to human depression, such as self-esteem and the ability to perceive the future, that are absent in mice (see[3,89]) Additionally, given the dearth of understanding concerning the causative factors, and the pathophysiology of the disease state in humans, this precludes basing animal models solely on etiology.[88]

Despite these limitations a number of diverse animal models of depression have been widely used and many show substantial predictive validity (i.e., antidepressant administration reverses the behavioral parameters assessed). As discussed earlier, these animal models have all been validated since the introduction of clinically approved monoamine-based medications.[10,95] This also renders the predictive validity of the models unclear until a novel acting compound from preclinical testing is successful applied in man. There have been numerous reviews written regarding the majority of these animal models, which are summarized in Table 7.1, and as such we will not discuss them individually in this review but direct the interested reader to the references.

The majority of the current tests are stressor based and while there is evidence for a link between stress and depression this does not always follow (see[10]). Another difficulty with animal models is the requirement for reproducibility between laboratories, which implies controlling all possible elements of the test.[96,97] Additionally, as was shown with the recent modifications introduced to the traditional forced swim test, a degree of flexibility is required to refine individual models.[88,98] Ultimately, validation of the utility of such animal models awaits the clinical approval of a novel compound, which is active in the models. An example of the limitation of traditional animal models is represented by the failure in clinical Phase II trials of flibanserin, a 5-HT_{1A} receptor agonist and a 5-HT_{2A} receptor antagonist.[99] This compound was found to be active in 10 out of 13 animal models tested.[99] It was active in the learned helpless test in rats, in the bulbectomized rat, in the chronic mild stress in rats and mice, in muricidal rats, in the amphetamine withdrawal and REM sleep latency in rats, in the forced swimming test in mice and in fixed ratio test in mice. However, flibanserin failed in the forced swimming test and in the differential reinforcement 72s test in

---

[viii] Please refer to Koob, The role of animal models in reward deficit disorders: Views from academia, in this volume; Large *et al.*, Developing therapeutics for bipolar disorder (BPD): From animal models to the clinic; Steckler *et al.*, Developing novel anxiolytics: Improving preclinical detection and clinical assessment in Volume 2, Psychiatric Disorders; Lindner *et al.*, Development, optimization and use of preclinical behavioral models to maximize the productivity of drug discovery for Alzheimer's disease; Wagner *et al.*, Huntington Disease, in Volume 3, Neurologic Disorders for further discussion regarding concepts of validity in animal models of behavioral disorders and differences in modeling behavioral disorders in animals and the procedures used to assess changes in behavior.

Table 7.1 Traditional animal models used in depression research

Animal model	Description	References
Forced swim test (rats and mice)	Rodents, placed in an inescapable container of water swim more following antidepressant administration.	188,189
Modified swim test (rats)	Same as above but swimming and climbing behaviors are separated and are increased with serotonergic or catecholaminergic antidepressants respectively.	98,190
Tail suspension test	Rodents, chiefly mice, when hung from the tail will adopt an immobile posture. antidepressants treatment increases the time animals spend in active behaviors.	191
Learned helplessness (rats and mice)	Animals exposed to inescapable shocks subsequently fail to escape when able to. Antidepressants treatment increases the number of escapes – not all animals develop this helpless behavior.	165
Olfactory bulbectomy (rats and mice)[a]	Removal of the olfactory bulbs causes a constellation of behavioral and neurochemical alterations, which are only reversed by chronic antidepressants treatment.	192–194
DRL-72[b] (rats)	Reinforcement of responses with inter-responses longer than 72 s. Antidepressant administration improves the number of reinforced trials.	195
Maternal deprivation	When animals are separated from the mother during early postnatal life they can develop a number of depression-like behavioral characteristics. These behaviors are not present in all animals subjected to this treatment.	196–198
Neonatal clomipramine administration (rats and mice)	When exposed to neonatal clomipramine adult animals display a number of symptoms analogous to depression, including decreased reward seeking, aggressiveness and sexual behavior. Antidepressants treatment can reverse behaviors.	199
Social stress in shrews	Tree shrews form stable dominant/subordinate relationship with subordinate showing behavioral and neurochemical alterations similar to depressed patients. A number of these alterations can be reversed with antidepressants treatment but model requires further validation.	200
Chronic mild stress	Animals are subjected to a variety of unpredictable stressors, which leads to a constellation of symptoms, which are reversed by antidepressant treatment.	201–203

Table 7.1 (Continued)

Animal model	Description	References
Agonistic behavior	Animals are subjected to repeated agonistic encounters; chronic (but not acute) antidepressant treatment will increase rodent aggressive behavior as an indicator of increased assertive behavior.	204
Flinders Sensitive rats	Rats bred for cholinergic sensitivity display a wide spectrum of behavioral alterations sensitive to reversal by antidepressants.	170

[a] *See Large et al., Developing therapeutics for bipolar disorder: From animal models to the clinic in this volume, for further discussion of the bulbectomized rat as a model of bipolar disorder-like behavior.*
[b] *Differential-reinforcement of low response rate 72 s (DRL-72).*

rats, and in the tail suspension in mice. Nevertheless, the data indicated that it could exert antidepressant action faster than imipramine (Tofranil®) or fluoxetine, as shown in chronic mild stress and learned helplessness tests.[99] However, flibanserin did not meet the expectations in clinical trials. In the same battery of animal models, the SSRIs citalopram (Celexa®) and escitalopram (Lexapro®) showed activity,[100,101] but in contrast to flibanserin, both of these drugs resulted demonstrated antidepressant potential in humans and these simple models were even able to differentiate these two drugs in terms of efficacy and time to effect. Thus, the use of a broad range of conventional models predictive of antidepressant activity is necessary, but not sufficient to ensure clinical success even for monoaminergic acting compounds. The question may arise whether addition of more translational preclinical measures (e.g., *in vivo* receptor occupancy, sleep EEG, etc.) could have predicted the clinical failure of flibanserin.

Animal Model of Depression or Test of Antidepressant Activity

The distinction between a model and a test is not always made clear and as a result sometimes a test is called a model.[ix] While a model is comprised of both an independent variable, known as the inducing manipulation, and a dependent variable,[10,95] that is a behavioral/neurochemical readout, a test simply comprises of the later variable. Since the underlying pathophysiology of mood disorders is poorly understood this has had a knock-on effect in choosing independent variables. However, in recent years,

---

[ix] As indicated by the authors, historically, there has been a good deal of confusion regarding the terms "models" and "tests or procedures" used in behavioral research. The interested reader is invited to consult Steckler *et al.*, Developing novel anxiolytics: Improving preclinical detection and clinical assessment in this volume; Lindner *et al.*, Development, optimization and use of preclinical behavioral models to maximize the productivity of drug discovery for Alzheimer's Disease; Wagner *et al.*, Huntington Disease, in Volume 2, Neurologic Disorders; Koob, The role of animal models in reward deficit disorders: Views from academia; Markou *et al.*, Contribution of animal models and preclinical human studies to medication development for nicotine dependence, in Volume 3, Reward Deficits Disorders for further discussion regarding "models" or procedures.

the increased clinical experimental evidence has provided preclinical researchers with more information with which to design the independent variable and therefore garner more information about the underlying etiology of mood disorders. This has also been aided by the relatively recent focus on an endophenotype-based approach to study psychiatric disorders.[3,10,102-104]

Endophenotype-style Approaches

The traditional models of depression rely mainly on a small number of final readouts following a stressor. However, given the lack of antidepressants with novel mechanisms being derived using this approach there has been a shift toward using alternative approaches to the study of depression. Recently, a more focused approach has been taken to study psychiatric disorders in preclinical laboratories, which attempts to assess only one symptom, or marker, of the disease.[105] This approach aims to identify putative endophenotypes characteristic of diseases and model them independently rather than the whole syndrome *per se*.[103,104] The term endophenotype, in a psychiatric context, was coined by Gottesman and Shields in the early 1970s,[106] where they described it as an internal phenotypes that emerges from the pathway between genes and the disease state. Fundamental to the concept is the assumption that the genetic basis of variations of the given endophenotypes between patients and control subjects are fewer than those involved in the manifestation of a complex disorder *per se*.[102,104] Thus employing endophenotypic approaches provides a means for identifying the genetic basis of specific clinical phenotypes, in addition to aiding the analysis of the phenotypic consequences of genes being turned on or off.[102,104] More recently, Hasler and colleagues have outlined the methods available to identify endophenotypes which may include neuropsychological, cognitive, neurophysiological, neuroanatomical, and biochemical measures.[104] [x]

This approach has the benefit of simplifying a complex disorder, such as depression, into individual behaviors, which are more easily defined and thus measurable in both patients and laboratory animals and which more likely, share a common genetic underpinning.[102,107] Such endophenotypes of depression that can be easily modeled in animals include psychomotor alterations, hedonic deficit (lowered response to rewarding and pleasurable stimuli), appetite and weight alterations, circadian and sleep disturbances, and cognitive deficits. However, care must be taken when using this approach for concerns of pseudospecificity may arise, as even those endophenotypes considered as "core" symptoms in depression can, and usually are, present in other diseases.[108] That said, there are those that argue that the pursuit of specific screens for testing drugs may be inappropriate, given the substantial comorbidity of psychiatric illness. There exist a number of criteria, which have been proposed to evaluate

---

[x] For further discussion regarding endophenotypes and their role in current model development, refer to Bartz *et al.*, Preclinical animal models of autistic spectrum disorders (ASD); Joel *et al.*, Animal models of obsessive-compulsive disorder: From bench to bedside via endophenotypes and biomarkers; Steckler *et al.*, Developing novel anxiolytics: Improving preclinical detection and clinical assessment; Tannock *et al.*, Towards a biological understanding of ADHD and the discovery of novel therapeutic approaches; Large *et al.*, Developing therapeutics for bipolar disorder: From animal models to the clinic, in this volume.

the relevance of different endophenotypes, including specificity to the disease of interest, heritability and biological relevance to the disease state.[104] Therefore, depression can be broken down to a number of symptomatic clusters and assessed independently in basic research. Here, we focus on three potential endophenotypes.

Anhedonia

One of the most studied potential endophenotypes of depression is anhedonia, the loss of pleasure or interest in normally rewarding stimuli. Anhedonia represents an extremely tractable, quantitative, symptom to study, both in human experimental medicine and in preclinical research. Anhedonia has been used as a behavioral endpoint for a number of the existing animal models of depression, such as chronic mild stress and maternal separation, with sucrose preference being measured.[88,108,109] Anhedonia can be easily monitored in rodents as an altered responding for appetitive stimuli.[108,109] Recently, Pizzagalli and colleagues used a signal detection task, which measures whether a subject perceives an ambiguous stimulus as being similar to an emotionally charged target stimulus to assess differentially reinforced stimuli, and found that depressed patients do not exhibit a normal bias for stimuli associated with higher reinforcement (rewarding stimuli).[110] It should be possible to devise analogous experiments in mice. Clinical studies are attempting to design approaches to assess anhedonia. Similar to these findings, Shestyuk *et al.*,[111] demonstrated that depressed patients display decreased brain activity when processing positive, but not negative, stimuli compared with controls during a working memory task. This study assessed the slow wave component of event-related potentials, which are proposed to relate to neural activity of sustained processing of information. These findings closely parallel to a positron emission tomography (PET) imaging study, which demonstrated that depressed patients show less activation of the orbitofrontal cortex to reward expectation.[112] This region has been shown in numerous human and primate studies to be important in reward expectation and value.[113,114] This suggests that depressed patients exhibit decreased cognitive processing of positive stimuli despite having intact behavioral responses in this relatively easy task.

It is possible to conceive of similar tasks, which could be applied in preclinical research to assess such response biases and brain activity. A task, which favored a reward for a particular stimulus could then be the final read-out following behavioral, genetic or pharmacological manipulations, which would enable greater insight into the circuitry involved and a closer correlation with human studies.

The brain reward system (BRS) has been extensively studied in preclinical research and began with the chance finding that rats would return to areas of their environment, in which they had received a direct intracranial stimulation.[115] Since this discovery, adaptation of the stimulus to be coupled to a lever press or wheel turn has greatly advanced our understanding of the reward processing.[xi] This technique, termed

---

[xi] Please refer to Koob, The role of animal models in reward deficit disorders: Views from academia; Markou *et al.*, Contribution of animal models and preclinical human studies to medication development for nicotine dependence; Rocha *et al.*, Development of medications for heroin and cocaine addiction and regulatory aspects of abuse liability testing in Volume 3, Reward Deficit Disorders for further discussion on ICSS and the BRS.

intracranial self-stimulation (ICSS) has shown that a number of structures will support this behavior, including the VTA, amygdala, nucleus accumbens, lateral hypothalamus and anterior cingulate cortex. ICSS represents a powerful technique with which to study the BRS as there is no satiation or tolerance to the stimulation, responding remains stable for long periods of time (weeks to months) and it by-passes sensory inputs.[116-119] A number of brain regions which support ICSS responding have been demonstrated from human neuroimaging studies to have altered activity in MDD patients and therefore ICSS responding may represent a novel behavioral measurement of the BRS with which to study depression preclinically. Indeed, in recent years, a number of studies have attempted to assess the effects of chronic mild stress[120] and drug withdrawal[121] using ICSS. More extensive use of the ICSS procedure in preclinical research would provide invaluable insights into the time-course of alterations to the reward pathways and anhedonic-like behavior. Although, there has not been substantial research of the reward pathway in depression, a number of recent studies have shown that this system appears to be hypersensitive in depressed patients.[122-124] Depression severity was closely correlated with the rewarding effects of d-amphetamine administration, with mild/moderate depressives reacting similarly to controls but severely depressed patients reacting much greater.[124] Similarly, two studies using d-amphetamine demonstrated a hypersensitivity in severely depressed patients.[122,123] The adaptation of a translational approach to study brain reward pathways in animals and humans can only help in the discovery of drugs for specific depression endophenotypes. However, as it has already been noted, anhedonia is not a specific endophenotypes for depression but is also a core feature of the negative symptoms of schizophrenia and may be a tractable endophenotypes of this disorder too.[125] One other concern arises in terms of developing therapies that directly target reward circuitry, as such treatments may be burdened with an abuse liability due to their ability to alter the same neurochemical pathways as abused drugs.[xii]

Cognitive Function

Cognitive impairments, including decreased ability to concentrate, decreased learning and memory and deficits in executive function (the ability to plan and participate in goal-directed behavior) are observed in depressed patients; indeed decreased concentration is a DSM-IV criteria of the disease.[14] Although impairments have been reported in attention, working memory, verbal fluency and planning in depressed patients, such findings are not consistent (see[126] for review). This is likely to represent the heterogeneity of the patients used in the tests and also to methodological differences between studies. The deficits in cognition can be partially explained from neuroimaging studies demonstrating decreased activity in many regions of the frontal cortex,[127] as executive function has been shown to be dependent on these regions.[126,128] For example, in the Stroop color-word test, when incongruent word and color are paired, activity in the anterior cingulate cortex is increased compared with a congruent trial and depressed

---

[xii] Please refer to Rocha *et al.*, Development of medications for heroin and cocaine addiction and regulatory aspects of abuse liability testing in Volume 3, Reward Deficit Disorders for further discussion regarding abuse liability of candidate drugs interacting with the BRS.

patients do worse in this test. Additionally, the hippocampus has been shown to be involved in long-term memory retrieval and decreased hippocampal volume is amongst one of the most consistent findings in studies of depressed patients.[129-133] The hippocampal volume loss is also dependent on the duration of MDD rather than the severity of the symptoms.[134] Repetitive stress in rodents has been shown to cause dendritic shortening in the CA3 field of the hippocampus, as well as in the medial prefrontal cortex but increased dendritic growth in the amygdala.[135] Increased understanding of the underlying molecular mechanisms of this phenomenon could lead to increased understanding of the volume loss and decreased activity seen in the frontal cortex, or increased activity in the amygdala of depressed patients. Thus a deeper biological understanding of the impaired neuronal plasticity associated with impaired cognition in depression and how antidepressants may modulate the molecular mechanisms linked to neuronal plasticity is likely to lead to novel and improved therapeutic approaches. The observation that apparently all antidepressant drugs and electroconvulsive shock therapy (ECT) as well as physical exercise stimulate hippocampal neurogenesis, and that chronic stress produces the opposite effect, has created a lot of interest in this field of research, though the functional significance in cognitive processing remains to be understood better in order to evaluate the potential for identification of novel drug targets.[136,137]

Sleep and Circadian Rhythm Disturbances

Sleep disturbance is a key aspect of depression, with 90% of patients suffering from MDD complaining about their sleep and these complaints are often the reason why they search out medical help.[138] Similarly pronounced disturbances of the circadian rhythms are closely associated with depression and there is a growing interest in understanding the role of the circadian clock in depression.[139] Although, sleep and circadian rhythm disturbances are common in numerous psychiatric illnesses, the high level of disturbance seen in MDD suggests that investigation of sleep architecture, circadian biology and the underlying biological processes in their regulation could shed light on aspects of the underlying pathophysiology of depression and lead to novel and improved therapeutic approaches.[140] [xiii] Additionally, almost every clinically approved antidepressant, as well as ECT, increases REM latency and decreases total REM sleep and has effects on the overall sleep architecture.[141] Development of the novel antidepressant drug, agomelatine (Valdoxan®), which is a melatonin receptor agonist and 5-HT$_{2C}$ receptor antagonist is the first initiative to target depression specifically with this approach in mind.[142-147] In addition to having some antidepressant properties in short-term trials agomelatine rapidly relieves sleep complaints.[23] Its approval as antidepressant in Europe is still pending as agomelatine was not shown to be sufficiently active on a long-term study (Doc. Ref. EMEA/267703/2006). Experience from clinical use of agomelatine in the future may provide further insight into the value of this strategy. Sleep deprivation research is another area that may bring

---

[xiii] Please refer to Doran *et al.*, Translational models of sleep and sleep disorders, in this volume for further discussion regarding sleep disturbances as risk factors for mood disorders.

forward novel therapeutics.[148] One night of total sleep deprivation reduces depressive symptoms in an estimated 50% of patients.[149] The decrease in REM sleep appears to be related to serotonin levels.[141,150,151] These findings have been replicated in 5-HT$_{1A}$ receptor knockout mice[152] and Rouen mice, which have altered 5-HT$_{1A}$ receptor activity and display decreased sleep latency.[153] In two other genetic models of depression, Flinders Sensitive Line and congenitally learned helpless rats, elevations in REM sleep and decreases in REM latency have been observed in the lines displaying depression-like behaviors. Another interesting line of research is focusing on understanding the functional role of the deep stages of non-REM sleep in depression.[154] It will be of interest to observe whether drugs that prolong this sleep stage may have antidepressant potential. Increased use of sleep monitoring using EEG techniques in behavioral paradigms may help to generate more confidence in the model and gain further insights into this potential depression endophenotype.[3] The ready availability of sleep EEG measurements in animals, facilitates the direct translational need between preclinical and clinical research.[155]

GENETIC APPROACHES: TOWARD NEW TARGETS

Over the past two decades efforts to gain a better understanding of the underlying pathophysiology of neuropsychiatric disorders are driven by technical advances in the field of molecular genetics.[156,157] Indeed, it is hoped that the recent elucidation and the ongoing functionalization of the human genome may provide new insights into the etiology, course and thence treatment strategies for psychiatric illnesses. One of the most important advances in understanding psychiatric disorders has been the development of mice with genetically altered expression of a specific protein, be it a receptor, transporter, enzyme or signal transduction molecule.[3,157,158] These new tools have the potential to examine novel targets for disorders for which few established pharmacological tools exist. Additionally, these mice will enable the better testing of the validity of current molecular theories of various psychiatric disorders. However, care must be taken when using knockout mice, as compensatory changes can occur due to the lifelong ablation of a protein and it may in fact be such alterations that result in the behavioral phenotype.[159,160] More recently, inducible and site-specific knock-outs have been generated, which enable the role of proteins to be assessed in adult mice negating the compensatory effects.[156,157] Similar strategies can also be used to knock-in specific genes, which lead to an over-expression of the protein. One novel strategy is the use of RNA interference which can be used in adult animals to knockdown specific genes *in vivo* thus overcoming the issue of developmental compensation and enhance target validation efforts in drug discovery.[161-165] The development and refinement of more mouse-specific behavioral models has also expanded the strength of genetically modified mice and as such they represent a powerful tool with which to study the role of specific proteins in depression.[3,166]

Coupled with advances in mouse genetics, there also has been a remarkable upsurge in the development of rodent models which have been genetically selected based on a specific behavioral response relevant to depression.[153,167-170] Further, increased focus is being placed on the molecular basis of resilience to stress-induced depression-like behaviors within a given population of rodent.[171] [xiv] Together with these selected lines such approaches are poised to serve as powerful substrates for understanding the neurobiological and genetic basis of behavioral processes and neuropsychiatric disorders.

Both genetically targeted and selectively bred rodent lines have also great potential[172,173] for delineating the complex gene X environment interactions that underpin predisposition to many behavioral traits and subsequently neuropsychiatric disorders.[174,175] The success of genetic approaches in basic psychiatric and neurological research is contingent on the usefulness of available behavioral models. Therefore, increasing research efforts have also been directed toward developing and refining specific behavioral tests for such analysis.[3,166,176,177]

PERSPECTIVES

Presently, with the advances in techniques to study affective disorders in humans, there is an opportunity to incorporate such findings into preclinical research. In this context, while translational medicine in basic research and drug discovery efforts necessitates valid animal models of human disease, this approach is a two-way bridge. While preclinical research to an increasing extent provides detailed information on the relation between pharmacodynamic and pharmacokinetic measures and occupancy at relevant drug targets and suggestions for relevant biomarkers and translational measures to facilitate the entry into clinical development, the converse is also essential.[108] The trend in clinical development programs for novel drug candidates is to conduct several small exploratory clinical studies in well-defined patient populations or healthy subjects and to include collection of blood samples and other measure for biomarker identification and validation. In addition to providing guidance to the design of the big confirmatory Phase III studies these initiatives may provide insight into basic biological mechanisms and thereby guide identification of novel drug targets. The development of clinical research tools that are informed by, and can parallel rather than specifically recapitulate, rodent models of depression may well be the most fruitful path to understanding these diseases. Additionally, the increased awareness of the need for cooperation between psychiatrists and behavioral neuroscientists has lead to a more endophenotype-based approach to study single symptomatic clusters. Such approaches have been employed by investigators assessing cognitive dysfunction in neuropsychiatric disorders such as schizophrenia and Huntington's disease with considerable success.[178] [xv]

One area of research where clinical research currently outpaces laboratory research is in the field of non-invasive brain imaging. There has been a recent explosion of data on the neural circuits underlying anxiety or mood disorders from the field of psychiatric neuroimaging.[179,180] These findings should serve to inform laboratory studies that use mouse models to allow for the testing of experimental questions that are

---

[xiv] Please refer to Klitgaard *et al.*, Animal and translational models of the epilepsies in Volume 2, Neurologic Disorders for further discussion on treatment resistance and how animal models are being developed to study them.

[xv] See also Jones *et al.*, Developing new drugs for schizophrenia: From animals to the clinic, in this volume and Wagner *et al.*, Huntington Disease, in Volume 2, Neurologic Disorders.

not feasible in human studies, including the influence of genetic manipulations on the function of these circuits and emotional behaviors they mediate.[181-183] It should be noted that there has been much headway made in developing small-animal imaging platforms within academic and industry settings to aid in translational approaches to CNS drug discovery.[184] Indeed, recent *in vivo* imaging studies have highlighted a stress-sensitive circuit within the hippocampus which responds to antidepressant therapy.[185]

Furthermore, genetic approaches are giving detailed insights into changes which occur throughout entire molecular cascades relevant to depression and the mechanisms of action of antidepressant drugs.[44] Initially, such efforts will provide a greater understanding of the pathophysiology of depression that in the long term we hope will lead to a biological-based diagnostic approach[186] which is the basis for developing novel, faster and more efficacious antidepressants. Novel therapeutic strategies for depression are emerging[5,6,187] these range from the peptide antagonists; $GABA_B$ receptor antagonists, glutamatergic ligands to compounds that alter neurogenic pathways. The development of both *in vitro* and *in vivo* technologies that will facilitate robust target validation, including the use of RNA interference technology,[163] coupled with endophenotype-defined animal models and robust clinical biomarkers will aid in future drug discovery efforts.

However, clinical strategies should also comprise direct studies to assure that plasma levels may guarantee sufficient central receptor occupancy. This is useful not only to understand if plasma concentrations are sufficient to exert pharmacological effects but also to bridge preclinical hypotheses with clinical findings. For example, bupropion (Wellbutrin®/Zyban®) is an antidepressant that is considered to exert its action through dopamine uptake blockade,[205] but in humans, at therapeutic doses, it only occupies by 22% the dopamine transporter.[206] [xvi] Buspirone (Buspar®), which is considered a 5-HT_{1A} receptor agonist in animals[207] shown to behave as antagonist in *in-vitro* human hippocampus,[208] does not occupy 5-HT_{1A} receptors, at therapeutically effective doses.[209] Likewise, the regimen of pindolol (Visken®), thought to potentiate antidepressant effects,[210] used in the vast majority of clinical trials did not achieve significant receptor occupancy.[211,212]

REFERENCES

1. Andlin-Sobocki, P., Jonsson, B., Wittchen, H.U., and Olesen, J. (2005). Cost of disorders of the brain in Europe. *Eur J Neurol*, 12(Suppl 1):1–27.
2. Murray, C.J. and Lopez, A.D. (1997). Alternative projections of mortality and disability by cause 1990–2020: Global burden of disease study. *Lancet*, 349(9064):1498–1504.
3. Cryan, J.F. and Holmes, A. (2005). The ascent of mouse: Advances in modelling human depression and anxiety. *Nat Rev Drug Discov*, 4(9):775–790.
4. Wong, M.L. and Licinio, J. (2001). Research and treatment approaches to depression. *Nat Rev Neurosci*, 2(5):343–351.
5. Wong, M.L. and Licinio, J. (2004). From monoamines to genomic targets: A paradigm shift for drug discovery in depression. *Nat Rev Drug Discov*, 3(2):136–151.

[xvi] See Markou *et al.*, Contribution of animal models and preclinical human studies to medication development for nicotine dependence, in Volume 3, Reward Deficit Disorders, for further discussion on bupropion and receptor occupancy.

6. Berton, O. and Nestler, E.J. (2006). New approaches to antidepressant drug discovery: Beyond monoamines. *Nat Rev Neurosci*, 7(2):137–151.

7. Keller, M., Montgomery, S., Ball, W., Morrison, M., Snavely, D., Liu, G. *et al.* (2006). Lack of efficacy of the substance p (neurokinin1 receptor) antagonist aprepitant in the treatment of major depressive disorder. *Biol Psychiatr*, 59(3):216–223.

8. Kramer, M.S., Cutler, N., Feighner, J., Shrivastava, R., Carman, J., Sramek, J.J. *et al.* (1998). Distinct mechanism for antidepressant activity by blockade of central substance P receptors. *Science*, 281(5383):1640–1645.

9. Rupniak, N.M. and Kramer, M.S. (1999). Discovery of the antidepressant and anti-emetic efficacy of substance P receptor (NK1) antagonists. *Trend Pharmacol Sci*, 20(12):485–490.

10. Cryan, J.F. and Slattery, D.A. (2007). Animal models of mood disorders: Recent developments. *Curr Opin Psychiatr*, 20(1):1–7.

11. Angst, J. (1995). The epidemiology of depressive disorders. *Eur Neuropsychopharmacol*, 5(Suppl):95–98.

12. Agid, Y., Buzsaki, G., Diamond, D.M., Frackowiak, R., Giedd, J., Girault, J.A. *et al.* (2007). How can drug discovery for psychiatric disorders be improved? *Nat Rev Drug Discov*, 6(3):189–201.

13. Pangalos, M.N., Schechter, L.E., and Hurko, O. (2007). Drug development for CNS disorders: Strategies for balancing risk and reducing attrition. *Nat Rev Drug Discov*, 6(7):521–532.

14. American Psychiatric Association (1994). *Diagnostic and Statistical Manual of Mental Disorders*, 4th edition. American Psychiatric Press, Washington, DC.

15. Kessler, R.C., Berglund, P., Demler, O., Jin, R., Koretz, D., Merikangas, K.R. *et al.* (2003). The epidemiology of major depressive disorder: Results from the National Comorbidity Survey Replication (NCS-R). *JAMA*, 289(23):3095–3105.

16. Evans, D.L., Charney, D.S., Lewis, L., Golden, R.N., Gorman, J.M., Krishnan, K.R. *et al.* (2005). Mood disorders in the medically ill: Scientific review and recommendations. *Biol Psychiatr*, 58(3):175–189.

17. Mayer, E.A., Craske, M., and Naliboff, B.D. (2001). Depression, anxiety, and the gastrointestinal system. *J Clin Psychiatr*, 62(Suppl 8):28–36. discussion 7

18. Penninx, B.W., Beekman, A.T., Honig, A., Deeg, D.J., Schoevers, R.A., van Eijk, J.T. *et al.* (2001). Depression and cardiac mortality: Results from a community-based longitudinal study. *Arch Gen Psychiatr*, 58(3):221–227.

19. Stunkard, A.J., Faith, M.S., and Allison, K.C. (2003). Depression and obesity. *Biol Psychiatr*, 54(3):330–337.

20. Licinio, J. and Wong, M.L. (2005). Depression, antidepressants and suicidality: A critical appraisal. *Nat Rev Drug Discov*, 4(2):165–171.

21. Connor, T.J. and Leonard, B.E. (2003). Biological markers of depression. In: Feighner, J.P., Preskorn, S.H., and Stanga, C.Y. (eds.), *Handbook of Experimental Pharmacology, Antidepressants: Current and Future Perspectives*, Springer-Verlag, Berlin.

22. Nestler, E.J. and Carlezon, W.A., Jr. (2006). The mesolimbic dopamine reward circuit in depression. *Biol Psychiatr*, 59(12):1151–1159.

23. Wirz-Justice, A. (2006). Biological rhythm disturbances in mood disorders. *Int Clin Psychopharmacol*, 21(Suppl 1):S11–S15.

24. Wade, T.D., Bulik, C.M., Neale, M., and Kendler, K.S. (2000). Anorexia nervosa and major depression: Shared genetic and environmental risk factors. *Am J Psychiatr*, 157(3):469–471.

25. Moffoot, A.P., O'Carroll, R.E., Bennie, J., Carroll, S., Dick, H., Ebmeier, K.P. *et al.* (1994). Diurnal variation of mood and neuropsychological function in major depression with melancholia. *J Affect Disord*, 32(4):257–269.

26. Williams, K. and Reynolds, M.F. (2006). Sexual dysfunction in major depression. *CNS Spectr*, 11(8 Suppl 9):19–23.

27. Brown, G.W., Bhrolchain, M.N., and Harris, T. (1975). Social-class and psychiatric disturbance among women in an urban population. *Sociology J Br Sociol Assoc*, 9(2):225–254.

28. Paykel, E.S., Brugha, T., and Fryers, T. (2005). Size and burden of depressive disorders in Europe. *Eur Neuropsychopharmacol*, 15(4):411–423.

29. Rossler, W., Salize, H.J., van Os, J., and Riecher-Rossler, A. (2005). Size of burden of schizophrenia and psychotic disorders. *Eur Neuropsychopharmacol*, 15(4):399–409.

30. Blehar, M.C. (2006). Women's mental health research: The emergence of a biomedical field. *Annu Rev Clin Psychol*, 2:135–160.

31. Slattery, D.A., Hudson, A.L., and Nutt, D.J. (2004). Invited review: The evolution of antidepressant mechanisms. *Fundam Clin Pharmacol*, 18(1):1–21.

32. Anderson, I.M. (2000). Selective serotonin reuptake inhibitors versus tricyclic antidepressants: A meta-analysis of efficacy and tolerability. *J Affect Disord*, 58(1):19–36.

33. Perry, P.J. (1996). Pharmacotherapy for major depression with melancholic features: Relative efficacy of tricyclic versus selective serotonin reuptake inhibitor antidepressants. *J Affect Disord*, 39(1):1–6.

34. Hamilton, M. (1970). A rating scale for depression. *J Neurol Neurosurg Psychiatr*, 23:51–56.

35. Montgomery, S.A. and Asberg, M. (1979). A new depression scale designed to be sensitive to change. *Br J Psychiatr*, 134:382–389.

36. Bieck, P.R. and Potter, W.Z. (2005). Biomarkers in psychotropic drug development: Integration of data across multiple domains. *Annu Rev Pharmacol Toxicol*, 45:227–246.

37. Downing, G.J. (2002). Enhancing pathways to therapeutic development with clinical biomarkers. *Am J Geriatr Psychiatr*, 10(6):646–648.

38. Fava, M. (2003). Diagnosis and definition of treatment-resistant depression. *Biol Psychiatr*, 53(8):649–659.

39. Carroll, B.J. (1982). The dexamethasone suppression test for melancholia. *Br J Psychiatr*, 140:292–304.

40. Holsboer, F., Bender, W., Benkert, O., Klein, H.E., and Schmauss, M. (1980). Diagnostic value of dexamethasone suppression test in depression. *Lancet*, 2(8196):706.

41. Rush, A.J., Giles, D.E., Schlesser, M.A., Orsulak, P.J., Parker, C.R., Jr., Weissenburger, J.E. et al. (1996). The dexamethasone suppression test in patients with mood disorders. *J Clin Psychiatr*, 57(10):470–484.

42. Anisman, H. and Zacharko, R.M. (1990). Multiple neurochemical and behavioral consequences of stressors: Implications for depression. *Pharmacol Ther*, 46(1):119–136.

43. Barden, N. (2004). Implication of the hypothalamic–pituitary–adrenal axis in the physiopathology of depression. *J Psychiatr Neurosci*, 29(3):185–193.

44. Charney, D.S. and Manji, H.K. (2004). Life stress genes, and depression: Multiple pathways lead to increased risk and new opportunities for intervention. *Sci STKE*, 2004(225):re5.

45. de Kloet, E.R., Joels, M., and Holsboer, F. (2005). Stress and the brain: from adaptation to disease. *Nat Rev Neurosci*, 6(6):463–475.

46. Dinan, T.G. (1994). Glucocorticoids and the genesis of depressive illness. A psychobiological model. *Br J Psychiatr*, 164(3):365–371.

47. Duman, R.S. (2004). Depression: A case of neuronal life and death? *Biol Psychiatr*, 56(3):140–145.

48. Nestler, E.J., Barrot, M., DiLeone, R.J., Eisch, A.J., Gold, S.J., and Monteggia, L.M. (2002). Neurobiology of depression. *Neuron*, 34(1):13–25.

49. Holsboer, F. (2000). The corticosteroid receptor hypothesis of depression. *Neuropsychopharmacology*, 23(5):477–501.

50. Pariante, C.M. and Miller, A.H. (2001). Glucocorticoid receptors in major depression: Relevance to pathophysiology and treatment. *Biol Psychiatr*, 49(5):391–404.

51. Steckler, T., Holsboer, F., and Reul, J.M. (1999). Glucocorticoids and depression. *Baillieres Best Pract Res Clin Endocrinol Metab*, 13(4):597–614.

52. Vale, W., Spiess, J., Rivier, C., and Rivier, J. (1981). Characterization of a 41-residue ovine hypothalamic peptide that stimulates secretion of corticotropin and beta-endorphin. *Science*, 213(4514):1394–1397.

53. Duvigneaud, V., Gish, D.T., and Katsoyannis, P.G. (1954). A synthetic preparation possessing biological properties associated with arginine–vasopressin. *J Am Chem Soc*, 76(18):4751–4752.

54. Scott, L.V. and Dinan, T.G. (1998). Vasopressin and the regulation of hypothalamic-pituitary-adrenal axis function: Implications for the pathophysiology of depression. *Life Sci*, 62(22):1985–1998.

55. Baylis, P.H. (1989). Regulation of vasopressin secretion. *Baillieres Clin Endocrinol Metab*, 3(2):313–330.

56. McKinley, M.J., Mathai, M.L., McAllen, R.M., McClear, R.C., Miselis, R.R., Pennington, G.L. *et al.* (2004). Vasopressin secretion: Osmotic and hormonal regulation by the lamina terminalis. *J Neuroendocrinol*, 16(4):340–347.

57. Murphy, D., Waller, S., Fairhall, K., Carter, D.A., and Robinson, I.C.A.F. (1998). Regulation of the synthesis and secretion of vasopressin. *Adv Brain Vasopressin*, 119:137–143.

58. deWied, D. (1997). Neuropeptides in learning and memory processes. *Behav Brain Res*, 83(1–2):83–90.

59. Whitnall, M.H., Smyth, D., and Gainer, H. (1987). Vasopressin coexists in 1/2 of the corticotropin-releasing factor axons present in the external zone of the median-eminence in normal rats. *Neuroendocrinology*, 45(5):420–424.

60. Scott, L.V. and Dinan, T.G. (2002). Vasopressin as a target for antidepressant development: An assessment of the available evidence. *J Affect Disord*, 72(2):113–124.

61. De Kloet, E.R., Vreugdenhil, E., Oitzl, M.S., and Joels, M. (1998). Brain corticosteroid receptor balance in health and disease. *Endocr Rev*, 19(3):269–301.

62. Ma, X.M., Lightman, S.L., and Aguilera, G. (1999). Vasopressin and corticotropin-releasing hormone gene responses to novel stress in rats adapted to repeated restraint. *Endocrinology*, 140(8):3623–3632.

63. Gold, P.W., Goodwin, F.K., and Reus, V.I. (1978). Vasopressin in affective-illness. *Lancet*, 1(8076):1233–1236.

64. Cole, M.A., Kim, P.J., Kalman, B.A., and Spencer, R.L. (2000). Dexamethasone suppression of corticosteroid secretion: Evaluation of the site of action by receptor measures and functional studies. *Psychoneuroendocrinology*, 25(2):151–167.

65. Vonbardeleben, U. and Holsboer, F. (1989). Cortisol response to a combined dexamethasone human corticotropin-releasing hormone challenge in patients with depression. *J Neuroendocrinol*, 1(6):485–488.

66. Heuser, I., Yassouridis, A., and Holsboer, F. (1994). The combined dexamethasone CRH test – A refined laboratory test for psychiatric-disorders. *J Psychiatr Res*, 28(4): 341–356.

67. Gjerris, A., Hammer, M., Vendsborg, P., Christensen, N.J., and Rafaelsen, O.J. (1985). Cerebrospinal-fluid vasopressin – Changes in depression. *Br J Psychiatr*, 147:696–701.

68. vanLonden, L., Goekoop, J.G., vanKempen, G.M.J., FrankhuijzenSierevogel, A.C., Wiegant, V. M., vanderVelde, E.A. *et al.* (1997). Plasma levels of arginine vasopressin elevated in patients with major depression. *Neuropsychopharmacology*, 17(4):284–292.

69. Inder, W.J., Donald, R.A., Prickett, T.C.R., Frampton, C.M., Sullivan, P.F., Mulder, R.T. *et al.* (1997). Arginine vasopressin is associated with hypercortisolemia and suicide attempts in depression. *Biological Psychiatr*, 42(8):744–747.

70. Purba, J.S., Hoogendijk, W.J.G., Hofman, M.A., and Swaab, D.F. (1996). Increased number of vasopressin- and oxytocin-expressing neurons in the paraventricular nucleus of the hypothalamus in depression. *Arch Gen Psychiatr*, 53(2):137–143.

71. Raadsheer, F.C., Hoogendijk, W.J.G., Stam, F.C., Tilders, F.J.H., and Swaab, D.F. (1994). Increased numbers of corticotropin-releasing hormone expressing neurons in the hypothalamic paraventricular nucleus of depressed-patients. *Neuroendocrinology*, 60(4):436–444.

72. Dinan, T.G., Lavelle, E., Scott, L.V., Newell-Price, J., Medbak, S., and Grossman, A.B. (1999). Desmopressin normalizes the blunted adrenocorticotropin response to corticotropin-releasing hormone in melancholic depression: Evidence of enhanced vasopressinergic responsivity. *J Clin Endocrinol Metab*, 84(6):2238–2240.

73. Muller, M.B., Landgraf, R., Preil, J., Sillaber, I., Kresse, A.E., Keck, M.E. *et al.* (2000). Selective activation of the hypothalamic vasopressinelgic system in mice deficient for the corticotropin-releasing hormone receptor 1 is dependent on glucocorticoids. *Endocrinology*, 141(11):4262–4269.

74. Debellis, M.D., Gold, P.W., Geracioti, T.D., Listwak, S.J., and Kling, M.A. (1993). Association of fluoxetine treatment with reductions in CSF concentrations of corticotropin-releasing hormone and arginine vasopressin in patients with major depression. *Am J Psychiatr*, 150(4):656–657.

75. Heuser, I., Bissette, G., Dettling, M., Schweiger, U., Gotthardt, U., Schmider, J. *et al.* (1998). Cerebrospinal fluid concentrations of corticotropin-releasing hormone, vasopressin, and somatostatin in depressed patients and healthy controls: Response to amitriptyline treatment. *Depress Anxiety*, 8(2):71–79.

76. van West, D., Del-Favero, J., Aulchenko, Y., Oswald, P., Souery, D., Forsgren, T. *et al.* (2004). A major SNP haplotype of the arginine vasopressin 1B receptor protects against recurrent major depression. *Mol Psychiatr*, 9(3):287–292.

77. Dempster, E.L., Burcescu, I., Wigg, K., Kiss, E., Baji, I., Gadoros, J. *et al.* (2007). Evidence of an association between the vasopressin V1b receptor gene (AVPR1B) and childhood-onset mood disorders. *Arch Gen Psychiatr*, 64(10):1189–1195.

78. Griebel, G., Stemmelin, J., Gal, C.S.L., and Soubrie, P. (2005). Non-peptide vasopressin V-1b receptor antagonists as potential drugs for the treatment of stress-related disorders. *Curr Pharmaceut Des*, 11(12):1549–1559.

79. Nielsen, D.M. (2006). Corticotropin-releasing factor type-1 receptor antagonists: The next class of antidepressants? *Life Sci*, 78(9):909–919.

80. Flores, B.H., Kenna, H., Keller, J., Solvason, H.B., and Schatzberg, A.F. (2006). Clinical and biological effects of mifepristone treatment for psychotic depression. *Neuropsychopharmacology*, 31(3):628–636.

81. Healy, D.G., Harkin, A., Cryan, J.F., Kelly, J.P., and Leonard, B.E. (1999). Metyrapone displays antidepressant-like properties in preclinical paradigms. *Psychopharmacology (Berl)*, 145(3):303–308.

82. Thakore, J.H. and Dinan, T.G. (1995). Cortisol synthesis inhibition – A new treatment strategy for the clinical and endocrine manifestations of depression. *Biol Psychiatr*, 37(6):346–348.

83. Arana, G.W., Santos, A.B., Laraia, M.T., Mcleodbryant, S., Beale, M.D., Rames, L.J. *et al.* (1995). Dexamethasone for the treatment of depression – A randomized placebo-controlled, double-blind trial. *Am J Psychiatr*, 152(2):265–267.

84. DiMasi, J.A., Hansen, R.W., and Grabowski, H.G. (2003). The price of innovation: New estimates of drug development costs. *J Health Econ*, 22(2):151–185.

85. Frantz, S. (2004). Therapeutic area influences drug development costs. *Nat Rev Drug Discov*, 3(6):466–467.

86. Lakoff, A. (2002). The mousetrap: Managing the placebo effect in antidepressant trials. *Mol Interv*, 2(2):72–76.

87 McArthur, R. and Borsini, F. (2006). Animal models of depression in drug discovery: A historical perspective. *Pharmacol Biochem Behav*, 84(3):436–452.

88. Cryan, J.F., Markou, A., and Lucki, I. (2002). Assessing antidepressant activity in rodents: Recent developments and future needs. *Trend Pharmacol Sci*, 23(5):238–245.

89. Cryan, J.F. and Mombereau, C. (2004). In search of a depressed mouse: Utility of models for studying depression-related behavior in genetically modified mice. *Mol Psychiatr*, 9(4):326–357.

90. Rupniak, N.M. (2003). Animal models of depression: Challenges from a drug development perspective. *Behav Pharmacol*, 14(5–6):385–390.

91. Chaki, S., Nakazato, A., Kennis, L., Nakamura, M., Mackie, C., Sugiura, M. *et al.* (2004). Anxiolytic- and antidepressant-like profile of a new CRF1 receptor antagonist, R278995/CRA0450. *Eur J Pharmacol*, 485(1–3):145–158.

92. Chaki, S., Yoshikawa, R., Hirota, S., Shimazaki, T., Maeda, M., Kawashima, N. *et al.* (2004). MGS0039: A potent and selective group II metabotropic glutamate receptor antagonist with antidepressant-like activity. *Neuropharmacology*, 46(4):457–467.

93. Cryan, J.F. and Kaupmann, K. (2005). Don't worry 'B' happy!: A role for GABA(B) receptors in anxiety and depression. *Trend Pharmacol Sci*, 26(1):36–43.

94. Swanson, C.J., Bures, M., Johnson, M.P., Linden, A.M., Monn, J.A., and Schoepp, D.D. (2005). Metabotropic glutamate receptors as novel targets for anxiety and stress disorders. *Nat Rev Drug Discov*, 4(2):131–144.

95. Geyer, M.A. and Markou, A. (1995). Animal models of psychiatric disorders. In Bloom, F.E. and Kupfer, D.J. (eds.), *Psychopharmacology: The Fourth Generation of Progress*. Raven Press, New York, pp. 787–798.

96. Crabbe, J.C., Wahlsten, D., and Dudek, B.C. (1999). Genetics of mouse behavior: Interactions with laboratory environment. *Science*, 284(5420):1670–1672.

97. Wahlsten, D., Metten, P., Phillips, T.J., Boehm II, S.L., Burkhart-Kasch, S., Dorow, J. *et al.* (2003). Different data from different labs: Lessons from studies of gene–environment interaction. *J Neurobiol*, 54(1):283–311.

98. Lucki, I. (1997). The forced swimming test as a model for core and component behavioral effects of antidepressant drugs. *Behav Pharmacol*, 8(6–7):523–532.

99. Borsini, F., Evans, K., Jason, K., Rohde, F., Alexander, B., and Pollentier, S. (2002). Pharmacology of flibanserin. *CNS Drug Rev*, 8(2):117–142.

100. Montgomery, S.A., Loft, H., Sanchez, C., Reines, E.H., and Papp, M. (2001). Escitalopram (S-enantiomer of citalopram): Clinical efficacy and onset of action predicted from a rat model. *Pharmacol Toxicol*, 88(5):282–286.

101. Sanchez, C. (2006). The pharmacology of citalopram enantiomers: The antagonism by R-citalopram on the effect of S-citalopram. *Basic Clin Pharmacol Toxicol*, 99(2):91–95.

102. Gottesman, I.I. and Gould, T.D. (2003). The endophenotype concept in psychiatry: Etymology and strategic intentions. *Am J Psychiatr*, 160(4):636–645.

103. Hasler, G., Drevets, W.C., Gould, T.D., Gottesman, I.I., and Manji, H.K. (2006). Toward constructing an endophenotype strategy for bipolar disorders. *Biol Psychiatr*, 60(2): 93–105.

104. Hasler, G., Drevets, W.C., Manji, H.K., and Charney, D.S. (2004). Discovering endophenotypes for major depression. *Neuropsychopharmacology*, 29(10):1765–1781.

105. Hyman, S.E. and Fenton, W.S. (2003). Medicine. What are the right targets for psychopharmacology?. *Science*, 299(5605):350–351.

106. Gottesman, I.I. and Shields, J. (1973). Genetic theorizing and schizophrenia. *Br J Psychiatr*, 122(566):15–30.

107. Gould, T.D. and Gottesman, I.I. (2006). Psychiatric endophenotypes and the development of valid animal models. *Gene Brain Behav*, 5(2):113–119.

108. Matthews, K., Christmas, D., Swan, J., and Sorrell, E. (2005). Animal models of depression: Navigating through the clinical fog. *Neurosci Biobehav Rev*, 29(4-5):503-513.

109. Geyer, M.A. and Markou, A. (2002). The role of preclinical models in the development of psychotropic drugs. In Bloom, F.E. and Kupfer, D.J. (eds.), *Psychopharmacology: The Fifth Generation of Progress*. Raven, New York.

110. Pizzagalli, D.A., Jahn, A.L., and O'Shea, J.P. (2005). Toward an objective characterization of an anhedonic phenotype: A signal-detection approach. *Biol Psychiatr*, 57(4):319-327.

111. Shestyuk, A.Y., Deldin, P.J., Brand, J.E., and Deveney, C.M. (2005). Reduced sustained brain activity during processing of positive emotional stimuli in major depression. *Biol Psychiatr*, 57(10):1089-1096.

112. Elliott, R. (1998). The neuropsychological profile in unipolar depression. *Trend Cogn Sci*, 2(11):447-454.

113. Hollerman, J.R., Tremblay, L., and Schultz, W. (2000). Involvement of basal ganglia and orbitofrontal cortex in goal-directed behavior. *Prog Brain Res*, 126:193-215.

114. Kringelbach, M.L. (2005). The human orbitofrontal cortex: Linking reward to hedonic experience. *Nat Rev Neurosci*, 6(9):691-702.

115. Olds, J. and Milner, P. (1954). Positive reinforcement produced by electrical stimulation of septal area and other regions of rat brain. *J Comp Physiol Psychol*, 47(6):419-427.

116. Kornetsky, C. (2004). Brain-stimulation reward, morphine-induced oral stereotypy, and sensitization: Implications for abuse. *Neurosci Biobehav Rev*, 27(8):777-786.

117. Markou, A. and Koob, G.F. (1992). Construct validity of a self-stimulation threshold paradigm: Effects of reward and performance manipulations. *Physiol Behav*, 51(1):111-119.

118. Phillips, A.G., Blaha, C.D., and Fibiger, H.C. (1989). Neurochemical correlates of brain-stimulation reward measured by ex vivo and in vivo analyses. *Neurosci Biobehav Rev*, 13(2-3):99-104.

119. Wise, R.A., Bauco, P., Carlezon, W.A., Jr., and Trojniar, W. (1992). Self-stimulation and drug reward mechanisms. *Ann N Y Acad Sci*, 654:192-198.

120. Moreau, J.L., Jenck, F., Martin, J.R., Mortas, P., and Haefely, W.E. (1992). Antidepressant treatment prevents chronic unpredictable mild stress-induced anhedonia as assessed by ventral tegmentum self-stimulation behavior in rats. *Eur Neuropsychopharmacol*, 2(1): 43-49.

121. Cryan, J.F., Hoyer, D., and Markou, A. (2003). Withdrawal from chronic amphetamine induces depressive-like behavioral effects in rodents. *Biol Psychiatr*, 54(1):49-58.

122. Tremblay, L.K., Naranjo, C.A., Graham, S.J., Herrmann, N., Mayberg, H.S., Hevenor, S. et al. (2005). Functional neuroanatomical substrates of altered reward processing in major depressive disorder revealed by a dopaminergic probe. *Arch Gen Psychiatr*, 62(11):1228-1236.

123. Tremblay, L.K., Naranjo, C.A., Cardenas, L., Herrmann, N., and Busto, U.E. (2002). Probing brain reward system function in major depressive disorder: Altered response to dextroamphetamine. *Arch Gen Psychiatr*, 59(5):409-416.

124. Naranjo, C.A., Tremblay, L.K., and Busto, U.E. (2001). The role of the brain reward system in depression. *Prog Neuropsychopharmacol Biol Psychiatr*, 25(4):781-823.

125. Crespo-Facorro, B., Paradiso, S., Andreasen, N.C., O'Leary, D.S., Watkins, G.L., Ponto, L.L. et al. (2001). Neural mechanisms of anhedonia in schizophrenia: A PET study of response to unpleasant and pleasant odors. *JAMA*, 286(4):427-435.

126. Rogers, M.A., Kasai, K., Koji, M., Fukuda, R., Iwanami, A., Nakagome, K. et al. (2004). Executive and prefrontal dysfunction in unipolar depression: A review of neuropsychological and imaging evidence. *Neurosci Res*, 50(1):1-11.

127. Phillips, M.L., Drevets, W.C., Rauch, S.L., and Lane, R. (2003). Neurobiology of emotion perception II: Implications for major psychiatric disorders. *Biol Psychiatr*, 54(5):515-528.

128. Dalley, J.W., Cardinal, R.N., and Robbins, T.W. (2004). Prefrontal executive and cognitive functions in rodents: Neural and neurochemical substrates. *Neurosci Biobehav Rev*, 28(7):771–784.

129. Bremner, J.D., Narayan, M., Anderson, E.R., Staib, L.H., Miller, H.L., and Charney, D.S. (2000). Hippocampal volume reduction in major depression. *Am J Psychiatr*, 157(1):115–118.

130. Campbell, S., Marriott, M., Nahmias, C., and MacQueen, G.M. (2004). Lower hippocampal volume in patients suffering from depression: A meta-analysis. *Am J Psychiatr*, 161(4):598–607.

131. MacQueen, G.M., Campbell, S., McEwen, B.S., Macdonald, K., Amano, S., Joffe, R.T. *et al.* (2003). Course of illness, hippocampal function, and hippocampal volume in major depression. *Proc Natl Acad Sci USA*, 100(3):1387–1392.

132. Rosso, I.M. (2005). Review: Hippocampal volume is reduced in people with unipolar depression. *Evid Based Ment Health*, 8(2):45.

133. Sheline, Y.I., Gado, M.H., and Kraemer, H.C. (2003). Untreated depression and hippocampal volume loss. *Am J Psychiatr*, 160(8):1516–1518.

134. Sheline, Y.I., Sanghavi, M., Mintun, M.A., and Gado, M.H. (1999). Depression duration but not age predicts hippocampal volume loss in medically healthy women with recurrent major depression. *J Neurosci*, 19(12):5034–5043.

135. Brown, E.S., Rush, A.J., and McEwen, B.S. (1999). Hippocampal remodeling and damage by corticosteroids: Implications for mood disorders. *Neuropsychopharmacology*, 21(4):474–484.

136. Santarelli, L., Saxe, M., Gross, C., Surget, A., Battaglia, F., Dulawa, S. *et al.* (2003). Requirement of hippocampal neurogenesis for the behavioral effects of antidepressants. *Science*, 301(5634):805–809.

137. Schmidt, H.D. and Duman, R.S. (2007). The role of neurotrophic factors in adult hippocampal neurogenesis, antidepressant treatments and animal models of depressive-like behavior. *Behav Pharmacol*, 18(5–6):391–418.

138. Nofzinger, E.A., Schwartz, R.M., Reynolds III, C.F., Thase, M.E., Jennings, J.R., Frank, E. *et al.* (1993). Correlation of nocturnal penile tumescence and daytime affect intensity in depressed men. *Psychiatr Res*, 49(2):139–150.

139. McClung, C.A. (2007). Circadian genes, rhythms and the biology of mood disorders. *Pharmacol Ther*, 114(2):222–232.

140. Lam, R.W. (2006). Sleep disturbances and depression: A challenge for antidepressants. *Int Clin Psychopharmacol*, 21(Suppl 1):S25–S29.

141. Wilson, S. and Argyropoulos, S. (2005). Antidepressants and sleep: A qualitative review of the literature. *Drugs*, 65(7):927–947.

142. Ghosh, A. and Hellewell, J.S. (2007). A review of the efficacy and tolerability of agomelatine in the treatment of major depression. *Expert Opin Investig Drug*, 16(12):1999–2004.

143. Banasr, M., Soumier, A., Hery, M., Mocaer, E., and Daszuta, A. (2006). Agomelatine, a new antidepressant, induces regional changes in hippocampal neurogenesis. *Biol Psychiatr*, 59(11):1087–1096.

144. Barden, N., Shink, E., Labbe, M., Vacher, R., Rochford, J., and Mocaer, E. (2005). Antidepressant action of agomelatine (S 20098) in a transgenic mouse model. *Prog Neuropsychopharmacol Biol Psychiatr*, 29(6):908–916.

145. Bertaina-Anglade, V., la Rochelle, C.D., Boyer, P.A., and Mocaer, E. (2006). Antidepressant-like effects of agomelatine (S 20098) in the learned helplessness model. *Behav Pharmacol*, 17(8):703–713.

146. Loiseau, F., Le Bihan, C., Hamon, M., and Thiebot, M.H. (2005). Antidepressant-like effects of agomelatine, melatonin and the NK1 receptor antagonist GR205171 in impulsive-related behaviour in rats. *Psychopharmacology (Berl)*, 182(1):24–32.

147. Zupancic, M. and Guilleminault, C. (2006). Agomelatine: A preliminary review of a new antidepressant. *CNS Drug*, 20(12):981–992.
148. Conti, B., Maier, R., Barr, A.M., Morale, M.C., Lu, X., Sanna, P.P. *et al.* (2007). Region-specific transcriptional changes following the three antidepressant treatments electro convulsive therapy, sleep deprivation and fluoxetine. *Mol Psychiatr*, 12(2):167–189.
149. Wu, J.C. and Bunney, W.E. (1990). The biological basis of an antidepressant response to sleep deprivation and relapse: Review and hypothesis. *Am J Psychiatr*, 147(1):14–21.
150. Moore, P., Gillin, C., Bhatti, T., DeModena, A., Seifritz, E., Clark, C. *et al.* (1998). Rapid trypto-phan depletion, sleep electroencephalogram, and mood in men with remitted depression on serotonin reuptake inhibitors. *Arch Gen Psychiatr*, 55(6):534–539.
151. Gillin, J.C., Jernajczyk, W., Valladares-Neto, D.C., Golshan, S., Lardon, M., and Stahl, S.M. (1994). Inhibition of REM sleep by ipsapirone, a 5HT1A agonist, in normal volunteers. *Psychopharmacology (Berl)*, 116(4):433–436.
152. Monaca, C., Boutrel, B., Hen, R., Hamon, M., and Adrien, J. (2003). 5-HT 1A/1B recep-tor-mediated effects of the selective serotonin reuptake inhibitor, citalopram, on sleep: Studies in 5-HT 1A and 5-HT 1B knockout mice. *Neuropsychopharmacology*, 28(5): 850–856.
153. El Yacoubi, M., Bouali, S., Popa, D., Naudon, L., Leroux-Nicollet, I., Hamon, M. *et al.* (2003). Behavioral, neurochemical, and electrophysiological characterization of a genetic mouse model of depression. *Proc Natl Acad Sci USA*, 100(10):6227–6232.
154. Germain, A., Nofzinger, E.A., Kupfer, D.J., and Buysse, D.J. (2004). Neurobiology of non-REM sleep in depression: Further evidence for hypofrontality and thalamic dysregulation. *Am J Psychiatr*, 161(10):1856–1863.
155. Antonijevic, I. (2007). HPA axis and sleep: Identifying subtypes of major depression. *Stress*, 11(1):15–27.
156. Bucan, M. and Abel, T. (2002). The mouse: Genetics meets behaviour. *Nat Rev Genet*, 3(2):114–123.
157. Tecott, L.H. (2003). The genes and brains of mice and men. *Am J Psychiatr*, 160(4):646–656.
158. Phillips, T.J., Belknap, J.K., Hitzemann, R.J., Buck, K.J., Cunningham, C.L., and Crabbe, J.C. (2001). Harnessing the mouse to unravel the genetics of human disease. *Gene Brain Behav*, 1(1):14–26.
159. Gerlai, R. (2001). Gene targeting: Technical confounds and potential solutions in behavioral brain research. *Behav Brain Res*, 125(1–2):13–21.
160. Pfaff, D. (2001). Precision in mouse behavior genetics. *Proc Natl Acad Sci USA*, 98(11):5957–5960.
161. Cryan, J.F., Thakker, D.R., and Hoyer, D. (2007). Emerging use of non-viral RNA interference in the brain. *Biochem Soc Trans*, 35(Pt 2):411–415.
162. Fendt, M., Schmid, S., Thakker, D.R., Jacobson, L.H., Yamamoto, R., Mitsukawa, K. *et al.* (2007). mGluR7 facilitates extinction of aversive memories and controls amygdala plastic-ity. *Mol Psychiatr*.
163. Thakker, D.R., Hoyer, D., and Cryan, J.F. (2006). Interfering with the brain: Use of RNA inter-ference for understanding the pathophysiology of psychiatric and neurological disorders. *Pharmacol Ther*, 109(3):413–438.
164. Thakker, D.R., Natt, F., Husken, D., Maier, R., Muller, M., van der Putten, H. *et al.* (2004). Neurochemical and behavioral consequences of widespread gene knockdown in the adult mouse brain by using nonviral RNA interference. *Proc Natl Acad Sci USA*, 101(49):17270–17275.
165. Thakker, D.R., Natt, F., Husken, D., van der Putten, H., Maier, R., Hoyer, D. *et al.* (2005). siRNA-mediated knockdown of the serotonin transporter in the adult mouse brain. *Mol Psychiatr*, 10(8):782–789.

166. Crawley, J.N. (2000). *What's Wrong with My Mouse? Behavioral Phenotyping of Transgenic and Knockout Mice.* Wiley-Liss, New York.

167. Landgraf, R., Kessler, M.S., Bunck, M., Murgatroyd, C., Spengler, D., Zimbelmann, M. *et al.* (2007). Candidate genes of anxiety-related behavior in HAB/LAB rats and mice: Focus on vasopressin and glyoxalase-I. *Neurosci Biobehav Rev*, 31(1):89–102.

168. Muigg, P., Hoelzl, U., Palfrader, K., Neumann, I., Wigger, A., Landgraf, R. *et al.* (2007). Altered brain activation pattern associated with drug-induced attenuation of enhanced depression-like behavior in rats bred for high anxiety. *Biol Psychiatr*, 61(6):782–796.

169. Neumann, I.D., Wigger, A., Kromer, S., Frank, E., Landgraf, R., and Bosch, O.J. (2005). Differential effects of periodic maternal separation on adult stress coping in a rat model of extremes in trait anxiety. *Neuroscience*, 132(3):867–877.

170. Overstreet, D.H., Friedman, E., Mathe, A.A., and Yadid, G. (2005). The Flinders Sensitive Line rat: A selectively bred putative animal model of depression. *Neurosci Biobehav Rev*, 29(4–5):739–759.

171. Krishnan, V., Han, M.H., Graham, D.L., Berton, O., Renthal, W., Russo, S.J. *et al.* (2007). Molecular adaptations underlying susceptibility and resistance to social defeat in brain reward regions. *Cell*, 131(2):391–404.

172. Fox, M.A., Andrews, A.M., Wendland, J.R., Lesch, K.P., Holmes, A., and Murphy, D.L. (2007). A pharmacological analysis of mice with a targeted disruption of the serotonin transporter. *Psychopharmacology (Berl)*, 195(2):147–166.

173. Hariri, A.R. and Holmes, A. (2006). Genetics of emotional regulation: The role of the serotonin transporter in neural function. *Trend Cogn Sci*, 10(4):182–191.

174. Gray, L. and Hannan, A.J. (2007). Dissecting cause and effect in the pathogenesis of psychiatric disorders: Genes, environment and behaviour. *Curr Mol Med*, 7(5):470–478.

175. Moffitt, T.E., Caspi, A., and Rutter, M. (2005). Strategy for investigating interactions between measured genes and measured environments. *Arch Gen Psychiatr*, 62(5):473–481.

176. Crabbe, J.C. and Morris, R.G. (2004). Festina lente: Late-night thoughts on high-throughput screening of mouse behavior. *Nat Neurosci*, 7(11):1175–1179.

177. Tecott, L.H. and Nestler, E.J. (2004). Neurobehavioral assessment in the information age. *Nat Neurosci*, 7(5):462–466.

178. Robbins, T.W. (1998). Homology in behavioural pharmacology: An approach to animal models of human cognition. *Behav Pharmacol*, 9(7):509–519.

179. Cannistraro, P.A. and Rauch, S.L. (2003). Neural circuitry of anxiety: Evidence from structural and functional neuroimaging studies. *Psychopharmacol Bull*, 37(4):8–25.

180. Mayberg, H.S., Lozano, A.M., Voon, V., McNeely, H.E., Seminowicz, D., Hamani, C. *et al.* (2005). Deep brain stimulation for treatment-resistant depression. *Neuron*, 45(5):651–660.

181. Bissiere, S., McAllister, K.H., Olpe, H.R., and Cryan, J.F. (2006). The rostral anterior cingulate cortex modulates depression but not anxiety-related behaviour in the rat. *Behav Brain Res*, 175(1):195–199.

182. Bissiere, S., Plachta, N., Hoyer, D., McAllister, K.H., Olpe, H.R., Grace, A. *et al.* (2008). The rostral anterior cingulate cortex modulates the efficiency of amygdala-dependent fear learning, *Biol Psychiatr*, 63(9):821–831.

183. Slattery, D.A. and Cryan, J.F. (2008). The infralimbic cortex modulates stress-induced coping behaviour in the rat. *Frontiers Behav Neurosci* (in press).

184. Rudin, M. and Weissleder, R. (2003). Molecular imaging in drug discovery and development. *Nat Rev Drug Discov*, 2(2):123–131.

185. Airan, R.D., Meltzer, L.A., Roy, M., Gong, Y.Q., Chen, H., and Deisseroth, K. (2007). High-speed imaging reveals neurophysiological links to behavior in an animal model of depression. *Science*, 317(5839):819–823.

186. Hyman, S.E. (2007). Can neuroscience be integrated into the DSM-V? *Nat Rev Neurosci*, 8(9):725–732.

187. Schechter, L.E., Ring, R.H., Beyer, C.E., Hughes, Z.A., Khawaja, X., Malberg, J.E. *et al.* (2005). Innovative approaches for the development of antidepressant drugs: Current and future strategies. *NeuroRx*, 2(4):590–611.

188. Petit-Demouliere, B., Chenu, F., and Bourin, M. (2005). Forced swimming test in mice: A review of antidepressant activity. *Psychopharmacology (Berl)*, 177(3):245–255.

189. Borsini, F. (1995). Role of the serotonergic system in the forced swimming test. *Neurosci Biobehav Rev*, 19(3):377–395.

190. Cryan, J.F., Valentino, R.J., and Lucki, I. (2005). Assessing substrates underlying the behavioral effects of antidepressants using the modified rat forced swimming test. *Neurosci Biobehav Rev*, 29(4–5):547–569.

191. Cryan, J.F., Mombereau, C., and Vassout, A. (2005). The tail suspension test as a model for assessing antidepressant activity: Review of pharmacological and genetic studies in mice. *Neurosci Biobehav Rev*, 29(4–5):571–625.

192. Harkin, A., Kelly, J.P., and Leonard, B.E. (2003). A review of the relevance and validity of olfactory bulbectomy as a model of depression. *Clin Neurosci Res*, 3:253–262.

193. Kelly, J.P., Wrynn, A.S., and Leonard, B.E. (1997). The olfactory bulbectomized rat as a model of depression: An update. *Pharmacol Ther*, 74(3):299–316.

194. Song, C. and Leonard, B.E. (2005). The olfactory bulbectomised rat as a model of depression. *Neurosci Biobehav Rev*, 29(4–5):627–647.

195. O'Donnell, J.M., Marek, G.J., and Seiden, L.S. (2005). Antidepressant effects assessed using behavior maintained under a differential-reinforcement-of-low-rate (DRL) operant schedule. *Neurosci Biobehav Rev*, 29(4–5):785–798.

196. Pryce, C.R., Ruedi-Bettschen, D., Dettling, A.C., Weston, A., Russig, H., Ferger, B. *et al.* (2005). Long-term effects of early-life environmental manipulations in rodents and primates: Potential animal models in depression research. *Neurosci Biobehav Rev*, 29(4–5): 649–674.

197. Pryce, C.R. and Feldon, J. (2003). Long-term neurobehavioural impact of the postnatal environment in rats: Manipulations, effects and mediating mechanisms. *Neurosci Biobehav Rev*, 27(1–2):57–71.

198. Pryce, C.R., Ruedi-Bettschen, D., Dettling, A.C., and Feldon, J. (2002). Early life stress: Long-term physiological impact in rodents and primates. *News Physiol Sci*, 17:150–155.

199. Vogel, G., Neill, D., Kors, D., and Hagler, M. (1990). REM sleep abnormalities in a new animal model of endogenous depression. *Neurosci Biobehav Rev*, 14(1):77–83.

200. Fuchs, E. (2005). Social stress in tree shrews as an animal model of depression: An example of a behavioral model of a CNS disorder. *CNS Spectr*, 10(3):182–190.

201. Ducottet, C., Griebel, G., and Belzung, C. (2003). Effects of the selective nonpeptide corticotropin-releasing factor receptor 1 antagonist antalarmin in the chronic mild stress model of depression in mice. *Prog Neuropsychopharmacol Biol Psychiatr*, 27(4):625–631.

202. Willner, P. (1997). Validity, reliability and utility of the chronic mild stress model of depression: A 10-year review and evaluation. *Psychopharmacology (Berl)*, 134(4):319–329.

203. Willner, P., Muscat, R., and Papp, M. (1992). Chronic mild stress-induced anhedonia: A realistic animal model of depression. *Neurosci Biobehav Rev*, 16(4):525–534.

204. Mitchell, P.J. (2005). Antidepressant treatment and rodent aggressive behaviour. *Eur J Pharmacol*, 526(1–3):147–162.

205. Cooper, B.R., Hester, T.J., and Maxwell, R.A. (1980). Behavioral and biochemical effects of antidepressant bupropion (Wellbutin): Evidence for selective blockade of dopamine uptake in vivo. *J Pharmacol Exp Ther*, 215(1):127–134.

206. Meyer, J.H., Goulding, V.S., Wilson, A.A., Hussey, D., Christensen, B.K., and Houle, S. (2002). Bupropion occupancy of the dopamine transporter is low during clinical treatment. *Psychopharmacology*, 163(1):102–105.

207. De Vivo and Maayani (1986). Characterization of the 5-hydroxytryptamine1a receptor-mediated inhibition of forskolin-stimulated adenylate cyclase activity in guinea pig and rat hippocampal membranes. *J Pharmacol Exp Ther*, 238(1):248–253.

208. Marazziti, D., Palego, L., Giromella, A., Mazzoni, M.R., Borsini, F., Mayer, N., Naccarato, A. G., Lucacchini, A., and Cassano, G.B. (2002). Region-dependent effects of flibanserin and buspirone in adenylyl cyclase activity in the human brain. *Int J Neuropsychopharmacol*, 5(2):131–140.

209. Rabiner, E.A., Gunn, R.N., Wilkins, M.R., Sargent, P.A., Mocaer, E., Sedman, W., Cowen, P.J., and Grasby, P.M. (2000). Drug action at 5-HT(1A) receptor in vivo: Autoreceptor and postsynaptic receptor occupancy examined with PET and [carbonyl-(11C)]WAY-100635. *Nucl Med Biol*, 27(5):509–513.

210. Artigas, F., Perez, V., and Alvarez, E. (1994). Pindolol induces a rapid improvement of depressed patients with serotonin reuptake inhibitors. *Arch Gen Psychiatr*, 51(3):248–251.

211. Cremers, T.I., Wiersma, L.J., Bosker, F.J., den Boer, J.A., Westrink, B.H., and Wikstrom, H.V. (2001). Is the beneficial antidepressant effect of coadministration of pindolol really due to somatodendritic autoreceptor antagonism? *Biol Psychiatr*, 50(1):13–21.

212. Rabiner, E.A., Bhagwagar, Z., Gunn, R.N., Sargent, P.A., Bench, C.J., Cowen, P.J., and Grasby, P.M. (2001). Pindolol augmentation of selective serotonin reuptake inhibitors: PET evidence that the dose used in clinical trials is too low. *Am J Psychiatr*, 158(12):2080–2082.

Developing New Drugs for Schizophrenia: From Animals to the Clinic

Declan N.C. Jones[1], Jane E. Gartlon[1], Arpi Minassian[2], William Perry[2] and Mark A. Geyer[3]

[1]New Frontiers Science Park, GlaxoSmithKline, Harlow, Essex, CM19 5AW, UK
[2]Department of Psychiatry, University of California, San Diego, CA 92103-8620, USA
[3]Department of Psychiatry, University of California, San Diego, La Jolla, CA 92093-0804, USA

Animal and Translational Models for CNS Drug Discovery,
Vol. 1 of 3: Psychiatric Disorders
Robert McArthur and Franco Borsini (eds), Academic Press, 2008

INTRODUCTION

Schizophrenia is typically a lifelong and often devastating, but relatively common (lifetime risk of 1%), psychiatric disorder which often begins in late adolescence or early adulthood.[i] Schizophrenia patients are 10 times more likely to commit suicide than the general population.[2] It is estimated that by ~2010 there will be over 270 million sufferers worldwide,[3] which represents an enormous societal and financial burden. Schizophrenia is characterized by a cluster of symptoms, which are heterogeneous between patients and generally do not remain stable within patients. These symptoms can be divided into positive (e.g., delusions, hallucinations, disorganized speech), negative (e.g., affective flattening, avolition, impoverishment of speech and language, social

---

[i] For a brief overview.[1]

withdrawal), cognitive (e.g., attention deficits, impaired executive function and working memory), and mood (e.g., anxiety and depression) symptoms.

A diagnosis of schizophrenia is based on the descriptions/criteria listed within DSM-IV-TR[4]; see also http://www.psychnet-uk.com/dsm_iv/schizophrenia_disorder. htm) or ICD-10.[5] Outlined below are the criteria listed in DSM-IV-TR.

Criterion A. Characteristic symptoms: Two or more of the following for a significant portion of time during a 1-month period:

1. Delusions (only one symptom is required if a delusion is bizarre)
2. Hallucinations (only one symptom is required if hallucinations are of at least two voices talking to one another or of a voice that keeps up a running commentary on the patient's thoughts or actions)
3. Speech that shows incoherence, derailment, or other disorganization
4. Severely disorganized or catatonic behavior
5. Negative symptom such as flat affect, reduced speech, or lack of volition.

Criterion B. Social/occupational dysfunction: For a significant portion of the time since onset of the disturbance, one or more major areas of functioning, for example, work, interpersonal relations, or self-care, are markedly below pre-onset levels.

Criterion C. Duration: The patient must show some evidence of the disorder for at least 6 continuous months. At least 1 month must include the symptoms of frank psychosis (Criterion A). During the balance of this time (either as a prodrome or as residual of the illness), the patient must show either or both:

1. Negative symptoms as mentioned above.
2. In attenuated form, at least two of the other symptoms described in Criterion A (e.g., odd beliefs, unusual perceptual experiences).

Criterion D. Schizoaffective and Mood Disorder exclusion: Either (1) no Major Depressive, Manic, or Mixed-Episodes have occurred concurrently with active-phase symptoms or (2) if mood episodes have occurred during active-phase symptoms, their total duration has been brief relative to the duration of the active and residual periods.

Criterion E. Substance/general medical condition exclusion: The disturbance is not due to substance abuse, effects of medication, or a general medical condition.

Criterion F. Relationship to a Pervasive Developmental Disorder (PDD): If there is a history of Autistic Disorder or another PDD, the additional diagnosis of schizophrenia is made only if there are prominent delusions or hallucinations also present for at least a month.

It is interesting to note that these criteria emphasize the psychotic features of the disorder, place significantly less emphasis on negative symptoms, and make little or no mention of cognitive symptoms.[6-8] Both DSM-IV and ICD-10 are currently undergoing revision, with the expectations of DSM-V being published in 2011. Hyman[9] discusses the shortcomings of using DSM-IV for research purposes, given the categorical approach adopted. He suggests that increased understanding of the neurobiology of psychiatric disorders, and schizophrenia in particular, should allow the adoption of a more dimensional approach in DSM-V. Further, Keefe and Fenton[10] outlined the rationale and potential mechanisms for including severe cognitive deficit as part of the DSM-V diagnostic criteria for schizophrenia.

This chapter will review the current drug treatments for schizophrenia, the outstanding unmet needs for patients, the current understanding of the neurobiology of schizophrenia, and strategies for drug discovery. This chapter will focus in particular on the development of appropriate animal models and translational approaches to aid in the understanding of the neurobiology of schizophrenia and to investigate the potential efficacy of novel pharmacological approaches. We will discuss the challenges in drug discovery from both a preclinical and clinical perspective. Finally, we will review the exciting advances in the understanding of this disorder and the various Academic/Government/Industry initiatives which are likely to make a major impact upon drug discovery in this area. It is not our intention to provide an exhaustive review of each of the topics listed above, or list all the novel pharmacological approaches. However, where appropriate, we will discuss in some detail approaches which exemplify novel strategies for drug discovery or clinical investigation which promise significant advances in this field.

HISTORY OF DRUG DISCOVERY AND CURRENT TREATMENTS

Drug treatment is the mainstay for therapeutic intervention in schizophrenia, but really only dates from the first description of the beneficial effects of chlorpromazine (Largactil™ or Thorazine™) in 1952 in schizophrenic patients (see[11]). Chlorpromazine was originally developed as an anesthetic agent, but side effects were noted, described as a "chemical lobotomy," which brought this drug to the attention of psychiatrists. It was only in the 1960s that the therapeutic benefit and appropriate dosing regimes were established. The discovery of chlorpromazine led to the identification of a range of structurally similar (phenothiazines, including fluphenazine [Prolixin™], trifluoperazine [Stelazine™ amongst others], thioridazine [Thioril™ amongst others]) and distinct including, butyrophenones (e.g., haloperidol [Haldol™ amongst others]), thioxanthenes (e.g., flupenthixol [Depixol™ or Fluanxol™]) antipsychotics, based on a chlorpromazine-like behavioral profile in animals (including reduced spontaneous motor activity, catalepsy, interference with classical conditioning[11]) Carlsson and Lindquest[12] proposed that the antipsychotic effects of these drugs were mediated by blockade of dopamine receptors.

The discovery of clozapine (Clozaril™ amongst others) in the 1960s opens the second major chapter in the pharmacological treatment of schizophrenia. Whilst demonstrating clear efficacy against positive symptoms, typical antipsychotics were also associated with a range of side effects, including acute extrapyramidal (EPS) side effects in 50-90% of patients (e.g., akathisia, dystonia, Parkinsonism), chronic extrapyramidal signs in 15-20% of patients (e.g., tardive dyskinesia) and hyperprolactinaemia. Further, negative and cognitive symptoms are relatively refractory to typical antipsychotics. In contrast, clozapine was demonstrated to be an effective antipsychotic with a markedly reduced risk of EPS, and thus, became the prototype of the *atypical* class of antipsychotics. This class of drugs is operationally defined as those antipsychotics with a reduced propensity for causing EPS in both animals (e.g., catalepsy) and man. In light of the purpose of this book, it is interesting to note that the launch of clozapine was apparently delayed by its challenge of the perceived wisdom that antipsychotic efficacy should

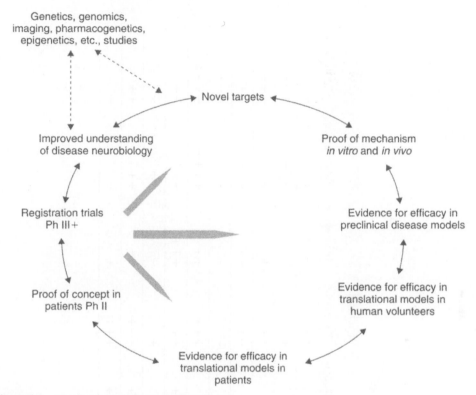

Figure 8.1 Idealized drug discovery flowchart

always be accompanied by EPS.[13] Unfortunately, clozapine was withdrawn from the clinic for a number of years because of a number of cases of fatal agranulocytosis, and was only reintroduced with appropriate blood monitoring and as third-line treatment.

In the 1980s and the next two decades, drug discovery shifted focus in an attempt to identify drugs that possessed the atypicality associated with clozapine, but without the white cell toxicity. Clozapine has a very "rich" pharmacology, targeting a wide range of dopaminergic, serotonergic, muscarinic, adrenergic, and other monoaminergic receptors[14-16] (Table 8.1). Therefore, designing a molecule that mimics the pharmacology responsible for the beneficial clinical effects of clozapine has been the aim of many pharmaceutical companies.[14,15] Using a mixture of *in vitro* and *in vivo* screening techniques, a number of atypical antipsychotics were identified which can be roughly categorized (see Table 8.1) as (1) relatively selective dopamine D_2/D_3 receptor antagonists, such as amisulpride (Solian™) and remoxipride; (2) mixed serotonin (5-hydroxytryptamine; 5-HT) 5-HT_2 and dopamine D_2/D_3 receptor antagonists, such as risperidone (Risperdal™ amongst others), paliperidone (Invega™), lurasidone; (3), mixed 5-HT_2 and dopamine D_2/D_3 receptor antagonists, but with a "richer" pharmacology, such as olanzapine (Zyprexa™), sertindole (Serdolect™), ziprasidone (Geodon™ or Zeldox™), quetiapine (Seroquel™); and (4) aripiprazole (Abilify™), a molecule with pharmacology similar to drugs in category (3), but with the significant exception of having low efficacy partial agonism at dopamine D_2 receptors

Table 8.1 Relative receptor pharmacology of antipsychotic drugs[a]

Receptor	Typical		Atypicals					
	Haloperidol	Amisulpride	Aripiprazole	Clozapine	Olanzapine	Quetiapine	Risperidone	Ziprasidone
D_1	++	−	+	++	++	+	+	+
D_2	++++	+++	++++	+	++	+	+++	+++
D_3	+++	+++	++++	+	++	+	+++	+++
D_4	+++	−	++	++	++	++	+++	++
$5\text{-}HT_{1A}$	−	−	+++	+	−	+	+	+++
$5\text{-}HT_{2A}$	−	−	+++	++	+++	++	++++	++++
$Alpha_1$	+++	−	++	+++	++	+++	++++	++
$Alpha_2$	−	−	−	+	+	−	++	−
H_1	++	−	−	+++	+++	++	++	++
M_1	−	−	−	+++	+++	+	−	−

[a] *Adapted from Abi-Dargham and Laruelle, 2005; GSK in-house data.*

(see[11,14,15,53]). The current drug discovery pipeline and strategies for schizophrenia are reviewed by Gray and Roth[54] and Wong *et al.*[55]

Atypicals show greater, albeit limited, benefit against both the negative and cognitive symptoms of this disease (see[56-58]). There is, however, recent evidence to suggest that at lower doses than were prescribed previously, typical antipsychotic medication such as haloperidol may also be effective in ameliorating negative symptoms.[59,60] In terms of tolerability, atypicals on the whole show a reduced propensity to cause hyperprolactinaemia and EPS (e.g.,[61]), but are associated with a number of significant additional side effects, such as weight gain and metabolic syndrome, including increased incidence of diabetes and hypercholesterolemia.[62-66]

Unmet Clinical Need

It is often forgotten that the introduction of antipsychotic drugs not only revolutionized the treatment of schizophrenia, but also encouraged the perception that schizophrenia was caused by an underlying pathological neurobiology. The newer atypical drugs have individual clinical characteristics and fewer or different side effects (see above), and offer the clinician a much wider choice of treatment options than were available even 10 years ago. Nevertheless, there remain very clear unmet needs for the treatment of schizophrenia and other psychotic disorders.

With the general exception of clozapine, which has demonstrated benefit against treatment resistance and suicidality and clear evidence for better efficacy (see[16,58]), there is a only a general trend from randomized controlled trials (RCT), but no absolute evidence, that atypicals have a greater efficacy against positive symptoms than typical antipsychotics.[58,67] Davis *et al.*[67] argue that atypicals are not a homogenous group, although there are still insufficient data to determine whether there are significant efficacy differences within the atypical class[58]). It should be noted that these meta-analyses lack data on important clinical dimensions such as cognition and quality of life, and that pharmaceutical company sponsorship of RCTs, the relatively short duration of trials and limited types of assessment used (e.g., last-observation-carried-forward analyses) limit the interpretation of these data (see[16]). Recent large-scale studies have compared treatment with atypical and typical antipsychotics in a less restrictive way than standard RCTs (e.g., Clinical Antipsychotic Trials of Intervention [CATIE], and Cost Utility of the Latest Antipsychotic Drugs in Schizophrenia Study [CUtLASS 1, see[68]). Despite some methodological questions about these studies, the overall conclusion from these trials was that atypicals, with the exception of clozapine, represent only an incremental progress over the older, cheaper typical drugs (see[58,68]).

Hagan and Jones[69] carried out a survey of the literature describing the effects of antipsychotics upon cognition in schizophrenia, and concluded that there is some support to the hypothesis that atypical antipsychotics, and to a lesser extent, typical antipsychotics, can improve cognition in schizophrenia across a number of domains. At present, the understanding of which cognitive domains are affected by which compound is poor. The relationship between medication and cognitive status is further complicated by the fact that many drug studies to date show a relationship between medication status and specific cognitive measures rather than cognitive domains.

Thus, further studies are clearly needed to better understand the efficacy of antipsychotic medication on cognitive status given that there is a moderate relationship at best between similar measures purported to assess the same cognitive function.[70,71] Further work is also required to explore the extent to which statistically significant effects in experimental studies translate into functional benefit for patients ([72] and see discussion below).

In summary, perhaps the clearest unmet needs are the incomplete efficacy against positive symptoms, and the relatively poor/negligible efficacy against negative and cognitive symptoms. Therefore, the current drugs are accurately described as antipsychotics, rather than anti-schizophrenia drugs. In addition, better tolerability may improve the very poor treatment compliance seen in this patient population.

CURRENT UNDERSTANDING OF THE NEUROBIOLOGY OF SCHIZOPHRENIA AND DISEASE HYPOTHESES

The historical approach to drug discovery in schizophrenia is best defined as a "top down" approach, as defined by Insel and Scolnick.[73] That is, serendipitous discovery of drugs such as chlorpromazine provoked intensive investigation of the mechanism of action of such drugs and the subsequent identification of pharmacologically "me too" drugs, which showed incremental improvements in terms of efficacy, tolerability, and/or safety. A better understanding of the neurobiology of schizophrenia will allow a conversion to a "bottom up" approach in drug discovery, that is, identify novel drug targets that are more closely associated with the underlying neuropathology (i.e., *novel target identification and validation*), design drugs to act at these targets and then test these drugs in clinical trials[73] (Figure 8.1). This is easier said than done give our relatively superficial current understanding of the neurobiology of schizophrenia.[74] However, the following section will briefly review the hypotheses that are currently driving drug discovery, including the development of new disease models, and the exciting ongoing approaches to expand our understanding of disease neurobiology that will influence drug discovery in the future.

Neurotransmitter Hypotheses of Schizophrenia

Dopamine Hypothesis

The hyperdopaminergic hypothesis of schizophrenia is derived from data generated over the last 50 years; including the findings that dopamine agonists, such as apomorphine and amphetamine, exacerbate psychosis and that all marketed antipsychotics have affinity for D_2 and D_3 receptors.[14,15,75,76] Further, schizophrenia patients show an exaggerated dopaminergic response to amphetamine inferred from imaging studies investigating displacement of radiotracers such as [11^C]raclopride or [123^I]IBZM (see[77]) and the clinical benefit of antipsychotics is associated with a threshold level of striatal dopamine D_2 receptor occupancy.[78] Given the inability of D_2 receptor antagonist antipsychotic drugs to treat all the symptoms of schizophrenia, and based on further clinical and preclinical work of many scientists, the dopaminergic hypothesis has been refined to suggest an imbalance between subcortical and cortical dopaminergic systems (see reviews by[77,79,80]). That is, the subcortical mesolimbic dopaminergic projections are hyperactive, causing excessive stimulation of D_2 receptors, and consequently, positive symptoms. In contrast, mesocortical dopaminergic projections to the prefrontal cortex are hypoactive, causing suboptimal stimulation of cortical D_1 receptors, and consequently, negative and cognitive symptoms. Therefore, despite a waxing and waning of the perceived importance of the dopamine hypothesis in schizophrenia research, there is very good reason to believe that a dysregulation of this system is fundamental in at least some of the most prominent symptoms of schizophrenia.

Glutamate or NMDA Receptor Hypofunction Hypothesis

This hypothesis is derived from data showing that open channel *N*-methyl-d-aspartate (NMDA) receptor blockers such as phencyclidine (PCP), ketamine, and dizocilpine (MK-801) produce transient psychotomimetic effects in healthy volunteers, including negative and cognitive symptoms as well as positive symptoms, and precipitate psychotic episodes in schizophrenic patients (see[74,79-85]). Further, adjunctive treatment with co-agonists at the NMDA receptor, albeit with suboptimal characteristics for clinical use, such as glycine, D-serine, and D-cycloserine appear to have some benefit in schizophrenics (see[86]). In addition, a prodrug for an mGluR$_{2/3}$ agonist, LY2140023, was as effective as olanzapine as monotherapy in a recent clinical trial.W[87] More directly, a recent paper investigating the functional role of neuregulin-1 and its receptor, erbB4, in post-mortem prefrontal cortex from schizophrenics demonstrated a significant reduction in NMDA receptor activation by NMDA/glycine compared with controls.[88] Therefore, there appears to be compelling evidence for a dysfunctional glutamatergic system in schizophrenia, and in particular hypofunction of NMDA receptors.

GABAergic Hypofunction Hypothesis

Our understanding of the dysregulation of GABAergic systems in schizophrenia has been primarily driven by the work of Francine Benes and others[74,89-91]; Guidotti *et al.*, 2000. GABAergic interneurons are a core component of the corticolimbic circuitry and provide inhibitory and disinhibitory modulation of cortical and hippocampal circuits and therefore, contribute to the control of network oscillations, information processing, and sensorimotor gating within the corticolimbic system (see[90]). All these processes are disturbed in schizophrenia.[40,93] Post mortem studies, although not always consistent on individual markers, in general show disruption of the GABAergic system in schizophrenia, including reduced glutamate acid decarboxylase 67 (GAD67) expression (see[89]), and other markers of GABAergic function such as parvalbumin,[94] and the GABA transporter, GAT-1.[95] Therefore, a disruption in GABAergic function will have profound impact upon the processes underlying complex behaviors and may give rise to the significant cognitive deficits seen in schizophrenia.

Serotonin System

There is evidence that abnormalities in serotonin and in 5-HT$_{2A}$ receptor function in particular, may play a role in some symptoms of schizophrenia. Some of the evidence comes from the hallucinogenic properties of 5-HT$_{2A}$ agonists, such as lysergic acid diethylamide (LSD) or psilocybin (see[96,97]), in that psilocybin induces psychotic symptoms, deficits in mismatch negativity and AX-continuous performance task, spatial working memory deficits,[96,98,99] and abnormalities in sensorimotor gating[100] in volunteers. Preclinically, 5-HT$_{2A}$ agonists also cause sensorimotor gating deficits.[101] In addition, there is good preclinical and clinical evidence to support the use of 5-HT$_{2A}$ antagonists as adjunctive therapy in schizophrenia. First, atypical antipsychotics generally have higher affinity for 5-HT$_{2A}$ receptors than D$_2$ receptors (see[15] and Table 8.1) and atypicals show greater occupancy of cortical 5-HT$_{2A}$ receptors compared with moderate/high basal ganglia D$_2$ receptor occupancy,[102,103] with the exception of aripiprazole.[104] Second, molecules such as M100,907, eplivanserin, and ritanserin have moderate efficacy in schizophrenia monotherapy trials,[105,106] albeit of insufficient size to justify progression as stand-alone therapy. Third, 5-HT$_{2A}$ receptor antagonists also exhibit some antipsychotic-like effects in preclinical tests, (e.g., suppression of conditioned avoidance response (CAR), inhibition of NMDA antagonist-induced behaviors)[106,107] and potentiate the effects of other antipsychotics against amphetamine- or MK-801-induced hyperactivity.[108] Finally, 5-HT$_{2A}$ receptor antagonists increase extracellular dopamine levels in the cortex at high doses and potentiate the effects of haloperidol upon cortical dopamine at lower doses (e.g., eplivanserin, ACP-103,[109]).

Integration of Neurochemical Hypotheses

Given the interrelationship between neurochemical systems in the CNS, a number of workers have attempted to integrate the data for individual neurotransmitter systems in order to obtain a more coherent understanding of the neurochemical dysregulation in schizophrenia (see[74,79,80,90]). For example, Laruelle et al.[79,80] and Carlsson et al.[81] propose a neuronal circuitry model of glutamate-dopamine interactions, incorporating a role for GABAergic systems, and describe how this may be altered in schizophrenia. Lewis and Gonzalez-Burgos[74] considered the integration of the neurochemical hypotheses and the effects upon working memory in schizophrenia concentrating on the dorsolateral prefrontal cortex (DLPFC). Specifically, they postulated that hypofunction of the NMDA receptors that mediate excitatory inputs to prefrontal pyramidal cells leads to decreased activity in cortical excitatory projections to mesencephalic dopamine cell nuclei resulting in decreased activity of dopamine neurons projecting to the DLPFC and increased activity of those that project to the basal ganglia. Cortical hypodopaminergia leads to compensatory, but functionally insufficient, upregulation of D$_1$ receptors. The NMDA hypofunction and altered D$_1$-mediated signaling may reduce the activity of parvalbumin containing chandelier neurons, causing a decrease in activity-dependent expression of GAD1 (which encodes for GAD67). Reduced GAD67 results in reduced GABA release, down regulation of GAT1 in chandelier cell cartridges and upregulation of GABA$_A$ receptor α_2 subunits in the axon initial segment of the DLPFC pyramidal cells. A consequence of these net changes is reduced gamma band oscillations, a marker of the synchronized firing of a network of neurons, putatively contributing to a deficit in working memory (see[92]).

Neurodevelopmental Hypotheses of Schizophrenia

The neurodevelopmental hypothesis of schizophrenia postulates that an early event disrupts normal brain maturation, resulting in the appearance of obvious clinical symptoms at puberty or young adulthood (e.g., see[6]). In her working model, Andreasen suggests that the etiologies may be multiple (e.g., obstetric complications, maternal viral infection, nutritional deficits, psychological experiences), but lead to relatively similar impairment in brain development, with consequent deficits in neuronal connectivity and cognitive impairments. This hypothesis has been built on by others to propose a "two hit hypothesis," which posits that a combination of genetic vulnerability and neurodevelopmental trauma[110,111] may be required for the impaired neurodevelopment sufficient to cause schizophrenia.

Evidence for a neurodevelopment hypothesis includes premorbid subtle, nonclinical abnormalities in cognitive and social functioning, and evidence for later attainment of development milestones (see[112]). Cytoarchitectural abnormalities also suggest neurodevelopment abnormalities, including abnormal laminar distribution of neurons in the cortex, disruption of cortical layers, decreased cortical volume, and aberrant invaginations of the cortical surface (see[90,112]). It has been suggested that the emergence of more overt symptoms in late adolescence/early adulthood may be related to abnormal pruning which reveal the underlying cytoarchitectural abnormalities (see[112]). Further, a number of the recently identified candidate genes associated with risk for schizophrenia code for proteins with a fundamental role in brain development (see below, e.g., neuregulin 1 (NRG-1), erbB4, DISC-1,[113,114]).

Structural and Molecular Changes in Schizophrenia

Ultrastructural Changes

The process of gliosis, a proliferation of astrocytes in areas of neuronal damage, is absent in post-mortem brains in schizophrenia, suggesting that neuronal death is not a major contributing factor to the regional volume loss.[115,116] Instead, evidence suggests that the observed changes in gray matter result from reduced neuropil density (dendrites, dendritic spines, axons, and pre- and postsynaptic terminals) and support the suggestion that schizophrenia is a disorder of synaptic connectivity. These observations include smaller cell bodies, fewer dendritic spines and reduced dendritic aborizations in pyramidal cells of the hippocampus and neocortex (reviewed in[114 and 16]). In agreement with these observations, an increased neuronal density of 13–21% is reported in the frontal cortex[117] with another group reporting no change in neuronal number in this region.[118] The spatial organization of neurons may also be altered in schizophrenia. In particular, aberrantly located neurons in the interstitial white matter immediately below the neocortex have been reported by several groups (see[119]). These neurons form part of the cortical subplate, a transitional structure formed in the second trimester in humans and involved in the formation of cortical connections. Therefore, abnormal migration in this region is likely to reflect a developmental abnormality.

N-*Acetylaspartate*

The functional "integrity" of neurons may also be affected. *N*-acetylaspartate (NAA) is an amino acid used as a neuronal marker as it is but distributed almost exclusively in neurons.[120] NAA deficits are linked to a number of diseases with a neural pathology,[121] and can normalize following treatment or recovery from brain injury.[122,123] The function of NAA is unknown, although roles in myelin synthesis,[124] osmoregulation,[125] and inflammation[126] have been demonstrated. In vivo magnetic resonance studies (MRS) studies in schizophrenia patients have shown reductions in NAA in frontal and temporal regions.[44,419] A recent meta-analysis of the MRS literature (1256 schizophrenia patients, 1209 normal controls) revealed consistent reductions in NAA with the hippocampus (medial temporal regions) and prefrontal lobe most affected[129]. Somewhat in agreement, post-mortem studies using a senstive high performance liquid chromatography (HPLC) method have demonstrated reductions in NAA in temporal cortex, striatum and hippocampus, but not in the frontal cortex.[43,128] Other studies have shown an association between regional deficits in NAA, particularly in the prefrontal cortex, and other aspects of schizophrenia, including cognitive deficits[130,131] and severity of negative symptoms.

Glial Cell Abnormalities

Further evidence for changes in neuronal function comes from reported changes in glial cell structure and function.[114] Glial cells are known to play an important role in neural development and support processes such as synaptic plasticity and synaptogenesis.[133,134] In schizophrenia, the number of oligodendrocytes are reduced in the neocortex, prefrontal, motor, and anterior cingulate cortices[133-137] along with decreased expression of glial fibrillary acidic protein (GFAP).[138] Other studies have shown a disruption in the expression of myelination genes and non-volumetric changes in the microstructure of white matter (reviewed in[139]).

Genetic Findings in Schizophrenia

There is a high degree of heritability in schizophrenia, estimated at between 24% and 80% (depending on the diagnostic criteria or the use of endophenotypes,[140-142]), although no single gene has been identified that represents a major risk factor for schizophrenia (see[113]). Nevertheless, some of the most exciting recent advances in schizophrenia research have been made in the field of genetics. A recent issue of Biological Psychiatry (Vol 60, 2006) detailed the findings over the previous 7 years since it last devoted an issue to genes and schizophrenia (1999). Straub and Weinberger[113] summarized the situation optimistically, detailing the surprising success of linkage studies in identifying genes such as dysbindin, neuregulin-1 (NRG-1), and G72/G30.

Many of the genes identified so far appear to be implicated in fundamental processes of brain development,[113,114] neuronal differentiation, synaptic function, and plasticity.[113] Further, these findings have broadened out from investigating individual genes to identifying additional genes in the candidate gene pathway in order to understand further the functional consequences of gene variation, and to identify points for therapeutic intervention (e.g., NRG1 and its receptor, erbB4). It is worthwhile to spend some time briefly reviewing the data associated with a number of these genes as examples of the processes that have been followed to begin to understand the biological implications of variation in genes (e.g., see[143]).

Example Genes: NRG1/ErbB4, COMT, and DISC-1

NRG1/ErbB4: The neuroregulins (NRG) are a family of four genes (NRG1-4) which activate the ErbB tyrosine kinase receptors inducing growth and differentiation of epithelial, neuronal, glial, and other cell types. NRG1 is a large complex gene which contains at least 25 alternatively spliced exons, which can produce multiple promoters upstream of the coding region (see[144,145]). NRG1 signaling via ErbB receptors has a variety of functions in the CNS and is implicated in neuronal differentiation and myelination and in the development and functioning of NMDA receptors, α7 nicotinic receptors, and migration of cortical GABA interneurons (see[144-146]).

NRG1 remains one of the best candidate genes for schizophrenia. Since the original report from a genome-wide linkage study of large Icelandic pedigrees that identified NRG1 as a risk factor for schizophrenia,[147] a number of studies have supported its potential role in disease risk[148-150] and see[144]. However, no single variant has been uniformly implicated and all of the putatively associated polymorphisms are in non-coding regions, making any conclusion regarding their biological influences more challenging. Subsequent association studies have implicated the tyrosine kinase receptor ErbB4 as a putative schizophrenia risk gene and a genetic interaction (epistasis) between variants at the ligand and receptor loci has been reported to increase risk in several studies.[150,151]

These genetic data have prompted extensive investigation of the expression and function of NRG1 and ErbB4 (see[144]). For example, a number of groups have shown differential expression of NRG1 mRNA isoforms (type I–IV) in schizophrenia (see[144]), including the brain specific Type IV mRNA whose expression is regulated by a schizophrenia risk-associated functional promoter or SNP.[146] Further, NRG1 stimulation suppresses NMDA receptor activation in rat prefrontal cortex slices, presumably via ErbB4 receptors.[152] This effect has also been demonstrated in post-mortem human prefrontal cortex, where the effects of NRG1 were exaggerated in tissue from schizophrenic patients.[88] Thus, aberrant NRG1–ErbB4 signaling might underlie NMDA receptor hypofunction and clinical phenotype (e.g., working memory impairments[74]) in schizophrenia. In further support of a biological role of variation in this gene, an associated NRG1 promoter allele was shown in an fMRI study to predict impaired frontal and temporal lobe activation, deficits in cognitive function and prevalence of psychotic symptoms.[153] Therefore, in less than 5 years since the initial report of the genetic finding for NRG1, there has been a wealth of biological data implicating altered NRG1-ErbB4 signaling in schizophrenia.

COMT: Catechol-*O*-methyltransferase (COMT) catalyses methyl conjugation and inactivation of catecholamines and is the main route of dopamine catabolism in the frontal cortex,[154] and indirectly alters dopaminergic function in subcortical areas (see[155]). A SNP at Val158Met alters COMT enzyme activity; Val/Val confers high-enzymatic activity; Met/Met confers low-enzymatic activity (and consequently, higher cortical dopamine function), while Val/Met confers intermediate activity (see[156]). There is relatively mixed and weak evidence for a genetic association of COMT with schizophrenia (see[156]), although there is some evidence for an interaction with other genetic and environmental risk factors to modulate schizophrenia risk[155] and some data suggesting that the Val allele is more frequently transmitted from the parents to their ill offspring than the Met allele (see[157]). There is stronger evidence for a role for genetic variation of COMT upon frontal cortical function and in cognitive tasks that rely upon this brain region, for example, Wisconsin Card Sorting Test (Egan *et al.*, 2001 and see[157]). However, the putative U-shaped relationship between dopamine levels and cortical function complicates the interpretation beyond the simple understanding that Val/Val is "bad" and Met/Met "good" for cognitive function (see[155]). The net effect of COMT activity will depend upon where on the U-shaped curve the person is during different circumstances (e.g., during times of elevated stress) and the test being carried out. Tunbridge *et al.*[155] summarized a complicated situation elegantly:

> *The Met COMT allele is associated with improved working memory and executive function compared with the Val allele, perhaps mediated by improved signal to noise ratio, resulting in improved cognitive stability. There may be an associated cost, however, in that Met also appears to be associated with impaired emotional processing.*

COMT inhibitors, in particular tolcapone, have been investigated preclinically and clinically for effects upon cognitive function (see[157]). For example, tolcapone altered cortical dopamine and improved performance in an attentional set shifting task in rats.[158] Clinically, tolcapone improved the performance of healthy volunteers of tasks which measure DLPFC function and improved the "information processing efficiency" during the n-back task, as inferred from the altered fMRI signal in response to the task (see[157]). Consequently, the use of COMT inhibitors to treat the cognitive deficits in schizophrenia has been proposed (see[157]) and www.clinicaltrials.gov lists an ongoing Phase 2 study evaluating the effects of tolcapone in schizophrenia (NCT00044083).

DISC-1: Multiple converging lines of evidence from cellular, mouse mutant and post-mortem brain studies implicate the disrupted-in-schizophrenia-1 gene (DISC1) in the pathophysiology of schizophrenia and other mental illnesses.[159-161] DISC1 was identified in the breakpoint of a chromosomal translocation present in schizophrenic and bipolar patients; and a non-synonymous SNP in DISC1 has been associated with altered hippocampal structure and function, gray matter volume and cognitive performance in healthy and affected subjects ([162] see also[160]).

DISC-1 is found in multiple cellular compartments and interacts with a wide variety of proteins (see[159]). Proteins that interact with DISC-1 have been investigated in order to understand the functional consequence of this disruption. The impaired interaction with binding partners, fasciculation and elongation protein zeta-1 (Fez1), DISC-1-binding zinc finger protein (DBZ) and Kendrin has been reviewed by Matsuzaki and Tohyama.[163] This group proposed that DISC-1 participates in neurite outgrowth through its interaction with either Fez1 or DISC1-DBZ or both and consequently, disruption of this interaction will result in an immature neural circuit formation. Kendrin is a giant centrosomal protein and disruption of the DISC-1-Kendrin interaction disturbs the development of neurons through the impaired maturation of the cytoskeleton system. Other interacting proteins include NudE-like (NUDEL), lissencephaly-1 (LIS1), growth factor receptor bound protein 2 (Grb2), and phosphodiesterase 4B (PDE4B).

There has been the greatest focus on the role of PDE4B, which perhaps reflects the availability of pharmacological and mutant mouse tools. Preclinically, drugs which inhibit PDE4 activity, including rolipram, influence NMDA receptor-mediated memory, and demonstrate an antipsychotic-like profile,[164] which mutant mouse studies tell us is dependent to some extent upon the presence of functional interaction of DISC-1 and PDE4B.[165,166] Therefore, targeting PDE4 inhibition may provide a novel approach to the treatment of schizophrenia.

Future of Genetic Studies

Although there is a high degree of heritability of schizophrenia, the difficulties inherent in genetic studies in schizophrenia and other psychiatric disorders is elegantly summarized by Craddock *et al.*,[167] who note that genetic susceptibility does not respect current diagnostic boundaries defined by DSM-IV or ICD-10. Indeed, DISC-1 appears to be more closely associated with major depressive disorder[168] and was originally discovered in an extended Scottish pedigree which suffered from a variety of psychiatric disorders. Further, given the broadness of the symptom spectrum within schizophrenia, there is no guarantee that comparison of genetic studies carried out in different cohorts of schizophrenic patients is not confounded by different frequencies of symptoms and/or diagnostic criteria, genetic differences between geographically or ethnically distinct populations, and ascertainment (i.e., sampling designs).[113,167,169] Craddock and colleagues[167] urge the use of more detailed measures of lifetime psychopathology and when possible endophenotypic markers, such as neuroimaging or cognitive testing, in order to define more homogenous patient cohorts.[169] Technical advances, including the availability of the International HapMap resource, dense genotyping chips and large (>1000 cases and control) well-characterized patient cohorts, have allowed whole genome-wide association (WGA) studies to be carried out in complex disorders.[170] There are a number of WGA studies ongoing for schizophrenia worldwide, carried out by various consortia of research groups (e.g., Consortium on the Genetics of Schizophrenia,[169,171]) which should report out in 2007/2008 and beyond and are likely to identify genes associated with a modest effect size. Although these studies are unlikely to provide obvious drug targets immediately, it is clear that they will generate findings that will help to drive basic biological studies over the next 5–10 years and provide novel avenues for drug discovery.

It is generally accepted that genes and environmental insults interact to influence the emergence of schizophrenia. While the literature is replete with genetic linkage studies of the disease as well as reports of neurodevelopmental or environmental trauma, few studies have examined the combined influence of genes and environment in the same cohort. Admittedly, as Jaffee and Price[172] describe, such studies are challenging because they require large sample sizes, and environmental and developmental events must be rigorously and accurately measured. Given that there are now promising candidate genes for schizophrenia, such as NRG-1 and others, as well as innovative methods of inducing controlled environmental conditions in preclinical species such as isolation rearing or introduction of a virus, it is now possible to carefully study the environmental events that may mediate genetic risk for schizophrenia (see below).

Epigenetics

A range of influences may contribute to define the etiology of complex psychiatric disorders, such as schizophrenia.[173-176] Phenotypic variation has been attributed to genetic and environmental variation[177] and gene–environment interaction studies have provided further evidence that both interact to determine the course of disease.[172] Epigenetics refers to features such as chromatin and DNA modifications that are stable over rounds of cell division but do not involve changes in the underlying DNA sequence of the organism.[178] The emerging field of psychiatric epigenetics explores the molecular mechanisms that may control gene–environment interactions.[179] Epigenetic factors are inherited and acquired modifications of DNA (methylation) and histones (acetylation, phosphorylation, methylation, and ubiquitination) which regulate genomic functions. They play a critical role in controlling gene expression, chromosome stability, genomic imprinting, and X chromosome inactivation. The significance of chromatin remodeling in psychiatric disorders is emerging. For example, membrane-bound catechol-*O*-methyltransferase (MB-COMT) over-expression due to promoter hypomethylation and/or a hyperactive allele of COMT may increase dopamine degradation in the frontal lobes, providing a possible molecular basis for some symptoms of schizophrenia.[180] Recent studies also suggest the possibility that epigenetic aberration from the normal DNA methylation status of the human RELN gene may confer susceptibility to psychiatric disorders.[181,182] Complementing genetic and functional genomic approaches with epigenetic strategies may help identify novel drug targets.

CURRENT DRUG DISCOVERY IN SCHIZOPHRENIA

Preclinical Models of Aspects of Schizophrenia

Understanding the neurobiology and drug discovery in schizophrenia require "fit for purpose" animal models and equally as important, suitable experimental medicine (translational) approaches in humans. Such approaches may demonstrate centrally mediated pharmacodynamic effects of novel drugs, proof of principle of the drug target, and ideally, potential for efficacy against individual symptoms before embarking on the massive expense of large-scale clinical trials which risk exposing a large number of patients to an unproven drug.

General Considerations re: Psychiatric Animal Models

It is not the intention of this Chapter to review in detail the history of animal model development in schizophrenia drug discovery, but to briefly discuss those models which are still used in drug discovery and the future direction of animal modeling in schizophrenia. It is worth spending some time discussing general concepts around animal models of psychiatric disorders. For the sake of brevity, we will concentrate in the most part on rodent models.

A model allows the testing of hypotheses as well as novel drugs (e.g., effects of genetic mutations, effects of environmental modifications, interactions between genes and the environment) which cannot be readily manipulated in man. An important concept to emphasize is that we should not expect a single animal model to provide the definitive answers on whether a particular gene or gene product is important in schizophrenia or whether a novel drug will be effective in schizophrenic patients. In a field outside of biology, George Box, the industrial statistician, is credited with the quote "all models are wrong, some are useful," which was subsequently expanded to "Remember that all models are wrong; the practical question is how wrong do they have to be to not be useful."[183] Therefore, any information obtained should be placed into the context of that obtained from other sources. Thus, a convergence of information from multiple animal models, genetic/genomic data, clinical studies with similar drugs, and other sources is useful to interrogate a given hypothesis, and define the next experiment to investigate the hypothesis.

Criteria used to evaluate models

In considering the validity of a model, both the independent (i.e., inducing manipulation, see below) and dependent (assays or measures) variables need to be evaluated (see[184-186]). The reliability and predictive validity of the model system are relevant to both the independent variable and the dependent measures and are the most important criteria to satisfy. The additional criteria relevant to the independent variable include etiological, construct, and face validity, with etiological validity being the most relevant. The criteria relevant to the dependent variable include construct, convergent, discriminant, and face validity. Face validity is useful heuristically particularly in the case of some disorders, such as schizophrenia, in which relatively little is known about the pathophysiology or etiology.

Reliability refers to the consistency and stability with which the variables of interest are observed.[185,187] Face validity refers to the phenomenological similarity between the behavior (i.e., dependent variable) exhibited by the animal model and the specific symptoms of the human condition.[188] Although face validity is an intuitively appealing criterion with which to validate models,[189,190] it is actually not necessary, can be misleading, and is difficult to defend rigorously. Face validity provides a heuristic starting point for the development of an animal model, but cannot be used to establish the validity of the model. Predictive validity refers to the ability of a model to make correct predictions about the human phenomenon of interest. The term predictive validity is often used in the narrow sense of the model's ability to identify drugs having therapeutic value in humans (i.e., pharmacological isomorphism,[191]). However, the identification of any variables that have similar influences in both the experimental preparation and the modeled phenomenon can demonstrate predictive value of the model and may enhance one's understanding of the phenomenon. Construct validity of a test is defined as the accuracy with which the test measures what it is intended to measure,[192] and does not necessarily have anything to do with the presumed etiology of an illness. Although difficult to establish, construct validity is considered to be the most important property of a test or measure.[192,193] Because theoretical constructs of a disease are constantly being refined, construct validation can never be the only type of validity met. Nevertheless, the process of construct validation is valuable in the continuing process of model development and refinement. The concepts of etiological validity and construct validity are often confused. A model has etiological validity if the etiologies of the phenomenon in the animal model and the human condition are identical. As such, assessing etiological validity involves an evaluation of the inducing conditions, and the implicit or explicit hypotheses about the etiology of the disease.[185]

Animal models-manipulations and measures

Development of any disease model includes two components, the manipulation which attempts to cause the disease-like phenomena and the ability to measure the response to that manipulation (i.e., the assay, test, or paradigm). Taking examples from Alzheimer's disease (AD) research, a variety of mice have been produced which express disease-associated gene mutations that cause abnormal processing of β amyloid (the *manipulation*) and subsequently shown to demonstrate impaired cognitive performance in variety of cognition assays (e.g., radial arm maze) and AD-like plaques (*the tests* or *paradigms*) (see[194]). Thus, taken together, some of these mice strains represent models of the cognitive deficits and/or the neuropathology seen in AD. However, there are specific challenges for the development of animal models of psychiatric disorders as briefly outlined by Eric Nestler.[195] First, psychiatric disorders are defined and diagnosed on the basis of behavioral and emotional abnormalities, some of which are impossible to measure in animals (e.g., delusions, paranoia, guilt, or worthlessness). Second, unlike AD, psychiatric disorders have no well-validated molecular or cellular markers (biomarkers). Third, although there is a clear genetic basis for psychotic disorders, the polygenic nature and the complicated interaction between genes and the environment have made the production of valid mutant mouse models difficult (see below).

Another important consideration is that, based on the understanding that schizophrenia is a uniquely human disorder with a subtle neuropathology and a poorly understood etiology, it is impossible to develop a model of all the aspects of schizophrenia in rodents or even primates. However, as our understanding of the underlying neurobiology of schizophrenia improves and as the concept emerges that schizophrenia may be a cluster of individual disorders defined by specific endophenotypes, then it may be possible to adequately mimic individual aspects of the disorder or hypotheses about etiology. This approach has gained considerable support over recent years. [184,196-202] Indeed, this difficulty is not restricted to animal models of schizophrenia symptoms. For example, it would not be considered sensible to try to recapitulate all the different clinical pain or hypertension conditions in a single animal model. Therefore, it should not be considered a "failure" that there is no single animal model of schizophrenia that recapitulates all aspects of this disorder. Indeed, the careful experimental scientist has probably always considered that their paradigms mimic only aspects of the disease, generally positive symptoms, and were perhaps more guilty of sloppy semantics in describing these as *animal models of schizophrenia* in the scientific literature. The limited efficacy of current drugs, including atypicals, against both negative and cognitive symptoms and the focus on symptoms other than positive symptoms has brought this issue into sharp focus.

Measures: Paradigms for preclinical testing

Therefore, starting with a consideration of the rodent tests or paradigms available to us, it is possible to construct a list of the available behavioral, physiological, neurochemical, neuroanatomical, and imaging paradigms in rodents and attempt to map these on to the corresponding symptoms or behavioral and phenomenological changes seen in schizophrenia (see Table 8.2).[200,201,203] One could also make a comment on whether these paradigms can be directly translated to human (Table 8.2). A number of the physiological measures with particular potential for cross-species use are described briefly below (e.g., PPI, P50 suppression).

From this exercise, it is clear that there is a variety of well-characterized paradigms in which measurements in man can be translated to those used in rodents. Alternatively, one can use a "reverse translational" approach where existing animal

Table 8.2 Examples of paradigms in rodents with mapping onto phenomena in schizophrenia

Symptom domain	Clinical descriptions/phenomena	Examples of animal paradigms (tests/assays)	Translatable to man[a]?	Example references
Positive symptoms	Delusions/Hallucinations	No	N/A	
	Disorganized speech	No	N/A	
	Grossly disorganized behavior	Changes in pattern of motor activity	Yes	17
	Psychomotor agitation	Basal locomotor activity and response to novelty	Yes	18,17
Negative symptoms	Affective flattening/Anhedonia	Saccharine/sucrose consumption test, ICSS	Yes	19–21
	Alogia	No	N/A	
	Avolition	Progressive ratio test	Yes	22,19,23
	Social withdrawal	Social Interaction in rats	Yes	24–30
		Social Interaction with a juvenile conspecific in rats and mice		
		Resident-Intruder test in mice		
		Nest building in mice		
		Home cage social behavior		
Physiological measures	Increased sensitivity to psychomotor stimulants (e.g., amphetamine, PCP)	Measurement of motor activation following psychomotor stimulants	Yes	18,31
	Impaired PPI	PPI of an acoustic or tactile startle response in rats and mice	Yes	32,33
	Impaired Auditory Evoked Potentials (AEP, i.e., P50 gating)	AEP measurement in mice	Yes	34,35
	Impaired Latent Inhibition (LI)	LI in rodents	Yes	36,37
	Impaired Mismatch Negativity (MMN)	MMN (EEG recording) in anesthetized rodents	Yes	38
	Impaired network oscillations	EEG recording in rodents	Yes	39,40
Other measures	Alterations in neurochemistry	Ex vivo measurements of neurochemistry or in vivo microdialysis	Yes	41–44
	Sleep disturbances	Sleep/Wake EEG assessment	Yes	45–47
	Self Care	Measurement of feeding, body weight, gross behavior, coat conditions, general health, SHIRPA etc	Yes	26,48,49
	Reduced cortical/hippocampal dendritic spine density	Post mortem assessment post Golgi staining	No	50
	Changes in cortical volume	Structural MRI or post-mortem assessment	Yes	51,52

models that are related to specific neurotransmitters can be adapted to study patients with schizophrenia. An example is the translation of the classic animal open field test to a parallel human paradigm, where exploratory activity in patients with psychiatric illness can be quantified and compared with rodent models of the same diseases.[17] However, the major challenge lies in developing the appropriate manipulations in animals, which can be paired with the tests outlined in Table 8.2 to create the models of individual disease symptoms or phenomena.

It is also possible to undertake a similar exercise when considering the cognitive domains outlined by the MATRICS initiative (see below) and map these on to the available rodent tests of cognition (Table 8.3,[69,204,386] and see detailed discussion of these assays by Lindner *et al.*, 2008[ii]). Non-human primates may be more appropriate than rodents for evaluating the cognitive effects of novel compounds due to the higher homology between human and non-human primate cortical architecture and function, higher cognitive capacities[205] and the availability of computerized test batteries analogous to those used for humans.[206,207] For example, in an fMRI study, performance of an identical attentional set-shifting task recruited homologous regions of the ventro-lateral prefrontal cortex in humans and macaques.[208] Hagan and Jones[69] reviewed the effects of antipsychotics upon the performance of normal animals in these tests and reached a number of broad conclusions. First, apart from paradigms such as prepulse inhibition of startle (PPI) and latent inhibition (LI), there have been few systematic preclinical investigations of the effects of typical and atypical antipsychotics on tests of attentional control, executive function, avoidance learning and retention, recognition memory, spatial learning, memory or recall. Second, apart from a few notable exceptions (e.g., iloperidone[209]), antipsychotics do not improve cognitive performance in the majority of these tests in normal animals. Indeed, in most studies antipsychotics impair task acquisition or performance. Thus, despite modest evidence for cognitive benefits in clinical studies the preclinical data for antipsychotics has so far failed to identify a convincing and robust signal for improved cognition in normal animals. However, a review of the effects of drugs which are designed to target cognitive processes specifically (e.g., AMPA positive modulators, muscarinic agonists, and nicotinic receptor agonists) yields a completely different answer (see[69,210]). Sarter[210] has recently proposed a strategy for more effective predictive preclinical studies of putative cognition enhancers and suggested that the investigation of reciprocal relationships among molecular, cellular, behavioral, and cognitive processes modulated by candidate drugs should represent the core of such research. A similar concept underlies the Cognitive Neuroscience-based Approaches to Measuring and Improving Treatment Effects on Cognition in Schizophrenia (CNTRICS) initiative (see below).

Physiological Measures Available for Translational Research

It is worth spending some time discussing some of those measures which may particularly lend themselves to cross-species translational research (see[93]).

[ii] Please refer to Lindner *et al.*, Development, optimization and use of preclinical behavioral models to maximize the productivity of drug discovery for Alzheimer's Disease, Volume 2 *Neurological Disorders*.

Table 8.3 MATRICS Cognitive domains and example corresponding preclinical and clinical cognition tests

Cognitive domain	Animal tests (models)	Clinical battery (beta version)
Sensorimotor gating/ pre-attentive processing	PPI (mouse/rats) PPI disrupted by NMDA antagonists PPI disrupted by isolation rearing	Not in MATRICS battery
Working memory	Operant or T-maze DNMTP/ DMTP Radial arm maze Spatial span task Odor span task Holeboard task	BACS WMS-III Spatial Span WAIS-III Letter-Number sequence UoM Letter-Number Span Spatial Delayed Response Task
Attention/vigilance/speed of processing	5-Choice Serial Reaction Time Task Latent Inhibition Sustained Attention Task Lateralized reaction-time task	3-7 CPT Identical pairs CPT Category fluency Trail making A WAIS-III Digit Symbol-Coding BACS – Symbol Coding
Verbal learning and memory	Not applicable	NAB- Daily Living Memory HVLT-Revised
Visual learning and memory	Novel Object Recognition Social Recognition T-maze alternation task Barnes circular maze Morris Water maze (mouse, rat) Radial arm maze Spatial span task	NAB – Shape Learning BVMT-Revised
Reasoning and problem solving	Attentional set shifting Maze tasks	WAIS-III Block design BACS- Tower of London NAB – Mazes
Social cognition	Social interaction/Social recognition	MSCEIT – Managing emotions MSCEIT – Perceiving emotions

Adapted from Hagan and Jones, 2005 and Geyer and Young, 2006 (http://www.turns.ucla.edu/preclinical-TURNS-report-2006b.pdf).

Prepulse inhibition and startle habituation

Prepulse inhibition (PPI) is a measure of sensorimotor gating used to identify deficits in early stage information processing. In mammalian species, PPI refers to the reduction in the response to a startle stimulus (pulse) when a lower intensity non-startling stimulus (prepulse) is presented shortly before the startle stimulus (neurobiology reviewed in[211,212]). The startle response is commonly measured using the eye blink response in humans and using the whole body startle response in rodents. A wide literature supports PPI deficits in schizophrenia patients and in non-affected relatives (reviewed in[213]). PPI is reduced in animals by administration of NMDA antagonists, dopamine agonists, serotonin receptor agonists, or various neurodevelopmental insults (reviewed in[32,211 and 214]), and is also altered in a number of transgenic mice having relevance to schizophrenia.[32] There is some controversy regarding the effects of antipsychotic treatments on PPI in schizophrenia patients, with some studies showing higher PPI levels in patients receiving atypicals,[215-217] and others[218,420] reporting no effect of drug treatment. A recent double-blind study showed that olanzapine increased PPI in schizophrenia patients during an 8-week period, whereas haloperidol did not.[219] Further, Minassian *et al.*[220] reported improved PPI in patients after 2 weeks of drug treatment. Thus, on balance, there is reasonable evidence that treatment with antipsychotics will improve impaired PPI in schizophrenic patients.

It is suggested that PPI deficits, and the resultant "sensory overload," may relate to other symptoms, for example perceptual distortion.[213,221] However, attempts to correlate PPI deficits with positive and negative symptoms in schizophrenia have yielded mixed findings.[222] Swerdlow *et al.*[223,224] found a correlation between PPI and functional impairments in schizophrenia patients, but not with cognitive function. Other studies, however, have observed correlations of reduced PPI with increases in thought disorder[216,225,226] or distractibility[227] in schizophrenia. Startle habituation, the reduction in response to a repeated stimulus, is also reduced in schizophrenia patients,[228,229] but this behavior is mediated via different neurobiological mechanisms.

P50 suppression

In the P50 sensory gating paradigm, two acoustic clicks are presented in rapid succession (~500 ms apart). Normal subjects show a suppressed P50 event-related potential to the second click, whereas patients with schizophrenia (and first degree relatives and subjects with schizotypal personality disorder) have diminished suppression of the P50 response.[40,93,221,230] Auditory gating can also be measured in animals using EEG recording of an analogous response (N40[34,35]), although some controversy exists over this suggestion for rodents.[217] Evidence suggests that PPI and P50 suppression are distinct measures of information processing in rodents[217,231] and the two are not correlated in schizophrenia patients.[169,232]

It has been reported that schizophrenics have impaired gating when acutely ill and medicated with typical antipsychotics, acutely ill and unmedicated, or when clinically stable and medicated with typical antipsychotics (see[233] for references). Adler *et al.*[234] evaluated P50 auditory gating in schizophrenic patients who were either unmedicated or treated with typical antipsychotics, clozapine, olanzapine, risperidone, or quetiapine in a naturalistic design. Only the mean gating ratio of the clozapine group was not statistically impaired compared with healthy controls. All remaining groups were significantly impaired compared with healthy controls, with the approximate order of impairment (mean P50 gating ratio): quetiapine = typicals > unmedicated schizophrenics = olanzapine = risperidone > clozapine > healthy controls. Similarly, in a double-blind trial of treatment resistant patients (no placebo or normal controls), neither 12 weeks of treatment with haloperidol/benztropine combination nor olanzapine improved the gating ratio compared with baseline levels.[235] However, there was no improvement in clinical symptoms in either group. In a longitudinal study in treatment refractory patients (10 subjects), sensory gating of P50 was first examined while still on typical antipsychotic medication (baseline) and in the same patients 1 month and 15 months after starting clozapine treatment.[236] Clozapine caused both clinical improvement (i.e., >20% reduction in total Brief Psychiatry Rating Scale (BPRS) score) and normalization of the gating of the P50 response in the majority of patients.[233] There was a clear relationship between clinical improvement and improved auditory gating in this study. A recent clinical study with the α7 nicotinic receptor partial agonists, DMXB-A, showed improved P50 gating and neurocognitive improvement in schizophrenic patients[237]; supporting previous suggestions of a role for this receptor (see[238]).

Measuring auditory gating in rodents is technically more difficult than PPI, which explains the much smaller preclinical dataset available for auditory gating. Maxwell *et al.*[421] demonstrated that continuous administration of olanzapine, but not haloperidol, improved upon auditory gating in C57/BL6j mice. Simosky *et al.*[34,239] showed that clozapine and olanzapine, but not haloperidol, improved the impaired auditory gating in DBA/2 mice. The effects of other antipsychotics have yet to be determined. However, the impaired auditory gating model in DBA/2 mice is increasingly being used in drug discovery.

Latent inhibition

During Latent Inhibition (LI) non-contingent presentation of a stimulus attenuates the ability of that stimulus to enter into subsequent associations and is considered an index of learned inattention or irrelevance.[240,241] Impaired LI has been reported in acute schizophrenic patients, but less often in chronic patients,[242] a reduction which some authors suggest results from chronic antipsychotic treatment (see[240,241,243]). However, consistency is poor as Williams *et al.*[244] reported intact LI in antipsychotic-naïve acute schizophrenics, but impaired LI in treated patients. Interestingly Leumann *et al.*[243] showed that patients who were treated with typical and atypical antipsychotics showed intact LI, but PPI was intact in only those patients treated with atypicals. The clinical literature suffers from a lack of longitudinal studies in which LI is measured before treatment and after appropriate treatment durations.

The preclinical pharmacology of LI has been reviewed in detail,[37,245] including evaluation of the effects of antipsychotics on weak LI and upon drug-induced impaired LI models (e.g., by amphetamine). Moser *et al.*[37] concluded that there is good evidence that haloperidol caused a robust and reproducible potentiation of weak LI. In contrast, the data for clozapine is much less robust, with a variety of findings described, including lack of effect, impaired or enhanced LI. However, methodological differences critically determine response and variations in methodology between studies may contribute to the variable findings with antipsychotics.[246] The limited number of LI studies conducted in man have been reviewed recently.[36,240,241] Studies of antipsychotic drug effects in normal volunteers have produced mixed results. Barrett *et al.*[36] reported that chlorpromazine, risperidone, and amisulpiride had no effect upon auditory LI, while risperidone and amisulpride disrupted visual LI. These findings contrast with the potentiation of low LI levels by haloperidol and chlorpromazine (see[36]). Therefore, the utility of LI studies in man in drug development is not clear.

Mismatch negativity

Mismatch negativity (MMN) is an auditory event-related potential that occurs when a sequence of repetitive sounds is interrupted by an occasional "oddball" sound that differs in frequency or duration. Schizophrenia patients have abnormal MMN compared to non-patients,[247] as do relatives of individuals in the schizophrenia spectrum.[248] Deviations in MMN are correlated with poor functional outcome in schizophrenia.[249] Furthermore, MMN is not dependent upon active engagement on the part of the subject. MMN-like evoked potentials have been observed in mice,[38] suggesting that this paradigm might be amenable to translational study. Further, the investigation of MMN in monkeys has shown that NMDA antagonists block the generation of the MMN response, suggesting that NMDA receptors play an important role in this index of information processing and working memory.[250] Consequently, MMN is one of a family of EEG signals that may hold promise as a translational biomarker for schizophrenia, as do other markers of neuronal network activity such as gamma-band oscillation that are aberrant in schizophrenia patients.[40] Network oscillations may be valuable tools in pharmacological and translational studies that are aimed at developing and refining new treatment interventions for schizophrenia.

Manipulations: Disease or Etiological Models-Defined by the Inducing Manipulation

Pharmacological isomorphism

An example of a more limited use of an animal model related to schizophrenia is the systematic study of the effects of antipsychotic treatments on specific behaviors or other endpoints. The principle guiding this approach has been termed "pharmacological isomorphism" because the explicit purpose of the model is to predict treatment efficacy.[191] This approach is limited by the fact that such models are developed and validated by reference to the effects of known therapeutic drugs. Hence this approach may limit the ability to identify drugs with novel mechanisms of action and discover new antipsychotics that might better treat the symptoms of schizophrenia that are refractory to current treatments, such as cognitive deficits. For example, blockade of dopamine agonist-induced behaviors such as amphetamine-induced hyperactivity may limit the target of antipsychotic screens to D_2 dopamine receptor antagonists (although see below). Other examples of approaches where an antipsychotic-like response has been established include conditioned avoidance responding (CAR) in rats,[251] regional CNS c-fos response,[252] or depolarization block of dopamine neurons in the ventral tegmental area (see[191]). Although these approaches may lead to the development of "me-too" molecules, they are not without merit (see below), given that a number of non-dopaminergic antipsychotic mechanisms have been identified in these assays.[253-256]

Drug-driven models

Animal models based on pharmacological challenges remain the most widely used in preclinical drug discovery in schizophrenia research.[257,258] The similar behavioral consequences of these drugs in humans and rodents, and their sensitivity to antipsychotic treatments in both species, are the basis, for example, for the dopamine and glutamate neurochemical hypotheses of schizophrenia (discussed above). Acutely administered drug-driven models have the main advantage that schizophrenia-like readouts are generated quickly and with relative ease. Although these models generally lack convincing etiological validity, they provide end-points which are sensitive to the effects of current antipsychotic treatments, and some novel approaches, and so are of particular use for drug screening.

Behavioral responses to dopamine receptor agonists   Dopamine agonists, such as amphetamine, apomorphine, or quinpirole, induce characteristic motor responses in rodents, which have been reviewed extensively by others.[258,259] The amphetamine-induced hyperlocomotor response is elicited, at least in part, by increased dopaminergic activity in the mesolimbic pathway, particularly in the nucleus accumbens and olfactory tubercle.[260-263] Given that hyperactivity in the same pathway is thought to underlie positive symptoms in the human condition,[77,264,265] amphetamine-induced hyperactivity is commonly used as positive symptom readout in animals. In terms of predictive validity, all currently marketed antipsychotic drugs inhibit amphetamine-induced hyperactivity[266] (C. Reavill, personal communication). This may be a circular argument, given that all marketed antipsychotics are dopamine D_2/D_3 receptor antagonists.[258] However, drugs with clinically demonstrated antipsychotic activity, which do not target dopamine receptors directly, including 5-HT$_{2A}$ receptors antagonists and mGluR$_{2/3}$ agonists, are able to inhibit amphetamine-induced hyperactivity in rodents (see[87,105,106,256]). In the case of 5-HT$_{2A}$ antagonists, the effects are not particularly robust when administered alone, but there is evidence for additive/synergistic effects when combined with other antipsychotic drugs.[108] Therefore, the behavioral response to dopamine agonists remains a useful manipulation in which to investigate novel mechanisms, although alterations in experimental design may be required.

Dopamine agonists such as amphetamine, quinpirole, and apomorphine also disrupt PPI,[211,267,268] as well as latent inhibition.[37,269] The predictive validity of such approaches is discussed in detail by others.[69,211,214] Behavioral responses induced by acute treatments with dopamine agonists are generally not useful for modeling negative and cognitive symptoms, which have been associated with dopamine hypofunction in the prefrontal cortex.[270] However, amphetamine is able to induce cognitive deficits in rodents.[271]

Behavioral responses to acute NMDA receptor antagonists   The use of NMDA receptor antagonists in preclinical species (see reviews by[84,272]) is driven by the many reports of transient psychotomimetic effects of these drugs in healthy volunteers and schizophrenia patients (reviewed in[273-275]). For example, acute administration of MK-801, PCP, or ketamine to adult rodents produces behavioral effects relevant to positive, negative, and cognitive symptom domains, including locomotor hyperactivity and stereotypy,[264,265,276] impaired PPI (reviewed in[211]), reduced social interaction,[28,277] increased immobility in the forced swim test,[278] and cognitive deficits across several domains (e.g., passive avoidance[279]; reversal learning[281,271]). As for the use of dopamine-agonist-induced behaviors, most drug evaluation has been in the most accessible assays such as the motor-activating and PPI-disruptive effects of PCP, MK-801, or ketamine in rodents. As reviewed elsewhere,[184,214,282] while the dopamine agonist-induced effects are sensitive to both typical and atypical antipsychotics, it is generally found that the effects of NMDA antagonists are relatively insensitive to typical and preferentially sensitive to atypical antipsychotics such as clozapine (although see[283]). These differential effects parallel those observed in patients with schizophrenia.[204]

Behavioral responses to subchronically administered NMDA receptor antagonists Although the fundamental NMDA antagonist model is based on the acute psychotogenic effects of drugs such as PCP, and there is little if any evidence that repeated PCP administration leads to enduring psychoses in humans, repeated administration of PCP in animals leads to long-term changes that include reductions in glutamatergic functions. Hence, subchronic administration of NMDA antagonists is often used in animals as a hypoglutamatergic model that leads to enduring behavioral abnormalities (see[272, 284]). In brief, these effects include increased hyperactivity response to psychostimulants,[285,427] decreased social interaction,[286] decreased motivation in the mouse forced swim test,[278] and persistent impaired cognitive function. For example, deficits in novel object recognition (NOR) are found up to six weeks following PCP administration to rats (Gartlon *et al.*, unpublished data). Long-lasting cognitive deficits are observed in those domains thought to be worst affected in schizophrenia,[287] including working memory (deficits in T-maze and radial arm maze tests[288-290]) learning and memory (reduced acquisition in the water maze task,[291] deficits in NOR[285,292]), and reasoning and problem-solving (executive function) (deficits in an attentional set shifting[280,293,294] and deficits in reversal learning of an operant task[295]). However, it should be noted that not all the cognitive deficits reported following subchronic PCP have been replicated (see[69,272,296]), which may be explained by the different dosing regimes used (i.e., doses of PCP, repeated versus intermittent dosing, duration of washout period).

Repeated PCP administration to rats causes neuroanatomical changes which mirror those found in schizophrenia patients to some degree (reviewed briefly in[272,297]) including parvalbumin deficits in the hippocampus and frontal cortex,[298,299] regionally specific reductions in NAA[300] and changes in BDNF expression.[301] In addition, subchronic PCP disrupts learning- or emotion-associated phosphorylation of intracellular signaling (calcium calmodulin kinase II and extracellular signaling-regulated kinase) in the prefrontal cortex, hippocampus, and amygdala of mice and significantly reduces prefrontal dendritic spine density in rats.[272] Metabolic hypofunction (i.e., reduced glucose utilization) has been shown in the prefrontal cortex, reticular nucleus of the thalamus and auditory system after chronic, intermittent PCP.[299] Thus, the changes listed above are consistent with the reported cognitive deficits in animals. Repeated dosing with higher doses of PCP (e.g., 5 mg/kg twice daily) may be associated with widespread neurodegeneration and increased astroglia process density[272]; therefore, it is important to use the lowest dose consistent with reproducible effects to avoid overt neurotoxicity.

This paradigm does not appear to provide a model of the positive symptoms, however, and there are marked differences in the readouts obtained following acute and repeated PCP dosing regimens. For example, in contrast to an acute challenge, repeat administration of PCP does not produce long lasting changes in PPI or baseline motor activity after washout.[285,302] However, subchronic PCP-induced cognitive deficits are attractive for drug testing because compounds are tested in the absence of a challenge dose of PCP, thereby eliminating potential confounds due to pharmacokinetic interactions. For example, atypical, but not typical, antipsychotics reverse sub-chronic PCP-induced deficits in NOR and reversal learning[292,295] (Gartlon *et al.* unpublished data), and social behavior,[303] while novel approaches, such as the PDE10 inhibitor papaverine, reverse the effects of repeated PCP upon attentional set shifting.[293] In primates, Jentsch *et al.*[304] showed that haloperidol impaired performance of an object retrieval/detour task in vervet monkeys, a test of fronto-striatal function, and potentiated the impairment caused by repeated PCP. In contrast, clozapine attenuated the effects of PCP in vervet monkeys.[288] Elsworth *et al.*[305] recently showed that clozapine "normalized" dopaminergic tone in the prefrontal cortex of subchronically treated vervet monkeys. Further evaluation of the predictive validity of this approach is required in order to understand the utility of this model of schizophrenia-like cognitive deficits in identifying molecules with potential to improve cognition in the disease.

Neurodevelopmental approaches

Neurodevelopmental models attempt to mimic the developmental nature of schizophrenia and, in some cases, mirror the emergence of symptoms post-puberty. For example, behaviors such as reduced PPI and dopamine hyper-responsiveness appear post-puberty in the social isolation and hippocampal lesion models.[306-308] Developmental models based on environmental manipulations may have further etiological relevance as the precipitating factors, such as stress or social isolation, may be relevant to the predisposing factors in humans.[418] Below is a brief summary of the most commonly used approaches broadly classified as: environmental "insults" (obstetric complications, viral infection, social isolation), or approaches involving a direct "insult" (ventral hippocampal lesion, neonatal NMDA antagonist administration).

Isolation rearing Rats reared in social isolation from weaning show profound behavioral changes including impaired PPI, locomotor hyperactivity, increased sensitivity to psychostimulants, increased timidity, neophobia, anxiogenesis, and cognitive deficits.[22,309-311] These behavioral changes are accompanied by alterations in dopamine and serotonin neurochemistry, volume loss in the prefrontal cortex, reduced NAA in the temporal cortex, reduced parvalbumin and calbindin immunoreactivity in the hippocampus, reduced prefrontal cortical GAT-1 immunoreactive chandelier cartridges, and reduced cortical and hippocampal dendritic spine density.[50,51,301,312-314] Thus, isolation rearing appears to model a number of the behavioral, neurochemical, and neuroanatomical phenomena seen in schizophrenia.

Isolation rearing-induced PPI deficits are reversed by atypical and typical antipsychotics (see[211,310,313,315]) and also by non-dopaminergic drugs, for example α7 nicotinic receptor agonists,[306,307] which are also reported to be efficacious against information-processing deficits in schizophrenia.[238] However, PPI deficits are not reversed by drugs such as chlordiazepoxide, diazepam, and amitriptyline.[313,316] Thus, the PPI deficit in the isolation-rearing model has a good degree of predictive validity and is the developmental manipulation most commonly used to model the deficits in sensorimotor gating observed in schizophrenia. We (DJ) have also recently demonstrated that chronic clozapine, but not haloperidol, restored the decreased dendritic spine density in the hippocampus of isolation-reared rats (H. Critchlow *et al.*, unpublished data).

Lesion models   Bilateral lesion of the ventral hippocampus,[317,318] is a well-characterized neurodevelopmental model (reviewed in[319,320]). In most cases ibotenic acid–induced lesions are carried out at postnatal day 7 (to achieve a permanent lesion,[317] or the sodium channel blocker tetrodotoxin to achieve a transient inactivation[321]). In rodents, long-term effects include deficits in PPI[308] together with hyperactivity responses to novelty, stress, and amphetamine which emerge post-puberty and are ameliorated by antipsychotic drugs.[317,322] Le Pen *et al.* have also shown PPI deficits which are improved by treatment with clozapine, olanzapine, risperidone, glycine and a glycine transporter (GlyT1) inhibitor (ORG 24598), but not haloperidol.[323] Other effects include neurochemical changes, gene expression and cognitive changes of relevance to schizophrenia.[321,324,325] One drawback to these models is the severity of the excitotoxic lesion, namely that the ventral hippocampus is completely inactivated. There has been significantly less investigation of the transient hippocampal inactivation approach.

Neonatal NMDA receptor antagonist treatment   Administration of NMDA antagonists such as PCP and MK- 801 to rats around postnatal day 7 causes a relatively subtle "lesion" by inducing a short burst of widespread apoptotic neurodegeneration in the developing brain.[326] This neurodegeneration response is distinct from the excitotoxic cell death seen after high doses of NMDA antagonists in adult brains.[327] NMDA receptors undergo a period of hypersensitivity in the first two weeks of life (corresponding to the brain growth spurt, which occurs in the third trimester in humans), during which time neurons expressing NMDA receptors are highly sensitive to both NMDA-mediated excitotoxicity[328] and NMDA hypofunction.[326] It is postulated that NMDA receptor hypofunction causes developing neurons to undergo apoptosis during critical stages of synaptogenesis.[329] The long-term consequences of early life NMDA receptor administration are particularly relevant to schizophrenia (reviewed in[330]) and include PPI deficits, cognitive deficits (spatial learning, object recognition, and social recognition), increased locomotor sensitivity to novelty and amphetamine and neuropathological changes of relevance to schizophrenia,[331-335] although there were no effects upon progressive ratio responding, a measure of avolition.[23] There has been limited pharmacological evaluation of this model, although some of these behavioral changes are sensitive to drug treatment, for example, social discrimination deficits are reversed by an mGluR2/3 agonist, LY-354740, and a mGluR2 receptor potentiator, LY-487379,[422] a D_2 receptor antagonist/5-HT$_{1A}$ receptor agonist, SSR181507,[333] while NOR deficits are attenuated by clozapine (Gartlon *et al.*, unpublished data) and SSR504734, GlyT1.[336]

Maternal methylazoxymethanol acetate treatment Systemic administration of the mitotic inhibitor methylazoxymethanol acetate (MAM) to pregnant rats during gestation (embryonic day 17) disrupts neurogenesis in the developing fetus.[337] When grown to adulthood, rats treated with MAM display behavioral effects, including increased locomotion in response to mild stress and psychomotor stimulants, social interaction deficits, PPI deficits, and cognitive deficits.[337-343] Neuroanatomical changes include reduced whole brain, hippocampus and pre-frontal cortex volume, thinning of the limbic cortices with increased neuronal density, and reduced parvalbumin expression in the hippocampus.[343,344] However, some of these effects, for example deficits in learning and memory in the water maze,[345] appear to be inconsistent. The predictive validity of these changes, in terms of sensitivity to antipsychotic treatments, has not yet been reported.

Obstetric complications Obstetric complications which have been associated with increased risk (by a factor of two[346] for schizophrenia include maternal malnutrition, maternal stress and hypoxic/ischemic events during birth.[347,348] Some of these events can be mimicked in animals, for example intrauterine hypoxia,[349] anoxia during caesarean birth[350] and exposure to low oxygen environment during the early postnatal period,[351] reviewed in Boksa *et al.*[418] Long-term effects in animal models include locomotor hyperactivity. However, further schizophrenia-relevant changes in behavior, brain structure, or neurochemistry have not been reported (Boksa *et al.* 2004). There has been limited investigation of the effects of drugs and consequently, the predictive validity of these models is not yet understood.

Viral infection There is a large body of evidence linking maternal infections during pregnancy with increased incidence of schizophrenia[352,423,424]; briefly (reviewed in[202]). In rodents, exposure to viral infection during the prenatal or early postnatal period leads to behavioral changes including PPI deficits, reduced social interaction, reduced exploratory behavior and altered responses to psychotomimetic drugs.[353] Similarly, injection of the viral mimic polyriboinosinic-polyribocytidilic acid (poly I:C)[354] or the bacterial endotoxin lipopolysaccharide (LPS)[355] in early life leads to long-term schizophrenia-relevant changes, most notably a deficit in PPI.[356] However, there has been insufficient investigation of the effects of drugs to understand the usefulness of this approach in drug discovery.

Genetic models

Given the polygenic nature of the disease, and the subtle and poorly understood interactions between genetics and environmental factors, the knockout (either full or partial) or over expression of a single gene in mice is unlikely to produce a validated animal model of aspects of schizophrenia.[200,258] However, manipulation of individual genes, particularly in the absence of suitable pharmacological tools, may provide insight into gene function. The various approaches adopted are discussed below.

Hypothesis driven The dopamine and glutamate hypotheses of schizophrenia are still the major drivers of hypothesis-driven models (reviewed in[258,266,357]). Thus, for schizophrenia, hypothesis-driven genetic models are largely based on conclusions drawn from the drug-driven models discussed in the previous section. As a consequence, they do not provide information on the genetic susceptibility to the illness but, nevertheless, can provide useful insight into the role of molecular components of neurotransmission. Examples of models based on a hyperdopaminergic hypothesis include the dopamine transporter (DAT) knockout[358] which produces PPI deficits and locomotor hyperactivity, both of which are sensitive to D_2 antagonist treatment[197,359] and D_1 and D_2 receptor knockouts.[360-362] Glutamatergic mouse models include the NMDA receptor hypomorph mouse, in which the NR1 subunit of the NMDA receptor is markedly reduced.[363] These mice display hyperactivity, reduced metabolic activity in the hippocampus and cortical areas, enhanced sensitivity to the stimulant effects of amphetamine, impaired social interaction and PPI (see[363] for references). Intracellular signaling has also been targeted, with the advantage of disrupting the convergent points of several neurotransmitters, for example, the knockout of dopamine and cyclic adenosine monophosphate (cAMP)-regulated phosphoprotein of 32 KDa (DARPP-32) which is involved in dopamine, glutamate, and serotonin signaling.[364]

Phenotype driven An alternative approach is to screen for schizophrenia-relevant phenotypes across a wide range of genetic mutants or animal strains. This approach offers potential for providing clues for new disease mechanisms and, conceptually, is the reverse of the hypothesis-driven approach. Phenotype screening requires a systematic process to identify between-strain/mutant behavioral and pathological characteristics (e.g., the SHIRPA screen[425]). Large-scale phenotypic screening projects, for example the NIH "Knockout Mouse Project" (KOMP[365]), are aimed at providing access to animals and information regarding the phenotypes of every gene knockout in the mouse genome. Phenotypic differences in existing strains or spontaneous mutants can also be informative. For example, Brown Norway rats have reduced PPI compared with Wistar or Sprague-Dawley rats,[366] and Brattleboro rats, a mutant variant of the Long Evans strain with no detectable plasma vasopressin, display a PPI deficit which is sensitive to antipsychotic treatment[367] (Cilia *et al.* – unpublished data). Such an approach has provided a useful model, the DBA/2 mouse model of impaired auditory gating[34] (see above).

Strain differences may also help in identifying the genetic basis underlying susceptibility to environmental or development events. For example, Lewis rats differ from Sprague-Dawley rats in that they show no PPI deficit following isolation rearing[368] or maternal deprivation.[198] However, this type of "multiple gene" approach has so far yielded relatively little insight into the contribution of specific genes or mechanisms, perhaps reflecting the complexity of this work.

Susceptibility genes The use of genetic animal models has allowed investigation of the functional significance of the susceptibility genes recently identified for schizophrenia (see above and reviewed in[114]). Many of the susceptibility genes identified are implicated in processes such as synaptic plasticity, neurotransmission, and neurodevelopment, which are also likely to be affected in schizophrenia.[114] Given that many of these genes were identified using cognitive dysfunction as a phenotype in linkage or association studies, most of the susceptibility genes are also implicated in cognitive function.[197] The phenotypic characterization of mutant mouse models for schizophrenia susceptibility genes is ongoing and has been recently reviewed.[200] In brief, mice with manipulations of susceptibility genes which display a schizophrenia-related phenotype include NRG1, Proline dehydrogenase (PRODH), and DISC1. Manipulation of other genes, such as COMT, Regulator of G protein signalling 4 (RGS4), and Dysbindin (DTNBP1), have not resulted in a phenotype mimicking aspects of schizophrenia ([200] and references therein). Initiatives such as the NIH "Knockout Mouse Project" (see above) are likely to intensify research in this area by allowing many more researchers in the field to gain access to mutant mouse models.

Genetic models-future directions As outlined above, the interactions between risk genes and the environment in schizophrenia are poorly understood. The current genetic models, although technically sophisticated, do not reflect the changes in gene function caused by variations in DNA or environment, or the interaction between risk genes. For example, a complete knock out of NRG1 in a mouse is lethal, but even the use of heterozygote mice is light years away from the incredibly complex interplay of the NRG1 isoforms demonstrated in schizophrenia.[144] Appropriate studies would require modelling of the dysregulation of gene expression rather than targeting individual genes *per se* given that changes in the regulation of gene expression are likely to play a role in disease susceptibility.[369]

In an attempt to address at least some of this complexity, future directions in this area are likely to investigate the "two hit hypothesis", that is, incorporating an environmental insult (e.g., viral infection, isolation rearing, neonatal NMDA antagonist treatment) in specific rodent strains with apparent increased sensitivity to these manipulations (e.g., DBA2/J mice), or in particular, in mutant mice strains with manipulations of candidate risk genes (reviewed in[202]).

Technological developments, including RNA interference (RNAi) techniques, may circumvent the need for the production of mutant mice in the investigation of novel proteins.[426] Although not used routinely yet and not without disadvantages, this approach makes region-specific expression changes possible in adult animals (generally), and allows manipulation of more than one gene target in the same animal. In the absence of suitable pharmacological tools, this method may provide a more efficient way to understand gene function, in the adult at least.

To summarize the discussion on animal models of aspects of schizophrenia, it is clear that there are exciting developments in this field and models are now available to us that reflect multiple characteristics of the disorder. Nevertheless, establishing the construct, etiological, and predictive validity of the current (and future) models is dependent upon a better understanding of the etiology and neuropathology of the disease itself. The increased acceptance that no individual paradigm will model the disease in its entirety and that we should strive to model particular aspects of the disorder parallels the "deconstruction of schizophrenia" discussion ongoing within the clinical community (see below).

There are some clear examples of useful models of the positive (e.g., amphetamine-induced hyperactivity, isolation rearing, acute PCP), and cognitive symptoms (e.g., acute, subchronic, or neonatal PCP treatments in rodents), and some of the physiological deficits in schizophrenia (e.g., strains of mice or rats having low P50 or PPI gating). However, there is a clear need for a focus on the development of useful models of negative symptoms, an area of clear unmet need in schizophrenia. Although there are examples of manipulations that alter social behavior described above (e.g., various mutant mice, acute or subchronic PCP treatment), there appears to be less confidence in these models, perhaps based on the lack of clinically validated positive controls for negative symptoms.

Experimental/Translational Medicine Approaches

The development of symptom models in either healthy volunteers, enriched populations (e.g., healthy volunteers with low PPI, first-degree relatives, see below), or patients would be a major advance in drug development in schizophrenia.[370] The most typical example is the use of a drug-induced response, exemplified by the use of ketamine which induces a state that mimics some aspects of schizophrenia in healthy volunteers,[257,371] (and see[275] introducing a special issue of *Journal of Psychopharmacology* focusing on this model). Using a variety of techniques (e.g., MRI, MEG, PET, psychological assessment, pharmacological investigation), this approach may provide a route into understanding the neurobiology of individual symptoms (see[184 and 275]). However, this model has not been used extensively in drug discovery given the apparent limited predictive validity, that is, relative resistance of the effects to reversal by current antipsychotics,[372] other than clozapine.[373] In this context, it is important to note that, as in patients with schizophrenia, clozapine, but not typical antipsychotics, is able to prevent the PPI-disruptive effects of NMDA antagonists in mice, rats, and monkeys.[282,374,375] Thus, it has been suggested that the acute effects of NMDA antagonists may serve as a cross-species model of the atypical effects of drugs such as clozapine.[204,214] Furthermore, recent findings indicate that agonists at mGluR2/3, which are antipsychotic, reverse ketamine-induced working memory deficits in healthy volunteers.[87,376]

Other candidates for biomarkers include imaging probes. Studies that investigate the occupancy of drugs at receptors where radiotracers exist are already common in experimental medicine studies (e.g., D_2, 5-HT_{2A} receptor occupancy via positron emission tomography [PET] or single photon emission computed tomography [SPECT]). Such studies provide evidence of CNS penetration, and where an understanding about target levels of receptor occupancy (e.g., D_2 receptors[102]), may provide very valuable information on appropriate doses for efficacy studies. However, this approach relies upon the novel agent having sufficient affinity for these target receptors, or causing neurochemical effects such that the radiotracer is displaced by an endogenous neurotransmitter. Whereas PET and SPECT studies have shown promise in understanding the pathophysiology of brain disorders, at present few radioligands have been sufficiently investigated to be available for functional imaging of target molecules. To this end, the National Institutes of Health (NIH) have created an initiative specifically for the development and testing of PET and SPECT imaging ligands, as discussed in an accompanying chapter.[377, iii]

Academic-Industry-Government Initiatives in Schizophrenia

The various Academic-Industry-Government initiatives are reviewed in detail by Winsky *et al.*[377] [iii]

MATRICS

The history and aims of the *MATRICS* (Measurement and Treatment Research to Improve Cognition in Schizophrenia) Program has been reviewed by Stephen Marder.[378] The Food and Drug Administration (FDA) in the US licenses drugs for use in schizophrenia only if they reduce the positive symptoms of psychosis (i.e., are anti-psychotics). Implicitly, the FDA operated from the assumption that to be registered as a new treatment for the cognitive deficits of schizophrenia, a drug should also treat the entire disorder, rather than attempt to treat specific clinical problems with specific compounds. This approach has been identified as a bottleneck preventing the identification and development of novel treatments for specific symptoms, such as cognitive deficits or negative symptoms (see[379]). In response to this issue, the US National Institute of Mental Health (NIMH) developed the MATRICS Program. MATRICS set out to develop a broad consensus regarding the nature of the cognitive impairments in schizophrenia and how they might best be assessed and treated[380] and in particular, begin to establish a clear path that would enable the FDA to consider registration of compounds intended to treat cognitive deficits in schizophrenia.

The MATRICS initiative consisted of a series of conferences seeking consensus opinion from leading NIH, FDA, as well as academic and industry representatives. With an unprecedented degree of success, the MATRICS group was able to establish agreement between these different constituencies in a number of key areas:

- The domains of cognition deemed most relevant in schizophrenia: working memory; attention/vigilance; verbal learning and memory; visual learning and memory; speed of processing; reasoning and problem-solving; and social cognition.[381]

- Identification of the most intriguing molecular targets, promising compounds, relevant human test measures, and potentially predictive animal models for use in the discovery of treatments that target basic mechanisms related to complex cognitive operations.[382]

- Established a MATRICS Consensus Cognitive Battery for Clinical Trials (listed on the MATRICS website, www.matrics.ucla.edu) and addressed the processes required for assessment of cognition as an endpoint in clinical trials,[383] which directly led to the TURNS initiative (Treatment Units for Research on Neurocognition and Schizophrenia[384]).

- Discussed the development of a research agenda that would foster improved methods for the discovery, validation, and assessment of pro-cognitive adjunctive treatments for schizophrenia (see special issue of Schizophrenia Bulletin, October 2005[379]). As results of this effort, two spin-off initiatives were started, TURNS and CNTRICS, as well as a number of other post-MATRICS programs[385] (see below).

[iii] Please refer to Winsky *et al.*, Drug discovery and development initiatives at the National Institute of Mental Health: From cell-based system to proof of concept in this volume.

TURNS

The *TURNS* Project (www.TURNS.ucla.edu) consists of a network of academic sites charged with selecting potential cognitive-enhancing agents and evaluating their potential efficacy in Phase 2 proof of concept trials.[384] As part of the TURNS program, a sub-group, chaired by Mark Geyer, is evaluating rodent and primate tests of each of the cognitive domains identified by MATRICS in order to provide better direction for preclinical scientists.[385,386]

CNTRICS

The *CNTRICS* (www.cntrics.ucdavis.edu) initiative was born of discussions during the MATRICS program about the desirability of utilizing tasks and tools derived from cognitive neuroscience to supplement the MATRICS cognitive test battery.[385,387] This supplementation could involve the use of additional physiological and behavioral measures, including event related potentials (ERPs) and PPI, or imaging technologies such as fMRI, MEG, PET, or MRS. The goal of this initiative, due to complete the final meeting in early 2008, is to fully integrate the tools and constructs of cognitive neuroscience to enhance translational research focusing on developing treatments that target impaired cognitive and emotional processing in schizophrenia. Carter and Barch[387] argued that a strong emphasis on understanding the neurobiology of cognition is required for the development of novel treatments, and that this understanding will depend upon the use of animals as well as man to identify novel molecular targets. The project aim is that the initial products of CNTRICS will have their most immediate impact in the earliest stage of clinical drug testing (Phases 1 and II) in order to provide evidence for efficacy as early as possible. In addition, the outcomes of CNTRICS may also interact with the product of other initiatives designed to improve measurement in preclinical species, by emphasizing the use of validated homologous animal and human paradigms during the drug discovery process.[387]

Other Post-MATRICS Initiatives

MATRICS CT (for co-primary selection and translation of the MATRICS test battery) reflects the international nature of drug discovery in schizophrenia and the requirement for translation from English and appropriate validation of the MATRICS test battery. Further, MATRICS CT will also consider the need for measures of functioning and functional capacity (see[385]). In addition, a MATRICS-style initiative to address the poor treatment of negative symptoms has begun (NIMH Initiative Regarding Treatment for Negative Symptoms[388]), with the aim of developing more sensitive instruments for measuring this symptom domain (see[385]).

FUTURE OF DRUG DISCOVERY IN SCHIZOPHRENIA AND DISCUSSION

Strategies for Drug Discovery

The environment for drug discovery for schizophrenia will be very different over the next 10 years, driven by exciting changes in our understanding of the neurobiology of the disease, but also by regulatory and pricing pressures. Pharmaceutical companies, and increasingly Academic/Government partnerships, will have to adopt multiple strategies for the development of treatments for this disease. For example, in order to develop a novel molecule, it should be defined in advance whether it is expected to be an antipsychotic, that is, it is expected to reveal its activity in acutely ill patients in standard 4–6 week trials, or it will be directed against individual symptoms and may only reveal efficacy after longer team adjunctive dosing in stabilized patients. This difference will have implications for the development package required for such studies, that is, will drug combination studies be required in the animal symptom models, or to determine pharmacokinetic or toxicological interactions.

The idealized flowchart for a drug discovery program is shown in Figure 8.1. It emphasizes that identification of drugs is not a linear process, but that each stage may provide information that can redefine the objectives of the program. The following sections discuss opportunities and challenges that the drug discoverer will meet. Perhaps the most important decision is the selection of the drug target(s). Already the change in our understanding of the neurobiology of this disease has influenced the selection of targets for drug discovery and the characterization and validation of animal models. An example discussed above, NRG1/ErbB4, illustrates the rapid progress that can be made in the biological understanding of a target when it catches the imagination of the scientific community. The promise of the ongoing whole genome association studies is that there will be additional similar examples that will provide druggable targets which are closer to the underlying pathophysiology of the disease in order the realize the ambition of a "bottom up" approach.[73]

The challenge for the drug discoverer is to configure *in vitro* screening and *in vivo* pharmacodynamic assays and appropriate chemical libraries in order to identify good tool molecules to interrogate targets further. Then molecules should be evaluated in appropriate models of the symptoms of schizophrenia in order to understand how to evaluate the molecule clinically in the most appropriate way either in experimental medicine studies or in Phase 2 trials in the disease population (Figure 8.1). Some of the issues and opportunities associated with the clinical aspects of this process are discussed below.

Development of Clinical Studies in Drug Discovery

Clinical trials have traditionally relied upon symptom-rating scales as primary measures of the efficacy of a new treatment. Instruments such as the Positive and Negative Syndrome Scale (PANSS)[389] and the BPRS[390] yield potentially informative ratings of symptom severity and improvement. The PANSS has typically been the instrument of choice for schizophrenia trials, as it has separate subscales for positive and negative symptoms as well as a "General" subscale for other indicators of psychopathology such as depression, anxiety, somatic concerns, and so on.

The usefulness of these measures is greatly dependent on, and is thus limited by, important factors. These include the skill and experience of the rater and the willingness or ability of the patient to accurately and honestly describe his or her symptoms. As McEvoy and Freudenreich[iv] describe in an accompanying chapter, techniques such

---

[iv] Please refer to McEvoy and Freudenreich, Issues in the Design and Conductance of Clinical Trials in this volume.

as videoconferencing are increasingly being used to train raters and improve consensus on ratings. The patient's capacity to accurately report symptoms, however, is a more challenging target. One can imagine, for example, that a schizophrenia patient with prominent negative symptoms may not be able to describe his thought content as eloquently as a patient who is verbose and interactive. Similarly, a highly suspicious patient may refrain from being forthcoming about the severity of her symptoms. Factors such as fatigue and sedation may confound symptom ratings. These limitations can be overcome when more objective, non-volitional indicators are used, underscoring the need for biologically based markers of clinical efficacy.

Thus, using biologically based measures of efficacy may result in a more objective evaluation of new drugs. Potential candidates for useful "biomarkers" that can be incorporated into clinical trials include EEG-based measures such as P50 suppression and MMN, as well as other psychophysiological probes such as PPI and visual scanning (see[93]). Whereas deficits in these indices of information processing have been traditionally considered stable endophenotypes of the illness, there is emerging evidence that the extent of the deficits may indeed fluctuate with illness state.

In the case of PPI, several studies have demonstrated that impaired PPI in schizophrenia patients improves to normal levels with treatment, and this improvement is in some cases correlated with improvement in symptoms.[216,220,391] Thus testing whether a novel compound can reverse PPI deficits among schizophrenia patients may be a useful means of screening antipsychotic medications. Recently, investigators have reported the effects of antipsychotics in healthy volunteers with low baseline PPI. When healthy volunteers are stratified in terms of low versus high PPI, atypical antipsychotics such as clozapine or quetiapine increase PPI in low responders while having no effect in high responders.[223,224,392] As with the reversal of PPI deficits in schizophrenia, this effect of clozapine-like drugs is not observed with haloperidol.[393] Further research is warranted to determine whether this use of "enriched" normal populations might provide a simple way to help identify either atypical antipsychotics or potentially procognitive adjunctive treatments.

MMN is an especially promising candidate in this regard given that, unlike PPI, deficits in MMN are relatively specific to schizophrenia,[394] and the effect sizes of the differences in MMN between schizophrenia patients and comparison subjects are large.[249] The recent evidence that abnormal MMN in schizophrenia is correlated with poor functional outcome also lends support to the potential value of this measure in assessing the efficacy of medications in improving cognitive and functional abilities.[249]

A less well-studied, but potentially useful, biomarker of schizophrenia is impairment in visual scanning. There are several scanning abnormalities that have been well documented in the literature. One is that of smooth pursuit eye movements (SPEM) and refers to prefrontally mediated visual tracking of stimuli. SPEM abnormalities have been reported to be an endophenotypic marker of schizophrenia.[395] Additionally, the visual scanning of a meaningful or relevant stimulus can provide a high-resolution index of how the brain processes environmentally salient information.[396] Schizophrenia patients show restricted and impoverished visual scanning of stimuli such as faces[397,398] and complex stimuli such as fractal images[399] and stimuli from the Rorschach test, a set of complex stimuli, which contain shading and color gradations.[428] This reduced ability to efficiently scan and process a visually complex environment may ultimately result in a repetitive and inflexible response to that environment. Thus visual scanning, which is relatively easy and inexpensive to measure,[399] may be a useful addition to a psychophysiology battery that can be used to test whether novel compounds can enhance cognitive deficits in schizophrenia, deficits that appear to have implications for daily functioning.

The Importance of Positive Symptoms in Designing Translational Models

One of the challenges in developing translational models of schizophrenia is how to model positive symptoms in animals. Whereas disorganized behavior and psychomotor agitation can be modeled in animal paradigms (see Table 8.2), the hallmark positive symptoms of the disease, hallucinations and delusions, are clearly difficult or impossible to recreate or measure in animals as well as in non-psychotic humans. This difficulty has led to creative efforts to cause psychotic-like states. For example, Hoffman[400] created a paradigm to study how non-schizophrenic humans attend to non-sensical auditory "babble" compared to schizophrenia patients who actively hallucinate.

The importance of attempting to model the positive symptoms of schizophrenia is underscored by schizophrenia patients' personal experience of their illness. Whereas scientists tend to regard positive symptoms and negative symptoms (cognitive deficits could arguably be included in the latter category) as clusters of symptoms that more or less develop independently from one another, the individual with schizophrenia will often identify more of a causal relationship between these problems. Many patients blame their positive symptoms for their decline in thinking, and for the withdrawal from social, occupational, or school activities. Thus in order to be able to understand the expression of schizophrenia and its impact on an individual's ability to manage his or her life, it is necessary to devote more effort to translational modeling of positive symptoms. Given the obvious challenges of mimicking hallucinations and delusions in animals, an alternative might be to focus on a surrogate phenotype that has been strongly associated with positive symptoms in humans. For example, delusions in schizophrenia have been related to alteration in the normal visual scanning of faces,[401] a measure that could be studied in non-human primates. The expression of thought disorder, a signature of schizophrenia, is moderately correlated with impaired PPI in schizophrenia patients[226] and is also associated with abnormal increases in brain activity in prefrontal and temporal areas.[402] These and other endophenotypes can serve as surrogate markers for thought disorder and can be studied in animals; to date little work has been done in this arena.

The Importance of Functional Outcome and Performance-based Assessment

Functional outcome itself is also a critical target for drug discovery. As mentioned above, what is largely missing in the study of the efficacy of antipsychotic medications is their impact on the day-to-day functional ability of the individual with schizophrenia.

Change in cognitive abilities can serve as a proxy for this measure, since functional deficits are correlated with neuropsychological impairment in schizophrenia patients.[403] However, the ideal way to measure whether antipsychotic medications have improved a patient's quality of life is through direct observation and tracking of everyday functioning in the patient's own environment. There have been efforts to move closer to this goal by assessing functioning using standardized, performance-based measures such as the UCSD Performance-Based Skills Assessment (UPSA),[404] which uses role-play situations to assess patients' skills in communication (using a telephone), household management (paying bills, going grocery shopping), travel (reading a bus schedule), and other domains. Measures such as the UPSA, however, are still laboratory based and cannot entirely replace the important role of direct subject observation in numerous "real-life" scenarios. Similarly, issues of cognitive and social resiliency have been overlooked when studying what baseline factors may influence medication efficacy in schizophrenia patients. While there is an extensive literature pertaining to resiliency in the general population, it has been widely overlooked in schizophrenia. Yet, resiliency may provide a protective factor and independently contribute to the ability to bounce back from the stressful events related to psychotic decompensated states.

Thus, there is room for new and creative approaches to monitoring schizophrenia patients as they negotiate tasks of everyday living that are specifically relevant to them and their own environmental demands. Very little work has been done to attempt to link functional ability in schizophrenia with potential genetic predictors, but there is promise that genes associated with planning and problem-solving, for example the COMT gene, may have an influence on the schizophrenia patient's day-to-day living.[405] From a translational perspective, it is challenging to design a comparable functional measure in animals, given that functional abilities are highly species specific. Evaluation of animal social behavior, grooming, hygiene, feeding, and so on, may hold some promise in this regard. With respect to clinical trials in humans, the FDA is taking its cue from initiatives such as MATRICS (see above) and is considering the incorporation of functional assessments in drug trials; research in this area is highly productive and is unfolding at a rapid pace.[406]

In order to develop better medications to treat schizophrenia, we must also have better tools to evaluate the often difficult-to-assess signs and symptoms of the disorder. Often researchers rely on global measures such as the Clinical Global Impression (CGI) or the Global Assessment of Function (GAF), which are overly broad and may not be sufficiently sensitive for testing the efficacy of compounds that are intended to target specific symptoms.[407] A more comprehensive assessment approach should target positive, negative, cognitive, social, and functional signs and symptoms of the disorder. However, the typical assessment of positive and negative symptoms and social and functional behavior is complicated by a host of factors that include: reliance on patient self report; rater-related bias; a lack of appreciation that these features vary across time and environmental conditions; consideration of secondary gain issues in patients who are assessed while in the hospital; etc. These complications may obscure our ability to detect subtle clinical signals. Consequently, effort needs to be made to develop objective "performance-based" measures of these signature characteristics of schizophrenia, similar to the well-validated neuropsychological measures used to objectively assess cognitive functioning. Improving our clinical measures will certainly enhance our ability to develop novel medications that may not ameliorate an entire domain (e.g., positive symptoms) but have powerful effects on debilitating features (e.g., misperception of easily identifiable objects).

Considering the Plasticity of Cognitive Deficits in Schizophrenia

It is understood by clinicians that the environment interacts with internal states to decrease or increase the manifestation of symptoms. For example, placing an agitated patient in a temporary state of seclusion with a reduction in environmental stimulation can help the patient to regain control and decrease symptoms of agitation. Conversely, affectively charged or cognitively challenging environments can increase symptoms of disorganization, lability, and delusional thinking. Yet, studies of cognition in schizophrenia rarely focus on whether changes in behavior, or phenotype, can be accomplished by changing the environment, for example, predictable versus novel environments, high versus low emotional content, high versus random versus low reinforcement. For example, the classic perseverative response pattern seen on the Wisconsin Card Sorting Test can be virtually eliminated by obligating schizophrenia patients to monitor their behavior and verbalize their problem-solving strategy.[70,71] Schizophrenia patients can modify their behavior in response to changes in environmental contingencies in the same way that non-patients do.[408] This behavior change can be observed in studies using a two-choice prediction task, where psychiatric populations can be distinguished based upon their responses to high versus low reinforcement rates.[409] In decision-making tasks where the anticipated outcome is obvious, reinforcement frequency and "payoff" principally determine selection of responses and are orchestrated by specific brain systems. In conditions where the outcome is more uncertain however, personality factors such as impulsivity influence a subject's response.[410] Furthermore, different regions of the brain are activated depending on whether decision-making is occurring in response to certain or uncertain outcomes, and this pattern of activation is altered in schizophrenia patients.[411] Thus, when attempting to model the cognitive features of schizophrenia, the influence of the environment as well as task-related demands should be taken into account.

Translational Models of Treatment in the Prodrome

Of late, there has been much interest in studying the schizophrenia prodrome, or the early, sub-syndromal state characterized by emergence of psychotic symptoms and the beginnings of disability and withdrawal from daily activities. The use of antipsychotic medications in this population at high risk for developing schizophrenia is increasingly considered a reasonable treatment option.[412] However, to date there have been very few placebo-controlled, double-blinded studies that test the efficacy of antipsychotics in prodromal individuals.[412] In fact, McGlashan and colleagues found that early treatment with olanzapine resulted in only a modest and not statistically significant decrease in the risk of conversion to schizophrenia. This is an area in need of further study and potentially amenable to translational research. Animal models of the prodrome include repeated amphetamine injections[413] and a variety of developmental manipulations.[414] For example, isolation rearing in rodents appears to lead to disruption of brain development as manifested by deficits in sensorimotor gating that emerge at or after puberty,[415] and which can be reversed by antipsychotic treatment (see above). Efforts are now underway to attempt to prevent the emergence of such delayed consequences of early developmental insults to assess the feasibility of animal models of prophylactic treatments.[414] Parallel treatment studies in high-risk humans and prodromal animal models may be an interesting approach to testing the efficacy of antipsychotic or, more likely, other medications in decreasing the risk for developing the illness.

Pharmacogenetics/Pharmacophenomics

In the near future, treatment strategies are likely to move away from a focus on treating a specific illness and more towards targeting symptoms and cognitive states. Treatment regimens will be determined not necessarily by a patient's diagnosis; rather patients will be treated with agents that are selective for their deficits or phenotype, a strategy that has been referred to as pharmacophenomics. Moreover, pharmacogenetics will increasingly play a role in influencing antipsychotic medication recommendations.[297,416] For example, schizophrenia patients carrying the dopamine D_2 (DRD2) TAQ1 allele have more severe side effects when treated with strong dopamine D_2 antagonist medications, suggesting that these individuals might be better treated with agents such as olanzapine or clozapine.[417] Genetic manipulations in animal models of schizophrenia may prove useful in further studying the interaction between genes, particularly those related to dopamine transport and regulation, as those genes influence the efficacy of existing antipsychotic agents.

CONCLUSION

In conclusion, it is an exciting time to be involved in schizophrenia research because the advances in this field provide novel opportunities for drug discovery and development. It is a time of unprecedented and productive collaboration between Industry, Academia, and Government, particularly for the treatment of cognitive symptoms, resulting in the testing of novel treatment approaches, including but not limited to, nicotinic agonists, NK3 antagonists, mGluR2/3 agonists, serotonin 5-HT$_6$ antagonists, phosphodiesterase inhibitors, and AMPA receptor positive modulators, as well as multi-target monoaminergic approaches, which may offer benefits in terms of improved efficacy and/or tolerability. This collaborative spirit needs to continue to focus our attention upon approaches which may improve the treatment of this debilitating and multi-syndromal disease.

ACKNOWLEDGEMENTS

This work was partially supported by a grant from the United States National Institute of Mental Health (1R01-MH071916).

REFERENCES

1. Picchioni, M.M. and Murray, R.M. (2007). Schizophrenia. *BMJ*, 335:91–95.
2. Heile, H., Haukka, J., Suvisaari, J., and Lonnqvist, J. (2005). Mortality among patients with schizophrenia and reduced psychiatric hospital care. *Psychol Med*, 35:725–732.
3. Gitkin, A., Harris, G., Birchenough, J. *et al.* (2001). *Nervous Breakdown. A Detailed Analysis of the Neurology Market*. UBS Warburg, New York, pp. 256–264.
4. American Psychiatric Association (2000). *Diagnostic and Statistical Manual of Mental Disorders, Fourth Edition, Text Revision*. Washington DC.
5. World Health Organisation (1992). *The ICD-10 Classification of Mental and Behavioural Disorders*, Geneva.
6. Andreasen, N.C. (2000). Schizophrenia: The fundamental questions. *Brain Res Rev*, 31:106–112.
7. Andreasen, N.C. (2007). DSM and the death of phenomenology in America: An example of unintended consequences. *Schiz Bull*, 33(1):108–112.
8. Lewis, R. (2004). Should cognitive deficits be a diagnostic criterion for schizophrenia. *Rev Psychiatr Neurosci*, 29(2):101–113.
9. Hyman, S.E. (2007). Can neuroscience be integrated into DSM-V. *Nat Rev Neurosci*, 8:725–732.
10. Keefe, R.S.E. and Fenton, W.S. (2007). How should DSM-V criteria for schizophrenia include cognitive impairment? *Schiz Bull*, 33(4):912–920.
11. Lehmann, H.E. and Ban, T.A. (1997). The history of the psychopharmacology of schizophrenia. *Can J Psych*, 42:152–162.
12. Carlsson, A. and Lindquist, M. (1963). Effect of chlorpromazine or haloperidol on the formation of 3-methoxytyramine and normetanephrine in mouse brain. *Acta Pharmacol Toxicol*, 20:140–144.
13. Ackenheil, M. and Hippius, H. (1977). Clozapine. In Usdin, E. and Forrest, I.S. (eds.), *Psychotherapeutic drugs: Part II*. Marcel Dekker, New York, pp. 923–956.
14. Roth, B.L., Sheffler, D.J., and Kroeze, W.K. (2004). Magic shotguns versus magic bullets: Selectively non-selective drugs for mood disorders and schizophrenia. *Nat Rev Drug Discov*, 3:353–359.
15. Garzya, V., Forbes, I.T., Gribble, A.D., Hadley, M.S., Lightfoot, A.P., Payne, A.H. *et al.* (2007). Studies towards the identification of a new generation of atypical antipsychotic agents. *Bioorg Med Chem Lett*, 17:400–405.
16. Jarskog, L.F., Miyamoto, S., and Lieberman, J.A. (2007). Schizophrenia: New pathological insights and therapies. *Annu Rev Med*, 58:49–61.
17. Young, J.W., Minassian, A., Paulus, M.P., Geyer, M.A., and Perry, W. (2007). A reverse-translational approach to bipolar disorder: Rodent and human studies in the Behavioral Pattern Monitor. *Neurosci Biobehav Rev*, 31(6):882–896.
18. Farrow, T.F., Hunter, M.D., Haque, R., and Spence, S.A. (2006). Modafinil and unconstrained motor activity in schizophrenia: Double-blind crossover placebo-controlled trial. *Br J Psychiatry*, 189:461–462.
19. Kirsch, P., Ronshausen, S., Mier, D., and Gallhofer, B. (2007). The influence of antipsychotic treatment on brain reward system reactivity in schizophrenia patients. *Pharmacopsychiatry*, 40(5):196–198.
20. Muscat, R. and Willner, P. (1992). Suppression of sucrose drinking by chronic mild unpredictable stress: A methodological analysis. *Neurosci Biobehav Rev*, 16(4):507–517.
21. Schaefer, G.J. and Michael, R.P. (1992). Schedule-controlled brain self-stimulation: Has it utility for behavioral pharmacology? *Neurosci Biobehav Rev*, 16(4):569–583.

22. Cilia, J., Piper, D.C., Upton, N., and Hagan, J.J. (2001). Clozapine enhances breakpoint in common marmosets responding on a progressive ratio schedule. *Psychopharmacology (Berl)*, 155(2):135–143.

23. Wiley, J.L. and Compton, A.D. (2004). Progressive ratio performance following challenge with antipsychotics, amphetamine, or NMDA antagonists in adult rats treated perinatally with phencyclidine. *Psychopharmacology (Berl)*, 177(1-2):170–177.

24. Deacon, R.M. (2006). Assessing nest building in mice. *Nat Protoc*, 1(3):1117–1119.

25. Hava, G., Vered, L., Yael, M., Mordechai, H., and Mahoud, H. (2006). Alterations in behavior in adult offspring mice following maternal inflammation during pregnancy. *Dev Psychobiol*, 48(2):162–168.

26. Harvey, P.D., Velligan, D.I., and Bellack, A.S. (2007). Performance-based measures of functional skills: Usefulness in clinical treatment studies. *Schizophr Bull*, 33(5):1138–1148.

27. Nadler, J.J., Moy, S.S., Dold, G., Trang, D., Simmons, N., Perez, A., Young, N.B., Barbaro, R.P., Piven, J., Magnuson, T.R., and Crawley, J.N. (2004). Automated apparatus for quantitation of social approach behaviors in mice. *Genes Brain Behav*, 3(5):303–314.

28. Sams-Dodd, F. (1995). Distinct effects of d-amphetamine and phencyclidine on the social behaviour of rats. *Behav Pharmacol*, 6(1):55–65.

29. Veenema, A.H. and Neumann, I.D. (2007). Neurobiological mechanisms of aggression and stress coping: A comparative study in mouse and rat selection lines. *Brain Behav Evol*, 70(4):274–285.

30. Bertrand, M.C., Sutton, H., Achim, A.M., Malla, A.K., and Lepage, M. (2007). Social cognitive impairments in first episode psychosis. *Schizophr Res*, 95(1-3):124–133.

31. Robbins, T.W., Jones, G.H., and Wilkinson, L.S. (1996). Behavioural and neurochemical effects of early social deprivation in the rat. *J Psychopharmacol*, 10:39–47.

32. Geyer, M.A., McIlwain, K.L., and Paylor, R. (2002). Mouse genetic models for prepulse inhibition: An early review. *Mol Psychiatry*, 7:1039–1053.

33. Geyer, M.A., Swerdlow, N.R., Mansbach, R.S., and Braff, D.L. (1990). Startle response models of sensorimotor gating and habituation deficits in schizophrenia. *Brain Res Bull*, 25:485–498.

34. Simosky, J.K., Stevens, K.E., Adler, L.E., and Freedman, R. (2003). Clozapine improves deficient inhibitory auditory processing in DBA/2 mice, via a nicotinic cholinergic mechanism. *Psychopharmacology (Berl)*, 165(4):386–396.

35. Stevens, K.E., Fuller, L.L., and Rose, G.M. (1991). Dopaminergic and noradrenergic modulation of amphetamine-induced changes in auditory gating. *Brain Res*, 555(1):91–98.

36. Barrett, S.L., Bell, R., Watson, D., and King, D.J. (2004). Effects of amisulpride, risperidone and chlorpromazine on auditory and visual latent inhibition, prepulse inhibition, executive function and eye movements in healthy volunteers. *J Psychopharmacol*, 18(2):156–172.

37. Moser, P.C., Hitchcock, J.M., Lister, S., and Moran, P.M. (2000). The pharmacology of latent inhibition as an animal model of schizophrenia. *Brain Res Brain Res Rev*, 33(2-3):275–307.

38. Umbricht, D., Vyssotki, D., Latanov, A., Nitsch, R., and Lipp, H.P. (2005). Deviance-related electrophysiological activity in mice: Is there mismatch negativity in mice? *Clin Neurophysiol*, 116(2):353–363.

39. Cunningham, M.O., Hunt, J., Middleton, S., LeBeau, F.E., Gillies, M.J., Davies, C.H. *et al.* (2006). Region-specific reduction in entorhinal gamma oscillations and parvalbumin-immunoreactive neurons in animal models of psychiatric illness. *J Neurosci*, 26(10):2767–2776.

40. Hajos, M. (2006). Targeting information-processing deficit in schizophrenia: A novel approach to psychotherapeutic drug discovery. *Trends Pharmacol Sci*, 27:391–398.

41. Heidbreder, C.A., Foxton, R., Cilia, J., Hughes, Z.A., Shah, A.J., Atkins, A. *et al.* (2001). Increased responsiveness of dopamine to atypical, but not typical antipsychotics in the medial prefrontal cortex of rats reared in isolation. *Psychopharmacology (Berl)*, 156(2-3):338–351.

42. Jones, G.H., Hernandez, T.D., Kendall, D.A., Marsden, C.A., and Robbins, T.W. (1992). Dopaminergic and serotonergic function following isolation rearing in rats: Study of behavioural responses and postmortem and in vivo neurochemistry. *Pharmacol Biochem Behav*, 43(1):17-35.

43. Reynolds, G.P. and Harte, M.K. (2007). The neuronal pathology of schizophrenia: Molecules and mechanisms. *Biochem Soc Trans*, 35(Pt 2):433-436.

44. Sigmundsson, T., Maier, M., Toone, B.K., Williams, S.C., Simmons, A., Greenwood, K. *et al.* (2003). Frontal lobe N-acetylaspartate correlates with psychopathology in schizophrenia: A proton magnetic resonance spectroscopy study. *Schizophr Res*, 64(1):63-71.

45. Deboer, T. (2007). Technologies of sleep research. *Cell Mol Life Sci*, 64(10):1227-1235.

46. Luthringer, R., Staner, L., Noel, N., Muzet, M., Gassmann-Mayer, C., Talluri, K. *et al.* (2007). A double-blind, placebo-controlled, randomized study evaluating the effect of paliperidone extended-release tablets on sleep architecture in patients with schizophrenia. *Int Clin Psychopharmacol*, 22(5):299-308.

47. Tafti, M. (2007). Quantitative genetics of sleep in inbred mice. *Dialogues Clin Neurosci*, 9(3):273-278.

48. Irwin, S. (1962). Drug screening and evaluative procedures. *Science*, 136:123-126.

49. Rogers, D.C., Fisher, E.M., Brown, S.D., Peters, J., Hunter, A.J., and Martin, J.E. (1997). Behavioral and functional analysis of mouse phenotype: SHIRPA, a proposed protocol for comprehensive phenotype assessment. *Mamm Genome*, 8(10):711-713.

50. Silva-Gomez, A.B., Rojas, D., Juarez, I., and Flores, G. (2003). Decreased dendritic spine density on prefrontal cortical and hippocampal pyramidal neurons in postweaning social isolation rats. *Brain Research*, 983(1-2):128-136.

51. Day-Wilson, K.M., Jones, D.N., Southam, E., Cilia, J., and Totterdell, S. (2006). Medial prefrontal cortex volume loss in rats with isolation rearing-induced deficits in prepulse inhibition of acoustic startle. *Neuroscience*, 141(3):1113-1121.

52. Molina, V., Reig, S., Sanz, J., Palomo, T., Benito, C., Sánchez, J., Pascau, J., and Desco, M. (2007). Changes in cortical volume with olanzapine in chronic schizophrenia. *Pharmacopsychiatry*, 40(4):135-139.

53. Shapiro, D.A., Renock, S., Arrington, E., Chiodo, L.A., Liu, L.-X., Sibley, D.R., Roth, B.L., and Mailman, R. (2003). Aripiprazole, a novel atypical antipsychotic drug with a unique and robust pharmacology. *Neuropsychopharmacology*, 28:1400-1411.

54. Gray, J.A. and Roth, R.H. (2007). The pipeline and future of drug development in schizophrenia. *Molecular Psychiatry*, 12:904-922.

55. Wong, E.H.F., Nikam, S.S., and Shahid, M. (2008). Multi- and single-target agents for major psychiatric diseases: Therapeutic opportunities and challenges. *Curr Opin Invest Drugs*, 9(1):28-36.

56. Buckley, P.F. and Stahl, S.M. (2007). Pharmacological treatment of negative symptoms of schizophrenia: Therapeutic opportunity or cul-de-sac?. *Acta Psychiatr Scand*, 115: 93-100.

57. Lublin, H., Eberhard, J., and Levander, S. (2005). Current therapy issues and unmet clinical needs in the treatment of schizophrenia: A review of the new generation antipsychotics. *Int Clin Psychopharmacol*, 20:183-198.

58. Tamminga, C.A. and Davis, J.M. (2007). The neuropharmacology of psychosis. *Schiz Bull*, 33(4):937-946.

59. Cuesta, M.J., Peralta, V., and Zarzuela, A. (2001). Effects of olanzapine and other antipsychotics on cognitive function in chronic schizophrenia: A longitudinal study. *Schizophr Res*, 48(1):17-28.

60. Liu, S.K., Chen, W.J., Chang, C.J., and Lin, H.N. (2000). Effects of atypical neuroleptics on sustained attention deficits in schizophrenia: A trial of risperidone versus haloperidol. *Neuropsychopharmacology*, 22(3):311-319.

61. Haro, J.M. and Salvador-Carulla, L. (2006). The SOHO (Schizophrenia Out-patient Health Outcomes) study: Implications for the treatment of schizophrenia. *CNS Drugs*, 20:293–301.

62. Allison, D.B., Mentore, J.L., Heo, M., Chandler, L.P., Cappelleri, J.C., Infante, M.C. *et al.* (1999). Antipsychotic-induced weight gain: A comprehensive research synthesis. *Am J Psychiatry*, 156(11):1686–1696.

63. American Diabetes Association, American Psychiatric Association, American Association of Clinical Endocrinologists, North American Association for the study of obesity. (2004). Consensus development conference on antipsychotics drugs and obesity. *Diabetes Care*, 27:596–601.

64. Nasrallah, H.A. (2008). Atypical antipsychotic-inducedmetabolic side effects: Insights from receptor-binding profiles. *Mol Psychiatry*, 13:27–35.

65. Newcomer, J.W. (2006). Medical risks in patients with bipolar disorder and schizophrenia. *J Clin Psychiatry*, 67(Suppl 9):25–30.

66. Newcomer, J.W. (2007). Metabolic considerations in the use of antipsychotic medications: A review of recent evidence. *J Clin Psychiatry*, 68(Suppl 1):20–27.

67. Davis, J.M., Chen, N., and Glick, I.D. (2003). A meta-analysis of the efficacy of second-generation antipsychotics. *Arch Gen Psychiatry*, 60(6):553–564.

68. Lieberman, J.A. (2006). Neurobiology and the natural history of schizophrenia. *J Clin Psychiatry*, 67(10):1555–2101.

69. Hagan, J.J. and Jones, D.N.C. (2005). Predicting drug efficacy for cognitive deficits in schizophrenia. *Schiz Bull*, 31:830–853.

70. Perry, W., Heaton, R.K., Potterat, E., Roebuck, T., Minassian, A., and Braff, D.L. (2001). Working memory in schizophrenia: Transient "online" storage versus executive functioning. *Schizophr Bull*, 27(1):157–176.

71. Perry, W., Potterat, E.G., and Braff, D.L. (2001). Self-monitoring enhances Wisconsin Card Sorting Test performance in patients with schizophrenia: Performance is improved by simply asking patients to verbalize their sorting strategy. *J Int Neuropsychol Soc*, 7(3): 344–352.

72. Harvey, P.D. and Keefe, R.S.E. (2001). Studies of cognitive change in patients with schizophrenia following novel antipsychotic treatment. *Am J Psych*, 158:176–184.

73. Insel, T.R. and Scolnick., E.M. (2006). Cure therapeutics and strategic prevention: Raising the bar for mental health research. *Mol Psychiatry*, 11:11–17.

74. Lewis, D.A. and Gonzalez-Burgos, G. (2006). Pathophysiologically based treatment interventions in schizophrenia. *Nature Medicine*, 12(9):1016–1022.

75. Creese, I., Burt, D.R., and Snyder, S.H. (1976). Dopamine receptor binding predicts clinical and pharmacological potencies of antischizophrenic drugs. *Science*, 19:481–483.

76. Seeman, P. and Lee, T. (1975). Antipsychotic drugs: Direct correlation between clinical potency and presynaptic action on dopamine neurons. *Science*, 188:1217–1219.

77. Guillin, O., Abi-Dargham, A., and Laruelle, M. (2007). Neurobiology of dopamine in schizophrenia. *Int Rev Neurobiol*, 78:1–39.

78. Kapur, S., Zipursky, R., Jones, C., Remington, G., and Houle, S. (2000). Relationship between dopamine (2) occupancy, clinical response, and side effects: A double-blind PET study of first episode schizophrenia. *Am J Psychiatry*, 157:514–520.

79. Laruelle, M., Kegeles, L.S., and Abi-Dargham, A. (2003). Glutamate, dopamine, and schizophrenia: From pathophysiology to treatment. *Ann NY Acad Sci*, 1003:138–158.

80. Laruelle, M., Kegeles, L.S., and Abi-Dargham, A. (2003). Glutamate, dopamine, and schizophrenia: From pathophysiology to treatment. *Ann NY Acad Sci*, 1003:138–158.

81. Carlsson, M.L., Carlsson, A., and Nilsson, M. (2004). Schizophrenia: From dopamine to glutamate and back. *Curr Med Chem*, 11(3):267–277.

82. Coyle, J.T., Tsai, G., and Goff, D. (2003). Converging evidence of NMDA receptor hypofunction in the pathophysiology of schizophrenia. *Ann NY Acad Sci*, 1003:318–327.

83. Halberstadt, A.L. (1995). The phencyclidine-glutamate model of schizophrenia. *Clin Neuropharmacol*, 18:237–249.
84. Large, C.H. (2007). Do NMDA receptor antagonist models of schizophrenia predict the clinical efficacy of antipsychotic drugs? *J Psychopharmacol*, 21(3):283–301.
85. Moghaddam, B. (2003). Bringing order to the glutamate chaos in schizophrenia. *Neuron*, 40:881–884.
86. Javitt, D.C. (2006). Is the glycine site half saturated or half unsaturated? Effects of glutamatergic drugs in schizophrenia patients. *Curr Opin Psychiatry*, 19:151–157.
87. Patil, S.T., Zhang, L., Martenyi, F., Lowe, S.L., Jackson, K.A., Andreev, B.V. *et al.* (2007). Activation of mGlu2/3 receptors as a new approach to treat schizophrenia: A randomized Phase 2 clinical trial. *Nat Med*, 13(9):1102–1107.
88. Hahn, C., Wang, H., Cho, D., Talbot, K., Gur, R.E., Berretini, W.H., Bakshi, K., Kamins, J., Borgmann-Winter, K.E., Siegel, S.J. *et al.* (2006). Altered neuregulin 1-erbB4 signaling contributes to NMDA receptor hypofunction in schizophrenia. *Nat Med*, 12(7):824–828.
89. Akbarian, A. and Huang, H. (2006). Molecular and cellular mechanism of altered GAD1/GAD67 expression in schizophrenia and related disorders. *Brain Res Rev*, 52:293–304.
90. Benes, F.M. and Berretta, S. (2001). GABAergic interneurons: Implications for understanding schizophrenia and bipolar disorders. *Neuropsychopharmacology*, 25(1):1–27.
91. Reynolds, G.P. and Beasley, C.L. (2001). GABAergic neuronal subtypes in the human frontal cortex – development and deficits in schizophrenia. *J Chem Neuroanat*, 22(1-2):95–100.
92. Ford, J.M., Krystal, J.H., and Mathalon, D.H. (2007). Neural synchrony in schizophrenia: From networks to new treatments. *Schiz Bull*, 33(4):848–852.
93. Javitt, D.C., Spencer, K.M., Thaker, G.K., Winterer, G., and Hajos, M. (2008). Neurophysiological biomarkers for drug development in schizophrenia. *Nat Rev Drug Discov*, 7:68–83.
94. Beasley, C.L. and Reynolds, G.P. (1997). Parvalbumin-immunoreactive neurons are reduced in the prefrontal cortex of schizophrenics. *Schizophr Res*, 24:349–355.
95. Pierri, J.N., Chaudry, A.S., Woo, T.U., and Lewis, D.A. (1999). Alterations in chandelier neuron axon terminals in the prefrontal cortex of schizophrenic subjects. *Am J Psychiatry*, 156:1709–1719.
96. Umbricht, D., Vollenweider, F.X., Schmid, L., Grubel, C., Skrabo, A., Huber, T., and Koller, R. (2003). Effects of the 5-HT2A agonist psilocybin on mismatch negativity generation and AX-continuous performance task: Implications for the neuropharmacology of cognitive deficits in schizophrenia. *Neuropsychopharmacology*, 28:170–181.
97. Vollenweider, F.X. and Geyer, M.A. (2001). A systems model of altered consciousness: Integrating natural and drug-induced psychoses. *Brain Res Bull*, 56:495–507.
98. Vollenweider, F.X., Leenders, K.L., Scharfetter, C., Maguire, P., Stadelmann, O., and Angst, J. (1997). Positron emission tomography and fluorodeoxyglucose studies of metabolic hyperfrontality and psychopathology in the psilocybin model of psychosis. *Neuropsychopharmacology*, 16:357–372.
99. Vollenweider, F.X., Vollenweider-Scherpenhuyzen, M.F., Babler, A., Vogel, H., and Hell, D. (1998). Psilocybin induces schizophrenia-like psychosis in humans via serotonin-2 agonist action. *Neuroreport*, 9:3897–3902.
100. Vollenweider, F.X., Csomor, P.A., Knappe, B., Geyer, M.A., and Quednow, B.B. (2007). The effects of the preferential 5-HT2A agonist psilocybin on prepulse inhibition of startle in healthy human volunteers depend on interstimulus interval. *Neuropsychopharmacology*, 32:1876–1887.
101. Geyer, M.A. (1998). Behavioral studies of hallucinogenic drugs in animals: Implications for schizophrenia research. *Pharmacopsychiatry*, 31(Suppl 2):73–79.
102. Kapur, S., Zipursky, R.B., and Remington, G. (1999). Clinical and theoretical implications of 5-HT2 and D2 receptor occupancy of clozapine, risperidone, and olanzapine in schizophrenia. *Am J Psychiatry*, 156(2):286–293.

103. Reimold, M., Solbach, C., Noda, S., Schaefer, J.E., Bartels, M., Beneke, M., Machulla, H.J., Bares, R., Glaser, T., and Wormstall, H. (2007). Occupancy of dopamine D(1), D (2) and serotonin (2 A) receptors in schizophrenic patients treated with flupentixol in comparison with risperidone and haloperidol. *Psychopharmacology*, 190(2):241–249.

104. Mamo, D., Graff, A., Mizrahi, R., Shammi, C.M., Romeyer, F., and Kapur, S. (2007). Differential effects of aripiprazole on D(2), 5-HT(2), and 5-HT(1A) receptor occupancy in patients with schizophrenia: A triple tracer PET study. *Am J Psychiatry*, 164(9):1411–1417.

105. Meltzer, H.Y., Arvanitis, L., Bauer, D., Rein, W., and Meta-Trial Study Group. (2004). Placebo-controlled evaluation of four novel compounds for the treatment of schizophrenia and schizoaffective disorder. *Am J Psychiatry*, 161(6):984, 975.

106. De Angelis, L. (2002). 5-HT2A antagonists in psychiatric disorders. *Curr Opin Invest Drugs*, 3(1):107–112.

107. Varty, G.B., Bakshi, V.P., and Geyer, M.A. (1999). M100907, a serotonin 5-HT2A receptor antagonist and putative antipsychotic, blocks dizocilpine-induced prepulse inhibition deficits in Sprague-Dawley and Wistar rats. *Neuropsychopharmacology*, 20:311–321.

108. Gardell, L.R., Vanover, K.E., Pounds, L., Johnson, R.W., Barido, R., Anderson, G.T. *et al.* (2007). ACP-103, a 5-hydroxytryptamine 2A receptor inverse agonist, improves the antipsychotic efficacy and side-effect profile of haloperidol and risperidone in experimental models. *J Pharmacol Exp Ther*, 322(2):862–870.

109. Li, Z., Ichikawa, J., Mei Huang, M., Adam, J., Prus, A.J., Jin Dai, J., and Meltzer, H.Y. (2005). ACP-103 a 5-HT2A/2C inverse agonist potentiates haloperidol-induced dopamine release in rat medial prefrontal cortex and nucleus accumbens. *Psychopharmacology*, 183:144–153.

110. Bayer, T.A., Falkai, P., and Maier, W. (1999). Genetic and non-genetic vulnerability factors in schizophrenia: The basis of the "two hit hypothesis". *J Psychiatr Res*, 33:543–548.

111. Lewis, D.A. and Lieberman, J.A. (2000). Catching up on schizophrenia: Natural history and neurobiology. *Neuron*, 28:325–334.

112. Wong, A.H.C. and Van Tol, H.H.M. (2003). Schizophrenia: From phenomenology to neurobiology. *Neurosci Biobehav Rev*, 27:269–306.

113. Straub, R.E. and Weinberger, D.R. (2006). Schizophrenia genes – famine to feast. *Biol Psychiatry*, 60:81–83.

114. Harrison, P.J. and Weinberger, D.R. (2005). Schizophrenia genes, gene expression, and neuropathology: On the matter of convergence. *Mol Psychiatry*, 10:40–68.

115. Roberts, G.W., Colter, N., Lofthouse, R., Johnstone, E.C., and Crow, T.J. (1987). Is there gliosis in schizophrenia? Investigation of the temporal lobe. *Biol Psychiatry*, 22(12):1459–1468.

116. Roberts, G.W., Colter, N., Lofthouse, R., Johnstone, E.C., and Crow, T.J. (1987). Is there gliosis in schizophrenia? Investigation of the temporal lobe. *Biol Psychiatry*, 22(12):1459–1468.

117. Selemon, L.D., Rajkowska, G., and Goldman-Rakic, P.S. (1998). Elevated neuronal density in prefrontal area 46 in brains from schizophrenic patients: Application of a three-dimensional, stereologic counting method. *J Comp Neurol*, 392(3):402–412.

118. Pakkenberg, B. (1993). Total nerve cell number in neocortex in chronic schizophrenics and controls estimated using optical dissectors. *Biol Psychiatry*, 34(11):768–772.

119. Eastwood, S.L. and Harrison, P.J. (2003). Interstitial white matter neurons express less reelin and are abnormally distributed in schizophrenia: Towards an integration of molecular and morphologic aspects of the neurodevelopmental hypothesis. *Mol Psychiatry*, 8(9):769–821, 831.

120. Urenjak, J., Williams, S.R., Gadian, D.G., and Noble, M. (1993). Proton nuclear magnetic resonance spectroscopy unambiguously identifies different neural cell types. *J Neurosci*, 13(3):981–989.

121. Tsai, G. and Coyle, J.T. (1995). N-acetylaspartate in neuropsychiatric disorders. *Prog Neurobiol*, 46(5):531–540.

122. Cendes, F., Andermann, F., Dubeau, F., Matthews, P.M., and Arnold, D.L. (1997). Normalization of neuronal metabolic dysfunction after surgery for temporal lobe epilepsy, Evidence from proton MR spectroscopic imaging. *Neurology*, 49(6):1525-1533.

123. Kalra, S., Cashman, N.R., Genge, A., and Arnold, D.L. (1998). Recovery of N-acetylaspartate in corticomotor neurons of patients with ALS after riluzole therapy. *Neuroreport*, 9(8):1757-1761.

124. Chakraborty, G., Mekala, P., Yahya, D., Wu, G., and Ledeen, R.W. (2001). Intraneuronal N-acetylaspartate supplies acetyl groups for myelin lipid synthesis: Evidence for myelin-associated aspartoacylase. *J Neurochem*, 78(4):736-745.

125. Baslow, M.H. (2003). N-acetylaspartate in the vertebrate brain: Metabolism and function. *Neurochem Res*, 28(6):941-953.

126. Rael, L.T., Thomas, G.W., Bar-Or, R., Craun, M.L., and Bar-Or, D. (2004). An anti-inflammatory role for N-acetyl aspartate in stimulated human astroglial cells. *Biochem Biophys Res Commun*, 319(3):847-853.

127. Auer, D.P., Wilke, M., Grabner, A., Heidenreich, J.O., Bronisch, T., and Wetter, T.C. (2001). Reduced NAA in the thalamus and altered membrane and glial metabolism in schizophrenic patients detected by 1H-MRS and tissue segmentation. *Schizophr Res*, 52(1-2):87-99.

128. Nudmamud, S., Reynolds, L.M., and Reynolds, G.P. (2003). N-acetylaspartate and N-Acetylaspartylglutamate deficits in superior temporal cortex in schizophrenia and bipolar disorder: A postmortem study. *Biol Psychiatry*, 53(12):1138-1141.

129. Steen, R.G., Hamer, R.M., and Lieberman, J.A. (2005). Measurement of brain metabolites by 1H magnetic resonance spectroscopy in patients with schizophrenia: A systematic review and meta-analysis. *Neuropsychopharmacology*, 30(11):1949-1962.

130. Galinska, B., Szulc, A., Tarasow, E., Kubas, B., Dzienis, W., Siergiejczyk, L. *et al.* (2007). Relationship between frontal N-acetylaspartate and cognitive deficits in first-episode schizophrenia. *Med Sci Monit*, 13(Suppl 1):11-16.

131. Ohrmann, P., Siegmund, A., Suslow, T., Pedersen, A., Spitzberg, K., Kersting, A. *et al.* (2007). Cognitive impairment and in vivo metabolites in first-episode neuroleptic-naive and chronic medicated schizophrenic patients: A proton magnetic resonance spectroscopy study. *J Psychiatr Res*, 41(8):625-634.

132. Callicott, J.H., Bertolino, A., Egan, M.F., Mattay, V.S., Langheim, F.J., and Weinberger, D.R. (2000). Selective relationship between prefrontal N-acetylaspartate measures and negative symptoms in schizophrenia. *Am J Psychiatry*, 157(10):1646-1651.

133. Cotter, D., Mackay, D., Chana, G., Beasley, C., Landau, S., and Everall, I.P. (2002). Reduced neuronal size and glial cell density in area 9 of the dorsolateral prefrontal cortex in subjects with major depressive disorder. *Cereb Cortex*, 12(4):386-394.

134. Cotter, D.R., Pariante, C.M., and Everall, I.P. (2001). Glial cell abnormalities in major psychiatric disorders: The evidence and implications. *Brain Res Bull*, 55(5):585-595.

135. Benes, F.M., Khan, Y., Vincent, S.L., and Wickramasinghe, R. (1996). Differences in the subregional and cellular distribution of GABAA receptor binding in the hippocampal formation of schizophrenic brain. *Synapse*, 22(4):338-349.

136. Rajkowska, G., Miguel-Hidalgo, J.J., Makkos, Z., Meltzer, H., Overholser, J., and Stockmeier, C. (2002). Layer-specific reductions in GFAP-reactive astroglia in the dorsolateral prefrontal cortex in schizophrenia. *Schizophr Res*, 57(2-3):127-138.

137. Hof, P.R., Haroutunian, V., Friedrich Jr, V.L., Byne, W., Buitron, C., Perl, D.P. *et al.* (2003). Loss and altered spatial distribution of oligodendrocytes in the superior frontal gyrus in schizophrenia. *Biol Psychiatry*, 53(12):1075-1085.

138. Johnston-Wilson, N.L., Sims, C.D., Hofmann, J.P., Anderson, L., Shore, A.D., Torrey, E.F. *et al.* (2000). Disease-specific alterations in frontal cortex brain proteins in schizophrenia, bipolar disorder, and major depressive disorder. The Stanley Neuropathology Consortium. *Mol Psychiatry*, 5(2):142-149.

139. Walterfang, M., Wood, S.J., Velakoulis, D., and Pantelis, C. (2006). Neuropathological, neuro-genetic and neuroimaging evidence for white matter pathology in schizophrenia. *Neurosci Biobehav Rev*, 30(7):918–948.

140. Cardno, A.G. and Gottesman, I.I. (2000). Twin studies of schizophrenia: From bow-and-arrow concordances to star wars Mx and functional genomics. *Am J Med Genet*, 97(1):12–17.

141. Greenwood, T.A., Braff, D.L., Light, G.A., Cadenhead, K.S., Calkins, M.E., Dobie, D.J. *et al.* (2007). Initial heritability analyses of endophenotypic measures for schizophrenia. The consortium on the genetics of schizophrenia. *Arch Gen Psychiatry*, 64(11):1242–1250.

142. Sullivan, P.F., Kendler, K.S., and Neale, M.C. (2003). Schizophrenia as a complex trait: Evidence from a meta-analysis of twin studies. *Arch Gen Psychiatry*, 60(12):1187–1192.

143. Gogos, J.A. and Gerber, D.J. (2006). Schizophrenia susceptibility genes: Emergence of positional candidates and future directions. *Trends Pharmacol Sci*, 27(4):226–233.

144. Harrison, P.J. and Law, A.J. (2006). Neuregulin I schizophrenia: Genetics, gene expression, neurobiology. *Biol Psychiatry*, 60:132–140.

145. Waddington, J.L., Corvin, A.P., Donohoe, G., O'Tuathaigh, C.M., Mitchell, K.J., and Gill, M. (2007). Functional genomics and schizophrenia: Endophenotypes and mutant models. *Psychiatric Clin North Am*, 30(3):365–399.

146. Tan, W., Wang, Y., Gold, B., Chen, J., Dean, M., Harrison, P.J., Weinberger, D.R., and Law, A.J. (2007). Molecular cloning of a brain-specific, developmentally regulated neuregulin I (NRG1) isoform and identification of a functional promoter variant associated with schizophrenia. *J Bio Chem*, 282(33):24343–24351.

147. Stefansson, H., Sigurdsson, E., Steinthorsdottir, V., Bjornsdottir, S., Sigmundsson, T., Ghosh, S. *et al.* (2002). Neuregulin 1 and susceptibility to schizophrenia. *Am J Hum Genet*, 71:877–892.

148. Stefansson, H., Sarginson, J., Kong, A., Yates, P., Steinthorsdottir, V., Gudfinnsson, E. *et al.* (2003). Association of neuregulin 1 with schizophrenia confirmed in a Scottish population. *Am J Hum Genet*, 72(1):83–87.

149. Li, D., Collier, D.A., and He, L. (2006). Meta-analysis shows strong positive association of the neuregulin 1 (NRG1) gene with schizophrenia. *Hum Mol Genet*, 15:1995–2002.

150. Benzel, I., Bansal, A., Browning, B.L., Galway, N.W., Maycox, P.R., McGinnis, R., Smart, D., St Clair, D., Yates, P., and Purvis, I. (2007). Interaction among genes in the ErbB-Neuregulin signalling network are associated with increased susceptibility to schizophrenia. *Behav Brain Funct*, 3:31–42.

151. Norton, N., Moskvina, V., Morris, D.W., Bray, N.J., Zammit, S., Williams, N.M., Williams, H.J., Preece, A.C., Dwyer, S., Wilkinson, J.C. *et al.* (2006). Evidence that interaction between neuregulin 1 and its receptor erbB4 increases susceptibility to schizophrenia. *Am J Med Genet B Neuropsychiatr Genet*, 141:96–101.

152. Gu, Z., Jiang, Q., Fu, A.K.Y., Ip, N.Y., and Yan, Z. (2005). Regulation of NMDA receptors by neuregulin signaling in prefrontal cortex. *J Neurosci*, 25(20):4974–4984.

153. Hall, J., Whalley, H.C., Job, D.E. *et al.* (2006). A neuregulin 1 variant associated with abnormal cortical function and psychotic symptoms. *Nat Neurosci*, 9:1477–1478.

154. Karoum, F., Chrapusta, S.J., and Egan, M.F. (1994). 3-Methoxytyramine is the major metabolite of released dopamine in the rat frontal cortex. *J Neurochem*, 63:972–979.

155. Tunbridge, E.M., Harrison, P.J., and Weinberger, D.R. (2006). Catechol-O-methyltransferase, cognition and psychosis: Val158Met and beyond. *Biol Psychiatry*, 60(2):141–151.

156. Hosak, L. (2007). Role of COMT gene Val158Met polymorphism in mental disorders: A review. *Eur Psychiatry*, 22:276–281.

157. Apud, J.A. and Weinberger, D.R. (2007). Treatment of cognitive deficits associated with schizophrenia. *CNS Drugs*, 21(7):535–557.

158. Tunbridge, E.M., Bannerman, D.M., Sharp, T., and Harrison, P.J. (2004). Catechol-o-methyltransferase inhibition improves set-shifting performance and elevates stimulated dopamine release in the rat prefrontal cortex. *J Neurosci*, 24(23):5331–5335.

159. Porteous, D.J.,Thomson, P., Brandon, N.J., and Millar, J.K. (2006).The genetics and biology of Disc1 - An emerging role in psychosis and cognition. *Biol Psychiatry*, 60:123-131.

160. Millar, J.K., Mackie, S., Clapcote, S.J., Murdoch, H., Pickard, B.S., Christie, S., Muir, W.J., Blackwood, D.H., Roder, J.C., Houslay, M.D. *et al.* (2007). Disrupted in schizophrenia 1 and phospodiesterase 4B: Towards an understanding of psychiatric disorders. *J Physiol*, 584:401-405.

161. Roberts, R.C. (2007). Schizophrenia in translation: Disrupted in schizophrenia (DISC1): Integrating clinical and basic findings. *Schizophr Bull*, 33(1):11-15.

162. Callicott, J.H., Straub, R.E., and Pezawas, L. (2005). Variation in DISC1 affects hippocampal structure and function and increases risk for schizophrenia. *Proc Natl Acad Sci USA*, 102(24):8627-8632.

163. Matsuzaki, S. and Tohyama, M. (2007). Molecular mechanism of schizophrenia with reference to disrupted-in-schizophrenia 1 (DISC1). *Neurochem Int*, 51:165-172.

164. Kanes, S.J.,Tokarczyk, J., Siegel, S.J., Bilker, W.,Abel,T., and Kelly, M.P. (2007). Rolipram:A specific phosphodiesterase 4 inhibitor with potential antipsychotic activity. *Neuroscience*, 144(1):239-246.

165. Clapcote, S.J., Lipina,T.V., Millar, J.K., Mackie, S., Christie, S., Ogawa, F., Lerch, J.P.,Trimble, K., Uchiyama, M., Sakuraba, Y. *et al.* (2007). Behavioral phenotypes of Disc1 missense mutations in mice. *Neuron*, 54(3):387-402.

166. Siuciak, J.A., Chapin, D.S., McCarthy, S.A., and Martin, A.N. (2007). Antipsychotic profile of rolipram: Efficacy in rats and reduced sensitivity in mice deficient in the phosphodiesterase-4B (PDE4B) enzyme. *Psychopharmacology*, 192(3):415-424.

167. Craddock, N., O'Donovan, M.C., and Owen, M.J. (2007). Phenotypic and genetic complexity of psychosis. *Br J Psych*, 190:200-201.

168. Blackwood, D.H., Fordyce, A.,Walker, M.T., St Clair, D.M., Porteous, D.J., and Muir, W.J. (2001). Schizophrenia and affective disorders - cosegregation with a translocation at chromosome 1q42 that directly disrupts brain-expressed genes: Clinical and P300 findings in a family. *Am J Hum Genet*, 69(2):428-433.

169. Braff, D.L., Freedman, R., Schork, N.J., and Gottesman, I.I. (2007). Deconstructing schizophrenia:An overview of the use of endophenotypes in order to understand a complex disorder. *Schiz Bull*, 33(1):21-32.

170. The Wellcome Trust Case Control Consortium (2007). Genome-wide association study of 14000 cases of seven common diseases and 3000 shared controls. *Nature*, 447: 661-678.

171. Calkins, M.E., Dobie, D.J., Cadenhead, K.S., Olincy, A., Freedman, R., Green, M.F. *et al.* (2007). The Consortium on the Genetics of Endophenotypes in Schizophrenia: Model recruitment, assessment, and endophenotyping methods for a multisite collaboration. *Schizophr Bull*, 33(1):33-48.

172. Jaffee, S.R. and Price,T.S. (2007). Gene-environment correlations:A review of the evidence and implications for prevention of mental illness. *Mol Psychiatry*, 12:432-442.

173. Petronis, A., Gottesman, I.I., Crow, T.J., DeLisi, L.E., Klar, A.J., Macciardi, F. *et al.* (2000). Psychiatric epigenetics:A new focus for the new century. *Mol Psychiatry*, 5:342-346.

174. Crow, T.J. (2007). How and why genetic linkage has not solved the problem of psychosis: Review and hypothesis. *Am J Psychiatry*, 164:13-21.

175. Tsankova, N., Renthal, W., Kumar, A., and Nestler, E.J. (2007). Epigenetic regulation in psychiatric disorders. *Nat Rev Neurosci*, 8:355-367.

176. van Vliet, J., Oates, N.A., and Whitelaw, E. (2007). Epigenetic mechanisms in the context of complex diseases. *Cell Mol Life Sci*, 64:1531-1538.

177. Richards, E.J. (2006). Inherited epigenetic variation - revisiting soft inheritance. *Nat Rev Genet*, 7:395-401.

178. Bird, A. (2007). Perceptions of epigenetics. *Nature*, 447:396-398.

179. Kaminsky, Z., Wang, S.C., and Petronis, A. (2006). Complex disease, gender and epigenetics. *Ann Med*, 38(8):530–544.

180. Abdolmaleky, H.M., Cheng, K.H., Faraone, S.V., Wilcox, M., Glatt, S.J., Gao, F. *et al.* (2006). Hypomethylation of MB-COMT promoter is a major risk factor for schizophrenia and bipolar disorder. *Hum Mol Genet*, 15(21):3132–3145.

181. Tamura, Y., Kunugi, H., Ohashi, J., and Hohjoh, H., (2007). Epigenetic aberration of the human REELIN gene in psychiatric disorders. *Mol Psychiatry*, 12(6):519, 593–600.

182. Veldic, M., Kadriu, B., Maloku, E., Agis-Balboa, R.C., Guidotti, A., Davis, J.M., and Costa, E. (2007). Epigenetic mechanism expressed in basal ganglia GABAergic neurons differentiate schizophrenia from bipolar disorder. *Schiz Res*, 91:51–61.

183. Box, G. and Draper, N. (1987). *Empirical Model Building and Response Surfaces.* John Wiley, New York. p. 74

184. Geyer, M.A. and Markou, A. (2002). The role of preclinical models in the development of psychotropic drugs. In Davis, K.L., Charney, D., Coyle, J.T., and Nemeroff, C. (eds.), *Neuropsychopharmacology: The Fifth Generation of Progress.* Lippincott Williams & Wilkins, Philadelphia, pp. 445–455. Chapter 33

185. Geyer, M.A. and Markou, A. (1995). Animal models of psychiatric disorders. In Bloom, F.E. and Kupfer, D. (eds.), *Psychopharmacology: The Fourth Generation of Progress.* Raven Press, New York, pp. 787–798.

186. Powell, S.B. and Geyer, M.A. (2007). Overview of animal models of schizophrenia, In Crawley, J.N. Skolnick, P. (eds.), *Current Protocols in Neuroscience*, John Wiley & Sons, New York.

187. Segal, D.S. and Geyer, M.A. (1985). Animal models of psychopathology. In Judd, L.L. and Groves, P.M. (eds.), *Psychobiological Foundations of Clinical Psychiatry.* J.B. Lippincott Co., Philadelphia, pp. 1–14.

188. Mosier, C.I. (1947). A critical examination of the concepts of face validity. *Educ Psychol Meas*, 7:191–205.

189. Ellenbroek, B.A. and Cools, A.R. (1990). Animal models with construct validity for schizophrenia. *Behav Pharmacol*, 1(6):469–490.

190. Wilner, P. (1986). Validation criteria for animal models of human mental disorders: Learned helplessness as a paradigm case. *Prog Neuropsychopharmacol Biol Psychiatry*, 10:677–690.

191. Matthysse, S. (1986). Animal models in psychiatric research. *Prog Brain Res*, 65:259–270.

192. Cronbach, L.J. and Meehl, P.E. (1955). Construct validity in psychological tests. *Psychol Bull*, 52(4):281–302.

193. Embretson (Whitely), S. (1983). Construct validity: Construct representation versus nomothetic span. *Psychol Bull*, 93:179–197.

194. Eriksen, J.L. and Janus, C.G. (2007). Plaques, tangles, and memory loss in mouse models of neurodegeneration. *Behav Genet*, 37:79–100.

195. Nestler, E.J. (2006). Editorial special issue: Animal models of mood and psychotic disorders *Biol Psychiatry*, 59:1103.

196. Arguello, P.A. and Gogos, J.A. (2006). Modeling madness in mice: One piece at a time. *Neuron*, 52:179–196.

197. Chen, J., Lipska, B.K., and Weinberger, D.R. (2006). Genetic mouse models of schizophrenia: From hypothesis-based to susceptibility gene-based models. *Biol Psychiatry*, 59:1180–1188.

198. Ellenbroek, B.A. and Cools, A.R. (2000). Animal models of negative symptoms of schizophrenia. *Behav Pharmacol*, 11:223–233.

199. Lipska, B.K. and Weinberger, D.R. (2000). To model a psychiatric disorder in animals: Schizophrenia as a reality test. *Neuropsychopharmacology*, 23(3):223–239.

200. O'Tuathaigh, C.M.P., Babovic, D., O'Meara, G., Clifford, J.J., Croke, D.T., and Waddington, J.L. (2007). Susceptibility genes for schizophrenia: Characterisation of mutant mouse models at the level of phenotypic behaviour. *Neurosci Biobehav Rev*, 31:60-78.

201. Powell, C.M. and Miyakawa, T. (2006). Schizophrenia - relevent behavioral testing in rodent models: A uniquely human disorder? *Biol Psychiatry*, 59:1198-1207.

202. Robertson, G.S., Hori, S.E., and Powell, K.J. (2006). Schizophrenia: An integrative approach to modelling a complex disorder. *J Psychiatry Neurosci*, 31(3):157-167.

203. Tordjam, S., Drapier, D., Bonnot, O., Graignic, R., Fortes, S., Cohen, D., Millet, B., Laurent, C., and Roubertoux, P.L. (2007). Animals models relevant to schizophrenia and autism: Validity and limitations. *Behav Genet*, 37:61-78.

204. Geyer, M.A. (2006). Are cross-species measures of sensorimotor gating useful for the discovery of procognitive cotreatments for schizophrenia? *Dialogues Clin Neurosci*, 8:9-16.

205. Castner, S.A., Goldman-Rakic, P.S., and Williams, G.V. (2004). Animal models of working memory: Insights for targeting cognitive dysfunction in schizophrenia. *Psychopharmacology*, 174(1):111-125.

206. Weed, M.R., Taffe, M.A., Polis, I., Roberts, A.C., Robbins, T.W., Koob, G.F., Bloom, F.E., and Gold, L.H. (1999). Performance norms for a rhesus monkey neuropsychological testing battery: Acquisition and long-term performance. *Brain Res Cogn Brain Res*, 8:185-201.

207. Katner, S.N., Davis, S.A., Kirsten, A.J., and Taffe, M.A. (2004). Effects of nicotine and mecamylamine on cognition in rhesus monkeys. *Psychopharmacol*, 175:225-240.

208. Nakahara, K., Hayashi, T., Konishi, S., and Mihashita, Y. (2002). Functional MRI of macaque monkeys performing a cognitive set-shifting task. *Science*, 295:1532-1536.

209. Gemperle, A.Y., McAllister, K.H., and Olpe, H.-R. (2003). Differential effects of iloperidone, clozapine and haloperidol on working memory of rats in the delayed non-matching-to-position paradigm. *Psychopharmacol*, 169:354-364.

210. Sarter, M. (2006). Preclinical research into cognition enhancers. *Trends I Pharmacol Sci*, 27(11):602-608.

211. Geyer, M.A., Krebs-Thomson, K., Braff, D.L., and Swerdlow, N.R. (2001). Pharmacological studies of prepulse inhibition models of sensorimotor gating deficits in schizophrenia: A decade in review. *Psychopharmacology (Berl)*, 156(2-3):117-154.

212. Swerdlow, N.R., Geyer, M.A., and Braff, D.L. (2001). Neural circuit regulation of prepulse inhibition of startle in the rat: Current knowledge and future challenges. *Psychopharmacology (Berl)*, 156(2-3):194-215.

213. Braff, D.L., Geyer, M.A., and Swerdlow, N.R. (2001). Human studies of prepulse inhibition of startle: Normal subjects, patient groups, and pharmacological studies 3. *Psychopharmacology (Berl)*, 156(2-3):234-258.

214. Geyer, M.A. and Ellenbroek, B. (2003). Animal behavior models of the mechanisms underlying antipsychotic atypicality. *Prog Neuropsychopharmacol Biolog Psychiatry*, 27(7):1071-1079.

215. Kumari, V., Soni, W., and Sharma, T. (2002). Prepulse inhibition of the startle response in risperidone-treated patients: Comparison with typical antipsychotics. *Schizophr Res*, 55(1-2):139-146.

216. Meincke, U., Mörth, D., Voß, T., Thelen, B., Geyer, M.A., and Gouzoulis-Mayfrank, E. (2004). Prepulse inhibition of the acoustically evoked startle reflex in patients with an acute schizophrenic psychosis - a longitudinal study. *Eur Arch Psychiatry clin Neurosci*, 254:415-421.

217. Oranje, B., Geyer, M.A., Bocker, K.B.E., Kenemans, J.L., and Verbaten, M.N. (2006). Prepulse inhibition and P50 suppression: Commonalities and dissociations. *Psychiatry Research*, 143:147-158.

218. Duncan, E., Szilagyi, S., Schwartz, M., Kunzova, A., Negi, S., Efferen, T. *et al.* (2003). Prepulse inhibition of acoustic startle in subjects with schizophrenia treated with olanzapine or haloperidol. *Psychiatry Res*, 120(1):1–12.

219. Wynn, J.K., Green, M.F., Sprock, J., Light, G.A., Widmark, C., Reist, C. *et al.* (2007). Effects of olanzapine, risperidone and haloperidol on prepulse inhibition in schizophrenia patients: A double-blind, randomized controlled trial. *Schizophr Res*, 95(1–3):134–142.

220. Minassian, A., Feifel, D., and Perry, W. (2007). The relationship between sensorimotor gating and clinical improvement in acutely ill schizophrenia patients. *Schiz Res*, 89(1–3): 225–231.

221. Braff, D.L. and Geyer, M.A. (1990). Sensorimotor gating and schizophrenia: Human and animal model studies. *Arch Gen Psychiatry*, 47:181–188.

222. Thaker, G.K. (2007). Schizophrenia endophenotypes as treatment targets. *Expert Opin Ther Targets*, 11(9):1189–1206.

223. Swerdlow, N.R., Geyer, M.A., Shoemaker, J.M., Light, G.A., Braff, D.L., Stevens, K.E., Sharp, R., Breier, M., Neary, A., and Auerbach, P.P. (2006). Convergence and divergence in the neurochemical regulation of prepulse inhibition of startle and N40 suppression in rats. *Neuropsychopharmacology*, 31:506–515.

224. Swerdlow, N.R., Talledo, J., Sutherland, A.N., Nagy, D., and Shoemaker, J.M. (2006). Antipsychotic effects on prepulse inhibition in normal "low gating" humans and rats. *Neuropsychopharmacology*, 31:2011–2021.

225. Perry, W. and Braff, D.L. (1994). Information-processing deficits and thought disorder in schizophrenia. *Am J Psychiatry*, 151(3):363–367.

226. Perry, W., Geyer, M.A., and Braff, D.L. (1999). Sensorimotor gating and thought disturbance measured in close temporal proximity in schizophrenic patients. *Arch Gen Psychiatry*, 56(3):277–281.

227. Karper, L.P., Freeman, G.K., Grillon, C., Morgan, C.A., Charney, D.S., and Krystal, J.H. (1996). Preliminary evidence of an association between sensorimotor gating and distractibility in psychosis. *J Neuropsychiatry Clin Neurosci*, 8:60–66.

228. Geyer, M.A. and Braff, D.L. (1987). Startle habituation and sensorimotor gating in schizophrenia and related animal models. *Schizophr Bull*, 13(4):643–668.

229. Meincke, U., Light, G.A., Geyer, M.A., Braff, D.L., and Gouzoulis-Mayfrank, E. (2004). Sensitization and habituation of the acoustic startle reflex in patients with schizophrenia. *Psychiatry Res*, 126:51–61.

230. Adler, L.E., Pachtman, E., Franks, R.D., Pecevich, M., Waldo, M.C., and Freedman, R. (1982). Neurophysiological evidence for a defect in neuronal mechanisms involved in sensory gating in schizophrenia. *Biolog Psychiatry*, 17(6):639–654.

231. Ellenbroek, B.A., van Luijtelaar, G., Frenken, M., and Cools, A.R. (1999). Sensory gating in rats: Lack of correlation between auditory evoked potential gating and prepulse inhibition. *Schizophr Bull*, 25(4):777–788.

232. Light, G.A. and Braff, D.L. (2001). Measuring P50 suppression and prepulse inhibition in a single recording session. *Am J Psychiatry*, 158(12):2066–2068.

233. Nagamoto, H.T., Adler, L.E., Hea, R.A., Griffith, J.M., McRae, K.A., and Freedman, R. (1996). Gating of auditory P50 in schizophrenics: Unique effects of clozapine. *Biol Psych*, 40: 181–188.

234. Adler, L.E., Olincy, A., Cawthra, E.M., McRae, K.A., Harris, J.G., Nagamoto, H.T., Waldo, M.C., Hall, M.-H., Bowles, A., Woodward, L. *et al.* (2004). Varied effects of atypical neuroleptics on P50 auditory gating in schizophrenic patients. *Am J Psych*, 161:1822–1828.

235. Arango, C., Summerfelt, A., and Buchanan, R.W. (2003). Olanzapine effects on auditory sensory gating in schizophrenia. *Am J Psych*, 160:2066–2068.

236. Nagamoto, H.T., Adler, L.E., McRae, K.A., Cawthra, E., Gerhardt, G., Hea, R.A., and Griffith, J. (1999). Gating of auditory P50 in schizophrenics: Unique effects of clozapine. *Neuropsychobiol*, 39:10-17.

237. Olincy, A., Harris, J.G., Johnson, L.L., Pender, V., Kongs, S., Allensworth, D. *et al.* (2006). Proof-of-concept trial of an alpha7 nicotinic agonist in schizophrenia. *Arch Gen Psychiatry*, 63(6):630-638.

238. Olincy, A. and Stevens, K.E. (2007). Treating schizophrenia symptoms with an alpha7 nicotinic agonist, from mice to men. *Biochem Pharmacol*, 74(8):1192-1201.

239. Simosky, J.K., Stevens, K.E., and Freedman, E.F. (2004). A novel element of the mechanism of action of atypical antipsychotic drugs: Clozapine and olanzapine activate α7 nicotinic receptors to produce improved inhibitory processing. *Soc for Neurosci*, 798:1.

240. Gray, N.S. and Snowden, R.J. (2005). The relevance of irrelevance to schizophrenia. *Neurosci Biobehav Rev*, 29(6):989-999.

241. Lubow, R.E. (2005). Construct validity of the animal latent inhibition model of selective attention deficits in schizophrenia. *Schiz Bull*, 31:139-153.

242. Swerdlow, N.R., Braff, D.L., Hartston, H., Perry, W., and Geyer, M.A. (1996). Latent inhibition in schizophrenia. *Schizophr Res*, 20:91-103.

243. Leumann, L., Feldon, J., Vollenweider, F.X., and Ludewig, K. (2002). Effects of typical and atypical antipsychotic on prepulse inhibition and latent inhibition in chronic schizophrenia. *Biol Psych*, 52:729-739.

244. Williams, J.H., Wellman, N.A., Geaney, D.P., Cowen, P.J., Feldon, J., and Rawlins, J.N. (1998). Reduced latent inhibition in people with schizophrenia: An effect of psychosis or of its treatment. *Br J Psychiatry*, 172:243-249.

245. Weiner, I., Gaisler, I., Schiller, D., Green, A., Zuckerman, L., and Joel, D. (2000). Screening of antipsychotic drugs in animal models. *Drug Develop Res*, 50:235-249.

246. Shadach, E., Schiller, D., Gaisler, I., and Weiner, I. (2000). The latent inhibition model dissociates between clozapine, haloperidol, and ritanserin. *Neuropsychopharm*, 23:151-161.

247. Braff, D.L. and Light, G.A. (2004). Preattentional and attentional cognitive deficits as targets for treating schizophrenia. *Psychopharmacology*, 174:75-85.

248. Michie, P.T., Innes-Brown, H., Todd, J., and Jablensky, A.V. (2002). Duration mismatch negativity in biological relatives of patients with schizophrenia spectrum disorders. *Biol Psychiatry*, 52:749-758.

249. Light, G.A. and Braff, D.L. (2005). Mismatch negativity deficits are associated with poor functioning in schizophrenia patients. *Arch Gen Psychiatry*, 62:127-136.

250. Javitt, D.C., Steinschneider, M., Schroeder, C.E., and Arezzo, J.C. (1996). Role of cortical N-methyl-D-aspartate receptors in auditory sensory memory and mismatch negativity generation: Implications for schizophrenia. *Proc Natl Acad Sci U S A*, 93(21):11962-11967.

251. Smith, A., Li, M., Becker, S., and Kapur, S. (2004). A model of antipsychotic action in conditioned avoidance: A computational approach. *Neuropsychopharmacology*, 29(6): 1040-1049.

252. Sumner, B.E., Cruise, L.A., Slattery, D.A., Hill, D.R., Shahid, M., and Henry, B. (2004). Testing the validity of c-fos expression profiling to aid the therapeutic classification of psychoactive drugs. *Psychopharmacology*, 171(3):306-321.

253. Hansen, H.H., Timmermann, D.B., Peters, D., Walters, C., Damaj, M.I., and Mikkelsen, J.D. (2007). Alpha-7 nicotinic acetylcholine receptor agonists selectively activate limbic regions of the rat forebrain: An effect similar to antipsychotics. *J Neurosci Res*, 85(8):1810-1818.

254. Marquis, K.L., Sabb, A.L., Logue, S.F., Brennan, J.A., Piesla, M.J., Comery, T.A. *et al.* (2007). WAY-163909 [(7bR,10aR)-1,2,3,4,8,9,10,10a-octahydro-7bH-cyclopenta-[b][1,4]diazepino [6,7,1hi]indole]: A novel 5-hydroxytryptamine 2C receptor-selective agonist with preclinical antipsychotic-like activity. *J Pharmacol Exp Ther*, 320(1):486-496.

255. Thomsen, M.S., Hansen, H.H., Kristensen, S.E., Timmerman, D.B. A. Hay-Schmidt, and J.D. Mikkelsen The selective alpha-7 nicotinic acetylcholine receptor agonists SSR180711 and A-582941 activate immediate early genes in limbic regions of the forebrain in juvenile and adult rats, *Soc for Neurosci.*

256. Woolley, M.L., Pemberton, D.J., Bate, S., Corti, C., and Jones, D.N.C. (2008). The mGlu2 but not mGlu3 receptor mediates the actions of the mGlu2/3 agonist, LY379268, in mouse models predictive of antipsychotic activity. *Psychopharmacology*, 196(3):431–440.

257. Krystal, J.H., D'Souza, D.C., Petrakis, I.L., Belger, A., Berman, R.M., Charney, D.S. *et al.* (1999). NMDA agonists and antagonists as probes of glutamatergic dysfunction and pharmacotherapies in neuropsychiatric disorders. *Harv Rev Psychiatry*, 7(3):125–143.

258. Geyer, M.A. and Moghaddam, B. (2002). Animal models relevant to schizophrenia disorders. In Davis, K.L., Charney, D., Coyle, J.T., and Nemeroff, C. (eds.), *Neuropsychopharmacology: The Fifth Generation of Progress*. Lippincott Williams &Wilkins, Philadelphia, pp. 689–701. Chapter 50

259. Cho, A.K. and Segal, D.S. (eds.). (1994). *Amphetamine and its Analogs: Neuropsychopharmacology Toxicology and Abuse*, Academic Press, New York, pp. 177–208.

260. Costall, B., Naylor, R.J., and Nohria, V. (1979). Hyperactivity response to apomorphine and amphetamine in the mouse: The importance of the nucleus accumbens and caudate-putamen. *J Pharm Pharmacol*, 31(4):259–261.

261. Cools, A.R. (1986). Mesolimbic dopamine and its control of locomotor activity in rats: Differences in pharmacology and light/dark periodicity between the olfactory tubercle and the nucleus accumbens. *Psychopharmacology (Berl)*, 88(4):451–459.

262. Struyker-Boudier, H.A. and Cools, A.R. (1984). (3,4-Dihydroxyphenylimino)-2-imidazoline (DPI): A stimulant of alpha-adrenoceptors and dopamine receptors. *J Pharm Pharmacol*, 36(12):859–860.

263. Swerdlow, N.R. and Koob, G.F. (1987). Dopamine, schizophrenia, mania, and depression: Toward a unified hypothesis of cortico-striato-pallido-thalamic function. *Behav Brain Sci*, 10:197–245.

264. Segal, D.S., Geyer, M.A., and Schuckit, A. (1981). Stimulant-induced psychosis: An evaluation of animal models. In Youdim, M.B.H., Lovenberg, W., Sharman, D.F., and Lagnado, J.R. (eds.), *Essays in Neurochemistry and Neuropharmacology*. John Wiley & Sons, New York, pp. 95–130.

265. Segal, S.A., Moerschbaecher, J.M., and Thompson, D.M. (1981). Effects of phencyclidine, d-amphetamine and pentobarbital on schedule-controlled behavior in rats. *Pharmacol Biochem Behav*, 15(5):807–812.

266. Ellenbroek, B.A. (2003). Animal models in the genomic era: Possibilities and limitations with special emphasis on schizophrenia. *Behav Pharmacol*, 14(5-6):409–417.

267. Mansbach, R.S., Geyer, M.A., and Braff, D.L. (1988). Dopaminergic stimulation disrupts sensorimotor gating in the rat. *Psychopharmacology*, 94:507–514.

268. Tenn, C.C., Fletcher, P.J., and Kapur, S. (2003). Amphetamine-sensitized animals show a sensorimotor gating and neurochemical abnormality similar to that of schizophrenia. *Schizophr Res*, 64(2-3):103–114.

269. Murphy, C.A., Fend, M., Russig, H., and Feldon, J. (2001). Latent inhibition, but not prepulse inhibition, is reduced during withdrawal from an escalating dosage schedule of amphetamine. *Behav Neurosci*, 115(6):1247–1256.

270. Abi-Dargham, A. and Moore, H. (2003). Prefrontal DA transmission at D1 receptors and the pathology of schizophrenia. *Neuroscientist*, 9(5):404–416.

271. Idris, N.F., Repeto, P., Neill, J.C., and Large, C.H. (2005). Investigation of the effects of lamotrigine and clozapine in improving reversal-learning impairments induced by acute phencyclidine and D-amphetamine in the rat. *Psychopharmacology*, 179(2):336–348.

272. Mouri, A., Noda, Y., Enomoto, T., and Nabeshima, T. (2007). Phencyclidine animal models of schizophrenia: Approaches from abnormality of glutamatergic neurotransmission and neurodevelopment. *Neurochem Int*, 51(2–4):173–184.

273. Coyle, J.T. (2006). Glutamate and schizophrenia: Beyond the dopamine hypothesis. *Cell Mol Neurobiol*, 26(4–6):365–384.

274. Lieberman, J.A., Kane, J.M., and Alvir, J. (1987). Provocative tests with psychostimulant drugs in schizophrenia. *Psychopharmacology (Berl)*, 91(4):415–433.

275. Riedel, W.J. (2007). The ketamine model of positive, negative and cognitive symptoms in schizophrenia: Facts and frictions. *J Psychopharmacology*, 21(3):235–236.

276. Kalinichev, M., Bates, S., Coggon, S.A., and Jones, D.N.C. (2008). Locomotor reactivity to a novel environment and sensitivity to MK-801 in five strains of mice. *Behav Pharmacol*, 19:71–75.

277. Sams-Dodd, F. (1996). Phencyclidine-induced stereotyped behaviour and social isolation in rats: A possible animal model of schizophrenia. *Behav Pharmacol*, 7(1):3–23.

278. Noda, Y., Yamada, K., Furukawa, H., and Nabeshima, T. (1995). Enhancement of immobility in a forced swimming test by subacute or repeated treatment with phencyclidine: A new model of schizophrenia. *Br J Pharmacol*, 116(5):2531–2537.

279. Nabeshima, T., Kozawa, T., Furukawa, H., and Kameyama, T. (1986). Phencyclidine-induced retrograde amnesia in mice. *Psychopharmacology (Berl)*, 89(3):334–337.

280. Egerton, A., Reid, L., McGregor, S., Cochran, S.M., Morris, B.J., and Pratt, J.A. (2008). Subchronic and chronic PCP treatment produces temporally distinct deficits in attentional set shifting and prepulse inhibition in rats. *Psychopharmacology*, 198(1):37–49.

281. Abdul-Monim, Z., Reynolds, G.P., and Neill, J.C. (2003). The atypical antipsychotic ziprasidone, but not haloperidol, improves phencyclidine-induced cognitive deficits in a reversal learning task in the rat. *J Psychopharmacol*, 17(1):57–65.

282. Brody, S.A., Conquet, F., and Geyer, M.A. (2004). Effect of antipsychotic treatment on the prepulse inhibition deficit of mgluR5 knockout mice. *Psychopharmacology*, 172:187–195.

283. Cilia, J., Hatcher, P., Reavill, C., and Jones, D.N. (2007). (+/−) Ketamine-induced prepulse inhibition deficits of an acoustic startle response in rats are not reversed by antipsychotics. *J Psychopharmacol*, 21(3):302–311.

284. Morris, B.J., Cochran, S.M., and Pratt, J.A. (2005). PCP: From pharmacology to modelling schizophrenia. *Curr Opin Pharmacol*, 5(1):101–106.

285. Gartlon, J.E., Barnes, S.A., and Jones, D.N.C. (2006). Comparison of sub-chronic PCP dosing regimes as animal models for schizophrenia. *J Psychopharmacol*, 20:A44.

286. Lee, P.R., Brady, D.L., Shapiro, R.A., Dorsa, D.M., and Koenig, J.I. (2005). Social interaction deficits caused by chronic phencyclidine administration are reversed by oxytocin. *Neuropsychopharmacology*, 30(10):1883–1894.

287. Nuechterlein, K.H., Barch, D.M., Gold, J.M., Goldberg, T.E., Green, M.F., and Heaton, R.K. (2004). Identification of separable cognitive factors in schizophrenia. *Schizophr Res*, 72(1):29–39.

288. Jentsch, J.D., Tran, A., Le, D., Youngren, K.D., and Roth, R.H. (1997). Subchronic phencyclidine administration reduces mesoprefrontal dopamine utilization and impairs prefrontal cortical-dependent cognition in the rat. *Neuropsychopharmacology*, 17(2):92–99.

289. Stefani, M.R. and Moghaddam, B. (2002). Effects of repeated treatment with amphetamine or phencyclidine on working memory in the rat. *Behav Brain Res*, 134(1–2):267–274.

290. Li, Z., Kim, C.H., Ichikawa, J., and Meltzer, H.Y. (2003). Effect of repeated administration of phencyclidine on spatial performance in an eight-arm radial maze with delay in rats and mice. *Pharmacol Biochem Behav*, 75(2):335–340.

291. Podhorna, J. and Didriksen, M. (2005). Performance of male C57BL/6 J mice and Wistar rats in the water maze following various schedules of phencyclidine treatment. *Behav Pharmacol*, 16(1):25–34.

292. Grayson, B., Idris, N.F., and Neill, J.C. (2007). Atypical antipsychotics attenuate a sub-chronic PCP-induced cognitive deficit in the novel object recognition task in the rat. *Behav Brain Res*, 184(1):31–38.

293. Rodefer, J.S., Murphy, E.R., and Baxter, M.G. (2005). PDE10A inhibition reverses sub-chronic PCP-induced deficits in attentional set-shifting in rats. *Eur J Neurosci*, 21(4): 1070-1076.

294. McLean, S.L., Beck, J.P., Wooley, M.L., and Neill, J.C. (2008). A preliminary investigation into the effects of antipsychotics on sub-chronic phencyclidine-induced deficits in attentional set-shifting in female rats. *Behav Brain Res*, 189(1):152–158.

295. Abdul-Monim, Z., Reynolds, G.P., and Neill, J.C. (2006). The effect of atypical and classical antipsychotics on sub-chronic PCP-induced cognitive deficits in a reversal-learning paradigm. *Behav Brain Res*, 169(2):263–273.

296. Fletcher, P.J., Tenn, C.C., Rizos, Z., Lovic, V., and Kapur, S. (2005). Sensitization to amphetamine, but not PCP, impairs attentional set shifting: Reversal by a D1 receptor agonist injected into the medial prefrontal cortex. *Psychopharmacology*, 183(2):190–200.

297. Reynolds, G.P. (2007). The impact of pharmacogenetics on the development and use of antipsychotic drugs. *Drug Discov Today*, 12(21–22):953–959.

298. Abdul-Monim, Z., Neill, J.C., and Reynolds, G.P. (2007). Sub-chronic psychotomimetic phencyclidine induces deficits in reversal learning and alterations in parvalbumin-immunoreactive expression in the rat. *J Psychopharmacol*, 21(2):198–205.

299. Cochran, S.M., Kennedy, M., McKerchar, C.E., Steward, L.J., Pratt, J.A., and Morris, B.J. (2003). Induction of metabolic hypofunction and neurochemical deficits after chronic intermittent exposure to phencyclidine: Differential modulation by antipsychotic drugs. *Neuropsychopharmacology*, 28(2):265–275.

300. Reynolds, G.P., Abdul-Monim, Z., Neill, J.C., and Zhang, Z.J. (2004). Calcium binding protein markers of GABA deficits in schizophrenia–postmortem studies and animal models. *Neurotox Res*, 6(1):57–61.

301. Harte, M.K., Powell, S.B., Swerdlow, N.R., Geyer, M.A., and Reynolds, G.P. (2007). Deficits in parvalbumin and calbindin immunoreactive cells in the hippocampus of isolation reared rats. *J Neural Transm*, 114(7):893–898.

302. Martinez, Z.A., Ellison, G.D., Geyer, M.A., and Swerdlow, N.R. (1999). Effects of sustained phencyclidine exposure on sensorimotor gating of startle in rats. *Neuropsychopharmacology*, 21:28–39.

303. Snigdha, S. and Neill, J.C. (2008). Improvement of phencyclidine-induced social behaviour deficits in rats: Involvement of 5-HT(1A) receptors. *Behav Brain Res*, 191(1):26–31.

304. Jentsch, J.D. and Roth, R.H. (1999). The neuropsychopharmacology of phencyclidine: From NMDA receptor hypofunction to the dopamine hypothesis of schizophrenia. *Neuropsychopharmacology*, 20(3):201–225.

305. Elsworth, J.D., Jentsch, J.D., Morrow, B.A., Redmond, D.E., Jr, and Roth, R.H. (2008). Clozapine normalizes prefrontal cortex dopamine transmission in monkeys subchronically exposed to phencyclidine. *Neuropsychopharmacology*, 33:491–496.

306. Cilia, J., Cluderay, J.E., Robbins, M.J., Reavill, C., Southam, E., Kew, J.N. *et al.* (2005). Reversal of isolation-rearing-induced PPI deficits by an alpha7 nicotinic receptor agonist. *Psychopharmacology (Berl)*, 182(2):214–219.

307. Cilia, J., Hatcher, P.D., Reavill, C., and Jones, D.N. (2005). Long-term evaluation of isolation-rearing induced prepulse inhibition deficits in rats: An update. *Psychopharmacology (Berl)*, 180(1):57–62.

308. Lipska, B.K., Swerdlow, N.R., Geyer, M.A., Jaskiw, G.E., Braff, D.L., and Weinberger, D.R. (1995). Neonatal excitotoxic hippocampal damage in rats causes post-pubertal changes in prepulse inhibition of startle and its disruption by apomorphine. *Psychopharmacology (Berl)*, 122(1):35–43.

309. Geyer, M.A., Wilkinson, L.S., Humby, T., and Robbins, T.W. (1993). Isolation rearing of rats produces a deficit in prepulse inhibition of acoustic startle similar to that in schizophrenia. *Biolog Psychiatry*, 34:361–372.

310. Powell, S.B. and Geyer, M.A. (2002). Developmental markers of psychiatric disorders as identified by sensorimotor gating. *Neurotox Res*, 4(5–6):489–502.

311. Weiss, I.C. and Feldon, J. (2001). Environmental animal models for sensorimotor gating deficiencies in schizophrenia: A review. *Psychopharmacology (Berl)*, 156(2–3):305–326.

312. Bloomfield, C., French, S.F., Jones, D.N.C., Reavill, C., Southam, E., Cilia, J., and Totterdell, S. (in press). Chandelier cartridges in the prefrontal cortex are reduced in isolation reared rats. *Synapse*.

313. Cilia, J., Reavill, C., Hagan, J.J., and Jones, D.N. (2001). Long-term evaluation of isolation-rearing induced prepulse inhibition deficits in rats. *Psychopharmacology (Berl)*, 156(2–3):327–337.

314. Harte, M.K., Powell, S.B., Reynolds, L.M., Swerdlow, N.R., Geyer, M.A., and Reynolds, G.P. (2004). Reduced N-acetylaspartate in the temporal cortex of rats reared in isolation. *Biolog Psychiatry*, 56(4):296–299.

315. Bakshi, V.P., Swerdlow, N.R., Braff, D.L., and Geyer, M.A. (1998). Reversal of isolation rearing-induced deficits in prepulse inhibition by Seroquel and olanzapine. *Biol Psychiatry*, 43(6):436–445.

316. Nakato, K., Morita, T., Wanibuchi, F., and Yamaguchi, T. (1997). Antipsychotics restored but antidepressants and anxiolytics did not restore prepulse inhibition (PPI) deficits in isolation-reared rats. *Soc Neurosci Abstr*, 23:1855.

317. Lipska, B.K., Jaskiw, G.E., and Weinberger, D.R. (1993). Postpubertal emergence of hyperresponsiveness to stress and to amphetamine after neonatal excitotoxic hippocampal damage: A potential animal model of schizophrenia. *Neuropsychopharmacology*, 9(1):67–75.

318. Schroeder, H., Grecksch, G., Becker, A., Bogerts, B., and Hoellt, V. (1999). Alterations of the dopaminergic and glutamatergic neurotransmission in adult rats with postnatal ibotenic acid hippocampal lesion. *Psychopharmacology (Berl)*, 145(1):61–66.

319. Lipska, B.K. and Weinberger, D.R. (2002). A neurodevelopmental model of schizophrenia: Neonatal disconnection of the hippocampus. *Neurotox Res*, 4(5–6):469–475.

320. Lipska, B.K. (2004). Using animal models to test a neurodevelopmental hypothesis of schizophrenia. *J Psychiatry Neurosci*, 29(4):282–286.

321. Lipska, B.K., Halim, N.D., Segal, P.N., and Weinberger, D.R. (2002). Effects of reversible inactivation of the neonatal ventral hippocampus on behavior in the adult rat. *J Neurosci*, 22(7):2835–2842.

322. Lipska, B.K. and Weinberger, D.R. (1994). Subchronic treatment with haloperidol and clozapine in rats with neonatal excitotoxic hippocampal damage. *Neuropsychopharmacology*, 10(3):199–205.

323. Le Pen, G., Kew, J., Alberati, D., Borroni, E., Heitz, M.P., and Moreau, J.L. (2003). Prepulse inhibition deficits of the startle reflex in neonatal ventral hippocampal-lesioned rats: Reversal by glycine and a glycine transporter inhibitor. *Biolog Psychiatry*, 54(11): 1162–1170.

324. Lillrank, S.M., Lipska, B.K., Bachus, S.E., Wood, G.K., and Weinberger, D.R. (1996). Amphetamine-induced c-fos mRNA expression is altered in rats with neonatal ventral hippocampal damage. *Synapse*, 23(4):292–301.

325. Lipska, B.K., Lerman, D.N., Khaing, Z.Z., and Weinberger, D.R. (2003). The neonatal ventral hippocampal lesion model of schizophrenia: Effects on dopamine and GABA mRNA markers in the rat midbrain. *Eur J Neurosci*, 18(11):3097–3104.

326. Ikonomidou, C., Bosch, F., Miksa, M., Bittigau, P., Vockler, J., Dikranian, K. *et al.* (1999). Blockade of NMDA receptors and apoptotic neurodegeneration in the developing brain. *Science*, 283(5398):70–74.

327. Olney, J.W., Labruyere, J., Wang, G., Wozniak, D.F., Price, M.T., and Sesma, M.A. (1991). NMDA antagonist neurotoxicity: Mechanism and prevention. *Science*, 254(5037):1515–1518.

328. Ikonomidou, C., Mosinger, J.L., Salles, K.S., Labruyere, J., and Olney, J.W. (1989). Sensitivity of the developing rat brain to hypobaric/ischemic damage parallels sensitivity to N-methylaspartate neurotoxicity. *J Neurosci*, 9(8):2809–2818.

329. Olney, J.W., Newcomer, J.W., and Farber, N.B. (1999). NMDA receptor hypofunction model of schizophrenia. *J Psychiatr Res*, 33(6):523–533.

330. du Bois, T.M. and Huang, X.F. (2007). Early brain development disruption from NMDA receptor hypofunction: Relevance to schizophrenia. *Brain Res Rev*, 53(2):260–270.

331. Gartlon, J.E., Harte, M.K., Reynolds, G.P., and Jones, D.N.C. (2007). PCP administration to neonatal rats results in long-term deficits in novel object recognition and reduced parvalbumin-immunoreactive neurons in the hippocampus. *J Psychopharmacol*, 21(7):A66.

332. Nemeth, H., Varga, H., Farkas, T., Kis, Z., Vecsei, L., Horvath, S. *et al.* (2002). Long-term effects of neonatal MK-801 treatment on spatial learning and cortical plasticity in adult rats. *Psychopharmacology (Berl)*, 160(1):1–8.

333. Terranova, J.P., Chabot, C., Barnouin, M.C., Perrault, G., Depoortere, R., Griebel, G. *et al.* (2005). SSR181507, a dopamine D(2) receptor antagonist and 5-HT(1A) receptor agonist, alleviates disturbances of novelty discrimination in a social context in rats, a putative model of selective attention deficit. *Psychopharmacology*, 181(1):134–144.

334. Wang, C., McInnis, J., Ross-Sanchez, M., Shinnick-Gallagher, P., Wiley, J.L., and Johnson, K.M. (2001). Long-term behavioral and neurodegenerative effects of perinatal phencyclidine administration: Implications for schizophrenia. *Neuroscience*, 107(4):535–550.

335. Wiseman-Harris, L., Sharp, T., Gartlon, J., Jones, D.N.C., and Harrison, P.J. (2003). Long-term behavioural, molecular and morphological effects of neonatal NMDA receptor antagonism. *Eur J Pharmacol*, 18:1706–1710.

336. Depoortere, R., Dargazanli, G., Estenne-Bouhtou, G., Coste, A., Lanneau, C., Desvignes, C. *et al.* (2005). Neurochemical, electrophysiological and pharmacological profiles of the selective inhibitor of the glycine transporter-1 SSR504734, a potential new type of antipsychotic. *Neuropsychopharmacology*, 30(11):1963–1985.

337. Talamini, L.M., Koch, T., Ter Horst, G.J., and Korf, J. (1998). Methylazoxymethanol acetate-induced abnormalities in the entorhinal cortex of the rat; parallels with morphological findings in schizophrenia. *Brain Res*, 789(2):293–306.

338. Flagstad, P., Mork, A., Glenthoj, B.Y., van Beek, J., Michael-Titus, A.T., and Didriksen, M. (2004). Disruption of neurogenesis on gestational day 17 in the rat causes behavioral changes relevant to positive and negative schizophrenia symptoms and alters amphetamine-induced dopamine release in nucleus accumbens. *Neuropsychopharmacology*, 29(11):2052–2064.

339. Goto, Y. and Grace, A.A. (2006). Alterations in medial prefrontal cortical activity and plasticity in rats with disruption of cortical development. *Biol Psychiatry*, 60(11):1259–1267.

340. Gourevitch, R., Rocher, C., Le Pen, G., Krebs, M.O., and Jay, T.M. (2004). Working memory deficits in adult rats after prenatal disruption of neurogenesis. *Behav Pharmacol*, 15(4):287–292.

341. Featherstone, R.E., Rizos, Z., Nobrega, J.N., Kapur, S., and Fletcher, P.J. (2007). Gestational methylazoxymethanol acetate treatment impairs select cognitive functions: Parallels to schizophrenia. *Neuropsychopharmacology*, 32(2):483–492.

342. Le Pen, G., Gourevitch, R., Hazane, F., Hoareau, C., Jay, T.M., and Krebs, M.O. (2006). Peripubertal maturation after developmental disturbance: A model for psychosis onset in the rat. *Neuroscience*, 143:395–405.

343. Moore, H., Jentsch, J.D., Ghajarnia, M., Geyer, M.A., and Grace, A.A. (2006). A neurobehavioral systems analysis of adult rats exposed to methylazoxymethanol acetate on E17: Implications for the neuropathology of schizophrenia. *Biol Psychiatry*, 60(3):253–264.

344. Penschuck, S., Flagstad, P., Didriksen, M., Leist, M., and Michael-Titus, A.T. (2006). Decrease in parvalbumin-expressing neurons in the hippocampus and increased phencyclidine-induced locomotor activity in the rat methylazoxymethanol (MAM) model of schizophrenia. *Eur J Neurosci*, 23(1):279–284.

345. Leng, A., Jongen-Relo, A.L., Pothuizen, H.H., and Feldon, J. (2005). Effects of prenatal methylazoxymethanol acetate (MAM) treatment in rats on water maze performance. *Behav Brain Res*, 161(2):291–298.

346. Geddes, J.R. and Lawrie, S.M. (1995). Obstetric complications and schizophrenia: A meta-analysis. *Br J Psychiatry*, 167(6):786–793.

347. Lewis, D.A. and Levitt, P. (2002). Schizophrenia as a disorder of neurodevelopment. *Annu Rev Neurosci*, 25:409–432.

348. Boog, G. (2004). Obstetrical complications and subsequent schizophrenia in adolescent and young adult offsprings: Is there a relationship? *Eur J Obstet Gynecol Reprod Biol*, 114(2):130–136.

349. El Khodor, B.F. and Boksa, P. (1997). Long-term reciprocal changes in dopamine levels in prefrontal cortex versus nucleus accumbens in rats born by Caesarean section compared to vaginal birth. *Exp Neurol*, 145(1):118–129.

350. Bjelke, B., Andersson, K., Ogren, S.O., and Bolme, P. (1991). Asphyctic lesion: Proliferation of tyrosine hydroxylase-immunoreactive nerve cell bodies in the rat substantia nigra and functional changes in dopamine neurotransmission. *Brain Res*, 543(1):1–9.

351. Tejkalova, H., Kaiser, M., Klaschka, J., and Stastny, F. (2007). Does neonatal brain ischemia induces schizophrenia-like behaviour in young adult rats? *Physiol Res*, 56(6): 815–823.

352. Barr, C.E., Mednick, S.A., and Munk-Jorgensen, P. (1990). Exposure to influenza epidemics during gestation and adult schizophrenia. A 40-year study. *Arch Gen Psychiatry*, 47(9):869–874.

353. Shi, L., Fatemi, S.H., Sidwell, R.W., and Patterson, P.H. (2003). Maternal influenza infection causes marked behavioral and pharmacological changes in the offspring. *J Neurosci*, 23(1):297–302.

354. Zuckerman, L., Rehavi, M., Nachman, R., and Weiner, I. (2003). Immune activation during pregnancy in rats leads to a postpubertal emergence of disrupted latent inhibition, dopaminergic hyperfunction, and altered limbic morphology in the offspring: A novel neurodevelopmental model of schizophrenia. *Neuropsychopharmacology*, 28(10): 1778–1789.

355. Borrell, J., Vela, J.M., Arevalo-Martin, A., Molina-Holgado, E., and Guaza, C. (2002). Prenatal immune challenge disrupts sensorimotor gating in adult rats. Implications for the etiopathogenesis of schizophrenia. *Neuropsychopharmacology*, 26(2):204–215.

356. Fortier, M.E., Luheshi, G.N., and Boksa, P. (2007). Effects of prenatal infection on prepulse inhibition in the rat depend on the nature of the infectious agent and the stage of pregnancy. *Behav Brain Res*, 181(2):270–277.

357. Gainetdinov, R.R., Mohn, A.R., and Caron, M.G. (2001). Genetic animal models: Focus on schizophrenia. *Trends Neurosci*, 24(9):527–533.

358. Giros, B., Jaber, M., Jones, S.R., Wightman, R.M., and Caron, M.G. (1996). Hyperlocomotion and indifference to cocaine and amphetamine in mice lacking the dopamine transporter. *Nature*, 379(6566):606–612.

359. Ralph, R.J., Paulus, M.P., Fumagalli, F., Caron, M.G., and Geyer, M.A. (2001). Prepulse inhibition deficits and perseverative motor patterns in dopamine transporter knockout mice: Differential effects of D1 and D2 receptor antagonists. *J Neurosci*, 21:305–313.

360. Baik, J.H., Picetti, R., Saiardi, A., Thiriet, G., Dierich, A., Depaulis, A. *et al.* (1995). Parkinsonian-like locomotor impairment in mice lacking dopamine D2 receptors. *Nature*, 377(6548):424–428.

361. Ralph, R.J., Varty, G.B., Kelly, M.A., Wang, Y.-M., Caron, M.G., Rubinstein, M., Grandy, D.K., Low, M.J., and Geyer, M.A. (1999). The dopamine D2 but not D3 or D4 receptor subtype is essential for the disruption of prepulse inhibition produced by amphetamine in mice. *J Neurosci*, 19:4627–4633.

362. Xu, M., Moratalla, R., Gold, L.H., Hiroi, N., Koob, G.F., Graybiel, A.M. *et al.* (1994). Dopamine D1 receptor mutant mice are deficient in striatal expression of dynorphin and in dopamine-mediated behavioral responses. *Cell*, 79(4):729–742.

363. Duncan, G.E., Moy, S.S., Lieberman, J.A., and Koller, B.H. (2006). Typical and atypical antipsychotic drug effects on locomotor hyperactivity and deficits in sensorimotor gating in a genetic model of NMDA receptor hypofunction. *Pharmacol Biochem Behav*, 85(3):481–491.

364. Rakhilin, S.V., Olson, P.A., Nishi, A., Starkova, N.N., Fienberg, A.A., Nairn, A.C. *et al.* (2004). A network of control mediated by regulator of calcium/calmodulin-dependent signaling. *Science*, 306(5696):698–701.

365. Austin, C.P., Battey, J.F., Bradley, A., Bucan, M., Capecchi, M., Collins, F.S. *et al.* (2004). The knockout mouse project. *Nat Genet*, 36(9):921–924.

366. Palmer, A.A., Dulawa, S.C., Mottiwala, A.A., Conti, L.H., Geyer, M.A., and Printz, M.P. (2000). Prepulse startle deficit in the Brown Norway rat: A potential genetic model. *Behav Neurosci*, 114(2):374–388.

367. Feifel, D., Melendez, G., Priebe, K., and Shilling, P.D. (2007). The effects of chronic administration of established and putative antipsychotics on natural prepulse inhibition deficits in Brattleboro rats. *Behav Brain Res*, 181(2):278–286.

368. Varty, G.B. and Geyer, M.A. (1998). Effects of isolation rearing on startle reactivity, habituation, and prepulse inhibition in male Lewis, Sprague-Dawley, and Fischer F344 rats. *Behav Neurosci*, 112(6):1450–1457.

369. Bray, N.J., Buckland, P.R., Owen, M.J., and O'Donovan, M.C. (2003). Cis-acting variation in the expression of a high proportion of genes in human brain. *Hum Genet*, 113(2):149–153.

370. Gilles, C. and Luthringer, R. (2007). Pharmacological models in healthy volunteers: Their use in the clinical development of psychotropic drugs. *J Psychopharmacology*, 21(3):272–282.

371. Malhotra, A.K., Pinals, D.A., Weingartner, H., Sirocco, K., Missar, C.D., Pickar, D., and Breier, A. (1996). NMDA receptor function and human cognition: The effects of ketamine in healthy volunteers. *Neuropsychopharmacology*, 14:301–307.

372. Krystal, J.H., D'Souza, D.C., Karper, L.P., Bennet, A., Abi-Dargham, A., Abi-Saab, D. *et al.* (1999). Interactive effects of subanesthetic ketamine and haloperidol in healthy humans. *Psychopharmacology*, 145:193–204.

373. Malhotra, A.K., Adler, C.M., Kennison, S.D., Elman, I., Pickar, D., and Breier, A. (1997). Clozapine blunts N-methyl-D-aspartate antagonist-induced psychosis: A study with ketamine. *Biol Psychiatry*, 42:664–668.

374. Bakshi, V.P., Swerdlow, N.R., and Geyer, M.A. (1994). Clozapine antagonizes phencyclidine-induced deficits in sensorimotor gating of the startle response. *J Pharmacol Exp The*, 271:787–794.

375. Linn, G.S., Negi, S.S., Gerum, S.V., and Javitt, D.C. (2003). Reversal of phencyclidine-induced prepulse inhibition deficits by clozapine in monkeys. *Psychopharmacol*, 169:234–239.

376. Krystal, J.H., Abi-Saab, W., Perry, E., D'Souza, D.C., Liu, N., Gueorguieva, R. *et al.* (2005). Preliminary evidence of attenuation of the disruptive effects of the NMDA glutamate receptor antagonist, ketamine, on working memory by pretreatment with the group II metabotropic glutamate receptor agonist, LY354740, in healthy human subjects. *Psychopharmacology*, 179(1):303–309.

377. Winsky, L., Driscoll, J., and Brady, L. (2008). Drug discovery and development initiatives at the National Institute of Mental Health: from cell-based systems to proof of concept. In McArthur, R.A. and Borsini, F. (eds.), *Animal and Translational Models of Behavioural Disorders Volume 1-Psychiatric Disorders*, Elsevier, San Diego.

378. Marder, S.R. (2006). The NIMH-MATRICS project for developing cognition-enhancing agents for schizophrenia. *Dialogues Clin Neurosci*, 8:109–113.

379. Geyer, M.A. and Heinssen, R. (2005). New approaches to measurement and treatment research to improve cognition in schizophrenia. *Schizophr Bull*, 31:806–809.

380. Marder, S.R. and Fenton, W. (2004). Measurement and Treatment Research to Improve Cognition in Schizophrenia: NIMH MATRICS initiative to support the development of agents for improving cognition in schizophrenia. *Schizophr Res*, 72:5–9.

381. Green, M.F., Nuechterlein, K.H., Gold, J.M. *et al.* (2004). Approaching a consensus cognitive battery for clinical trials in schizophrenia: The NIMH-MATRICS conference to select cognitive domains and test criteria. *Biol Psychiatry*, 56:301–307.

382. Geyer, M.A. and Tamminga, C.A. (2004). Measurement and treatment research to improve cognition in schizophrenia: Neuropharmacological aspects. *Psychopharmacology*, 174:1–2.

383. Buchanan, R.W., Davis, M., Goff, D. *et al.* (2005). A summary of the FDA-NIMH-MATRICS workshop on clinical trial design for neurocognitive drugs for schizophrenia. *Schizophr Bull*, 31:5–19.

384. Buchanan, R.W., Freedman, R., Javitt, D.C., Abi-Dargham, A., and Lieberman, J.A. (2007). Recent advances in the development of novel pharmacological agents for the treatment of cognitive impairments in schizophrenia. *Schizophr Bull*, 33(5):1120–1130.

385. Stover, E.L., Brady, L., and Marder, S.R. (2007). New paradigms for treatment development. *Schiz Bull*, 33(5):1093–1099.

386. J. Young, Y. M.A. Geyer, and the TURNS Preclinical Subcommittee (2007). Cognitive task list and preclinical task survey. http://www.turns.ucla.edu/preclinical-TURNS-report-2006b.pdf

387. Carter, C.S. and Barch, D.M. (2007). Cognitive neuroscience-based approaches to measuring and improving treatment effects on cognition in schizophrenia: The CNTRICS initiative. *Schizophr Bull*, 33(5):1131–1137.

388. Buchanan, R.W. (2007). Persistent negative symptoms in schizophrenia: An overview. *Schizophr Bull*, 33(4):1013–1022.

389. Kay, S.R., Fiszbein, A., and Opler, L.A. (1987). The positive and negative syndrome scale (PANSS) for schizophrenia. *Schizophr Bull*, 13(2):261–276.

390. Overall, J.R. and Gorham, D.R. (1980). The brief psychiatric rating scale. *J Oper Psychiatry*, 11:48–64.

391. Quednow, B.B., Wagner, M., Westheide, J., Beckmann, K., Bliesener, N., Maier, W., and Kuhn, K.U. (2006). Sensorimotor gating and habituation of the startle response in schizophrenic patients randomly treated with amisulpride or olanzapine. *Biol Psychiatry*, 59(6):536–545.

392. Vollenweider, F.X., Barro, M., Csomor, P.A., and Feldon, J. (2006). Clozapine enhances prepulse inhibition in healthy humans with low but not with high prepulse inhibition levels. *Biol Psychiatry*, 60:597–603.

393. Csomor, P.A., Stadler, R.R., Feldon, J., Yee, B.K., Geyer, M.A., and Vollenweider, F.X. (2008). Haloperidol differentially modulates prepulse inhibition and P50 gating in healthy humans stratified for low and high gating levels. *Neuropsychopharmacology*, 33: 497–512.

394. Umbricht, D., Koller, R., Schmid, L., Skrabo, A., Grubel, C., Huber, T., and Stassen, H. (2003). How specific are deficits in mismatch negativity generation in schizophrenia? *Biol Psychiatry*, 53:1120–1131.

395. Kathmann, N., Hochrein, A., Uwer, R., and Bondy, B. (2003). Deficits in gain of smooth pursuit eye movements in schizophrenia and affective disorder patients and their unaffected relatives. *Am J Psychiatry*, 160(4):696–702.

396. Manor, B.R., Gordon, E., Williams, L.M., Rennie, C.J., Bahramali, H., Latimer, C.R., Barry, R.J., and Meares, R.A. (1999). Eye movements reflect impaired face processing in patients with schizophrenia. *Biolog Psychiatry*, 46:963–969.

397. Loughland, C.M., Williams, L.M., and Gordon, E. (2002). Schizophrenia and affective disorder show different visual scanning behavior for faces: A trait versus state-based distinction? *Biolog Psychiatry*, 52(4):338–348.

398. Loughland, C.M., Williams, L.M., and Harris, A.W. (2004). Visual scanpath dysfunction in first-degree relatives of schizophrenia probands: Evidence for a vulnerability marker? *Schizophr Res*, 67:11–21.

399. Benson, P.J., Leonards, U., Lothian, R.M., St Clair, D.M., and Merlo, M.C. (2007). Visual scan paths in first-episode schizophrenia and cannabis-induced psychosis. *J Psychiatry Neurosci*, 32(4):267–274.

400. Hoffman, R.E. (1999). New methods for studying hallucinated 'voices' in schizophrenia. *Acta Psychiatr Scand*, 395:89–94.

401. Phillips, M.L. and David, A.S. (1998). Abnormal visual scan paths: A psychophysiological marker of delusions in schizophrenia. *Schizophr Res*, 29(3):235–245.

402. Kuperberg, G.R., Deckersbach, T., Holt, D.J., Goff, D., and West, W.C. (2007). Increased temporal and prefrontal activity in response to semantic associations in schizophrenia. *Arch Gen Psychiatry*, 64(2):38–151.

403. Twamley, E.W., Doshi, R.R., Nayak, G.V. *et al.* (2002). Generalized cognitive impairments, ability to perform everyday tasks, and level of independence in community living situations of older patients with psychosis. *Am J Psychiatry*, 159:2013–2020.

404. Patterson, T.L., Goldman, S., McKibbin, C.L., Hughs, T., and Jeste, D.V. (2001). UCSD Performance-Based Skills Assessment: Development of a new measure of everyday functioning for severely mentally ill adults. *Schizophr Bull*, 27:235–245.

405. Bosia, M., Bechi, M., Marino, E. *et al.* (2007). Influence of catechol-O-methyltransferase Val158Met polymorphism on neuropsychological and functional outcomes of classical rehabilitation and cognitive remediation in schizophrenia. *Neurosci Lett*, 417:271–274.

406. Green, M.F., Nuechterlein, K.H., Kern, R.S., Baade, L.E., Fenton, W.S., Gold, J.M., *et al.* (2008). Functional Co-Primary Measures for Clinical Trials in Schizophrenia: Results From the MATRICS Psychometric and Standardization Study. *Am J Psychiatry*, 165(2):221–228.

407. Moos, R.H., McCoy, L., and Moos, B.S. (2000). Global assessment of functioning (GAF) ratings: Determinants and role as predictors of one-year treatment outcomes. *J Clin Psychol*, 56(4):449–461.

408. Ludewig, K., Paulus, M.P., and Vollenweider, F.X. (2003). Behavioral Dysregulation of decision-making in deficit but not nondeficit schizophrenia patients. *Psychiatry Res*, 119(3):293–306.

409. Minassian, A., Paulus, M., Lincoln, A., and Perry, W. (2004). Increased sensitivity to error during decision-making in bipolar disorder patients with acute mania. *J Affective Disorders*, 82(2):203–208.

410. Wittmann, M. and Paulus, M.P. (2008). Decision making, impulsivity and time perception. *Trends Cogn Sci*, 12(1):7–12.

411. Paulus, M.P., Frank, L., Brown, G.G., and Braff, D.L. (2003). Schizophrenia subjects show intact success-related neural activation but impaired uncertainty processing during decision-making. *Neuropsychopharmacology*, 28(4):795–806.

412. McGlashan, T.H., Addington, J., Cannon, T., Heinimaa, M., McGorry, P., O'Brien, M. *et al.* (2007). Recruitment and treatment practices for help-seeking "prodromal" patients. *Schizophr Bull*, 33:715–726.

413. Tenn, C.C., Fletcher, P.J., and Kapur, S. (2005). A putative animal model of the "prodromal" state of schizophrenia. *Biol Psychiatry*, 57(6):586–593.

414. Powell, S.B., Risbrough, V.B., and Geyer, M.A. (2003). Potential use of animal models to examine antipsychotic prophylaxis for schizophrenia. *Clin Neurosci Res*, 3:289–296.

415. Bakshi, V.P. and Geyer, M.A. (1999). Ontogeny of isolation rearing-induced deficits in sensorimotor gating in rats. *Physiol Behav*, 67:385–392.

416. Arranz, M.J. and de Leon, J. (2007). Pharmacogenetics and pharmacogenomics of schizophrenia: A review of last decade of research. *Mol Psychiatry*, 12(8):707–747.

417. Alenius, M., Wadelius, M., Dahl, M., Hartvig, P., Lindstrom, L., and Hammarlund-Udenaes, M. (2007). Gene polymorphism influencing treatment response in psychotic patients in a naturalistic setting, *J Psychiat Res*, doi: 10.1016/j.psychires.2007.10.07.

418. Boksa, P. (2004). Animal models of obstetric complications in relation to schizophrenia. *Brain Res Brain Res Rev*, 45(1):1–17.

419. Rowland, L., Bustillo, J.R., and Lauriello, J. (2001). Proton magnetic resonance spectroscopy (H-MRS) studies of schizophrenia. *Semin. Clin. Neuropsychiatry*, 6:121–130.

420. Mackeprang, T., Kristiansen, K.T. and Glenthoj, B.Y. (2002). Effects of antipsychotics on prepulse inhibition of the startle response in drug-naïve schizophrenic patients. *Biol Psych*, 52:863–873.

421. Maxwell, C.R., Liang, Y., Weightman, B.D., Kanes, S.J., Abel, T., Gur, R.E., Turetsky, B.I., Bilker, W.B., Lenox, R.H., and Siegel, S.J. (2004). Effects of chronic olanzapine and haloperidol differ on the mouse N1 auditory evoked potential. *Neuropsychopharm*, 29:739–746.

422. Harich, S., Gross, G., and Bespalov, A. (2007). Stimulation of the metabotropic glutamate 2/3 receptor attenuates social novelty discrimination deficits induced by neonatal phencyclidine treatment. *Psychopharmacology*, 192(4):511–519.

423. Meyer, U., Yee, B.K., and Feldon, J. (2007). The neurodevelopmental impact of prenatal infections at different times of pregnancy: the earlier the worse? *Neuroscientist*, 13:241–256.

424. McGrath, J.J., Pemberton, M.R., Welham, J.L., and Murray, R.M. (1994). Schizophrenia and the influenza epidemics of 1954, 1957 and 1959: a southern hemisphere study. *Schizophr. Res*, 14:1–8.

425. Rogers, D.C., Fisher, E.M., Brown, S.D., Peters, J., Hunter, A.J., and Martin, J.E. (1997). Behavioral and functional analysis of mouse phenotype: SHIRPA, a proposed protocol for comprehensive phenotype assessment. *Mammalian Genome*, 8(10):711–713.

426. Mello, C.C. and Conte, D., Jr. (2004). Revealing the world of RNA interference. *Nature*, 431:338–342.

427. Jentsch, J.D., Taylor, J.R., and Roth, R.H. (1998). Subchronic phencyclidine administration increases mesolimbic dopaminergic system responsivity and augments stress- and psychostimulant-induced hyperlocomotion. *Neuropsychopharmacology*, 19(2):105–113.

428. Minassian, A., Granholm, E., Verney, S., and Perry, W. (2005). Visual scanning deficits in schizophrenia and their relationship to executive functioning impairment. *Schizophr Res*, 74:69–79.

Developing Therapeutics for Bipolar Disorder (BPD): From Animal Models to the Clinic

Charles H. Large[1], Haim Einat[2] and Atul R. Mahableshwarkar[3,4,5]

[1]Department of Neuropharmacology, Psychiatry CEDD, GlaxoSmithKline SpA, Via A Fleming 4, 37135, Verona, Italy
[2]College of Pharmacy, University of Minnesota, 123 Life Science, 1110 Kirby Drive, Duluth, MN 55812, USA
[3]Neurosciences Medical Development Center, GlaxoSmithKline Research and Development, Five Moore Drive, MAI-C2421, Research Triangle Park, NC 27709, USA
[4]Rosalind Franklin University of Health Sciences/The Chicago Medical School, 3333 Greenbay Road, North Chicago, IL 60064, USA
[5]Clinical Sciences, Takeda Global Research and Development, One Takeda Parkway, Deerfield, Illinois, 60015, USA

Animal and Translational Models for CNS Drug Discovery,
Vol. 1 of 3: Psychiatric Disorders
Robert McArthur and Franco Borsini (eds), Academic Press, 2008

INTRODUCTION

The Clinical Diagnosis and Management of Bipolar Disorder

Mania and depression, or melancholia, have been recognized and their clinical presentations described since the time of Hippocrates dating back to 400 BC. The Greek, Galen (ca. AD 130–201) was one of the earliest to suggest that symptoms of depression or mania might have a psychogenic origin. Around the same time, Aretaeus of Cappadocia in Turkey recognized symptoms of mania and depression occurring in the same individuals, and suggested that they might be linked. Much later in 1854, the French physician, Jules Falret introduced the term *folie circulaire*, again proposing a link between depression and mania. He identified in his patients distinct episodes of depression and euphoric mood and recognized that this illness was different from simple depression. This led, in 1875 to the classification of Manic-Depressive Psychosis to describe what Falret more loosely termed bipolar disorder. During the same period, Francois Baillarger, described bipolar disorder, which he called *folie à double forme*. His particular contribution was to distinguish bipolar disorder from schizophrenia, allowing bipolar disorder to receive a classification separate from other mental disorders. The distinction was reinforced early in the 20th century by Emil Kraeplin, who proposed that manic-depressive insanity and dementia praecox (now schizophrenia) were indeed two distinct diseases with differing signs, symptoms, and outcomes.[1] As early as 1952, the possibility that bipolar disorder was an inherited illness was proposed,[2] strengthening the case that it was a discreet disorder.

Despite a backlash against all medical diagnoses of psychiatric illness in the 1960s and early 1970s, the concept of bipolar disorder as a unique illness was widely accepted amongst psychiatrists, although a separation in diagnosis and treatment between Europe and the United States was evident, with a narrower definition of bipolar disorder and a much broader definition of schizophrenia in the United States compared to Europe.[3] However, following the publication of the *Diagnostic and Statistical Manual of Mental Disorders, Third Edition* (DSM-III) in 1980 and, more recently, DSM-IV Text Revision (DSM-IV-TR)[4] the EU–US diagnostic difference has been largely eliminated. The aim of DSM was to provide criteria for the diagnosis of psychiatric disorders that were empirical and evidence based. An alternative, although similar system endorsed by the World Health Organization is the International Classification of Diseases[5] currently in its 10th version (ICD-10). The success of these systems of diagnosis is not in question, but in the context of the present review, it is important to understand that both DSM and ICD are intended for practicing physicians whose primary goal is the reliable pairing of diagnosis with treatment in a manner that is recognized by government or insurance reimbursement agencies. DSM and ICD were not explicitly intended as the basis from which to conduct research.

In the next paragraph, we provide an overview of the DSM-IV-TR diagnostic criteria for bipolar disorder (BPD) and later in this chapter, we consider those elements that can or should be used as the basis for animal models.

DSM-IV-TR proposes three criteria that should be considered to provide a diagnosis of BPD. The primary diagnostic criterion (Criterion A) specifies symptoms and signs that must be present to attract the diagnosis of a major depressive or manic episode, and in addition stipulates that the symptoms must have been present for a minimum duration (1 week for mania, 2 weeks for depression). An episode of major depression requires the presence of sad mood or loss of interest or pleasure, and in addition, four other core symptoms, which could include somatic symptoms (e.g., weight change, loss of energy, reduced activity level, and altered sleep patterns) or psychic symptoms (e.g., reduced ability to concentrate, feelings of worthlessness or guilt, recurrent thoughts of death, and suicidal ideation). An episode of mania requires the presence of euphoric or irritable mood, and in addition, three or four core symptoms, which may be somatic (e.g., increased energy, decreased need for sleep or excessive involvement in high-risk activities), or psychic symptoms (e.g., inflated self-esteem or grandiosity, or a subjective experience of racing thoughts). An objective indication of mania that may also be evaluated by the physician is that the patient is more talkative than usual and is difficult, if not impossible to interrupt. Indeed, interviews with relatives or caregivers can be extremely valuable in identifying mania, since often the patients themselves will not recognize their symptoms of mania as abnormal. Criterion A establishes the presence of a mood episode; however, the patient will attract a diagnosis of BPD only if that episode is an episode of mania, or if a manic episode has been diagnosed in the past.

Criterion B states simply that mixed episodes of BPD (episodes in which criteria for both mania and depression are met) are not classified as episodes of depression and mania separately. Criterion C considers social and/or occupational dysfunction associated with the illness, providing an index of severity of impairment. Finally, additional criteria are provided to exclude a diagnosis of BPD if the symptoms can be accounted for by exogenous influences; for example, substance abuse, a general medical condition, or a life event such as bereavement.

It should be noted that BPD with psychotic features is explicitly distinguished from schizophrenia in DSM-IV-TR, since the presence of mood symptoms excludes a diagnosis of schizophrenia. However, the arguments here could be construed as circular, and leave a significant gray area in which schizoaffective disorder or BPD with psychotic symptoms seem to indicate a continuum rather than the existence of sharply defined illnesses. In a similar manner, episodes of elevated mood may occur that are not sufficiently severe to cause significant social or occupational dysfunction and do not meet the duration criteria for mania. These are classified as hypomanic episodes. Patients having hypomanic episodes together with episodes of major depression are classified as Bipolar II, to differentiate them from patients with full manic and depressive episodes, identified as Bipolar I. Importantly, these bipolar II patients may not recognize their periods of hypomania as episodes of illness, instead considering them periods of "normal" or even elevated functioning.

In the case that episodes of hypomania are interspersed with periods of depressive symptoms that, over the course of at least 2 years do not meet the criteria for major depression, the DSM-IV-TR diagnosis given is "cyclothymia." A curiosity of DSM-IV-TR is that if an episode of full mania occurs in a patient with an existing diagnosis of cyclothymia then he/she could attract the diagnosis of bipolar I disorder in addition to the diagnosis of "cyclothymia." Finally, patients whose symptoms do not meet the full criteria for a mood episode, and which do not fall into any of the classifications described above may attract a catch-all diagnosis of "Bipolar Disorder Not Otherwise Specified." Thus DSM-IV-TR intentionally provides a diagnosis for any eventuality in order to allow for reimbursable prescription of medications where needed. However, the wide range of diagnoses from bipolar I through cyclothymia to BPD Not Otherwise Specified belie the difficulty in providing a clear-cut classification of illness in the case of real patients. This is illustrated further by the brief description of real patient symptoms that follow. An alternative personal account of BPD by the researcher, Kay Redfield Jamison[6] provides an illuminating description of the disorder and its impact on a person's life.

Mood during a manic episode often appears to be cheerful, euphoric, unusually happy, and may have an infectious quality,[7-9] although these moods may be noticeably intense and may change rapidly to irritability and anger. Elevated mood is typically accompanied by inflated self-esteem, which with increasing severity of the episode can reach delusional proportions. An increase in energy is another hallmark of a manic episode that is manifested by increased involvement in a multitude of activities and decreased need for sleep. Cognitive and/or speech disturbances are also common in mania and may consist of rapid, pressured speech, the flight of ideas,[10] and loosening of associations. Associated with inflated self-esteem and increased energy, the patient may engage in high-risk activities, such as gambling, spending sprees, or liberal sexual relationships. These often lead to negative and potentially life-changing consequences, such as loss of employment, breakdown of a marriage, or criminal charges. When the symptoms of mania are severe, the patient typically requires hospitalization for their own protection and sometimes the protection of others.

Conversely, the mood during an episode of major depression is evidently depressed with a significant loss of interest or pleasure in activities that were previously interesting or pleasurable.[9,11] Patients describe the mood as sad or blue, or of feeling "down in the dumps." Activities that were previously fun and enjoyable no longer elicit any joy or interest. There is a marked decrease in energy levels and complaints of fatigue are often accompanied by decreased or interrupted sleep, and sleep that is not restful. Patients may complain of physical aches and pains, altered appetite, which may be accompanied by weight loss or gain. Speech may be decreased in output and volume,[12] and may be accompanied by poor memory and difficulties at work. There may be excessive self-blame or guilt, which could be delusional and psychotic.[9] Thoughts of death and dying are common and suicidal ideation or attempted suicide may follow. Many of these symptoms, and in particular suicidal ideation, often require hospitalization of the patient.

A further complexity may be the occurrence of mixed states, defined as episodes meeting the criteria for both major depression and mania. Reported rates of mixed states vary from a low of 13%[13] to a high of 65%[14] of the bipolar population. These patients are often difficult to treat and receive multiple medications. However, for the researcher, the existence of mixed states highlights a perspective on BPD as a disorder of mood instability that the distinct diagnoses of manic or depressive episodes in DSM-IV-TR tend to mask. This perspective is strengthened by considering the longitudinal course of BPD in which patients swing between the two symptomatic poles of mania and depression, enjoying symptom-free periods of normal social and occupational function at intervals in between. Thus another polarity emerges separated not by symptoms and signs, but by level of functioning, and characterized by discrete episodes of poor functioning and episodes which are symptom-free and associated with normal functioning. Kraeplin originally conceptualized manic-depressive illness as having a course of episodes of mania or depression with good interepisodic functioning and contrasted this with dementia praecox (schizophrenia), whose progressive deteriorating course ended in a cognitively dysfunctional state. However, this distinction was perhaps not emphasized and the longitudinal course of BPD not fully described. Indeed, Kraeplin's observations were limited, since in 45% of his bipolar cases he followed the patient through only one episode, and more than three episodes in only 28% of his patients. Modern review, however, reveals a somewhat different picture. Percentages of patients experiencing relapse range from 18% per year over a 4-year period reported by Tohen *et al.*,[15] a cumulative 73% over 5 years according to Gitlin *et al.*,[16] or ranging from 81 to 91% according to the National Institute of Mental Health's Collaborative Studies Program on the Psychobiology of Depression-Clinical Studies.[17] Systematic prospective evaluation of the presence of symptoms, with follow-up ranging from 1 year to 12.8 years, reveals the presence of symptoms at any given time in 44–47% of patients.[18,19] Suicide and other causes of mortality in bipolar patients is 2.3 times greater when compared to the expected rate in the general population, and ranks high among causes of morbidity measured by Disability Adjusted Life Years.[9] Unfortunately, significant side effects of current medications for BPD, leading to noncompliance, do little to reduce rates of relapse.[20] Overall, the picture is of a chronic and highly morbid disorder, characterized by tantalizing periods of normal functioning and periods of significant illness that are not well controlled by current medications. With this in mind and for the purposes of this chapter, we may consider that animal models should be less focused on reproducing symptoms of mania or depression and more focused on the underlying mood instability inherent in BPD.

Currently Indicated Medications for Bipolar Disorder

US Food and Drug Administration (FDA)-indicated medications for BPD are listed in Table 9.1 below and are representative of treatments used in Europe and other countries. Most of the drugs were originally used to treat other psychiatric conditions and were subsequently found to have utility in the management of BPD. Five of the ten are atypical antipsychotics, used primarily to treat schizophrenia; three are anticonvulsants. Only lithium, discovered serendipitously by Cade in 1949[21] was used for the treatment of BPD from the outset. Very few of the available treatments adequately address symptoms of bipolar depression, with antidepressant drugs, such as the selective serotonin reuptake inhibitors still widely used, despite concerns that they may switch patients into mania. Current treatment guidelines in Europe, the United Kingdom, and the United States emphasize the need to combine antidepressant treatment with drugs that may stabilize mood, such as lithium, lamotrigine (Lamictal®), or sodium valproate (Depakote®).[22,23]

In addition to pharmaceutical intervention, guidelines emphasize the need for psychosocial treatment to provide a complete package of care for sufferers of BPD.[22,23] In particular, there is a need to educate patients, relatives, and caregivers about the triggers for new mood episodes, such as stressful life events, drug or alcohol abuse, or disruption of normal daily routines. Furthermore, patients should be informed about

Table 9.1 List of FDA approved medications for bipolar disorder

Medication	Depression	Mania and mixed	Maintenance (mood stabilization)
Abilify® (aripiprazole)[a]	No	Yes	Yes
Equetro® (carbamazepine)[b]	No	Yes	No
Depakote® (valproate)[b]	No	Yes	No (but widely used)
Lamictal® (lamotrigine)[b]	No	No	Yes
Eskalith® (lithium)	No	Yes	Yes
Zyprexa® (olanzapine)[a,c]	No	Yes	Yes
Symbyax® (olanzapine-fluoxetine combination)	Yes	No	No
Risperdal® (risperidone)[a,c]	No	Yes	No
Seroquel® (quetiapine)[a,c]	Yes	Yes	Yes
Geodon® (ziprasidone)[a]	No	Yes	No

[a]Antipsychotic.
[b]Anticonvulsant.
[c]These are also indicated for the treatment of manic and mixed states in combination with lithium and Depakote.

the risks associated with not taking mood-stabilizing drugs, even during periods when symptoms are absent.

Unmet Needs in Bipolar Disorder

Bipolar disorder imposes a significant burden on patients, their families who suffer along with them, and society as a whole. The burden ranges from suffering and disability due to the disease, increased use of medical services, inability of patients to reach their full potential and consequent loss of earnings, and adverse impact on family members.[24] Bipolar illness generates a substantial economic burden, with reports of the direct and indirect costs totaling $28 to 45 billion in the United States.[25,26] In direct measures, such as private insurance costs are almost four-times greater for patients with BPD when compared to those with other disorders.[27] Potentially there are many unmet needs in BPD against which improved medications could be targeted:

1. Episode relapse
2. Interepisodic symptoms
3. Incomplete resolution of episodes
4. Medication side effects

5. Disability
6. Suicide
7. Excessive mortality
8. Comorbid disorders, in particular substance abuse

In addition, a significant unmet need is the early diagnosis of BPD and early intervention with appropriate treatments.[22,28] Given the often delayed emergence of manic symptoms, patients are often misdiagnosed with unipolar depression and receive treatment with classical antidepressant drugs for up to 10 years before a correct diagnosis of BPD is obtained and a mood-stabilizing drug is introduced.[29]

Approaches to Drug Discovery for the Treatment of Bipolar Disorder

It is reasonable to assume, given the heritability of BPD[30-32] that the illness has a neurobiological origin that might be ameliorated by the modification of brain function using drugs or other medical procedures; for example, transcranial magnetic stimulation. However, in the absence of knowledge regarding the neurobiological origin, our choice of means to modulate brain function is determined by other factors; in particular, what has worked in the past and what is safe. There have been significant advances in our understanding of the etiology of BPD at a holistic level: epidemiological and genetic studies confirm the heritability of the disorder,[30-32] as well as the influence of environment and lifestyle.[33,34] However, they also suggest that multiple etiologies can give rise to similar symptoms; emphasizing the *caveat* that one pill may not fit all. This is supported by clinical experience showing that response rates for an "effective" treatment such as lithium can be as low as 40–50%.[35,36] The many "flavors" of BPD identified in DMS-IV-TR provide further evidence of the heterogeneity across patients.

Conceptually, there are two approaches to the discovery of novel pharmacological treatments for BPD. The classical top down or "syndromal" approach seeks to identify drugs that modify behaviors in animals or in humans that might predict efficacy versus specific clinical symptoms of BPD. The alternative is a bottom up approach that seeks to identify and exploit genes that predispose to BPD. Drug development pipelines tend to be dominated by the fruits of the former approach, since in practice it is difficult to determine what intervention might lead to a beneficial effect for the patient when starting from a gene. For example, Alzheimer's disease is a disorder with a well-established genetic component; however, despite a significant and reproducible association between the apolipoprotein E4 allele and age of onset of the disease it has taken 15 years for related drugs to reach clinical trials.[37]

Recently, there has been increasing interest in a third approach that aims to develop drugs that can manipulate endophenotypes associated with BPD.[38-40] [i] This approach

---

[i] For further discussion of endophenotypes, please see Tannock *et al.*, towards a biological understanding of ADHD and the discovery of novel therapeutic approaches, Bartz *et al.*, Preclinical animal models of autistic spectrum disorders (ASD), Cryan *et al.*, Developing more efficacious antidepressant medications: improving and aligning preclinical detection and clinical assessment tools, or Joel *et al.*, Animal models of obsessive–compulsive disorder: from bench to bedside via endophenotypes and biomarkers in this volume.

allows a fresh look at the disorder unconstrained by the diagnostic criteria laid down in DSM-IV-TR or ICD-10, permitting researchers to escape the blunt nosology of clinical symptomatology and take advantage of advances in human biometric technologies, such as neuroimaging and proteomics. The importance of this approach will become particularly evident once a drug reaches clinical trial, since efficacy of the drug in humans should be readily measurable using the same endophenotype against which it was developed in the first place. This advantage should not be underestimated in the case of BPD, where there are significant hurdles to demonstrating efficacy, particularly versus depressive symptoms or in the case of mood prophylaxis.[41] However, despite providing more objective clinical endpoints, it may be some time before endophenotypes will be considered acceptable in pivotal trials of drug efficacy. Consequently, the use of endophenotypes in the development of novel treatments for BPD is likely to remain an area for exploratory medicine for the foreseeable future. Nevertheless, the pharmaceutical industry will be motivated to use endophenotypes as additional endpoints in clinical studies. In the event that the test drug does not show efficacy on primary endpoints of the disorder such as reduction in depressive or manic symptoms, efficacy in modifying the endophenotype would demonstrate the drug's ability to modify CNS function in measurable ways that might predict efficacy in other psychiatric or neurological disorders.

As with all other psychiatric disorders that rely on DSM-IV-TR or ICD-10, a psychological, in addition to a biological cause of BPD cannot be ruled out. In practice, the two may be difficult or even impossible to separate, and the division reflects our inability to superimpose subjective psychiatric symptoms onto a biological substrate. However, as argued by Hayes and Delgado,[42] failure to differentiate the symptoms of BPD in this way could undermine our ability to develop successful animal models, since some symptoms might arise through a dysfunction that occurs at a level of complexity that is present only in humans. For example, if BPD were a disorder or speech, would it be reasonable to try to model the dysfunction in non-humans? It is no surprise that most researchers steer away from the "higher" symptoms of BPD, preferring instead to focus on those that can be most easily recognized in other species, such as hyperactivity, inactivity, or sleep disturbance. In a later section of this chapter, the distinction between human symptoms that can be translated downwards and those that cannot will be discussed further.

In conclusion, regardless of the approach taken for the discovery of novel medicines for BPD, there is no doubt that there is a huge unmet need for better treatments. The pragmatic approach is to develop drugs that in some way modify CNS function and then determine whether they benefit patients with BPD. Alternatively, examination of the genes associated with BPD may help identify treatments that may help at least a subset of patients. Whichever approach is taken, animal models can help us to understand how novel treatments affect CNS function, which in turn should help to identify translational measures that can aid dose-selection in clinical trials, and provide the basis for objective clinical endpoints to complement psychiatric rating scales. More than that may be too much to ask until we have a clearer idea of the etiology of the disorder.

CURRENT ANIMAL MODELS

The development of animal models of BPD should start from the essential diagnostic features of the illness: recurrent episodes of depression and mania. However, animal models of BPD have tended to focus on the most superficial features of mania and depression: hyperactivity and immobility, respectively. Perhaps less attention has been placed on modeling the "recurrence" of episodes. Animal models will necessarily reflect better those components of the human disorder that can be reliably translated downwards. More complex or subjective features of BPDs, such as grandiosity, flight of ideas, or feelings of worthlessness are likely to remain beyond the reach of non-human models. Having said that, hopelessness, that might be considered a highly subjective human symptom, is commonly attributed to animals in models of depression such as the forced swim test, which evoke "learned helplessness," and which are backed up by a long history of research originating from studies of the effects of inescapable shock on dogs.[43,44] Thus, it may be premature to rule out future models that claim grandiosity, for example, in the behavior of rats or other animals.

The cornerstones of a model are face, construct, and predictive validity. Models with face validity for symptoms of BPD have been established, although in many cases they may not be specific to BPD.[ii] For example, hyperactivity does not appear only in manic patients but is common in individuals afflicted with attention deficit hyperactivity disorder (ADHD) and can be a normal personality trait in some individuals.[iii] Construct validity requires knowledge of the etiology and pathophysiology of the disorder being modeled; our understanding of the etiology of BPD is still in its infancy. The predictive validity of models of BPD necessarily relies upon the efficacy in the models of clinically active drugs (pharmacological isomorphism); in addition, the model should be insensitive to drugs proven to be ineffective in the treatment of BPD. A limitation is that the models may be valid only for novel drugs with a mechanism of action similar to the clinically active drug. Lithium is the standard most commonly used to provide validation for new animal models of BPD. This is a reasonable choice, since, unlike most other drugs used in the treatment of BPD, lithium is relatively specific in its efficacy (e.g., it is apparently neither anticonvulsant nor antipsychotic[45]). Most drugs used in the treatment of BPD were used primarily in the treatment of psychiatric disorders such as schizophrenia and unipolar depression, or a neurological disorder such as epilepsy. Ideally, a well-validated model would be sensitive to each of the different agents that are also effective at treating the symptom of BPD being modeled. For example, a model of mania should be responsive to lithium, atypical antipsychotic drugs, and sodium valproate, but not antidepressant drugs; a model of bipolar depression might respond to lamotrigine, quetiapine, and perhaps lithium, but less or not at all to valproate. Although this method of validation is considered crucial, reliance on pharmacological isomorphism has been criticized, as it is more likely to lead to the development and use of animal models sensitive to detecting drugs with a similar mechanism of

---

[ii] For further and detailed discussions regarding criteria of validity, the reader is invited to refer to discussions by Steckler *et al.*, Developing novel anxiolytics: improving preclinical detection and clinical assessment; Joel *et al.*, Animal models of obsessive–compulsive disorder: from bench to bedside via endophenotypes and biomarkers, in this volume; Lindner *et al.*, Development, optimization and use of preclinical behavioral models to maximize the productivity of drug discovery for Alzheimer's Disease in Volume 2, *Neurologic Disorders*; Koob, The role of animal models in reward deficit disorders: views from academia, Markou *et al.*, Contribution of animal models and preclinical human studies to medication development for nicotine dependence, in Volume 3, *Reward Deficits Disorders*.

[iii] For further discussion of ADHD, please see Tannock *et al.*, towards a biological understanding of ADHD and the discovery of novel therapeutic approaches, in this volume.

action to existing treatments. Considering the limited efficacy of existing pharmacological treatments for BPD,[36] models validated with known clinical standards can perhaps fail to detect potentially more efficacious drugs that are developed with very different mechanisms of action.[iv] To guard against this bias, it is important to keep in mind that there is no one current model that is accepted to represent the entire disorder and standard practice should be to use a number of different models for depression and mania in the evaluation of novel drugs.[46]

Mania

Hyperactivity is considered the simplest feature of mania that can be readily modeled in animals. However, a potential problem with the interpretation of studies using hyperactivity as the dependent measure is that the behavior of laboratory animals can be readily regulated by a plethora of environmental or pharmacological stimuli that may or may not be considered pathological. For example, the transfer of a rat from its home cage to an apparently similar, but novel cage will produce a brief surge in exploratory activity. Similarly, transfer to a cage that contains a variety of novel objects or compartments will also lead to an increase in activity. It is perhaps debatable whether a treatment for mania should or should not affect these increases, but fortunately, there have been attempts to explore the underlying dimensions of hyperactivity and identify those that relate most closely to symptoms of mania. For example, genetically modified mice that lack the dopamine transporter show characteristic repetitive movement near the perimeter of a novel environment that can be compared to the behavior of human patients with mania using a human "Behavioral Pattern Monitor."[47] This approach will be invaluable for homing in on models in rodents that most closely resemble the human disorder.

Psychostimulant Challenge

Amphetamine has been the most frequently used agent for pharmacological induction of mania.[48-54] The history and rationale of amphetamine-induced behavior as a model of mania has been recently reviewed.[50] Briefly, low doses of amphetamine have effects primarily on open field activity, whereas higher doses cause stereotypy.[55,56] Psychostimulants are known to induce mania in susceptible individuals,[57] and lithium has been reported to prevent the effects of psychostimulants in humans.[58] However, there is a long history of contradictory results in this field. Several studies in rats and mice have reported prevention of amphetamine-induced hyperactivity by acute and chronic lithium.[56,59,60] Whereas other publications report an absence of effect of lithium in the model.[61,62] New data indicate that lithium's effects on amphetamine hyperactivity may be related to genetic background, with

---

[iv] Please refer to Steckler *et al.*, Developing novel anxiolytics: improving preclinical detection and clinical assessment in this volume, or to Lindner *et al.*, Development, optimization and use of preclinical behavioral models to maximize the productivity of drug discovery for Alzheimer's Disease, in Volume 2, *Neurological Disorders* for further discussion of the strengths and limitations of pharmacological isomorphism in establishing model validity.

different susceptibility observed in different strains of mice[52,63,64,65] or in mice which have been genetically manipulated.[66-68]

A related pharmacological model combines administration to rodents of d-amphetamine with an anxiolytic dose of the benzodiazepine, chlordiazepoxide (Librium®).[70-77] The resulting hyperactivity can be measured as the total distance traveled in an open field, or from more complex measures, such as the exploration of holes in the floor of the arena,[75] or entry into arms of a Y-maze.[76,77] The mixture of d-amphetamine with chlordiazepoxide is suggested to evoke a qualitatively different "compulsive" hyperactivity compared to the hyperactivity induced by d-amphetamine alone.[72] The authors speculated that low doses of chlordiazepoxide reduce the anxiety associated with a novel environment and thus facilitate exploratory behavior, while d-amphetamine simply drives undirected locomotion through disinhibition of the basal ganglia. However, the behavioral effects of the combination of d-amphetamine and chlordiazepoxide in the human volunteers have not been described, although the two drugs have been administered to healthy human volunteers to investigate their combined effects on cortisol levels.[78,79]

The sensitivity of the hyperactivity induced by the mixture of d-amphetamine and chlordiazepoxide to drug treatment has been examined, and could be prevented by prior administration of lithium,[72,76] magnesium valproate,[75] carbamazepine,[70,77] levetiracetam (Keppra®)[77] and lamotrigine.[70] In several of these studies the ability of the drugs to prevent hyperactivity induced by amphetamine alone was investigated in parallel. Lithium, valproate, lamotrigine, carbamazepine, and levetiracetam were distinguished by their efficacy against hyperactivity induced by the mixture and their lack of efficacy against hyperactivity induced by d-amphetamine alone. In contrast haloperidol (Haldol®) was able to prevent hyperactivity in both cases. However, as discussed earlier, there have been mixed reports of the ability of lithium to prevent amphetamine-induced hyperactivity. Studies of this type provide useful information regarding spectrum of efficacy and conform to the recommendation to use multiple models in the evaluation of novel drugs.[46]

A concern with psychostimulant models and the d-amphetamine/chlordiazepoxide model in particular is the risk for drug-drug interactions that might confound interpretation. For example, careful choice of the dose of chlordiazepoxide was required to avoid inducing sedation rather than hyperactivity when combining with d-amphetamine: Arban *et al.*[70] found that an intraperitoneal (ip) dose of chlordiazepoxide of 6.25 mg/kg consistently increased the hyperactivity induced by 1.25 mg/kg ip of d-amphetamine to male CD1 mice, whereas a higher dose of 12.5 mg/kg did not. This suggests a bell-shaped dose-response curve for chlordiazepoxide in which any shift in the curve following addition of the test drug might lead to an apparent reduction in hyperactivity. Indeed, valproate and carbamazepine, but not lamotrigine, significantly reduced basal locomotor activity when in combination with a 6.25 mg/kg dose of chlordiazepoxide, suggesting that the apparent efficacy of the two drugs versus hyperactivity induced by d-amphetamine/chlordiazepoxide might be due to the potentiation of the sedative effects of chlordiazepoxide. Given that benzodiazepines have limited clinical value as primary treatments for bipolar mania,[80,81] this is a serious potential confound for the d-amphetamine/chlordiazepoxide model and highlights a danger of using pharmacological challenge models in isolation.

Repeated Challenge with Psychostimulants: Sensitization

Repeated administration of some psychostimulants, such as cocaine or amphetamine leads to a sensitization to the drug's effects.[82-84] Animals show an increasing response to the drug after multiple treatments compared to the first treatment. Beyond the similarities between the acute effects of psychostimulants and mania, it has been suggested that sensitized behavior has additional validity as a model for BPD, since it requires some chronic adaptation of the nervous system that could resemble pathological changes underlying the human disease.[84] The sensitization model also acquires greater face validity, since the sensitized behavior can represent the increasing intensity of mood episodes across the life span of untreated patients and the increased susceptibility to a variety of environmental stressors that can trigger an episode.[1] Moreover, some researchers suggest that specific oscillatory responses that appear across the process of sensitization may represent the cyclic nature of BPD.[16] Psychostimulant-induced sensitized behavior is now frequently explored in the context bipolar research,[17-19] although it is not clear whether for practical goals of identifying neuroactive drugs this model has any clear advantages compared with acute psychostimulant administration models.

Ouabain Challenge

An additional pharmacological method that has been suggested to model BPD is the inhibition of Na-K-ATPase ion pump using ouabain (for a recent review see[85]). The rationale for this model is that the neurochemical effects of ouabain may be similar to a decreased Na-K-ATPase activity and associated imbalance in electrolyte levels reported in some patients with BPD.[86] Additionally, in animals, the administration of subconvulsive doses of ouabain results in mania-like hyperactivity that is preventable with chronic lithium pretreatment.[85] As a result, this model appears to have face, predictive, and construct validity for mania. Yet, as all other models, the ouabain model also has limitations. The reported change in electrolytes in human is not strongly supported as part of the basic pathology of BPD, and furthermore, the effects of lithium to reduce ouabain-induced hyperactivity may be the result of a mechanism that is unrelated to the drug's effects in patients with BPD. It will be important to examine the effects of other drugs used in the treatment of BPD in the model. In the meantime, the ouabain model could be considered as part of a battery of tests to examine the mood-stabilizing activity of novel drugs.[85]

Sleep Deprivation and Manipulation of the Circadian Rhythm

Altered sleep patterns and loss of sleep is a common and possibly fundamental symptom of BPD.[87] In addition, sleep disturbance can induce mania in susceptible patients with BPD.[88,89] A possible explanation for both of these observations is that there is an underlying disruption of circadian mechanisms in BPD that predisposes to disrupted sleep patterns[90] and reciprocal sensitivity to imposed sleep disturbance.[91-93] As a result, elements of the circadian machinery, such as proteins involved in setting daily rhythms, have been proposed as targets for novel drugs to treat BPD.[94] Furthermore, sleep deprivation and manipulation of the sleep-wake cycle has been evaluated as a possible treatment for patients with BPD.[95-97] Mechanisms underlying circadian rhythm and the sleep-wake cycle are likely to be conserved between humans and non-human species, increasing the probability that models based on these measures will have reasonable predictive and perhaps even construct validity. Both sleep disturbance[98] and manipulation of the circadian machinery[99,100] have been shown to produce behavioral hyperactivity in rodents. Chronic dietary lithium has been shown to reduce hyperactivity associated with sleep deprivation in rats[98] and mutation of the *clock* gene in mice,[100] although there have been few studies confirming these findings. These initial studies targeting the sleep-wake cycle show promise for developing models that will allow researchers to explore the link with BPD and perhaps develop drugs specifically to treat this aspect of the disorder.[v]

Depression

Whereas psychostimulants provide the basis for many of the current models of mania, agents that depress the nervous system to produce hypoactivity have not been developed to provide models of depression. However, some form of hypoactivity is a feature in many of the existing animal models of depression,[39] although in each case the challenge is either environmental or surgical, rather than pharmacological. This relative sophistication in the modeling of depression may be due to the greater attention paid to psychological aspects of unipolar depression[101] compared to BPD.[102,103] [vi] Researchers evaluating novel treatments for bipolar depression have tended to adopt methods used to model unipolar depression. However, bipolar depression should not be considered equivalent to unipolar depression. Drugs used to treat unipolar depression are still heavily used in the treatment of bipolar depression, but clinicians are warned not to use them in the absence of a mood stabilizer, such as lithium, lamotrigine, or valproate, due to the risk of switching patients into mania.[23] In comparison to patients diagnosed with unipolar depression, patients with bipolar depression tend to show greater motor retardation, a higher rate of psychotic features, more frequent episodes, earlier age of onset, and are more likely to have a family history of psychiatric illness.[104] The strong heritability of BPD also sets it apart from unipolar depression and hints at a different biological cause. With this in mind, it seems clear that animal models of bipolar depression should be different to animal models of unipolar depression.[105] Models such as the forced swim test or other similar models based on theories of learned helplessness may be least appropriate if bipolar depression is the result of endogenous rather than environmental factors. It is notable that lamotrigine, one of the few drugs thought to be useful in the treatment of bipolar depression[106] was ineffective in the forced swim test (R. Arban, personal communication), although other groups have reported that it can be effective.[107] The development of drugs for the treatment of bipolar depression will rely on developing specific animal models of this facet of BPD.

---

[v] For further discussion regarding behavioral effects of sleep deprivation, please refer to Doran, Translational models of sleep and sleep disorders, in this volume.

[vi] Please refer to Cryan *et al.*, Developing more efficacious antidepressant medications: improving and aligning preclinical detection and clinical assessment tools, in this volume for further discussion of models of depressed-like behaviors.

Olfactory Bulbectomy

Bilateral destruction of the olfactory bulb in rats is considered a validated model of major depression.[108] The surgical procedure leads to a wide variety of behavioral, neuroanatomical, and neurochemical changes. At a behavioral level, olfactory bulbectomy appears to produce symptoms with face validity for mania, such as hyperactivity and increased exploration. However, other changes are perhaps more akin to depressive symptoms; for example, reduced impulsivity when faced with a food choice, reduced sexual activity, increased sensitivity to environmental stress, and cognitive impairment.[108] Anhedonia, considered a central feature of major depression, does not appear to be a stable feature of bulbectomized rats, although there does appear to be a disruption of central reward mechanisms,[109] suggesting a possible relevance to comorbid substance abuse. Bulbectomized rats show reduced levels of noradrenaline and serotonin, and these neurochemical changes provide construct validity and particular support for classification of the procedure as a model of depression. Consistent with this, chronic, but not acute, treatment with a wide range of antidepressant drugs can reverse most aspects of the bulbectomy phenotype. Importantly, lithium has also been shown to ameliorate at least some of the biochemical effects of olfactory bulbectomy.[110] Methylphenidate, commonly used for the treatment of ADHD in children, has also been shown to be effective at reducing the hyperactivity of bulbectomized rats, suggesting possible relevance for impulse control disorders. Given the wide range of drugs that can influence the phenotype of bulbectomized rats, and given the profound neurochemical, neuroanatomical, and behavioral changes induced by the procedure, it is not clear how well the model might predict clinical efficacy. However, the model merits consideration given that the phenotype includes behaviors resembling both depressive and manic symptoms.

Stress Challenge

A strong genetic and biological contribution to the development of BPD is well accepted, but the role of environmental factors and in particular stressful life events in triggering mood episodes is also clear and remains an important consideration for those seeking to provide a complete package of care for patients with the disorder. Thus psychosocial intervention is widely considered an integral part of treatment.[22,23] Furthermore, clinical research continues to explore the link between stressful events and the onset and course of the illness.[111,112] Evidence suggests that stress early in life leads to an earlier onset of BPD, and subsequently a lower threshold for the induction of manic or depressive episodes by later adverse events.[111] Stress may therefore be an important challenge to employ in animal models of BPD, although most models involving stress have been developed with unipolar depression in mind. The most common approaches are to use either chronic mild stress (CMS), in which animals are subjected to repeated minor stressors over a period of time, typically at least three weeks,[113-115] vii or resident-intruder stress, in which

---

vii For a detailed description of the CMS procedure, please refer to Koob, The role of animal models in reward deficit disorders: views from academia, Markou *et al.*, Contribution of animal models and preclinical human studies to medication development for nicotine dependence, in Volume 3, *Reward Deficits Disorders*.

animals are introduced into the home cage of a dominant male and suffer so-called "social defeat."[116,117] In both models, modification of the behavior of the animals may include a greater sensitivity to subsequent stressors, disrupted sleep pattern, anhedonia, as measured by reduced interest in preferred foods, and reduced locomotor activity.[118] Marked activation of the hypothalamic-pituitary-adrenal axis (HPA) also occurs.[119,120] Antidepressant drugs have been shown to prevent some of the behavioral and neurochemical consequences of CMS (reviewed in[113]) and social defeat.[121-123] In some respects, these models of chronic stress resemble the models of sensitization to psychostimulant challenge described earlier. It could be valuable to explore the combination of chronic stress with administration of psychostimulants as an approach to providing an integrated model of bipolar depression and mania.[viii] The increased sensitivity of animals subjected to chronic stress or repeated psychostimulant administration could model the underlying sensitivity and instability characteristic of BPD.

Mood Instability

A defining feature of BPD is the recurrence of mood episodes over the lifetime of the patient, with more than 90% of patients having a first manic episode going on to have further episodes.[17,124] In addition, there is a tendency for the frequency and severity of episodes to increase over time, particularly in the absence of treatment, with many patients eventually reaching the criteria for rapid cycling BPD (more than four mood episodes within a year). The prevalence of rapid cycling in the bipolar patient population has been estimated at between 13% and 56%,[125] with a higher percentage of female patients meeting the criteria. The high proportion of patients that go on to experience rapid cycling may be taken as evidence that bipolar illness is a progressive disorder, although some patients may display patterns of rapid cycling from the onset of their illness, whereas others may experience a period of rapid cycling followed by a later reduction in episode frequency. Whatever the pattern of mood episodes of an individual patient with BPD, it is well accepted that early treatment with mood-stabilizing drugs, such as lithium, valproate, or lamotrigine, is associated with a better prognosis.[22] There is evidence that response to treatment may be influenced by the number of previous manic or depressive episodes, with lithium response in the treatment of mania decreasing as a function of the number of previous manic episodes and valproate efficacy increasing with the number of prior episodes.[126] The early diagnosis and appropriate treatment of BPD is considered a major unmet need.[28,29]

As discussed earlier in the context of models of bipolar depression, stress is considered an important trigger for new mood episodes, leading to a well-developed hypothesis of sensitization of the brains of patients with BPD that can account for cycle acceleration and increasing severity of symptoms.[34,127-129] Heuristic comparisons have been drawn with the course of seizure disorders, such as temporal lobe epilepsy, the development of tolerance to anticonvulsant drugs, and the development of

---

[viii] For further discussion of effects of stress and changes in the HPA in other behavioral disorders, please refer to Cryan et al., Developing more efficacious antidepressant medications: improving and aligning preclinical detection and clinical assessment tools, Steckler et al. Developing novel anxiolytics: improving preclinical detection and clinical assessment, Tannock et al., towards a biological understanding of ADHD and the discovery of novel therapeutic approaches; in this volume.

sensitization to drugs such as cocaine. It was originally suggested that these models might serve to investigate and predict the efficacy of novel mood-stabilizing drugs, many of which happen also to be anticonvulsant; however, these models are now seen as providing a means to conceptualize illness recurrence without necessarily having construct validity for BPD.[129] Thus, as already highlighted in the previous section, the combination of chronic stress with repeated administration of psychostimulant drugs could provide the basis for a model of mood instability that may have greater construct validity for BPD.

Evaluation of Dose–Response, Safety, and Tolerability

A frequent problem with animal models of psychiatric disorders, including BPD, is a poor correlation between doses and schedules of administration used for patients and those used in the models. Ideally, dosing in animals should achieve serum and brain concentrations that are likely to be achievable in humans such that effects seen preclinically can be correlated with effects seen in patients. This is relevant for both efficacy signals and side effects. However, there is a tendency for higher doses to be used in animal models, reaching higher plasma and brain concentrations than could safely be used in humans. These higher doses may be required to observe acute efficacy in the model of interest. For example, in some recent studies conducted with lamotrigine in an animal model of cognitive dysfunction associated with psychosis,[130] a range of doses of lamotrigine was explored; a significant block of the disruption caused by phencyclidine was observed 60 min after an intraperitoneal dose of at least 20 mg/kg of lamotrigine. This dose of lamotrigine is associated with a plasma concentration of approximately 10 μg/mL in rats. Concentrations in this range are achieved in the clinical use of lamotrigine,[131-133] at least in the treatment of epilepsy, but more typical concentrations for the treatment of BPD are in the range of 2–4 μg/mL. Assuming that there are no major differences in the brain penetration of lamotrigine between rat and human, the higher plasma concentration required for efficacy in the animal model compared to the human disorder might suggest that the former is not predictive of the latter. This type of analysis provides a means to go beyond the face validity of a given model and explore the practical utility of the model in predicting drug efficacy in humans.

This consideration leads to the following key question: is the comparison between efficacy in the animal model and efficacy in human clinical trials fair? In the case of the animal model mentioned above, a 50% reduction in the disruptive effect of phencyclidine could be achieved with the 20 mg/kg ip dose of lamotrigine;[130] subsequently it was found that a slightly higher dose of 25 mg/kg ip was sufficient to completely prevent the disruptive effect of phencyclidine (N. Idris, personal communication). The effect size in this model, achieved after just 60 min with a single dose of lamotrigine, is huge in comparison to the reduction in depressive symptoms that might be observed after 6–8 weeks in patients, and difficult to compare in the case of clinical studies where the endpoint is individual patient recovery,[134] or the emergence of new episodes of depression in mood-prophylaxis studies.[135] The point is that clinical trial design rarely resembles the design of the animal model, making extrapolation of concentration-dependent efficacy from one to the other very difficult. In cases where the clinical measure more closely resembles the animal model response, such as in temporal lobe epilepsy,[136] much better extrapolations have been possible.[ix] For example, it has been repeatedly shown that the lowest plasma concentration of lamotrigine or other anticonvulsant drugs achieving a statistically significant increase in seizure threshold in a rodent electroshock seizure model is similar to the plasma concentration required for clinical efficacy in patients with epilepsy.[137] As will be discussed later, attempts to design early phase clinical trials in line with animal models used in drug development will be an important step forward in drug discovery for psychiatric disorders. In the meantime, careful attention to the doses of novel drugs used in animal models, particularly in acute studies, will be important to avoid generating false-positive results that will not be reproduced in patients, in part due to the intervention of dose-limiting side effects.[x]

Safety and tolerability have a significant impact on the extrapolation of results from animals to humans. Very often humans are more sensitive to side effects, limiting the range of doses that can be explored to achieve efficacy. In the example given above, doses of lamotrigine associated with plasma concentrations of 10 μg/mL or above were required for full efficacy in the reversal-learning model.[130] No apparent adverse effects of these doses of lamotrigine were observed in the study. However, plasma concentrations of lamotrigine of 10 μg/mL can be associated with CNS side effects such as dizziness, headache, and ataxia,[131] which could be a limiting factor in patients with BPD, and perhaps more so than in patients with epilepsy. Careful assessment of side effect liability alongside studies of efficacy in animals is essential in order to establish a likely therapeutic window for the drug. Predictions of clinical efficacy based on doses that are also associated with side effects are likely to be over-optimistic.

Lithium is perhaps a special case, since its narrow therapeutic window is well recognized. It is poorly tolerated in all species and doses must be carefully adjusted to ensure that plasma levels remain with the recommended therapeutic range (typically 0.4–0.8 mmol/L).[138] Behavioral and toxicological effects of excessive doses of lithium can severely confound the interpretation of animal model data.[139] Similarly, there is a suggestion that effects of lithium should be considered relevant to clinical use only after chronic dosing in animal models (typically at least 3 days of treatment), although effects can be observed following acute doses and may be equally informative as long as plasma concentrations remain within the therapeutic range.[140]

In summary, the design and development of animal models of BPD requires that careful attention is also paid to the choice of dose and dosing schedule used to test known or novel drugs. Issues of pharmacokinetics, drug metabolism, penetration into the brain, and differences in receptor affinity across species should all be carefully considered in the design of the study and interpretation the results.[xi]

[ix] See also, Klitgaard *et al.*, Animal and translational models of the epilepsies, in Volume 2, *Neurologic Disorders*.

[x] Please refer to Markou *et al.*, Contribution of animal models and preclinical human studies to medication development for nicotine dependence, in Volume 3, *Reward Deficit Disorders*, for further discussion of false negative and false-positive results, and the consequences thereof on drug discovery.

[xi] Please refer to Markou *et al.*, Contribution of animal models and preclinical human studies to medication development for nicotine dependence, in Volume 3, *Reward Deficit Disorders*, for further discussion of species differences on absorption, distribution, metabolism, and excretion profiles of drugs.

PROSPECTS FOR NEW MODELS

Models based on diagnostic biological markers would be ideal, since they would, by definition allow a novel treatment to be tested against the same biological lesion that is present in the patient. However, to date there are no diagnostic markers for BPD, so models in this category remain hypothetical, although to some extent transgenic mice generated to reflect a genetic association with BPD may be reasonable examples. Endophenotypes offer a middle ground for animal models that may have some construct validity, but they would require the same iterative process of clinical validation as symptom-based models in order to achieve acceptance. As a result, the focus of attention for the development of new animal models remains on the clinical symptoms of patients with BPD as defined by DSM-IV-TR or ICD-10. Despite this apparent impasse, there are aspects of the clinical presentation of BPD, such as sleep disturbance, vulnerability to drugs of abuse, and metabolic abnormalities that may lie more proximal to the underlying disorder, and which may offer an easier starting point for the development of better animal models and better targets for novel drugs. Assessment of mood in non-human animals is fraught with difficulty, whereas physiological functions such as sleep, circadian rhythm, reward mechanisms, and metabolic control are more likely to be homologous between humans and non-human animals. Thus research focused on these functions may be easier to translate into the clinic. In this context, it is worth considering animal models of epilepsy. The fidelity of some of these models with respect to specific human epilepsies is exemplary, with the major concern being the choice of the most appropriate model for the type of human epilepsy under consideration.[141] Simple models such as the electroshock seizure model in rats are sufficiently well understood and well characterized with a wide range drugs with different mechanisms of anticonvulsant action, that they can be used not only to predict efficacy versus human generalized seizures, but also to predict the appropriate human dose.[137] The strength of these models derives from the translational fidelity from human to animal and back again. The substrate and mechanisms underlying seizures in either case are very similar: disinhibition, axonal sprouting, neuroplasticity, necrosis, and excitotoxicity are common to human and animal brains. Considering BPD in a similar way, which may require that "higher" symptoms relating to mood or cognition are de-emphasized, may seem risky, but has distinct advantages and could be the paradigm shift that is required to make progress in the field. There may also be an immediate benefit from this approach for sufferers of BPD. Reclassification of BPD as more neurological than psychiatric could do much to remove the stigma associated with the diagnosis.

A Battery of Symptom-Based Models

Many of the models described earlier focus on specific symptoms or symptom clusters of BPD; they provide an indication that a novel drug might be capable of reducing these symptoms in a human patient. However, they require clinical validation for each new drug mechanism; furthermore, they carry a significant risk of false negative results, may not be specific for BPD, and risk giving results that consign a potential new medicine to the waste bin. Therefore, for these and other mainly practical reasons, the development of a battery of models related to BPD has been recently introduced.[46] In brief, the idea is to combine a number of models representing different facets of the disorder to provide a composite comprehensive model. It is desirable to concentrate on procedures that are simple to set up and behaviors that are simple to measure.[xii]

For example, the behavioral expression of mania in patients includes features such as increased energy, activity or restlessness, extreme irritability, reduced sleep, provocative, intrusive, or aggressive behavior, increased sexual drive, abuse of drugs, distractibility, reduced ability to concentrate, and risk taking.[142] Simple models in which these behaviors can be induced have been suggested previously in the literature either in the context of mania or other areas of psychiatry. Some of these are quite simple and so could be used as part of a screening battery (reviewed by[143]). Whereas each individual model should not be presumed to model mania, it is possible that the combination of several models can provide sufficient evaluation of the potential clinical efficacy of a new medication.

In a similar manner, simple models for other facets of BPD might be incorporated into the battery. For example, a simplified version of the resident-intruder paradigm was recently suggested to model aggression observed in BPD[46]; risk-taking behavior can be induced by a variety of drugs or environmental manipulations and can be easily measured in any of the anxiety-related tests (as risk taking can be considered a mirror image of anxiety); models for hedonia have been developed in the context of unipolar depression and models of susceptibility to drugs have been developed in the context of drug addiction. The task in hand is now to explore the predictive validity of these models for BPD and attempt to combine them into a simple battery with which a new drug can be evaluated.

Insights from the Mechanism of Action of Existing Drugs

The investigation of the molecular interactions of mood stabilizers such as lithium and valproate has identified a number of specific molecules and biochemical pathways that may be important for therapeutic effect.[144-152] These include protein kinase C (PKC), the Erk-MAP kinase pathway, GSK-3β, BCL-2, and mTOR. Interestingly, these molecules and pathways appear to be mostly related to cellular plasticity and resilience. The molecular findings have been followed up in animal studies, with findings that may support their relevance to changes in emotional behavior and response to mood-stabilizing drugs. For example, following the observation that both lithium and valproic acid inhibit the enzyme GSK-3β *in vitro*,[153,154] a mutation in a gene related to GSK-3β was found to be linked to lithium responses in patients.[155] Subsequently, administration of a GSK-3β specific inhibitor to animals resulted in mania-like behavioral changes.[156-158] Furthermore, mice with GSK-3β haploinsufficiency[159] or overexpressing with the beta-catenin transgene[160] were demonstrated to behave in a similar manner to animals treated with lithium. However, not all studies support a link between GSK-3β and BPD. For example, several groups have been unable to replicate the biochemical effect of lithium on

---

[xii] Please refer to Tannock *et al.*, towards a biological understanding of ADHD and the discovery of novel therapeutic approaches in this volume for further discussion regarding the difficulty of recapitulating all aspects of a multi-behavioral disorder in a single animal model.

GSK-3β activity and expression,[161] or the behavioral changes associated with GSK-3β haploinsufficiency (Belmaker, personal communication). Despite this, the exploration of GSK-3β and its relationship with BPD has included human genetics, biochemistry, and animal behavior, and could lead to the establishment of new animal models based on altered GSK-3β function in which to evaluate novel drugs. To the best of our knowledge, there are no clinical trials with drugs that specifically target GSK-3β yet in progress so it is too early to determine whether this approach will be valid in patients.

Protein kinase C is another molecule identified from studies of the effects of lithium *in vitro*. Behavioral studies in rodents are supportive of a role for the enzyme in the efficacy of lithium,[19] and in this case a drug was already available to test the hypothesis in humans: a small open clinical trial with the PKC inhibitor tamoxifen (Novaldex®) showed encouraging results,[162] as did a more recent double-blind placebo controlled study.[163] A larger clinical trial is now in progress. A spin off from these successful trials is likely to be the development of new animal models in which PKC or the associated biochemical cascade is modified to mimic what might be hypothesized to occur in the human disorder. These models may contribute to the evaluation of novel drugs and could point to other molecular targets that might be more tractable than PKC. These new approaches represent real progress in understanding and treating BPD; however, it should not be forgotten that the approach is based on mechanisms that confer efficacy of specific drugs, mechanisms that may not be feature of the underlying disorder.

Endophenotype-Based Models

Endophenotypes, as discussed in the introduction, are a hot topic of research in the field of psychiatric disease. They have emerged partly from an appreciation of the complex interplay between genes of susceptibility and environmental factors, which generate a disease phenotype. The exploration of endophenotypes will promote the development of tests in animals that model biological features that, whilst not necessarily causally related to BPD, may track the progression and/or resolution of symptoms during treatment. Modeling endophenotypes should be easier than modeling BPD, since they are by definition objective measures that could be observable in animals as well as in humans. Endophenotypes for BPD include attention deficit, instability of circadian rhythm, abnormal modulation of motivation and reward, structural changes within the brain, and increased sensitivity to stress or stimulant medications.[20] In many cases, endophenotypes may also be linked by genetic associations to BPD.[38] Examples of established endophenotypes for BPD are described below.

Dysfunction of the HPA Axis

There is considerable support for malfunction of the limbic-HPA axis in BPD.[164] However, the HPA axis has also been demonstrated to be hyperactive in many patients afflicted with major depression.[165] Thus, levels of cortisol (a marker for HPA axis activity) and left amygdala metabolism (a neuroanatomical marker of elevated HPA function) may be correlated in patients with either disorder.[166] Interestingly, HPA axis activation is most apparent in patients with hippocampal volume reduction,[167,168] consistent with the observation that stress can affect dendritic arborization in the medial prefrontal cortex,[169,170] (reviewed by[148]). The monitoring of HPA axis function and structural and functional brain imaging in humans might provide a means to follow the course and treatment of bipolar illness. This approach could lead to markers that could be studied in animal models and against which drug effects could be measured. Clearly, these markers may be most appropriate in animals models based on acute or chronic stress.

Neural Plasticity and Brain Derived Neurotrophic Factor

A polymorphism in brain derived neurotrophic factor (BDNF), a possible susceptibility gene for BPD, has been linked to anatomic variations in the hippocampus and prefrontal cortex,[171] as well as to cognitive performance associated with these same brain areas[172,173] in humans. BDNF has been shown to contribute to neuronal growth and plasticity associated with learning and memory,[172] and manipulation of the BDNF – Erk-MAP kinase pathway has been reported to lead to mood relevant behavioral changes.[174] Changes in expression of BDNF or associated proteins induced by a novel drug in animals could therefore predict drug efficacy in patients with BPD; however, it should be recognized that altered expression of BDNF is also a hallmark of antidepressant treatment (reviewed by[175]). Moving from animals to humans, effects of a novel drug on BDNF expression might be followed by monitoring anatomical variation in patients using structural magnetic resonance imaging. In practice, this is unlikely to be straightforward, although there are already examples where this approach has been successfully applied.[176,177]

Psychostimulant Sensitivity and Disruption of Reward Systems

Hypersensitivity to dopaminergic drugs has been suggested as an endophenotype of BPD[38]; indeed there is a high comorbidity with substance abuse in BPD patients. Given this relationship, it should be possible to extend measures of locomotor's activity following administration of psychostimulants to animals and examine additional behavioral effects such as risk taking or hedonia. Moreover, it should be possible to identify specific strains of animals that are particularly susceptible to psychostimulants, or to test for individual variability within groups of animals in the context of these measures.[64] Individual animals or strains that show increased vulnerability to a number of behaviors related to dopaminergic stimulation may provide an animal model for this specific endophenotype in BPD and may permit the study of related genetic differences.

Circadian Disturbance

Sleep disruption as a model and treatment approach for BPD was discussed earlier. There is good reason to suggest that a disruption of circadian mechanisms might underlie the effects of sleep disruption and may even underlie the emergence of the symptoms of BPD. Shifts in circadian pattern often precede episodes of mania[178]; sleep disturbance is present even during periods of euthymia[179] and is commonly observed in adolescent patients with BPD,[180] suggesting an early or even causal relationship with the disorder. Consistent with a possible circadian dysfunction in BPD, some patients with the illness show a greater sensitivity to season and a greater improvement in mood following exposure to sunshine.[181] A combination of lithium with manipulation of the sleep-wake cycle or deliberate sleep disturbance may be a valuable treatment approach for patients with bipolar depression.[182] This approach is supported by evidence that a polymorphism in the *clock* gene that regulates circadian rhythm may be associated with the recurrence of mood episodes in patients with BPD,[183] and a polymorphism in the promoter region of GSK-3β, which is also involved in circadian control, may influence the age of onset of the disorder.[184] Since both lithium and valproate can inhibit GSK-3β, the study of drug effects on circadian control would seem a potentially fruitful area of research for novel treatments for BPD. Animal models in which circadian control is modified by genetic or behavioral means could provide a useful testing ground for these treatments.

CLINICAL TESTING AND TRANSLATIONAL INITIATIVES FOR BIPOLAR DISORDER

New drugs reaching patients with BPD should have been shown to be safe after repeated administration to healthy volunteers over a defined range of doses associated with a known range of plasma concentrations.[185] Furthermore, the drugs will have been shown to be safe in animals at higher doses that achieve multiples of the highest plasma concentration that will be tested in humans. Ideally, the drug will also have been shown to be effective in animal models with some relevance to BPD, although currently it is more likely that they will have been tested only in models that predict efficacy in diseases other than BPD (e.g., seizure models that predict the anticonvulsant efficacy of sodium channel blockers, or models using psychostimulants that are used to predict antipsychotic efficacy). A common route to trials in patients with BPD has been to demonstrate first that the new drug is effective in patients with epilepsy or schizophrenia. This is the case for the vast majority of drugs that have received approval for the treatment of BPD including quetiapine, olanzapine, lamotrigine, and valproate; all of which were first approved for the treatment of either epilepsy[186,187] or schizophrenia.[188] To date, no drug has been developed and approved by first intent specifically for the treatment of BPD. If we make the reasonable assumption that the etiology of BPD differs from that of epilepsy and schizophrenia, then we may conclude that a significant breakthrough in the treatment of BPD is unlikely to happen if only drugs effective in these other disorders are ever tested in patients with BPD. Incidentally, this argument continues to motivate research into the mechanism of action of lithium, which is neither anticonvulsant nor antipsychotic.[45] The development of new drugs primarily for the treatment of BPD would ideally be based on the use of predictive animal models; furthermore, clinical trials should build on animal models and should allow a systematic incremental demonstration of efficacy that is consistent with the huge costs and difficulties associated with trials in BPD. For example, it is unlikely that an organization would fund a large 18-month multi-centre trial to demonstrate mood-prophylaxis with a novel drug without first having demonstrated acute efficacy versus symptoms of mania or depression and prior to that, having demonstrated efficacy of the drug in appropriate animal and human models.

Table 9.2 Pharmacodynamic models in which a dose-effect relationship for a novel drug might be investigated

Measure	Drugs class	Reference
Dopamine D_2 receptor occupancy (measured using a radiolabeled ligand with PET[a])	Risperidone, olanzapine, quetiapine, amisulpride, ziprasidone, aripiprazole, antipsychotic drugs in general	189,190
Changes in resting motor threshold assessed using TMS[a] applied to the motor cortex	Lamotrigine, carbamazepine, sodium channel blockers in general	191,192
Cortical silent period assessed using paired TMS pulses applied to the motor cortex	Tiagabine, some benzodiazepines	192,193
TMS over frontal cortex in combination with BOLD fMRI	Lamotrigine	194

[a] *TMS – transcranial magnetic stimulation; PET – positron emission tomography.*

The design of any clinical trial, as with any other scientific experiment, should be driven by a hypothesis.[xiii] Eventually the hypothesis may be that the drug will produce a clinically meaningful reduction in HAM-D or MADRS score (for bipolar depression), Young Mania Rating Scale (for mania), or will significantly delay episode recurrence; however, early on the hypothesis being tested is more likely to reflect aspects of the drug's known, or presumed, mechanism of action and theories developed from studies using animal models. These so-called "experimental medicine" or "proof-of-concept" studies may not provide pivotal results on which to base regulatory approval, but they can provide confidence to commit to larger Phase IIb trials. Furthermore, these approaches can often start during Phase I in trials with healthy volunteers.

Exploring Dose–Effect Relationships

Experimental medicine studies may be designed to increase knowledge of the efficacy of a new drug in relation to its expected mechanism of action, or may be designed simply to demonstrate that the drug interacts with its target protein in the central nervous system to a degree deemed sufficient for future efficacy. In each case, the degree of relationship between effect or receptor occupancy with the dose administered and the plasma concentration achieved is fundamental, providing a crucial basis for dose-selection for future trials. Examples of studies that contribute confidence in mechanism-of-action and support dose-selection for drugs used in the treatment of BPD are shown in Table 9.2.

In each case, there is no intent to demonstrate efficacy versus symptoms of BPD, and the studies may be conducted just as well in healthy volunteers. The intent is

---

[xiii] Please refer to McEvoy and Freudenreich, Issues in the design and conductance of clinical trials of psychiatric candidate drugs, in this volume for an overview of clinical development phases.

Table 9.3 Challenge models used for early evaluation of potential efficacy of novel treatments for BPD in patients or healthy human volunteers (?)

Model	Drugs evaluated	Reference
Amphetamine-induced euphoria	None	195
Ketamine-induced psychosis	Lamotrigine	196
Monoamine depletion	SSRIs, NRIs (note that several of these studies examined the response to monoamine depletion as a function of the prior treatment used, rather than examining the ability of the drugs to prevent or reverse the symptoms induced by depletion)	197–200
Sleep disturbance	This may be a therapeutic intervention in its own right as well as a means to induce manic symptoms. Some evidence that lithium can stabilise the beneficial effects of sleep deprivation in patients with bipolar depression.	38,201,202

to demonstrate a relationship between dose and interaction with the target protein. Results from this type of study will allow a further relationship to be examined in the patient population: the relationship between the degree of interaction of a drug with its target protein and its therapeutic effect.

Disease Models in Humans

Following the demonstration of a dose–effect relationship for a novel drug in an appropriate model in healthy volunteers, it may be desirable to investigate the efficacy of the drug in a model with some face or construct validity for BPD. In practice for ethical reasons, studies of this type may not be easy to set up, although there are examples of protocols in which an acute response to a challenge might be used to investigate the potential efficacy of a test compound. Examples of challenge models with some relevance to BPD are shown in Table 9.3. Ideally, the choice of challenge model should reflect the known mechanism of the test drug and perhaps follow on from a similar challenge model studied in animals.

In each case, the demonstration of efficacy provides further confidence in the CNS activity of a novel drug and provides additional information about the dose–effect relationship that may be helpful in planning clinical trials in patients.

Approaches to Evaluating Efficacy in Patients with Bipolar Disorder

Gathering evidence of efficacy in bipolar patients is a complex, costly, and time-consuming process. Since a novel treatment for BPD can be registered separately for the treatment of mania, bipolar depression, or prevention of mood episodes, the approach to efficacy trials should certainly reflect the likely spectrum of efficacy of the drug, based on its known mechanism of action and its efficacy in preclinical or healthy volunteer models. However, the intended indication should also reflect the unmet need in BPD and analysis of the risk-benefit of the drug in relation to that indication. This is particularly important given the current emphasis on assessment of cost-effectiveness of new treatments at the point of registration or approval for national use.[203] Currently, given the greater unmet need for an effective treatment for bipolar depression compared to mania, the risk-benefit hurdle for novel treatments for the former is likely to be lower than for the latter. Furthermore, reimbursement, once on the market, is likely to be greater for a novel treatment for bipolar depression compared to mania. Debate about the probability of success in terms of demonstrating efficacy of a novel treatment for a particular phase of BPD is likely to happen early on in clinical development and before committing to Phase II patient studies.

Clinical trials to demonstrate the efficacy of a novel treatment in patients with BPD are fraught with difficulty and subject to a high failure rate. First and foremost is the high placebo response in patients with BPD, which is likely to be related to the use of concomitant medications and psychotherapy, cessation of substance abuse upon enrollment,[xiv] frequent hospital visits as part of the trial protocol, and the spontaneous improvement in symptoms typical of an episodic illness.[204] In this latter case, inclusion criteria might stipulate that patients have only recently entered a manic or depressed phase. In the case of mood-prophylaxis studies, patients may be recruited during a mood episode and then started in the blinded part of the trial once they become euthymic.[135] The inclusion of a placebo arm in acute bipolar mania or depression studies remains a subject of ethical debate and may be particularly difficult in the case of long-term mood-prophylaxis studies. However, appropriate trial design and choice of endpoints, with the availability of rescue medication in the case of mood-prophylaxis studies can make the inclusion of a placebo arm tolerable, although this may still have an adverse effect on recruitment, which itself can be particularly slow in the case of bipolar mania trials.

Selection of a homogenous patient population for clinical trials, at least during the early phase of efficacy studies, is another critical area that can affect the probability of success. The selection of BPD patients necessarily considers first the target phase of illness (manic, depressed, or euthymic), and then considers whether to include or exclude subclasses of BPD (bipolar I, bipolar II, cyclothymic, or rapid cycling). Selection up to this point must rely on DSM-IV-TR or ICD-10. These diagnostic tools reliably diagnose BPD and differentiate it from other disorders; they also provide good inter-rater reliability such that a similar population of patients will be selected across multi-site trials. However, in the absence of definitive knowledge of the etiology and pathophysiology of BPD, DSM-IV-TR, and ICD-10 cannot adequately ensure that a biologically homogenous group of patients will be recruited into a clinical trial. Careful

---

[xiv] Please refer to McEvoy and Freudenreich, Issues in the design and conductance of clinical trials of psychiatric candidate drugs, in this volume and to Rocha *et al.*, Development of medications for heroin and cocaine addiction and regulatory aspects of abuse liability testing, in Volume 3, *Reward Deficit Disorders* for further discussion regarding patient selection, failed and negative clinical trial outcome, and problems of substance abuse as a confounding factor in clinical trial conductance.

phenomenological assessment of each patient and the use of endophenotypes may be alternative ways to increase biological homogeneity across the trial population.

Thus early Phase II studies may take advantage of additional sub-classification of bipolar patients, other markers, endophenotypes, and past-treatment response to try to pick out subgroups of patients in which the study drug may be more likely to be efficacious. The choice of these additional criteria should reflect knowledge about the mechanism of action of the study drug and its efficacy in animal and healthy volunteer models. Past-treatment response is likely to be a valuable basis on which to select patients where the study drug has a similar mechanism to an existing treatment. For example, for initial studies of the efficacy of a novel drug-targeting PKC, such as tamoxifen, it may be advisable to enrich for patients that have previously responded well to lithium. However as it happens, this approach was not explicitly taken in the case of the two studies so far conducted with tamoxifen.[162,163] Enrichment based on past-treatment response may be less attractive for a new drug with a novel mechanism of action. Sub-classifications of BPD into bipolar I or II, patients with mixed states, psychotic symptoms, or rapid cycling can also be useful basis to include or exclude subjects according to predicted efficacy or past experience with the study drug. These approaches certainly could help to improve the chance of demonstrating efficacy of a study drug, but in current practice, these measures are more likely to be applied *post hoc* during the analysis of larger trials. Similarly, most new BPD trials include blood draws for *post hoc* genotyping, rather than choosing study populations *a priori* based on candidate genes potentially linked to BPD or to the mechanism of action of the study drug;[205] although a Phase III trial in patients with unipolar depression has been completed recently with vilazodone using a genetic test that has reportedly identified candidate biomarkers to predict treatment response (news release by Clinical Data, September 4, 2007). *Post hoc* genotyping is conducted with the hope of identifying alleles of candidate genes that are associated with treatment response; alternatively, whole genome scans can be conducted looking for association of any genetic marker with treatment response.

The selection of a homogeneous patient population for early efficacy trials should also pay attention to comorbid disorders, such substance abuse or anxiety,[206] both of which have been shown to influence drug response. However, in practice these and other exclusion criteria are often relaxed due to the remarkably high percentage of bipolar patients that fall into this category, leading to a dramatic impact on recruitment. In conclusion, there are good reasons for constraining the patient population to pick out a homogeneous group of "ideal" subjects most likely to respond to the anticipated effects of a new drug, this approach should be exploited at least during Phase II studies. However, for later studies, selection of the patient population based strictly on DSM-IV-TR criteria is likely to remain essential for pivotal studies intended to be used for registration and approval. It can be appreciated that these studies may be limiting and may introduce a more heterogeneous patient group with a more heterogeneous response to the study drug.

Aside from patient selection, other more practical aspects of trial design can have a strong influence on the success of the study. Early in Phase II, carefully monitored studies using single sites may be preferable to large multi-centre trials in which sensitivity to a treatment effect can be reduced by increased heterogeneity of the patient population, variable physician care, and greater likelihood of deviations from the study protocol. One approach to ensuring greater consistency across sites during recruitment may be to include patient self-rating in addition to physician rating.

Choice of study sites may also influence the type of analysis that can be conducted on results. Classical study designs typically follow an intent-to-treat population over a fixed duration, accounting for dropouts by carrying forward the last observation of the subject before he or she retired from the study. Statistical analysis of the primary and any secondary endpoints for the trial is carried out comparing between treatment groups. An alternative analysis that can be useful in the case of a heterogeneous illness such as BPD is to evaluate treatment effect *within subjects*. This approach may be particularly useful for identifying subgroups of patients that respond better to the drug. However, in the case of multi-centre trials, each site must contribute a reasonable number of subjects for the approach to be effective, since in the event that just one or two subjects are available from a given site, then response or lack of response could be due to factors associated with the site rather than the subjects themselves. Irrespective of the number of sites, this analysis approach requires that greater attention is paid to the natural course of each subject's illness, excluding rapid cyclers and ensuring recruitment early in the mood episode to reduce the probability of a spontaneous remission of symptoms.

Finally, adaptive study designs and the use of Bayesian statistics are becoming increasingly popular during the early phases of clinical development. These designs include an interim analysis and hypothesis-driven statistical approach that can be used to steer the trial towards a successful outcome[207]; although these approaches have yet to have a major impact on trial design in BPD, there could be potential benefits in particular for long, expensive mood-prophylaxis trials in which survival in the trial is the primary endpoint.[208,209]

CONCLUSIONS

It is often the case that a field of research will experience a period of inflation before collapsing down to a new realization or level of understanding. Over the last decade, the awareness of BPD has dramatically increased, with the number of research projects focusing specifically on this disorder increasing in step. BPD is a chronic and highly debilitating illness, characterized by periods of normality and periods of illness that are not well controlled by current treatments. BPD imposes a huge burden on patients, their families, and society as a whole. The unmet need for better treatments is perhaps greater than for any other psychiatric illness.

An overview of the status of animal models of BPD suggests that there has been a period of inflation here too, but many of the models are still "borrowed" or adapted from other disorders, notably unipolar depression and schizophrenia. This reflects the fact that a large proportion of drugs that are used to treat BPD were first developed for other illnesses. To date no diagnostic biological markers for BPD have been identified, consequently the development of new drugs for the treatment of BPD and the parallel development of animal models to test them will remain largely focused on clinical symptoms defined by DSM-IV-TR or ICD-10. These systems of diagnosis are empirical and evidence based, giving rise to a reliable classification of the patients encountered in the physician's office. However, DSM and ICD were not explicitly intended as the basis from which to conduct research. Therefore, as a rule of thumb, scientists should always look for objective biological measures on which to base their research in preference, or at least in parallel, to the use of symptoms specified by DSM or ICD. In practice, symptoms that can be most easily translated down from humans to animals will tend to be favored, but to compensate there should at least be attempts to translate methods used in animal testing back up to humans; a good example of this is the "Behavioral Pattern Monitor."[47] [xv] Where possible, animal models should target the underlying nature of BPD, mood instability, rather than target specific manic or depressed symptoms. It should be kept in mind that pharmacological validation of models, necessarily dependent on the current pharmacopoeia for BPD, can lock drug discovery into a closed loop. Once again, the parallel use of alternative models or experimental markers of efficacy should accompany drug development using the more traditional approaches.

Despite the apparent circularity of research based on DSM or ICD criteria, there are now signs that BPD might be approached directly; notably through genetic associations and endophenotypes that may differentiate BPD from unipolar depression or schizophrenia. It will be important to extract features of BPD that are both unique and biological, and to use these in the design of new animal models. From there, further progress is likely to be iterative well into the future, with small advances in knowledge allowing novel treatments to be tested and the insights gained in clinical studies feeding back to preclinical research. The use of batteries of symptom-based models together with new genetic or endophenotype-based models may allow us to gather sufficient information about a new drug to permit progression into clinical studies. Where novel areas of biology are proposed, the availability of drugs from other areas of medicine that might allow a novel hypothesis to be explored in humans (e.g., tamoxifen[163]) will be essential to make progress.

Finally, more practical aspects of drug testing, such as dose–effect determination or side effect profiling, should not be ignored. Ideally, drug testing in animals should be mindful of concentrations that can be reached safely in humans. The predominant use of acute dosing and acute models in animals remains a major discrepancy between preclinical and clinical research. Attempts to bridge this gap with greater use of chronic animal models or the use of acute challenge models in humans should be encouraged. In summary, clinical approaches should always aim to build on the results of studies in animals, and hypothesis testing should be the foundation of clinical experimentation, as much as it is for animal studies.

REFERENCES

1. Kraeplin, E. (1921). *Manic-Depressive Insanity and Paranoia*. E & S Livingston, Edinburgh, UK.
2. Campbell, J.D. (1952). Manic depressive psychosis in children. *J Nerv Ment Dis*, 116(5):424–439.
3. Andreasen, N.C. (2007). DSM and the death of phenomenology in America: An example of unintended consequences. *Schizophr Bull*, 33(1):108–112.

[xv] Please refer to Lindner *et al.*, for an example of cross species testing instruments (Cambridge Neuropsychological Test Automated Battery, CANTAB) helping to bridge the translational gap in cognitive assessment.

4. American Psychiatric Association. (2000). *Diagnostic and Statistical Manual of Mental disorders, Fourth Edition, Text Revision*. American Psychiatric Press, Washington, DC, USA.

5. World Health Organization. (2007). *International Statistical Classification of Diseases and Related Health Problems (The) ICD-10 Second Edition 2007*. World Health Organization, Geneva, Switzerland.

6. Jamison, K.R. (1995). *An Unquiet Mind*. Alfred A. Knopf, a division of Random House, Inc.

7. Jaspers, K. (1968). *General Psychopathology*. Translated by Honeig, J. and Hamilton, M.W. (Ed.), University of Chicago Press, Chicago, USA. Republished by Johns Hopkins University Press, 1997.

8. Rush, B. (1812). *Medical Inquiries and Observations upon the Diseases of the Mind*. Kimber and Richardson, Philadelphia, USA.

9. Goodwin, F.K. and Jamison, K.R. (2007). *Manic-Depressive Illness; Bipolar Disorders and Recurrent Depression*, Oxford University Press, Oxford, UK.

10. Winokur, G., Clayton, P.J., and Reich, T. (1969). *Manic Depressive Illness*. CV Mosby, St. Louis, USA.

11. Deckersbach, T., Perlis, R.H., Frankle, W.G., Gray, S.M., Grandin, L., Dougherty, D.D. *et al.* (2004). Presence of irritability during depressive episodes in bipolar disorder. *CNS Spectr*, 9(3):227-231.

12. Andreasen, N.C. (1979). Thought, language, and communication disorders. I. Clinical assessment, definition of terms, and evaluation of their reliability. *Arch Gen Psychiatry*, 36(12):1315-1321.

13. Cassidy, F., Ahearn, E., and Carroll, B.J. (2001). A prospective study of inter-episode consistency of manic and mixed subtypes of bipolar disorder. *J Affect Disord*, 67(1-3):181-185.

14. Kotin, J. and Goodwin, F.K. (1972). Depression during mania: Clinical observations and theoretical implications. *Am J Psychiatry*, 129(6):679-686.

15. Tohen, M., Waternaux, C.M., and Tsuang, M.T. (1990). Outcome in mania. A 4-year prospective follow-up of 75 patients utilizing survival analysis. *Arch Gen Psychiatry*, 47(12):1106-1111.

16. Gitlin, M.J., Swendsen, J., Heller, T.L., and Hammen, C. (1995). Relapse and impairment in bipolar disorder. *Am J Psychiatry*, 152(11):1635-1640.

17. Keller, M.B., Lavori, P.W., Coryell, W., Endicott, J., and Mueller, T.I. (1993). Bipolar I: A five-year prospective follow-up. *J Nerv Ment Dis*, 181(4):238-245.

18. Judd, L.L., Akiskal, H.S., Schettler, P.J., Endicott, J., Maser, J., Solomon, D.A. *et al.* (2002). The long-term natural history of the weekly symptomatic status of bipolar I disorder. *Arch Gen Psychiatry*, 59(6):530-537.

19. Joffe, R.T., MacQueen, G.M., Marriott, M., and Trevor, Y.L. (2004). A prospective, longitudinal study of percentage of time spent ill in patients with bipolar I or bipolar II disorders. *Bipolar Disord*, 6(1):62-66.

20. Keck, P.E., Jr, McElroy, S.L., Strakowski, S.M., Bourne, M.L., and West, S.A. (1997). Compliance with maintenance treatment in bipolar disorder. *Psychopharmacol Bull*, 33(1):87-91.

21. Cade, J.F. (2000). Lithium salts in the treatment of psychotic excitement. 1949. *Bull World Health Organ*, 78(4):518-520.

22. American Psychiatric Association. (2002). *Practice Guidelines for the Treatment of Patients with Bipolar Disorder*, American Psychiatric Association, Arlington, VA.

23. Goodwin, G.M. and Young, A.H. (2003). The British Association for Psychopharmacology guidelines for treatment of bipolar disorder: A summary. *J Psychopharmacol*, 17(4 Suppl):3-6.

24. Calabrese, J.R., Hirschfeld, R.M., Reed, M., Davies, M.A., Frye, M.A., Keck, P.E. *et al.* (2003). Impact of bipolar disorder on a U.S. community sample. *J Clin Psychiatry*, 64(4):425-432.

25. Wyatt, R.J. and Henter, I. (1995). An economic evaluation of manic-depressive illness - 1991. *Soc Psychiatry Psychiatr Epidemiol*, 30(5):213-219.

26. Begley, C.E., Annergers, J.F., and Swann, A.C. (2001). The lifetime cost of Bipolar disorder in the US: An estimate for new cases in 1998. *Pharmacoeconomics*, 9:483–495.

27. Bryant-Comstock, L., Stender, M., and Devercelli, G. (2002). Health care utilization and costs among privately insured patients with bipolar I disorder. *Bipolar Disord*, 4(6):398–405.

28. Sachs, G.S. (2003). Unmet clinical needs in bipolar disorder. *J Clin Psychopharmacol*, 23(3 Suppl 1):S2–S8.

29. Hirschfeld, R.M., Lewis, L., and Vornik, L.A. (2003). Perceptions and impact of bipolar disorder: How far have we really come? Results of the national depressive and manic-depressive association 2000 survey of individuals with bipolar disorder. *J Clin Psychiatry*, 64(2):161–174.

30. Hayden, E.P. and Nurnberger, J.I., Jr (2006). Molecular genetics of bipolar disorder. *Genes Brain Behav*, 5(1):85–95.

31. Kato, T. (2007). Molecular genetics of bipolar disorder and depression. *Psychiatry Clin Neurosci*, 61(1):3–19.

32. Farmer, A., Elkin, A., and McGuffin, P. (2007). The genetics of bipolar affective disorder. *Curr Opin Psychiatry*, 20(1):8–12.

33. Sherazi, R., McKeon, P., McDonough, M., Daly, I., and Kennedy, N. (2006). What's new? The clinical epidemiology of bipolar I disorder. *Harv Rev Psychiatry*, 14(6):273–284.

34. Post, R.M. and Leverich, G.S. (2006). The role of psychosocial stress in the onset and progression of bipolar disorder and its comorbidities: The need for earlier and alternative modes of therapeutic intervention. *Dev Psychopathol*, 18(4):1181–1211.

35. Bowden, C.L. (2004). Making optimal use of combination pharmacotherapy in bipolar disorder. *J Clin Psychiatry*, 65(Suppl 15):21–24.

36. Post, R.M., Ketter, T.A., Pazzaglia, P.J., Denicoff, K., George, M.S., Callahan, A. *et al.* (1996). Rational polypharmacy in the bipolar affective disorders. *Epilepsy Res Suppl*, 11:153–180.

37. Roses, A.D. (2006). On the discovery of the genetic association of Apolipoprotein E genotypes and common late-onset Alzheimer disease. *J Alzheimers Dis*, 9(3 Suppl):361–366.

38. Hasler, G., Drevets, W.C., Gould, T.D., Gottesman, I.I., and Manji, H.K. (2006). Toward constructing an endophenotype strategy for bipolar disorders. *Biol Psychiatry*, 60(2):93–105.

39. Cryan, J.F. and Slattery, D.A. (2007). Animal models of mood disorders: Recent developments. *Curr Opin Psychiatry*, 20(1):1–7.

40. Lenox, R.H., Gould, T.D., and Manji, H.K. (2002). Endophenotypes in bipolar disorder. *Am J Med Genet*, 114(4):391–406.

41. Chou, J.C. and Fazzio, L. (2006). Maintenance treatment of bipolar disorder: Applying research to clinical practice. *J Psychiatr Pract*, 12(5):283–299.

42. Hayes, L.J. and Delgado, D. (2007). Invited commentary on animal models in psychiatry: Animal models of non-conventional human behavior. *Behav Genet*, 37(1):11–17.

43. Seligman, M.E., Maier, S.F., and Geer, J.H. (1968). Alleviation of learned helplessness in the dog. *J Abnorm Psychol*, 73(3):256–262.

44. Seligman, M.E. and Maier, S.F. (1967). Failure to escape traumatic shock. *J Exp Psychol*, 74(1):1–9.

45. Leucht, S., Kissling, W., and McGrath, J. (2007). Lithium for schizophrenia. *Cochrane Database Syst Rev*, 3:CD003834.

46. Einat, H. (2007). Establishment of a battery of simple models for facets of bipolar disorder: A practical approach to achieve increased validity, better screening and possible insights into endophenotypes of disease. *Behav Genet*, 37(1):244–255.

47. Young, J.W., Minassian, A., Paulus, M.P., Geyer, M.A., and Perry, W. (2007). A reverse-translational approach to bipolar disorder: Rodent and human studies in the Behavioral Pattern Monitor. *Neurosci Biobehav Rev*, 31(6):882–896.

48. Antelman, S.M., Caggiula, A.R., Kucinski, B.J., Fowler, H., Gershon, S., Edwards, D.J., Austin, M.C., Stiller, R., Kiss, S., and Kocan, D. (1998). The effects of lithium on a potential cycling model of bipolar disorder. *Prog Neuropsychopharmacol Biol Psychiatry*, 22(3):495–510.

49. Eckermann, K., Beasley, A., Yang, P., Gaytan, O., Swann, A., and Dafny, N. (2001). Methylphenidate sensitization is modulated by valproate. *Life Sci*, 69(1):47–57.

50. Einat, H., Shaldubina, A., Bersudskey, Y., and Belmaker, R.H. (2007). Prospects for the development of animal models for the study of bipolar disorder. In Soares, J.C. and Young, A.H. (eds.), *Bipolar Disorders: Basic Mechanisms and Therapeutic Implications*. Taylor & Francis, New York.

51. Einat, H., Yuan, P., Szabo, S.T., Dogra, S. and Manji, H.K. (2007). Protein kinase C inhibition by tamoxifen antagonizes manic-like behavior in rats: Implications for the development of novel therapeutics for bipolar disorder. *Neuropsychobiology*, 55(3–4):123–131.

52. Hamburger-Bar, R., Robert, M., Newman, M. and Belmaker, R.H. (1986). Interstrain correlation between behavioural effects of lithium and effects on cortical cyclic AMP. *Pharmacol Biochem Behav*, 24(1):9–13.

53. Namima, M., Sugihara, K., Watanabe, Y., Sasa, H., Umekage, T., and Okamotom, K. (1999). Quantitative analysis of the effects of lithium on the reverse tolerance and the c-Fos expression induced by methamphetamine in mice. *Brain Res Brain Res Protoc*, 4(1):11–18.

54. Post, R.M. and Weiss, S.R. (1989). Sensitization, kindling, and anticonvulsants in mania. *J Clin Psychiatry*, 50(Suppl):23–30; discussion 45–47.

55. Belmaker, R.H., Lerer, B., Klein, E., and Hamburger, R. (1982). The use of behavioral methods in the search for compounds with lithium-like activity. In Levy, A. and Spiegelstein M.Y. *Behavioral Models and the Analysis of Drug Action*. Amsterdam, Elsevier: 343–356.

56. Borison, R.L., Sabelli, H.C., Maple, P.J., Havdala, H.S., and Diamond, B.I. (1978). Lithium prevention of amphetamine-induced 'manic' excitement and of reserpine-induced 'depression' in mice: possible role of 2-phenylethylamine. *Psychopharmacology (Berl)*, 59(3):259–262.

57. Murphy, D.L., Brodie, H.K., Goodwin, F.K., and Bunney, W.E., Jr. (1971). Regular induction of hypomania by L-dopa in "bipolar" manic-depressive patients. *Nature*, 229(5280):135–136.

58. Van Kammen, D.P. and Murphy, D.L. (1975). Attenuation of the euphoriant and activating effects of d- and l-amphetamine by lithium carbonate treatment. *Psychopharmacologia*, 44(3):215–224.

59. Berggren, U., Tallstedt, L., Ahlenius, S., and Engel, J. (1978). The effect of lithium on amphetamine-induced locomotor stimulation. *Psychopharmacology (Berl)*, 59(1):41–45.

60. Gould, T.J., Keith, R.A., and Bhat, R.V. (2001). Differential sensitivity to lithium's reversal of amphetamine-induced open-field activity in two inbred strains of mice. *Behav Brain Res*, 118(1):95–105.

61. Cappeliez, P. and Moore, E. (1990). Effects of lithium on an amphetamine animal model of bipolar disorder. *Prog Neuropsychopharmacol Biol Psychiatry*, 14(3):347–358.

62. Ebstein, R.P., Eliashar, S., Belmaker, R.H., Ben-Uriah, Y., and Yehuda, S. (1980). Chronic lithium treatment and dopamine-mediated behavior. *Biol Psychiatry*, 15(3):459–467.

63. Gould, T.D., O'Donnell, K.C., Picchini, A.M., and Manji, H.K. (2007). Strain differences in lithium attenuation of d-amphetamine-induced hyperlocomotion: a mouse model for the genetics of clinical response to lithium. *Neuropsychopharmacology*, 32(6):1321–1333.

64. Hiscock, K., Linde, J., and Einat, H. (2007). Black Swiss mice as a new animal model for mania: a preliminary study. *J Med Biol Sci*, 1(2).

65. Ralph, R.J., Paulus, M.P., and Geyer, M.A. (2001). Strain-specific effects of amphetamine on prepulse inhibition and patterns of locomotor behavior in mice. *J Pharmacol Exp Ther*, 298(1):148–155.

66. Beaulieu, J.M., Sotnikova, T.D., Yao, W.D., Kockeritz, L., Woodgett, J.R., Gainetdinov, R.R., and Caron, M.G. (2004). Lithium antagonizes dopamine-dependent behaviors mediated by an AKT/glycogen synthase kinase 3 signaling cascade. *Proc Natl Acad Sci USA*, 101(14):5099–5104.

67. Le-Niculescu, H., McFarland, M.J., Ogden, C.A., Balaraman, Y., Patel, S., Tan, J., Rodd, Z.A., Paulus, M., Geyer, M.A., Edenberg, H.J., Glatt, S.J., Faraone, S.V., Nurnberger, J.I., Kuczenski, R., Tsuang, M.T., and Niculescu, A.B. (2008). Phenomic, convergent functional

genomic, and biomarker studies in a stress-reactive genetic animal model of bipolar disorder and co-morbid alcoholism. *Am J Med Genet B Neuropsychiatr Genet*, 147(2):134–166.

68. Ralph, R.J., Paulus, M.P., Fumagalli, F., Caron, M.G., and Geyer, M.A. (2001). Prepulse inhibition deficits and perseverative motor patterns in dopamine transporter knock-out mice: Differential effects of D1 and D2 receptor antagonists. *J Neurosci*, 21(1):305–313.

69. Ralph, R.J., Varty, G.B., Kelly, M.A., Wang, Y.M., Caron, M.G., Rubinstein, M. *et al*. (1999). The dopamine D2, but not D3 or D4, receptor subtype is essential for the disruption of prepulse inhibition produced by amphetamine in mice. *J Neurosci*, 19(11):4627–4633.

70. Arban, R., Maraia, G., Brackenborough, K., Winyard, L., Wilson, A., Gerrard, P. *et al*. (2005). Evaluation of the effects of lamotrigine, valproate and carbamazepine in a rodent model of mania. *Behav Brain Res*, 158(1):123–132.

71. Armitage, P., Rushton, R., and Steinberg, H. (1968). Interactions of chlordizepoxide and dexamphetamine in rats. *Naunyn Schmiedebergs Arch Exp Pathol Pharmakol*, 259(2):150–151.

72. Aylmer, C.G., Steinberg, H., and Webster, R.A. (1987). Hyperactivity induced by dexamphetamine/chlordiazepoxide mixtures in rats and its attenuation by lithium pretreatment:A role for dopamine? *Psychopharmacology (Berl)*, 91(2):198–206.

73. Rushton, R. and Steinberg, H. (1966). Combined effects of chlordiazepoxide and dexamphetamine on activity of rats in an unfamiliar environment. *Nature*, 211(5055):1312–1313.

74. Serpa, K.A. (1999). Chlordiazepoxide/d-d-amphetamine induced hyperactivity in rats: assessment as mania model using automated activity chambers. Meltzer, L.T. (Ed.) *Soc Neurosci Abstr*, 25, 533.13.

75. Cao, B.J. and Peng, N.A. (1993). Magnesium valproate attenuates hyperactivity induced by dexamphetamine-chlordiazepoxide mixture in rodents. *Eur J Pharmacol*, 237(2–3):177–181.

76. Vale, A.L. and Ratcliffe, F. (1987). Effect of lithium administration on rat brain 5-hydroxyindole levels in a possible animal model for mania. *Psychopharmacology (Berl)*, 91(3):352–355.

77. Lamberty, Y., Margineanu, D.G., and Klitgaard, H. (2001). Effect of the new antiepileptic drug levetiracetam in an animal model of mania. *Epilepsy Behav*, 2(5):454–459.

78. Butler, P.W., Besser, G.M., and Steinberg, H. (1968). Changes in plasma cortisol induced by dexamphetamine and chlordiazepoxide given alone and in combination in man. *J Endocrinol*, 40(3):391–392.

79. Besser, G.M. and Steinberg, H. (1967). The interaction of chlordiazepoxide and dexamphetamine in man. *Therapie*, 22(5):977–990.

80. Ashton, H. and Young, A.H. (2003). GABA-ergic drugs: Exit stage left, enter stage right. *J Psychopharmacol*, 17(2):174–178.

81. Ketter, T.A. and Wang, P.W. (2003). The emerging differential roles of GABAergic and antiglutamatergic agents in bipolar disorders. *J Clin Psychiatry*, 64(Suppl 3):15–20.

82. Kalivas, P.W., Sorg, B.A., and Hooks, M.S. (1993). The pharmacology and neural circuitry of sensitization to psychostimulants. *Behav Pharmacol*, 4(4):315–334.

83. Pierce, R.C. and Kalivas, P.W. (1997). A circuitry model of the expression of behavioral sensitization to amphetamine-like psychostimulants. *Brain Res Brain Res Rev*, 25(2):192–216.

84. Post, R.M., Weiss, S.R., and Pert, A. (1988). Cocaine-induced behavioral sensitization and kindling: Implications for the emergence of psychopathology and seizures. *Ann N Y Acad Sci*, 537:292–308.

85. Herman, L., Hougland, T., and El Mallakh, R.S. (2007). Mimicking human bipolar ion dysregulation models mania in rats. *Neurosci Biobehav Rev*, 31(6):874–881.

86. Looney, S.W. and El Mallakh, R.S. (1997). Meta-analysis of erythrocyte Na,K-ATPase activity in bipolar illness. *Depress Anxiety*, 5(2):53–65.

87. Jones, S.H. (2001). Circadian rhythms, multilevel models of emotion and bipolar disorder – an initial step towards integration? *Clin Psychol Rev*, 21(8):1193–1209.

88. Wehr, T.A. (1989). Sleep loss: A preventable cause of mania and other excited states. *J Clin Psychiatry*, 50(Suppl):8–16.

89. Perlman, C.A., Johnson, S.L., and Mellman, T.A. (2006). The prospective impact of sleep duration on depression and mania. *Bipolar Disord*, 8(3):271–274.

90. Laposky, A., Easton, A., Dugovic, C., Walisser, J., Bradfield, C., and Turek, F. (2005). Deletion of the mammalian circadian clock gene BMAL1/Mop3 alters baseline sleep architecture and the response to sleep deprivation. *Sleep*, 28(4):395–409.

91. Manev, H. and Uz, T. (2006). Clock genes: Influencing and being influenced by psychoactive drugs. *Trends Pharmacol Sci*, 27(4):186–189.

92. Wirz-Justice, A. (2006). Biological rhythm disturbances in mood disorders. *Int Clin Psychopharmacol*, 21(Suppl 1):S11–S15.

93. McClung, C.A. (2007). Circadian genes, rhythms and the biology of mood disorders. *Pharmacol Ther*, 114(2):222–232.

94. Kaladchibachi, S.A., Doble, B., Anthopoulos, N., Woodgett, J.R., and Manoukian, A.S. (2007). Glycogen synthase kinase 3, circadian rhythms, and bipolar disorder: A molecular link in the therapeutic action of lithium. *J Circadian Rhythms*, 5:3.

95. Benedetti, F., Barbini, B., Fulgosi, M.C., Colombo, C., Dallaspezia, S., Pontiggia, A. *et al.* (2005). Combined total sleep deprivation and light therapy in the treatment of drug-resistant bipolar depression: Acute response and long-term remission rates. *J Clin Psychiatry*, 66(12):1535–1540.

96. Papadimitriou, G.N., Dikeos, D.G., Soldatos, C.R., and Calabrese, J.R. (2007). Non-pharmacological treatments in the management of rapid cycling bipolar disorder. *J Affect Disord*, 98(1–2):1–10.

97. Riemann, D., Voderholzer, U., and Berger, M. (2002). Sleep and sleep-wake manipulations in bipolar depression. *Neuropsychobiology*, 45(Suppl 1):7–12.

98. Gessa, G.L., Pani, L., Fadda, P., and Fratta, W. (1995). Sleep deprivation in the rat: An animal model of mania. *Eur Neuropsychopharmacol*, 5(Suppl):89–93.

99. Easton, A., Arbuzova, J., and Turek, F.W. (2003). The circadian Clock mutation increases exploratory activity and escape-seeking behavior. *Genes Brain Behav*, 2(1):11–19.

100. Roybal, K., Theobold, D., Graham, A., Dinieri, J.A., Russo, S.J., Krishnan, V. *et al.* (2007). Mania-like behavior induced by disruption of CLOCK. *Proc Natl Acad Sci USA*, 104(15):6406–6411.

101. Frazer, A. and Morilak, D.A. (2005). What should animal models of depression model? *Neurosci Biobehav Rev*, 29(4–5):515–523.

102. Jones, S.H. and Tarrier, N. (2005). New developments in bipolar disorder. *Clin Psychol Rev*, 25(8):1003–1007.

103. Jones, S.H., Sellwood, W., and McGovern, J. (2005). Psychological therapies for bipolar disorder: The role of model-driven approaches to therapy integration. *Bipolar Disord*, 7(1):22–32.

104. Bowden, C.L. (2005). A different depression: Clinical distinctions between bipolar and unipolar depression. *J Affect Disord*, 84(2–3):117–125.

105. Machado-Vieira, R., Kapczinski, F., and Soares, J.C. (2004). Perspectives for the development of animal models of bipolar disorder. *Prog Neuropsychopharmacol Biol Psychiatry*, 28(2):209–224.

106. Goodnick, P.J. (2007). Bipolar depression: A review of randomised clinical trials. *Expert Opin Pharmacother*, 8(1):13–21.

107. Bourin, M., Masse, F., and Hascoet, M. (2005). Evidence for the activity of lamotrigine at 5-HT(1A) receptors in the mouse forced swimming test. *J Psychiatry Neurosci*, 30(4):275–282.

108. Song, C. and Leonard, B.E. (2005). The olfactory bulbectomised rat as a model of depression. *Neurosci Biobehav Rev*, 29(4–5):627–647.

109. Slattery, D.A., Markou, A., and Cryan, J.F. (2007). Evaluation of reward processes in an animal model of depression. *Psychopharmacology (Berl)*, 190(4):555–568.

110. Song, C., Killeen, A.A., and Leonard, B.E. (1994). Catalase, superoxide dismutase and glutathione peroxidase activity in neutrophils of sham-operated and olfactory-bulbectomised rats following chronic treatment with desipramine and lithium chloride. *Neuropsychobiology*, 30(1):24–28.

111. Dienes, K.A., Hammen, C., Henry, R.M., Cohen, A.N., and Daley, S.E. (2006). The stress sensitization hypothesis: Understanding the course of bipolar disorder. *J Affect Disord*, 95(1–3):43–49.

112. Johnson, S.L. and Roberts, J.E. (1995). Life events and bipolar disorder: Implications from biological theories. *Psychol Bull*, 117(3):434–449.

113. Willner, P. (2005). Chronic mild stress (CMS) revisited: Consistency and behavioural-neurobiological concordance in the effects of CMS. *Neuropsychobiology*, 52(2):90–110.

114. Willner, P. (1997). Validity, reliability and utility of the chronic mild stress model of depression: A 10-year review and evaluation. *Psychopharmacology (Berl)*, 134(4):319–329.

115. Willner, P., Muscat, R., and Papp, M. (1992). Chronic mild stress-induced anhedonia: A realistic animal model of depression. *Neurosci Biobehav Rev*, 16(4):525–534.

116. Koolhaas, J.M., De Boer, S.F., De Rutter, A.J., Meerlo, P., and Sgoifo, A. (1997). Social stress in rats and mice. *Acta Physiol Scand Suppl*, 640:69–72.

117. Razzoli, M., Roncari, E., Guidi, A., Carboni, L., Arban, R., Gerrard, P. *et al.* (2006). Conditioning properties of social subordination in rats: Behavioral and biochemical correlates of anxiety. *Horm Behav*, 50(2):245–251.

118. Rygula, R., Abumaria, N., Flugge, G., Fuchs, E., Ruther, E., and Havemann-Reinecke, U. (2005). Anhedonia and motivational deficits in rats: Impact of chronic social stress. *Behav Brain Res*, 162(1):127–134.

119. Keeney, A., Jessop, D.S., Harbuz, M.S., Marsden, C.A., Hogg, S., and Blackburn-Munro, R.E. (2006). Differential effects of acute and chronic social defeat stress on hypothalamic-pituitary-adrenal axis function and hippocampal serotonin release in mice. *J Neuroendocrinol*, 18(5):330–338.

120. Razzoli, M., Carboni, L., Guidi, A., Gerrard, P., and Arban, R. (2007). Social defeat-induced contextual conditioning differentially imprints behavioral and adrenal reactivity: A time-course study in the rat. *Physiol Behav*, 92(4):734–740.

121. Rygula, R., Abumaria, N., Domenici, E., Hiemke, C., and Fuchs, E. (2006). Effects of fluoxetine on behavioral deficits evoked by chronic social stress in rats. *Behav Brain Res*, 174(1):188–192.

122. Rygula, R., Abumaria, N., Flugge, G., Hiemke, C., Fuchs, E., Ruther, E. *et al.* (2006). Citalopram counteracts depressive-like symptoms evoked by chronic social stress in rats. *Behav Pharmacol*, 17(1):19–29.

123. von Frijtag, J.C., van den, B.R., and Spruijt, B.M. (2002). Imipramine restores the long-term impairment of appetitive behavior in socially stressed rats. *Psychopharmacology (Berl)*, 162(3):232–238.

124. Sachs, G.S. and Rush, A.J. (2003). Response, remission, and recovery in bipolar disorders: What are the realistic treatment goals? *J Clin Psychiatry*, 64(Suppl 6):18–22.

125. Coryell, W. (2005). Rapid cycling bipolar disorder: Clinical characteristics and treatment options. *CNS Drugs*, 19(7):557–569.

126. Swann, A.C., Bowden, C.L., Calabrese, J.R., Dilsaver, S.C., and Morris, D.D. (2000). Mania: Differential effects of previous depressive and manic episodes on response to treatment. *Acta Psychiatr Scand*, 101(6):444–451.

127. Post, R.M. (1992). Transduction of psychosocial stress into the neurobiology of recurrent affective disorder. *Am J Psychiatry*, 149(8):999–1010.

128. Post, R.M., Weiss, S.R., Smith, M., Rosen, J., and Frye, M. (1995). Stress, conditioning, and the temporal aspects of affective disorders. *Ann N Y Acad Sci*, 771:677–696.

129. Post, R.M. (2007). Kindling and sensitization as models for affective episode recurrence, cyclicity, and tolerance phenomena. *Neurosci Biobehav Rev*, 31(6):858–873.

130. Idris, N.F., Repeto, P., Neill, J.C., and Large, C.H. (2005). Investigation of the effects of lamotrigine and clozapine in improving reversal-learning impairments induced by acute phencyclidine and D-amphetamine in the rat. *Psychopharmacology (Berl)*, 179(2):336-348.

131. Hirsch, L.J., Weintraub, D., Du, Y., Buchsbaum, R., Spencer, H.T., Hager, M. *et al.* (2004). Correlating lamotrigine serum concentrations with tolerability in patients with epilepsy. *Neurology*, 63(6):1022-1026.

132. Rambeck, B. and Wolf, P. (1993). Lamotrigine clinical pharmacokinetics. *Clin Pharmacokinet*, 25(6):433-443.

133. Rambeck, B., Jurgens, U.H., May, T.W., Pannek, H.W., Behne, F., Ebner, A. *et al.* (2006). Comparison of brain extracellular fluid, brain tissue, cerebrospinal fluid, and serum concentrations of antiepileptic drugs measured intraoperatively in patients with intractable epilepsy. *Epilepsia*, 47(4):681-694.

134. Nierenberg, A.A., Ostacher, M.J., Calabrese, J.R., Ketter, T.A., Marangell, L.B., Miklowitz, D.J. *et al.* (2006). Treatment-resistant bipolar depression: A STEP-BD equipoise randomized effectiveness trial of antidepressant augmentation with lamotrigine, inositol, or risperidone. *Am J Psychiatry*, 163(2):210-216.

135. Goodwin, G.M., Bowden, C.L., Calabrese, J.R., Grunze, H., Kasper, S., White, R. *et al.* (2004). A pooled analysis of 2 placebo-controlled 18-month trials of lamotrigine and lithium maintenance in bipolar I disorder. *J Clin Psychiatry*, 65(3):432-441.

136. Nissinen, J. and Pitkanen, A. (2007). Effect of antiepileptic drugs on spontaneous seizures in epileptic rats. *Epilepsy Res*, 73(2):181-191.

137. Castel-Branco, M.M., Falcao, A.C., Figueiredo, I.V., and Caramona, M.M. (2005). Lamotrigine pharmacokinetic/pharmacodynamic modelling in rats. *Fundam Clin Pharmacol*, 19(6):669-675.

138. Schou, M. (2001). Lithium treatment at 52. *J Affect Disord*, 67(1-3):21-32.

139. Lenox, R.H., McNamara, R.K., Papke, R.L., and Manji, H.K. (1998). Neurobiology of lithium: An update. *J Clin Psychiatry*, 59(Suppl 6):37-47.

140. Ong, J.C., Brody, S.A., Large, C.H., and Geyer, M.A. (2005). An investigation of the efficacy of mood stabilizers in rodent models of prepulse inhibition. *J Pharmacol Exp Ther*, 315(3):1163-1171.

141. Fisher, R.S. (1989). Animal models of the epilepsies. *Brain Res Brain Res Rev*, 14(3):245-278.

142. Sadock, J. and Kaplan, H. (2002). *Synopsis of Psychiatry*. Lippincott and Williams, UK.

143. Einat, H. (2006). Modelling facets of mania – new directions related to the notion of Endophenotypes. *J Psychopharmacol*, 20(5):714-722.

144. Gould, T.D., Picchini, A.M., Einat, H., and Manji, H.K. (2006). Targeting glycogen synthase kinase-3 in the CNS: Implications for the development of new treatments for mood disorders. *Curr Drug Targets*, 7(11):1399-1409.

145. Shaltiel, G., Chen, G., and Manji, H.K. (2007). Neurotrophic signaling cascades in the pathophysiology and treatment of bipolar disorder. *Curr Opin Pharmacol*, 7(1):22-26.

146. Manji, H.K., Quiroz, J.A., Payne, J.L., Singh, J., Lopes, B.P., Viegas, J.S. *et al.* (2003). The underlying neurobiology of bipolar disorder. *World Psychiatry*, 2(3):136-146.

147. Chen, G. and Manji, H.K. (2006). The extracellular signal-regulated kinase pathway: An emerging promising target for mood stabilizers. *Curr Opin Psychiatry*, 19(3):313-323.

148. Carlson, P.J., Singh, J.B., Zarate, C.A., Jr, Drevets, W.C., and Manji, H.K. (2006). Neural circuitry and neuroplasticity in mood disorders: Insights for novel therapeutic targets. *NeuroRx*, 3(1):22-41.

149. Zarate, C.A., Jr, Singh, J., and Manji, H.K. (2006). Cellular plasticity cascades: Targets for the development of novel therapeutics for bipolar disorder. *Biol Psychiatry*, 59(11):1006-1020.

150. Bachmann, R.F., Schloesser, R.J., Gould, T.D., and Manji, H.K. (2005). Mood stabilizers target cellular plasticity and resilience cascades: Implications for the development of novel therapeutics. *Mol Neurobiol*, 32(2):173-202.

151. Gould, T.D. and Manji, H.K. (2005). Glycogen synthase kinase-3: A putative molecular target for lithium mimetic drugs. *Neuropsychopharmacology*, 30(7):1223–1237.

152. Gould, T.D., Quiroz, J.A., Singh, J., Zarate, C.A., and Manji, H.K. (2004). Emerging experimental therapeutics for bipolar disorder: Insights from the molecular and cellular actions of current mood stabilizers. *Mol Psychiatry*, 9(8):734–755.

153. Chen, G., Huang, L.D., Jiang, Y.M., and Manji, H.K. (1999). The mood-stabilizing agent valproate inhibits the activity of glycogen synthase kinase-3. *J Neurochem*, 72(3):1327–1330.

154. Stambolic, V., Ruel, L., and Woodgett, J.R. (1996). Lithium inhibits glycogen synthase kinase-3 activity and mimics wingless signalling in intact cells. *Curr Biol*, 6(12):1664–1668.

155. Benedetti, F., Serretti, A., Pontiggia, A., Bernasconi, A., Lorenzi, C., Colombo, C. *et al.* (2005). Long-term response to lithium salts in bipolar illness is influenced by the glycogen synthase kinase 3-beta -50 T/C SNP. *Neurosci Lett*, 376(1):51–55.

156. Gould, T.D., Einat, H., Bhat, R., and Manji, H.K. (2004). AR-A014418, a selective GSK-3 inhibitor, produces antidepressant-like effects in the forced swim test. *Int J Neuropsychopharmacol*, 7(4):387–390.

157. Gould, T.D., Picchini, A.M., Einat, H., and Manji, H.K. (2006). Targeting glycogen synthase kinase-3 in the CNS: Implications for the development of new treatments for mood disorders. *Curr Drug Targets*, 7(11):1399–1409.

158. Kaidanovich-Beilin, O., Milman, A., Weizman, A., Pick, C.G., and Eldar-Finkelman, H. (2004). Rapid antidepressive-like activity of specific glycogen synthase kinase-3 inhibitor and its effect on beta-catenin in mouse hippocampus. *Biol Psychiatry*, 55(8):781–784.

159. O'Brien, W.T., Harper, A.D., Jove, F., Woodgett, J.R., Maretto, S., Piccolo, S. *et al.* (2004). Glycogen synthase kinase-3beta haploinsufficiency mimics the behavioral and molecular effects of lithium. *J Neurosci*, 24(30):6791–6798.

160. Gould, T.D., Einat, H., O'donnell, K.C., Picchini, A.M., Schloesser, R.J., and Manji, H.K. (2007). Beta-Catenin overexpression in the mouse brain phenocopies lithium-sensitive behaviors. *Neuropsychopharmacology*, 32(10):2173–2783.

161. Kozlovsky, N., Nadri, C., Belmaker, R.H., and Agam, G. (2003). Lack of effect of mood stabilizers or neuroleptics on GSK-3 protein levels and GSK-3 activity. *Int J Neuropsychopharmacol*, 6(2):117–120.

162. Bebchuk, J.M., Arfken, C.L., Dolan-Manji, S., Murphy, J., Hasanat, K., and Manji, H.K. (2000). A preliminary investigation of a protein kinase C inhibitor in the treatment of acute mania. *Arch Gen Psychiatry*, 57(1):95–97.

163. Zarate, C.A., Jr, Singh, J.B., Carlson, P.J., Quiroz, J., Jolkovsky, L., Luckenbaugh, D.A. *et al.* (2007). Efficacy of a protein kinase C inhibitor (tamoxifen) in the treatment of acute mania: A pilot study. *Bipolar Disord*, 9(6):561–570.

164. Gottesman, I.I. and Gould, T.D. (2003). The endophenotype concept in psychiatry: Etymology and strategic intentions. *Am J Psychiatry*, 160(4):636–645.

165. Hasler, G., Drevets, W.C., Manji, H.K., and Charney, D.S. (2004). Discovering endophenotypes for major depression. *Neuropsychopharmacology*, 29(10):1765–1781.

166. Drevets, W.C., Ongur, D., and Price, J.L. (1998). Reduced glucose metabolism in the subgenual prefrontal cortex in unipolar depression. *Mol Psychiatry*, 3(3):190–191.

167. Sapolsky, R.M. (2000). Glucocorticoids and hippocampal atrophy in neuropsychiatric disorders. *Arch Gen Psychiatry*, 57(10):925–935.

168. Watson, S., Gallagher, P., Ritchie, J.C., Ferrier, I.N., and Young, A.H. (2004). Hypothalamic-pituitary-adrenal axis function in patients with bipolar disorder. *Br J Psychiatry*, 184:496–502.

169. Brown, S.M., Henning, S., and Wellman, C.L. (2005). Mild, short-term stress alters dendritic morphology in rat medial prefrontal cortex. *Cereb Cortex*, 15(11):1714–1722.

170. Cook, S.C. and Wellman, C.L. (2004). Chronic stress alters dendritic morphology in rat medial prefrontal cortex. *J Neurobiol*, 60(2):236–248.

171. Pezawas, L., Verchinski, B.A., Mattay, V.S., Callicott, J.H., Kolachana, B.S., Straub, R.E. *et al.* (2004). The brain-derived neurotrophic factor val66met polymorphism and variation in human cortical morphology. *J Neurosci*, 24(45):10099–10102.

172. Egan, M.F., Kojima, M., Callicott, J.H., Goldberg, T.E., Kolachana, B.S., Bertolino, A. *et al.* (2003). The BDNF val66met polymorphism affects activity-dependent secretion of BDNF and human memory and hippocampal function. *Cell*, 112(2):257–269.

173. Hariri, A.R., Goldberg, T.E., Mattay, V.S., Kolachana, B.S., Callicott, J.H., Egan, M.F. *et al.* (2003). Brain-derived neurotrophic factor val66met polymorphism affects human memory-related hippocampal activity and predicts memory performance. *J Neurosci*, 23(17):6690–6694.

174. Einat, H., Manji, H.K., Gould, T.D., Du, J., and Chen, G. (2003). Possible involvement of the ERK signaling cascade in bipolar disorder: Behavioral leads from the study of mutant mice. *Drug News Perspect*, 16(7):453–463.

175. Post, R.M. (2007). Role of BDNF in bipolar and unipolar disorder: Clinical and theoretical implications. *J Psychiatr Res*, 41(12):979–990.

176. Glitz, D.A., Manji, H.K., and Moore, G.J. (2002). Mood disorders: Treatment-induced changes in brain neurochemistry and structure. *Semin Clin Neuropsychiatry*, 7(4):269–280.

177. Moore, G.J., Bebchuk, J.M., Wilds, I.B., Chen, G., and Manji, H.K. (2000). Lithium-induced increase in human brain grey matter. *Lancet*, 356(9237):1241–1242.

178. Jackson, A., Cavanagh, J., and Scott, J. (2003). A systematic review of manic and depressive prodromes. *J Affect Disord*, 74(3):209–217.

179. Harvey, A.G., Schmidt, D.A., Scarna, A., Semler, C.N., and Goodwin, G.M. (2005). Sleep-related functioning in euthymic patients with bipolar disorder, patients with insomnia, and subjects without sleep problems. *Am J Psychiatry*, 162(1):50–57.

180. Harvey, A.G., Mullin, B.C., and Hinshaw, S.P. (2006). Sleep and circadian rhythms in children and adolescents with bipolar disorder. *Dev Psychopathol*, 18(4):1147–1168.

181. Hakkarainen, R., Johansson, C., Kieseppa, T., Partonen, T., Koskenvuo, M., Kaprio, J. *et al.* (2003). Seasonal changes, sleep length and circadian preference among twins with bipolar disorder. *BMC Psychiatry*, 3:6.

182. Benedetti, F., Barbini, B., Campori, E., Fulgosi, M.C., Pontiggia, A., and Colombo, C. (2001). Sleep phase advance and lithium to sustain the antidepressant effect of total sleep deprivation in bipolar depression: New findings supporting the internal coincidence model? *J Psychiatr Res*, 35(6):323–329.

183. Benedetti, F., Serretti, A., Colombo, C., Barbini, B., Lorenzi, C., Campori, E. *et al.* (2003). Influence of CLOCK gene polymorphism on circadian mood fluctuation and illness recurrence in bipolar depression. *Am J Med Genet B Neuropsychiatr Genet*, 123(1):23–26.

184. Benedetti, F., Serretti, A., Colombo, C., Lorenzi, C., Tubazio, V., and Smeraldi, E. (2004). A glycogen synthase kinase 3-beta promoter gene single nucleotide polymorphism is associated with age at onset and response to total sleep deprivation in bipolar depression. *Neurosci Lett*, 368(2):123–126.

185. Fletcher, A.J., Edwards, L.D., Fox, A.W., Stonier, P. (2002). *Principles and Practice of Pharmaceutical Medicine*, John Wiley & Sons, Ltd, London.

186. Rogawski, M.A. and Loscher, W. (2004). The neurobiology of antiepileptic drugs for the treatment of nonepileptic conditions. *Nat Med*, 10(7):685–692.

187. Bowden, C.L. and Karren, N.U. (2006). Anticonvulsants in bipolar disorder. *Aust N Z J Psychiatry*, 40(5):386–393.

188. Bowden, C.L. (2001). Novel treatments for bipolar disorder. *Expert Opin Investig Drugs*, 10(4):661–671.

189. Hiemke, C., Dragicevic, A., Grunder, G., Hatter, S., Sachse, J., Vernaleken, I. *et al.* (2004). Therapeutic monitoring of new antipsychotic drugs. *Ther Drug Monit*, 26(2):156–160.

190. Seeman, P. (2002). Atypical antipsychotics: Mechanism of action. *Can J Psychiatry*, 47(1):27–38.

191. Tergau, F., Wischer, S., Somal, H.S., Nitsche, M.A., Mercer, A.J., Paulus, W. *et al.* (2003). Relationship between lamotrigine oral dose, serum level and its inhibitory effect on CNS: Insights from transcranial magnetic stimulation. *Epilepsy Res*, 56(1):67–77.

192. Ziemann, U. (2004). TMS and drugs. *Clin Neurophysiol*, 115(8):1717–1729.

193. Rossini, P.M. and Rossi, S. (2007). Transcranial magnetic stimulation: Diagnostic, therapeutic, and research potential. *Neurology*, 68(7):484–488.

194. Li, X., Teneback, C.C., Nahas, Z., Kozel, F.A., Large, C., Cohn, J. *et al.* (2004). Interleaved transcranial magnetic stimulation/functional MRI confirms that lamotrigine inhibits cortical excitability in healthy young men. *Neuropsychopharmacology*, 29(7):1395–1407.

195. Drevets, W.C., Gautier, C., Price, J.C., Kupfer, D.J., Kinahan, P.E., Grace, A.A. *et al.* (2001). Amphetamine-induced dopamine release in human ventral striatum correlates with euphoria. *Biol Psychiatry*, 49(2):81–96.

196. Anand, A., Charney, D.S., Oren, D.A., Berman, R.M., Hu, X.S., Cappiello, A. *et al.* (2000). Attenuation of the neuropsychiatric effects of ketamine with lamotrigine: Support for hyperglutamatergic effects of N-methyl-D-aspartate receptor antagonists. *Arch Gen Psychiatry*, 57(3):270–276.

197. Norra, C. (2007). Challenge tests of monoaminergic systems: Neurophysiological aspects. *Clin EEG Neurosci*, 38(2):66–73.

198. Booij, L., Van der Does, A.J., and Riedel, W.J. (2003). Monoamine depletion in psychiatric and healthy populations: Review. *Mol Psychiatry*, 8(12):951–973.

199. Booij, L., Van der Does, A.J., Haffmans, P.M., and Riedel, W.J. (2005). Acute tryptophan depletion in depressed patients treated with a selective serotonin-noradrenalin reuptake inhibitor: Augmentation of antidepressant response? *J Affect Disord*, 86(2–3):305–311.

200. Van der Does, A.J. and Booij, L. (2005). Cognitive therapy does not prevent a response to tryptophan depletion in patients also treated with antidepressants. *Biol Psychiatry*, 58(11):913–915.

201. Wirz-Justice, A. and Van den Hoofdakker, R.H. (1999). Sleep deprivation in depression: What do we know, where do we go? *Biol Psychiatry*, 46(4):445–453.

202. Giedke, H. and Schwarzler, F. (2002). Therapeutic use of sleep deprivation in depression. *Sleep Med Rev*, 6(5):361–377.

203. Cohen, J., Cairns, C., Paquette, C., and Faden, L. (2006). Comparing patient access to pharmaceuticals in the UK and US. *Appl Health Econ Health Policy*, 5(3):177–187.

204. Vieta, E. and Carne, X. (2005). The use of placebo in clinical trials on bipolar disorder: A new approach for an old debate. *Psychother Psychosom*, 74(1):10–16.

205. Wang, S.J., O'Neill, R.T., and Hung, H.M. (2007). Approaches to evaluation of treatment effect in randomized clinical trials with genomic subset. *Pharm Stat*, 6(3):227–244.

206. Tohen, M., Calabrese, J., Vieta, E., Bowden, C., Gonzalez-Pinto, A., Lin, D. *et al.* (2007). Effect of comorbid anxiety on treatment response in bipolar depression. *J Affect Disord*, 104(1–3):137–146.

207. Maloney, A., Karlsson, M.O., and Simonsson, U.S. (2007). Optimal adaptive design in clinical drug development: A simulation example. *J Clin Pharmacol*, 47(10):1231–1243.

208. Desseaux, K. and Porcher, R. (2007). Flexible two-stage design with sample size reassessment for survival trials. *Stat Med*, 26(27):5002–5013.

209. Schmidli, H., Bretz, F., and Racine-Poon, A. (2007). Bayesian predictive power for interim adaptation in seamless phase II/III trials where the endpoint is survival up to some specified timepoint. *Stat Med*, 26(27):4925–4938.

Towards a Biological Understanding of ADHD and the Discovery of Novel Therapeutic Approaches

Rosemary Tannock[1,4], Brian Campbell[2], Patricia Seymour[2], Daniele Ouellet[3], Holly Soares[2], Paul Wang[2] and Phillip Chappell[2]

[1]Human Development and Applied Psychology, The Ontario Institute for Studies in Education, University of Toronto, Room 9-288, 252 Bloor Street West, Toronto ON M5S 1V6 Canada
[2]Pfizer Global Research and Development, Eastern Point Road, MS 8220–4012, Groton, CT 06340, USA
[3]GlaxoSmithKline, Five Moore Drive, Research Triangle Park, NC 27709, USA
[4]Neurosciences and Mental Health Research Program, Research Institute of the Hospital for Sick Children, Toronto, Ontario M5G 1X8, Canada

Animal and Translational Models for CNS Drug Discovery,
Vol. 1 of 3: Psychiatric Disorders
Robert McArthur and Franco Borsini (eds), Academic Press, 2008

INTRODUCTION

Attention-deficit/hyperactivity disorder (ADHD) is recognized as a priority clinical and public health concern because of its prevalence, chronicity, and associated morbidity and impairment in children, adolescents, and adults[1] (Report of the Surgeon General, US Public Health Service). Recent meta-analyses confirm that ADHD is one of the most common neurobehavioral disorders of childhood with worldwide prevalence rates conservatively estimated at 4–10%[2,3] (also, for recent epidemiological studies in Africa[4,5]). ADHD is also common in adults. Recent epidemiological studies using validated survey instruments indicate that about 3–4% of adults meet the DSM-IV diagnostic criteria for ADHD in North and South America, Europe, and the Middle East.[6,7] In general, ADHD affects more males than females (ratio of 3:1), but gender ratios vary substantially as a function of age (child, adolescent, adult) and whether the sample was derived from a clinic or the community.[3,8,9]

ADHD is one of the most extensively investigated mental health disorders of childhood and adolescence.[10] Nonetheless, it lacks specific biomarkers and remains underspecified. Moreover, ADHD is undergoing reconceptualization and the emerging neuroscientific understanding of ADHD challenges current targets for treatment.

In this chapter, we first provide an update on the clinical and neuroscientific perspectives on ADHD and then highlight the historical and current development of pharmacological treatment approaches. The chapter concludes with a discussion of the potential utility of biomarkers in drug development and the clinical challenges in pursuing novel pharmacological approaches for ADHD, given its primacy as a pediatric disorder.

CLINICAL AND NEUROSCIENTIFIC UPDATE OF ADHD: AN ACADEMIC PERSPECTIVE

Current Clinical Concepts of ADHD

From a clinical perspective, ADHD continues to be conceptualized and described as a mental health disorder, although its neurobiological features (described below) are generally acknowledged. It is characterized and defined by a persistent and pervasive pattern of symptoms of inattention, impulsivity, and hyperactivity, which first manifest in early childhood and are developmentally inappropriate and impairing.[11] The definition and diagnostic criteria for ADHD have changed considerably over the past century and are expected to continue to evolve over the next. For example, the essential clinical features of disorders of inattention (inconsistency of attention, which included both poor concentration and hyperfocusing) were first proposed by Dr. Alexander Crichton in 1798[12] and still map well to current descriptions of inattention and predominantly inattentive subtype.[11] The distinction between inattention and disruptive symptomatology (hyperactivity, impulsivity, non-compliance) was preserved in Heinrich Hoffman's descriptions of children seen in his clinic,[13] but this early recognition of the clinical significance of inattention was somewhat overshadowed by Dr. George Still's[14-16] emphasis on the disruptive symptomatology, which he interpreted as an "abnormal defect in moral control." Subsequent descriptions throughout the various iterations of the DSM and ICD taxonomies (International Classification of Diseases, WHO 1993) have continued to vacillate in their relative emphasis on inattention versus hyperactivity and impulsivity. Moreover, neuroscientific advances, based upon categorical and dimensional approaches to the investigation of ADHD and its comorbid disorders, may well change the current conceptualization and understanding of the behavioral phenotype and thus also change the treatment targets and approaches.

Clinical Phenomenology

The DSM-IV-TR diagnostic criteria for ADHD, which are currently applied to all ages and both genders, require the individual to demonstrate a minimum of six symptoms of hyperactivity or inattention that have persisted for a minimum of 6 months and are maladaptive plus inconsistent with developmental level. In addition, the following criteria must be met for a diagnosis: (1) identified symptoms must be evident before

7 years of age; (2) some impairment from the symptoms must be present in two or more settings (e.g., at school [or work] and at home); (3) there must be clear evidence of clinically significant impairment in social, academic, or occupational functioning; and (4) the symptoms do not occur exclusively during the course of a pervasive developmental disorder, schizophrenia, or other psychotic disorder and are not better accounted for by another mental disorder (e.g., mood disorder, anxiety disorder, dissociative disorder, or personality disorder).[i]

The clinical symptoms listed in the DSM-IV are heterogeneous and tend to manifest differently as a function of age, gender, comorbidity, and environmental context. Moreover as a clinical category, ADHD is highly heterogeneous in terms of its clinical presentation and treatment response, as well as in its probable pathophysiology and etiology.[17]

One of the most striking clinical characteristics, albeit not formally included in the diagnostic criteria, is the marked variability and inconsistency in behavioral symptoms and task performance.[18,19] Symptoms and performance fluctuate moment-to-moment and appear to be context-specific and vary as a function of the cognitive complexity and demand of the specific task. Rapid, flexible adaptation to changing demands of academic and social situations is rarely observed. In other words, one striking feature of ADHD is the consistency of inconsistency in behavior, regardless of whether the term "behavior" is used in the narrow sense of observable movements, or more broadly to include reaction times, errors, cognitive function, and eye-fixations etc. Until recently, intra-individual variability has been viewed as uninformative "noise" and largely ignored. However, as indicated in a later subsection, this type of moment-to-moment variability is now the focus of current theoretical and empirical work.[19-21]

Symptom Dimensions of ADHD, Subtypes: Age and Gender Differences

Factor analyses and latent class models have generally confirmed two separate symptom dimensions of ADHD (inattentive, hyperactive/impulsive) that can occur alone or in combination, but with marked variability in severity.[22-24] Findings generally hold across informants, cultures and gender in child and adolescent populations[24,25]: they may not hold for preschoolers.[26] Moreover, the DSM criteria have not been validated for adults: they do not include developmentally appropriate symptoms and threshold for adults, and fail to identify some adults who are nonetheless significantly impaired.[27]

Notably, the two dimensions are associated with different forms of functional impairment, developmental trajectories, and patterns of comorbidity. For instance, research has confirmed a differential rate of symptomatic decline of inattention versus hyperactive/impulsive symptoms across adolescence and adulthood, with the latter declining at a faster rate than the former.[28,29] Also, the inattentive dimension (but not the hyperactivity dimension) has been linked with marked academic impairments in reading, writing, and mathematics,[30-33] as well as chronic smoking in adolescence.[34-36] Moreover the inattention dimension has been linked with poor executive function, with findings holding for children, adolescents and adults,[30,37-41] with early inattention predicting later executive function impairments.[42] By contrast, the hyperactivity/impulsivity dimension has been linked with more global impairment, altered reinforcement

---

[i] Please refer to DSM-IV-TR for current definitions of these other behavioral disorders.

mechanisms, and comorbidity with disruptive behavior disorders and significant social impairments.[40,43]

By contrast, attempts to differentiate the three subtypes of ADHD, defined according to the relative predominance of one or both symptoms clusters, have yielded inconsistent findings. The discrepant findings may be attributable to inherent weaknesses in the diagnostic criteria which may not be applicable equally across different stages of development, as well as to the differential impact of changing context-dependent demands with increasing age (e.g., home, school, work).

Evidence for gender differences in the clinical phenotype of ADHD is equivocal. Previously reported gender differences[8,44] may reflect referral biases, since studies of non-referred community samples generally fail to find major differences between boys and girls in terms of core symptoms, DSM-IV subtypes of ADHD, comorbidity, or treatment history.[45-47] A few exceptions are that school suspensions are more common in boys[45] and that boys with combined type ADHD tend to be more impaired in terms of social problems and school performance.[47] Also, gender differences may arise as a function of informant: teachers rate boys as showing more problems at school compared to girls, although parents do not report differences in the home setting.[48] The higher level of teacher reported problem behavior at school may explain the high male–female ratio for ADHD in clinical settings.

Collectively, these findings suggest that a focus on the dimensions of ADHD or its impairments (rather than solely on its categorical subtypes), along with consideration of environmental and genetic risk factors, may be fruitful for developing novel treatment approaches.

Comorbidity

ADHD shows marked overlap with both internalizing and externalizing disorders as well as with other neurodevelopmental disorders and later substance abuse disorders. Similar rates of comorbidity are found in both clinical and community samples of ADHD, as well as in pediatric and psychiatric samples.[49,50] Comorbidity rates are similar in adults with ADHD, except that diagnosis of antisocial personality disorder replaces oppositional defiant and conduct disorders and the rate of mood disorders increase.[51,52] The available data underestimate the extant rates of co-existing problems, particularly in clinic populations, in which it is not unusual for an individual to meet diagnostic criteria for two or more "disorders" in addition to ADHD. Moreover, clinicians and researchers rarely take into consideration sub-threshold levels of other DSM-IV disorders, which nonetheless cause additional impairments and negative outcomes. Comorbidity poses critical issues for treatment. For example, comorbid conditions may alter the ADHD phenotype in clinically meaningful ways, such as cognitive correlates, clinical course, impairments, or response to treatment. Also, additional treatment may be required for the comorbid conditions, or if the comorbid condition differs in its etiology, it may need a different treatment approach.

Clinical Course and Outcomes

ADHD persists into adolescence and adulthood in the majority of cases, although the rates of remission versus persistence are unclear, in part because of differences in the definition of remission and in the number of symptoms and level of impairment required for the diagnostic threshold.[28,53,54] Distinctions between syndromatic remission (full loss of diagnostic status), symptomatic remission (loss of partial diagnostic status), and functional remission (loss of partial diagnostic status, plus a full recovery) are important, since syndromatic remission would mean loss of eligibility for pharmacological treatment, and perhaps access to other services, despite ongoing impairment. According to these definitions, a recent clinical follow-up study found that only 40% of cases met full criteria for ADHD by about age 20 (i.e., 60% showed syndromatic remission), but 90% had at least five symptoms of ADHD plus marked impairment as indexed by a Global Assessment of Functioning score below 60 (i.e., only 10% showed symptomatic remission).[28] Thus, most individuals with ADHD are at risk for continuing impairment and symptoms that will require treatment.

Left untreated, ADHD does not have a benign clinical course: impairments are evident across the lifespan.[55] ADHD is associated with an increased risk for injuries (particularly in childhood) and motor vehicle accidents in adolescence and young adulthood.[54,56,57] Also, ADHD increases the risk for poor academic achievement, grade retention, and dropping out before high-school graduation.[42,58,59] Adults with ADHD are less likely to gain and retain full-time employment, have a lower income and experience more marital difficulties.[7,60] ADHD is also associated with an increased risk for teen pregnancy, and higher than expected rates of antisocial and criminal behavior.[61] Not surprisingly, therefore, ADHD is associated with substantial socioeconomic costs.[62-65]

Current Neuroscientific Concepts of ADHD

Despite the widespread public skepticism concerning the legitimacy of ADHD as a "real" disorder,[66,67] the scientific community views ADHD as a mental health disorder of neurobiological origin arising from a complex interaction of genetic and environmental factors that alter brain structure, function, and neurochemistry.[68,69]

Neuroscientific Theories

A shift in focus from hyperactivity to attention deficits as a defining feature of ADHD occurred in the 1970s, triggered by studies of vigilance deficits in children with ADHD.[70] Around this time, advances in scientific understanding of the functions of the prefrontal cortex (PFC), led to observations that behavioral problems evident in ADHD resembled those of patients with frontal lobe lesions,[71] and more recently to the hypothesis that ADHD is associated with impairments in prefrontal-striatal neural networks that give rise to poor executive functioning.[72,73] Accordingly, most current theories of ADHD converge on the central role of dopamine (DA) and dysregulation of the prefrontal cortex (PFC) and striatum in the pathophysiology and treatment of ADHD.[74] For example, Wender[75] proposed that subtle alterations in the dopaminergic and noradrenergic neurotransmitter systems might account for the core behavioral symptoms of ADHD and that the therapeutic mechanism of stimulant medication may be via its regulatory action on these neurotransmitter systems. More recently, Sagvolden and colleagues[76] proposed that hypodopaminergic pathways interact with environmental factors and other neurotransmitter systems to produce the core symptoms of ADHD and their variation across development. However, other biological theories have been forwarded that suggest the involvement of serotonergic,[77,78] noradrenergic,[79,80] cholinergic,[81] and glutamatergic[21,82] systems in the pathophysiology and treatment of ADHD. For instance, recent theories propose a disturbed interaction between DA and glutamatergic systems.[21,76,83]

Neurobiology of ADHD

Converging findings suggest a pathway that links genetic and environmental influences to structural and functional brain abnormalities in ADHD, which in turn lead to age-dependent behavioral manifestations that include cognitive impairments as well as the observable behavioral symptoms of inattention, hyperactivity, and impulsivity.

Genetic Risk Factors

ADHD is highly heritable as indicated by family, adoption, and twin studies, with the latter converging in their estimation of a heritability of around 77%.[84] Two approaches are used to investigate genetic factors in ADHD: the candidate gene approach which focuses on one or more genes and is driven *a priori* by theory and empirical evidence; and the genome scan, in which all chromosomal locations are studied without constraints of theory or prior empirical evidence.

Candidate gene studies have focused primarily on genes within the DA system, consistent with the prevailing DA theories of ADHD and the DA sites of action of drugs used to treat ADHD. To date, 7 genes for which the same variant has been studied in at least 3 case-control or family-based studies, show a significant relationship with ADHD: dopamine D_4 receptor (DRD4) gene, dopamine D_5 receptor (DRD5) gene, dopamine transporter (DAT) gene, dopamine-hydroxylase (DBH) gene, the serotonin transporter (5-HTT) gene, the serotonin receptor $5-HT_{1B}$ (HTR1B) gene, and the synaptosomal-associated protein 25 (SNAP-25) gene (see reviews in[74,85]). Also, variations in glutamatergic genes (GRIN2B) have also been associated with ADHD, but require replication.[86] Moreover, emergent pharmacogenetic approaches suggest a relationship between some of these gene markers and treatment response. For example, both the DRD4-7-repeat and the DAT-10-repeat alleles have been associated with a diminished response to methylphenidate, but findings are inconsistent, indicating the need for replication in larger-scale studies.[85]

To date, published genome scans have revealed only weak signals (i.e., LOD scores ≤4), but suggest that regions 5p, 17p11, and 16p13 may contain genes associated with ADHD.[87,88] However, the combination of genome scan plus candidate gene approaches appear promising. For example, preliminary evidence suggests that genetic variation at the DAT1 locus may underlie the ADHD linkage peak on chromosome 5.[87]

In general, however, results suggest that the genetic architecture of ADHD is complex, may vary across subgroups of patients, will interact in complex ways with environmental factors, and that each gene is likely to have very small effects.

Environmental Risk Factors: Gene–Environmental Interactions

Pre- and peri-natal exposure to environmental neurotoxins has been the primary focus of research on environmental risk factors in ADHD, as well as in other disorders.[89] Here, we focus on pre- and postnatal exposure to nicotine via maternal smoking during pregnancy and environmental exposure to tobacco smoke, for several reasons. First, preclinical studies provide robust evidence that nicotine is a neurodevelopmental neurotoxin.[90] For instance, in rodents, prenatal exposure to nicotine stimulates nicotinic acetylcholine receptors (nACHRs), which play a key role in brain development (e.g., cell replication and differentiation, synaptic development), produces persistent cholinergic and serotonergic hypoactivity, and disrupts auditory processing and learning in later life.[91,92] Second, maternal smoking during pregnancy has been shown to increase the risk for ADHD (or symptoms of ADHD) in the offspring, in both clinical and populations-based studies.[93,94] Third, pre- and peri-natal exposure to nicotine is associated with fetal growth restriction, prematurity and low birth weight, which in turn is associated with developmental disorders in the offspring, particularly ADHD.[95-97] Fourth, both prenatal and adolescent exposure to nicotine via tobacco smoke has been found to alter the development of white matter microstructure in the internal capsule, which contains auditory corticofugal fibers.[98] This latter finding might partly account for the link between pre- and peri-natal exposure to nicotine and poor auditory processing and reading.[99,100] ii

Gene–environment interactions involving prenatal smoking exposure have been demonstrated. One study found that children exposed prenatally to nicotine and homozygous for the DAT1-10-repeat allele were at greater risk for ADHD than children with only one of those risk factors.[101] More recently, findings from a twin study confirmed the role of gene–environment interactions in modulating the risk for ADHD: the strength of the associations between ADHD and polymorphisms of the DAT1 or DRD4 genes were increased if the child had also been exposed prenatally to nicotine.[102] Furthermore, these findings were extended to the neural nicotinic acetylcholine receptor alpha 4 subunit gene (CHRNA4), which is located on presynaptic dopaminergic neurons.[103] Specifically, not only was a significant interaction found between prenatal exposure to nicotine and CHRNA4 for severe combined type of ADHD (defined by latent class analysis), but also that prenatal nicotine exposure interacted with genotypes at three loci (CHRNA4, DAT1, and DRD4) in further increasing the risk for severe combined type ADHD.[103]

Structural and Functional Brain Abnormalities

Structural brain imaging studies conducted over the last two decades provide convincing evidence of overall and regional reductions in brain volumes in children and adolescents with ADHD, particularly in the PFC region. Meta-analysis of these studies demonstrated reliable regional reductions in caudate, cerebellar vermis, and corpus callosum, as well as the PFC.[104] Importantly, findings from a large-scale longitudinal study (which permitted repeated scans of participants) suggest that the neuroanatomical abnormalities are present early in childhood, are non-progressive, reveal a delay in cortical maturation, and probably reflect early environmental and/or genetic effects.[105-107] Notably, the delay in cortical maturation (as indexed by cortical thickness) was most pronounced in the prefrontal brain regions,[106] which support an array of critical cognitive control functions, such as the ability to inhibit inappropriate thoughts and actions, executive control of attention,

---

ii Please refer to Markou *et al.*, Contribution of animal models and preclinical human studies to medication development for nicotine dependence, in Volume 3, *Reward Deficit Disorders*, for a review of nicotine and nicotine dependence.

working memory, high-order motor control, and evaluation of reward contingencies.[108] Deficits in these cognitive functions have been linked with ADHD.[20,109]

Meta-analysis and systematic reviews of functional neuroimaging studies suggests reduced activation primarily in the left PFC and striatum, and to some extent in temporal and parietal cortices (i.e., outside the frontal-striatal regions) during performance on tasks tapping attention processes, inhibition, working memory, and motor control.[110,111] For example, youngsters with ADHD were found to manifest dysfunctional attentional networks (alerting, orienting, executive control) in terms of both behavioral and neural (functional magnetic resonance imaging [fMRI]) measures, indicative of poor cortical control.[112] Moreover, reduced activity in the striatum, which is a major site of action of stimulant medication, correlated negatively with the severity of hyperactivity/impulsivity symptoms.[112]

Investigations of connectivity within and between brain regions reveal anomalies in white matter in prefrontal regions that influence attention and executive function, indicative of reduced frontostriatal connectivity.[113,114] Moreover, variation in the frontostriatal white matter tracts in individuals with ADHD was found to be related to their cognitive performance on an inhibition (go/no-go) task.[114] Also, preliminary evidence of an association between white matter integrity in the PFC in children with ADHD and their first-degree relatives, suggest heritability of factors associated with myelination.[114,115]

Intriguingly, a novel investigation of resting state in adult ADHD, revealed decreased functional connectivity in long-range connections between the anterior cingulate and two posterior regions (precuneous, posterior cingulate) comprising the so-called "default-mode" network.[116] Recent work suggests that the "resting-state" or "default-mode" network of brain regions, which shows strong coherent activation at rest, is negatively correlated with task-positive networks, which show coherent activation during attention-demanding tasks.[117,118] Individual differences in the correlations between these two networks has been found to relate to individual differences in response time variability,[119] which is a hallmark of ADHD.[20]

Findings from these brain-imaging studies are consistent with the proposed dysfunction in frontosubcortical pathways in ADHD as well as with the DA hypothesis. The frontosubcortical pathways are rich in catecholamines that are involved in the mechanism of action of stimulant medications, known to be effective in suppressing (*albeit* temporarily) the core behavioral symptoms of ADHD.

Neurocognitive Impairments

Given the preceding genetic and brain-imaging evidence supportive of the dopaminergic frontal-striatal hypothesis, it is not surprising that meta-analyses of cognitive studies have confirmed an association between ADHD and executive function deficits.[39,41] Executive function (EF) deficits refer to high-order cognitive processes that underlie self-regulation and goal-directed behavior. Thus research indicates that ADHD is associated with impairments in response inhibition, working memory, set-shifting and other aspects of EF.[109] However there is marked heterogeneity within ADHD in terms of EF deficits: only about 50% of individuals with ADHD manifest impaired performance on EF tasks.[120] These findings suggest that executive function deficits are neither necessary nor sufficient to play a causal role in ADHD. Moreover, these EF measures show poor diagnostic utility, in that abnormal scores on EF measures are generally good predictors of the diagnosis, but normal scores on one of more EF tasks cannot rule out the diagnosis of ADHD.[121] However, there is converging evidence that EF impairments are closely linked with inattention symptoms, whereas altered reinforcement mechanisms are linked with the hyperactivity symptoms,[40,122] suggesting that dimensional approaches might be more useful than categorical approaches in considering treatment approaches.

Search for Endophenotypes

Despite the high heritability of ADHD, it is clearly a heterogeneous and genetically complex disorder. Moreover, candidate gene and genome scan studies have yielded mixed results, suggesting that the categorical diagnosis of ADHD and its subtypes are not optimal for genetic analysis. Accordingly, the search for putative endophenotypes for ADHD is burgeoning.[20,123,124] This approach aims to reduce complex disorders into components, which may be neurophysiological, biochemical, endocrinological, neuroanatomical, or neuropsychological.[125,126] Endophenotypes are distinguished from "biomarkers" (or other related concepts, including "intermediate phenotype," "subclinical trait," or "vulnerability marker"), which do not necessarily have genetic underpinnings. Various criteria for valid endophenotypes have been proposed,[124,125] however, there is general agreement that measures of putative endophenotypes should: (1) have biological plausibility; (2) have sound psychometric properties, including being normally distributed in the general population; (3) show state-independence (will not vary with disease progression or vary as a function of measurement technique); (4) show sensitivity (common in affected individuals) and specificity (uncommon in non-affected individuals); (5) show heritability and genetic sensitivity and specificity; and (6) show family aggregation (occur in relatives of affected individuals, and in unaffected family members).[iii,125,127]

Neuropsychological Measures

The search for putative neuropsychological endophenotypes (particularly executive function deficits) has yielded mixed results.[123,128-130] To date, the only EF measure that meets virtually all of the validity criteria is that of response inhibition: the key measure of stop-signal reaction time (SSRT) correlates with ADHD in the population, shows greater deficits in ADHD probands than in unaffected relatives, and greater deficits in unaffected relatives than in controls, and is moderately correlated in siblings, suggesting familiality.[128-131] Other promising endophenotypes include measures of effort and activation (specifically, response variability and processing speed). For example, intraindividual response variability, which refers to short-term fluctuations in performance in the time scale of seconds, is a behavioral marker of CNS integrity.[132,133] It appears

---

[iii] For further discussion of endophenotypes, please see Bartz *et al.*, Preclinical animal models of autistic spectrum disorders (ASD), Cryan *et al.*, Developing more efficacious antidepressant medications: improving and aligning preclinical detection and clinical assessment tools, Joel *et al.*, Animal models of obsessive–compulsive disorder: from bench to bedside via endophenotypes and biomarkers, or Large *et al.*, Developing therapeutics for bipolar disorder: from animal models to the clinic in this volume.

to be a unitary and stable construct: individuals with ADHD who show high variability on one task tend to show it on other tasks.[18] It differentiates ADHD from reading disorder[134] and from high-functioning autism,[135] and shows modest (about .5) heritability estimates.[136] Moreover, intra-individual response variability has been associated with compromised neural connectivity as indexed by smaller white matter volume in the frontal lobe[137] and smaller corpus callosum area.[138]

On the negative side, although universality is not a validity criterion for an endophenotype, none of the candidate neuropsychological impairments are found in more than 50% of the ADHD population,[128] which raises questions about the utility of this approach for genetic studies or for the development of novel treatments. In summary, the limited available data and the modest reliability of many EF measures preclude firm conclusions and warrant further rigorous investigations of putative cognitive endophenotypes.

Structural and Functional Neuroimaging Measures

Neurophysiological processes have been proposed as potential endophenotypes of complex behavior and psychopathology.[139,140] As summarized previously, findings from neuroanatomical and functional neuroimaging as well as neurophysiological studies indicate several anomalies in groups of individuals with ADHD compared to control groups. However, there is a dearth of studies investigating whether these neuroimaging measures meet the validity criteria for endophenotypes. To date, twin studies have revealed evidence of heritability for some anatomic brain abnormalities associated with ADHD; specifically for volumetric reductions in frontal regions,[141,142] particularly orbitofrontal subdivisions,[143] in the posterior corpus callosum,[143] and in the cerebellum.[143,144] Automated measures of cortical thickness may also be useful as an imaging biomarker of ADHD.[145] This approach has revealed a delay in cortical maturation in ADHD, particularly in the prefrontal cortex, which has consistently shown structural anomalies and been implicated in the pathogenesis of ADHD.[106] Moreover, slower development of peak cortical thickness was related to poorer clinical outcomes.[107] Alterations in neurotrophins (required for the proliferation, differentiation, and survival of neuronal and non-neuronal cells) and/or in brain-derived neurotrophic factor and nerve growth factor (which have been found to have some linkage with ADHD, may play an etiological role.[146-150]

CURRENT TREATMENT STRATEGIES

Targets for Treatment

The primary treatment goal has been (and continues to be) the reduction of core behavioral symptoms (inattention, impulsivity, hyperactivity). However, consistent with the emergent reconceptualization of ADHD as a neurobiologically based disorder characterized by anomalies in frontal-striatal networks and impairments in attention regulation and executive function, alternative treatment approaches are discernible in the literature, which target the neural or cognitive impairments rather than the behavioral symptoms *per se*.

Pharmacological Strategies

The primary approach used in the symptomatic treatment of ADHD has been to target the DA system. Stimulants (methylphenidate, amphetamines), which are approved by the US Food and Drug Administration (FDA) and other international drug regulatory agencies for the treatment of ADHD, continue to be the predominant class of medications for the treatment of this disorder. Although the precise mechanisms of action are not yet fully specified, stimulants are believed to exert their therapeutic effects on the brain (and hence on core symptoms) via the dopamine and norepinephrine (NE) pathways. Methylphenidate (MPH) blocks the reuptake of DA and NE, thereby increasing the concentration of these neurotransmitters in the synapse; amphetamines stimulate the release of these neurotransmitters as well as blocking their reuptake.

One major drug development strategy evident over the past decade has been the development and FDA approval of longer-acting preparations of methylphenidate and amphetamine. The main goals of this drug development program have been to develop novel delivery systems for the stimulants, to (1) eliminate the need for multiple doses per day (particularly the need for a mid-day dose, which is problematic both for children at school and adults at work); (2) minimize the roller coaster-like on-off effect of the short-acting, immediate-release formulations; and (3) enhance the clinical utility of the longer-acting preparations. The current long-acting formulations extend the action of the stimulants to as long as 8–12 h.

Stimulant medications have demonstrated therapeutic efficacy and effectiveness in providing temporary reduction in the core behavioral symptoms, as well as some associated problems, such as non-compliance, academic productivity, and social functioning, etc. They also have an acceptable safety and tolerability profile. The primary concerns include the adverse effects of stimulants on cardiovascular safety, sleep disturbance, appetite suppression, growth, as well as the risk for misuse and diversion and increased risk for substance abuse. The latter problem appears to be primarily one of diversion of prescribed drugs rather than abuse risk in patients with ADHD *per se*.[151] Non-medical use of prescription ADHD medications has been documented in 2–9% of the general adolescent and adult population in the United States.[152,153] However, meta-analysis reveals that there is an almost twofold reduction in risk for later substance abuse disorder in patients with ADHD who have received treatment.[154] Nonetheless, the one adverse effect that remains controversial, of concern, and under ongoing surveillance is that of possible growth suppression.[155] Moreover, a substantial proportion of patients (~20%) discontinue medication because of intolerable adverse effects. An additional concern is poor long-term adherence to stimulant treatment. For example, despite the chronicity of ADHD and its marked lifespan impairments, most studies estimate the average duration of pharmacological treatment to be less than 1 or 2 years across children, adolescents, and adults.[156-159] In general, compliance with and adherence to pharmacological treatment is better with extended-release formulations of stimulant medication compared to immediate-release.[160,161]

A second major pharmacological approach has been the development of alternatives to stimulant medication. Atomoxetine (Strattera®), which is a NE reuptake inhibitor, has been approved in many countries for the treatment of ADHD in children, adolescents, and adults. In contrast to stimulants, atomoxetine is not a controlled substance because it does not have abuse potential, and so it is clinically useful because physicians can provide samples and provide refills easily. It also has demonstrated therapeutic efficacy and effectiveness for reducing the core behavioral symptoms of ADHD. This compound also has an acceptable safety and tolerability profile.[162] By contrast to the immediate therapeutic effects of stimulants, the full benefit of atomoxetine may not be discernible for weeks or longer. However, it may have the advantage of providing good coverage across the day with once daily dosing for many patients, having little or no effect on growth[163] and shows effectiveness for treating comorbid oppositional defiant disorder, depression, tics, and probably comorbid anxiety.[162]

Other pharmacological strategies include: (1) polypharmacy (e.g., use of stimulants and atomoxetine) and (2) off-label use of medications (e.g., use of drugs approved for treatment of disorders other than ADHD, such as tricyclic antidepressants, selective serotonin reuptake inhibitors, antihypertensives, and cholinergic agents). The available databases for these pharmacological agents are generally small and most of the studies do not meet standards for evaluating efficacy and effectiveness.

Non-pharmacological Strategies

The predominant intervention approach is psychosocial intervention, which includes parent training in effective behavior management techniques, and teacher training in effective classroom management techniques. Recent reviews of these approaches indicate there is sufficient evidence to classify psychosocial intervention as an empirically validated treatment for ADHD, although the effects appear to be short-term and often limited to the period of treatment.[164]

Emergent approaches aim to remediate impairments in thinking or in cognitive processes, rather than focusing on the core behavioral symptoms *per se*. For example, cognitive-behavioral interventions focus on strategy and meta-cognitive strategy training; cognitive interventions provide direct skills training (e.g., working memory, attention), and neural-based interventions aim to normalize neural deficiencies via neurofeedback. Notably, several of these approaches (e.g., computerized progressive training of working memory or attention) suggest therapeutic effects may extend to the cognitive and academic realm as well as reducing behavioral symptoms.[165,166] However, a recent review of these approaches suggest that findings from efficacy studies show promise, but further research is required to evaluate their effectiveness in real-world settings.[167]

Combined Modality Strategies

The combination of pharmacological and psychosocial treatments has garnered considerable attention, particularly with the advent of the largest randomized controlled trial of combined modality treatments (Multimodal Treatment Study of Children with ADHD [MTA], 1999). The basic logic of these approaches is that given the understanding of multiple factors involved in the pathogenesis of ADHD, different treatments are likely required to target the neurobiological substrate and remediate peripheral features. This premise was supported in general by the findings from the MTA study: carefully managed medication significantly decreased ADHD symptoms compared to the behavior program alone and any interventions available in the community. In general, the combined modality approach was not more beneficial than carefully managed medication alone – in terms of suppressing the behavioral symptoms – but it was advantageous in terms of effects on peripheral features, such as anxiety symptoms and social skills.

Meta-Analyses of Treatment Effects

Meta-analysis provides a useful and systematic framework for assessing the effects of various treatments by computing a standardized mean difference between a specific treatment and its control (e.g., placebo, alternative treatment) for each outcome measure. The effect size standardizes the unit of measurement across studies so that a change in one point on the effect-size scale has the same meaning in each study. Methodologies and statistical approaches vary widely in treatment studies and in meta-analytic studies. The effect sizes given below are aggregated across these studies, often without weighting, and thus are tentative and must be interpreted with great caution.

Recent meta-analyses of treatment effects indicate that the effect sizes for the core behavioral symptoms of ADHD are about: (1) 0.9 for immediate-release, short-acting stimulants; (2) 0.9 for longer-acting formulations of stimulants; (3) 0.7 for atomoxetine; (4) 1.27 for multi-modal approaches; (5) 0.4 for cognitive-behavioral training; (6) 0.35 for cognitive skills training; and (8) 1.0 for neurofeedback training.[167-169]

Effect sizes for other domains of function show a different pattern across the different intervention approaches. For example, effects sizes of treatments on academic performance are in the range of 0.19 for combined modality treatment, and 0.4 for stimulant treatment[169,170]; for cognitive skills, such as working memory, inhibition, and sustained attention, effect sizes range from 0.16 to 1.0 for cognitive-behavioral treatments, from 0.46 to 1.16 for cognitive skills training, and from 0.07 to 0.8 for neurofeedback.[167]

Need for Novel Treatment Approaches

Currently available medications show effectiveness for core behavioral symptoms in the majority of individuals with ADHD, but the effects are temporary and do not span the whole waking day. Moreover, it is rare that pharmacological treatments normalize or lead to complete remission of symptoms throughout the day. None of the available treatment strategies shows robust effects on the cognitive aspects of ADHD, underscoring the need for new therapeutics. Moreover, the emerging reconceptualization of ADHD as a genetically based, neurodevelopmental and heterogeneous disorder, suggests that multiple approaches will be needed, since "one size will not fit all." Future approaches might also consider targeting mechanisms underlying brain development (e.g., myelination, synaptic pruning), which is ongoing from conception to young adulthood, or targeting risk factors, such as prenatal smoking and nicotine addiction in adulthood.

DISCOVERY OF PHARMACEUTICAL TREATMENTS FOR ADHD – FROM SERENDIPITY TO RATIONAL DRUG DESIGN

Although a variety of medications exist to treat ADHD, the most widely used (>75% of prescriptions), and arguably most effective treatments to date are psychostimulants. The discovery of efficacy by stimulant medications in treating ADHD, similar to many medical treatments in early psychiatry, was largely serendipitous. The first published report of the use of stimulants to treat children with ADHD-like symptoms came in 1937 when Dr. Charles Bradley, working at the Emma Pendleton Bradley Home, first gave Benzedrine®, a racemic mixture of D- and L-amphetamine, to children hospitalized for a variety of behavioral abnormalities.[171] The rationale behind this treatment was not disclosed in the original publication, but later revealed to have been the result of a fortuitous observation.[172] As part of a thorough neurological exam designed to help understand the underlying causes of the behavioral abnormalities in some of the children at the hospital a pneumoencephalogram was performed. However, a common side effect of this procedure was severe headaches. Dr. Bradley, acting under the hypothesis that a stimulant would help to alleviate the headaches, gave the children Benzedrine. While the medication did not prevent the headaches as predicted, a striking improvement in the behavior of the children was seen including a paradoxical calming effect. This observation was later replicated using a larger cohort of patients with similar positive results.[171] It is of particular interest that in these early studies the children who responded to Benzedrine treatment showed a marked improvement in school performance, specifically an increase in attention and motivation to complete tasks, as well as a decrease in disruptive and aggressive behaviors. Although Dr. Bradley continued to treat patients with Benzedrine in his clinic, the use of psychostimulant medications in children was not widely accepted by the medical community for several decades and continues to bear a social stigma to this day.

Following the discovery that psychostimulants improve behavioral symptoms in ADHD both clinical and preclinical studies have focused on understanding the mechanism of action of these drugs. Evaluation of biological fluids from clinical studies including urine, plasma, and CSF demonstrated that psychostimulants alter dopamine (DA) and norepinephrine (NE) turnover with little evidence for changes in serotonin (5-HT) release.[173-176] Preclinical studies using a variety of animal species have demonstrated similar findings and allow for a more detailed understanding of the neural circuitry involved. Whereas high doses of psychostimulants typically associated with generalized behavioral activation increase DA efflux throughout the brain, lower drug doses that result in exposures similar to those used clinically elevate DA levels within the cortex while having less impact on sub-cortical DA pathways.[177,178] Importantly, at these same clinically relevant doses, amphetamine and MPH also cause significant increases in the synaptic availability of NE within the prefrontal cortex.

As mentioned previously, the prefrontal cortex is a region of the brain that is highly important for performing tasks requiring working memory and attention. Within the prefrontal cortex catecholamines such as DA and NE modulate information processing required for normal executive function (EF). These findings have been demonstrated through the use of animal model systems in which normal spatial and working memory has been disrupted following the application of neurotoxins into the prefrontal cortex which deplete DA and NE content.[179] These findings were further supported by studies demonstrating that improvements in attentional processing by MPH are inhibited by idazoxan or SCH-23390, α-adrenergic and DA D_1/D_5 receptor antagonists respectively.[180] Finally, a broad body of literature shows that in both preclinical animal models and within clinical populations drugs acting as agonists at adrenergic α_{2A}-receptors improve performance in tasks requiring working memory and vigilance.[181]

With a growing understanding of the role of NE in attention and vigilance, physicians in the early 1970s began testing NE reuptake inhibitors (NRIs) in an effort to identify alternative drug treatments for ADHD. Clinical studies tested tricyclic antidepressants such as imipramine (Tofranil®[182]) and more recently desipramine (Norpramin®[154]) and[183] tomoxetine (Strattera®[184]), all of which are potent NRIs. These trials successfully demonstrated the efficacy of NRIs in treating the core symptoms of ADHD, *albeit* to a lesser degree than stimulant medications. Currently, the only first line non-stimulant medication approved for treating ADHD is Strattera®, though it was originally developed as an antidepressant. Similar to stimulant medications, atomoxetine raises levels of extracellular NE and DA within the PFC; however, it does not significantly impact DA levels within the nucleus accumbens even at relatively high doses.[185] This is an important distinction since the nucleus accumbens is part of a sub-cortical DA system involved in reward, motivation, and abuse potential, and likely impacts attention and vigilance.

Given the evidence that direct and indirect adrenergic receptor activation enhances performance in attentional tasks in animal models and NRIs improve behavioral symptoms in ADHD it was rationally hypothesized that development of direct-acting agonists could also be effective in ADHD. In fact, clonidine (Catapres®), an antihypertensive medication that acts as a relatively non-selective agonist at α_2-adrenergic receptors has been tested clinically and found to improve ADHD symptoms.[186] While the outcome of these studies were encouraging, clonidine is poorly tolerated by patients causing adverse events including sedation, irritability, significant drops in blood pressure, and hypotension among its most common side effects. Additionally, clonidine has a poor pharmacokinetic profile resulting in unreliable predictions in patient to patient drug exposures making it less than ideal for treating ADHD especially considering that a large portion of the patient population are children and adolescents. Additional studies have evaluated guanfacine (Tenex®), a more selective α_2-adrenergic receptor agonist that also improves responses in spatial memory tasks in primate studies.[187,188] As with clonidine, guanfacine demonstrated therapeutic benefits in ADHD patients, *albeit* with a relatively poor safety and tolerability profile. More recent work focusing on adrenergic α_2-receptor agonists for treating ADHD have attempted to circumvent tolerability issues by developing new delivery systems including a drug patch to allow for a more stable pharmacokinetic profile thus limiting side effects associated with peaks and troughs in drug exposure.

The Search for Novel Therapeutic Targets

Although a variety of compounds targeting novel mechanisms are currently being evaluated by the pharmaceutical industry for efficacy in treating symptoms of ADHD (e.g., nicotinic acetylcholine agonists, glutamatergic agents, etc.)[189,190] all of the marketed compounds and most of those in late stage clinical development directly or indirectly manipulate catecholamine systems. The fundamental reason for this has been a general lack of understanding of the biology sub-serving the behavioral deficits in ADHD beyond what is known of the catecholamine systems and a reliance on retrospective analysis of neurochemical responses to medications that worked through trial and error in clinical settings. With the growth of genomic and proteomic biology over the past two decades, scientific understanding of this disorder has greatly improved (see Genetic risk factors). However, it is important to note that given the heterogeneity of ADHD in terms of genetic and environmental risk factors it has not been possible to delineate a role for individual genetic markers directly in specific behavioral manifestations of the disorder. Therefore, it is necessary to have model systems with which to test the role of genes and proteins experimentally that have been associated with ADHD in order to develop more reliable hypotheses and in turn discover more effective medications. To this end, there is a need for reliable and predictive animal models to test for efficacy by novel mechanisms especially where no clinically viable reference tools exist.

Needed Improvements in Current Pharmaceutical Agents

In ADHD there are four primary areas in which current drug therapies can be improved; abuse liability, onset of action, magnitude of efficacy (specifically for core behavioral symptoms in regards to non-stimulant medicines as well as untreated impairments and comorbid symptoms), and safety/tolerability. While stimulant medications are effective in treating the core behavioral symptoms in ~75% of ADHD patients, they carry a strong abuse liability resulting in diversion for illicit use, and as such carry a high administrative burden to both physicians and patients. In contrast, Strattera is a non-scheduled, non-abused medicine as previously noted but has a slower onset of action for full efficacy while peak responses are generally less than found with stimulant medicines, particularly in adult patients.[168,169] While both types of medications have issues regarding tolerability, often improvements in tolerability are insufficient motivating factors to convince physicians and drug formularies to switch patients to a new prescription, particularly where an adverse event is non-life threatening (e.g., insomnia, dizziness, weight loss, etc.). This may be in part due to the ability of physicians to start patients on low drug doses and increase exposure to therapeutic levels over time, thus limiting side effects associated with acute drug exposure. Furthermore, abuse liability is a matter of regulatory management relating to the potential for dependence and illicit diversion which cannot necessarily be determined prior to human testing. Therefore having the means to predict a greater magnitude of efficacy and/or onset of action of novel mechanisms in treating symptoms of ADHD are of critical importance in a preclinical drug discovery program.[iv]

MODELS AVAILABLE IN PRECLINICAL DRUG DISCOVERY

A few of the benefits of working with animal models include simpler central nervous systems with more direct access, better control over experimental environments including housing and history, and more genetic homogeneity. In addition, animal models allow for manipulation of variables and endpoints not possible in

---

[iv] Please refer to Rochas *et al.*, Development of medications for heroin and cocaine addiction and regulatory aspects of abuse liability testing, in Volume 3, *Reward Deficits Disorders*, for further discussion regarding schedule classification and regulatory considerations of drugs with abuse potential.

human populations such as altering genetics to elucidate the functions of genes and their impact on behavior. Conversely, the drawbacks of using animal models to understand ADHD include trying to mimic a complex human disorder in animals whose executive functions are not the same as humans, lack of behavioral intervention treatments that are often helpful in clinical populations, an inability to mimic the entire disorder in a single model and thus the need to develop multiple models to evaluate behavioral domains that mimic symptoms or deficits observed in ADHD, and difficulties associated with modeling poly-genetic disorders in genetically homogeneous animal populations.

Ideally, animal models of psychiatric disorders should be similar to the modeled disorder in terms of etiology, development, symptomology, underlying neurochemistry and treatment efficacy. A number of animal models of ADHD have been described and recently reviewed,[83,191,192] most notably the spontaneously hypertensive rat (SHR) model, but all fail to model all aspects of the disorder successfully. In addition, since ADHD is a clinically heterogeneous disorder that is only poorly understood, it is proposed that it is virtually impossible at present to model the disorder itself successfully. Thus, preclinical drug discovery programs currently rely on animal models of the various behavioral symptoms or deficits observed in ADHD. Some of these models use intact or normal animals, while others use animals that have been genetically, neurochemically, or pharmacologically manipulated, in an attempt to produce behavioral deficits that resemble those in patients.

Since ADHD is characterized by symptoms of hyperactivity, impulsivity, inattention and other cognitive deficits, these symptom domains have been a primary focus of drug discovery programs. In addition, drug discovery programs rely heavily on the pharmacological predictive validity (i.e., pharmacological isomorphism) of the various symptom domain models, but the predictive validity of the various models that are available is not yet firmly established. What is needed is a comprehensive pharmacological evaluation of each of the animal models using drugs that are known to be efficacious in ADHD patients, as well as others that are known to be not efficacious (i.e., negative controls). Regarding the cognitive deficits observed in the disorder, compounds that are clinically effective versus cognitive symptoms have not been firmly established, rendering it impossible at this time to establish the predictive validity of preclinical cognition assays for efficacy. For these reasons, drug discovery programs are often forced to rely on the demonstration of proof of mechanism (*in vivo*) for the proposed molecular target, followed by proof of efficacy in patients in the clinic.

ANIMAL MODELS OF ADHD

Although no single animal model exists that can fully mimic ADHD, a wide variety have been postulated to manifest behaviors that resemble aspects of the disorder.[v] Some animal strains have been characterized that innately express ADHD-like traits

---

[v] Please refer to Large *et al.*, Developing therapeutics for bipolar disorder (BPD): From animal models to the clinic in this volume for further discussion regarding the difficulty of recapitulating all aspects of a multi-behavioral disorder in a single animal model.

whereas others have been genetically modified through targeted gene manipulation. Still others attempt to induce ADHD-like behavioral patterns following neurochemical lesions or environmental insults during early development of the organisms. While a comprehensive review is beyond the scope of this chapter, several of the more widely used models are discussed below.

Genetic Models

The SHR genetic model of ADHD has been claimed to be the only model shown to demonstrate all of the behavioral characteristics of ADHD: hyperactivity, impulsivity, and sustained attention deficits.[21] Originally derived through targeted breeding from normotensive Wistar-Kyoto rats, this strain reportedly shows hyperactivity in a variety of behavioral paradigms depending on the parameters (e.g., in free- versus forced-open fields, duration of testing, illumination of the field) and an impaired ability to withhold responses, an indication of impulsivity.[193,194] In addition, the observed hyperactivity is claimed not to be present initially, but develops over time and after exposure to the same environment as in childhood ADHD.[195] Low doses of amphetamine and methylphenidate have been shown to reduce the hyperactivity and impulsivity observed in SHR rats,[196,197] and since both of these agents are effective in ADHD, this model may be a predictive tool for testing the efficacy of novel medication in a preclinical drug discovery setting. However, it is worth noting that the SHR model is not universally accepted since the behavior of these animals are often compared to Wistar-Kyoto rats which respond poorly on tasks of attention[198] and there is some controversy regarding the efficacy of stimulant medications across a range of behavioral models when compared to strains other than Wistar-Kyoto.[199,200]

Genetic manipulation of mouse strains through targeted disruption of DNA sequences has become an increasingly valuable tool to delineate the role of specific proteins in otherwise normal animals. As mentioned above (Genetic Risk Factors), several independent groups have identified an association between polymorphisms in the synaptosomal-associated protein-25 (SNAP-25) gene and ADHD in humans,[201] a nerve terminal protein involved in neurotransmitter release. The mouse mutant coloboma (Cm/+) has been produced by a semidominant deletion mutation on chromosome 2 in a region that includes the SNAP-25 gene. Mice that are heterozygous for this mutation produce a 50% reduction in the expression of SNAP-25 compared to wild-type controls and exhibit significant hyperactivity[202] that does not decline with age.[203] Hess *et al.*[202] has shown that the spontaneous hyperactivity of SNAP-25 mutant mice is markedly reduced by amphetamine, at doses which significantly increase activity in the wild type mice.[202] Administration of atomoxetine was also shown to decrease the hyperactivity in the coloboma mice, while having no effect on the controls. However, unlike amphetamine, methylphenidate increased locomotor activity in both coloboma and control mice.[204] The underlying reasons for this disparity between psychostimulant drug treatment efficacy is unknown, but bears further investigation. More recently, the coloboma mouse strain has been tested in latent inhibition and delayed reinforcement paradigms designed to measure inattention and impulsivity respectively, and found to be impaired.[205] To date, though, no reports have tested the efficacy of ADHD medications on these endpoints in coloboma mice.

Another promising genetic model is DA transporter knock-out (DAT-KO) mice. Throughout much of the brain, DA is cleared from the synaptic cleft via presynaptic DA transporters, one of the primary sites of action for psychostimulant medications. While extracellular DA levels in these mice are five times greater than normal, total DA content within the brain is significantly reduced,[206] likely as a compensatory mechanism. Behaviorally these animals show normal levels of activity in their home cages, but exhibit marked hyperactivity in novel environments.[206,207] The hyperactivity in this case has been reported to respond to amphetamine and methylphenidate as well as to direct DA agonists such as apomorphine and quinpirole. The efficacy of these latter compounds versus the hyperactivity symptoms in ADHD patients, however, is unknown. The efficacy of psychostimulants on hyperactivity symptoms in these animals would seem to be in conflict with the neurobiology of the DAT-KO model given a lack of DA transporters and an already high level of extracellular DA. However, two additional points to consider may help to explain these findings. First, psychostimulants also target NE transporters which presumably remain intact in this system and in fact do contribute to the efficacy of current ADHD medications. Second, as a compensatory mechanism it is possible that synaptic DA receptors are down regulated or desensitized since the opposite is true in model systems where DA is depleted.[208]

Neurotoxicity Models

A common means of generating model systems to study behavioral abnormalities in psychotherapeutic research is through pharmacological or toxicologic manipulation of otherwise normal animals. A variety of neurochemical insults and environmental challenges during early postnatal development have been demonstrated to induce hyperactivity in adolescent animals as well as to induce deficits in behavioral assays that measure memory and attention.[209,210] In general, these models have in common a requirement for the induction of early postnatal developmental changes. While some models have targeted the development of specific brain structures thought to be impacted in ADHD such as with the cerebellar stunting model which relies on early postnatal chemical challenges to reduce the total cerebellar volume, these models have not generally proven useful in eliciting either the anticipated behavioral deficits found in ADHD or in demonstrating predictive validity through reversal of behavioral abnormalities using stimulant medications.[211,212] Other models that damage selective neurotransmitter systems (e.g., catecholamines) such as the 6-hydroxydopamine (6-OHDA) model, or that target more global neuronal insults such as the neonatal hypoxia model have been more successful and are discussed in further detail below.

6-OHDA is a neurotoxin that destroys the cell when taken up into presynaptic terminals through DA (or other catecholamine) transporters. In the 6-OHDA model of ADHD, rats are subjected to this neurotoxin during early postnatal development (generally prior to postnatal day 10) resulting in the destruction of the majority of DA projections to the forebrain.[213] Importantly, NE terminals are also lost unless pharmacologically protected by a blocking agent such as desipramine. As these animals develop into adolescence they display signs of increased spontaneous locomotor activity compared to their non-treated littermates. This enhanced locomotor activity gradually declines as rats mature; a developmental change similarly observed in ADHD.

Importantly, this hyperactivity is reversed by low doses of D-amphetamine or methyl-phenidate.[214] Moran-Gates *et al.*[215] recently showed that atomoxetine also decreases the hyperactivity in 6-OHDA-lesioned rats while producing only a transient sedative effect in sham controls. Furthermore, although limited, there is evidence that rats injected with 6-OHDA during the early postnatal period develop learning and memory deficits,[216,217] but the efficacy of ADHD medication in treating these effects has not been tested. It is also important to note that while this model appears to demonstrate predictive validity, at least in terms of efficacy for hyperactivity symptoms, no studies have reported widespread catecholamine depletion in ADHD similar to what is found in this model (up to >99% reduction). As new medications are developed and tested in the clinic a retrospective analysis of those that are effective, as well as those that are not, will ultimately determine the continued predictive utility of this model for ADHD.

A second promising neurologic model is the rat neonatal hypoxia model. Although the etiology of ADHD has not been linked to hypoxic damage, the neonatal hypoxia model in rats displays a striking number of behavioral abnormalities that seem to mimic ADHD symptoms. Rats subjected to 100% nitrogen (thus eliminating oxygen) shortly after birth[218] or during the early postnatal period[219] develop hyperactivity and learning impairments. As with the 6-OHDA model, hyperactivity attenuates as rats develop into adolescence, however, the learning impairments persist into adulthood.[219,220] Pharmacological evaluation of this model has been limited, but where tested, D-amphetamine[218] was able to reverse hyperactivity. Continued characterization of the rat neonatal hypoxia model could result in a useful tool for preclinical drug discovery efforts, particularly as attention and impulsivity endpoints are pharmacologically evaluated.

Behavioral Assays

Regardless of the model system being used, be it genetically modified, chemically challenged, or normal animals, the assays used to predict preclinical efficacy of novel medications for ADHD often rely on either innate or learned behavioral endpoints. While hyperactivity is rather easy to conceptualize and is modeled well in animal systems the attention and impulsivity domains of ADHD are more difficult to evaluate. Within this section, we will review the challenges of developing behavioral assays in preclinical species that require the assessment and interpretation of complex interactions between the animals and their environment. In the course of this, we will highlight a few of the models which are commonly used today.

Assessment of Attention

As in humans, attention in animals has been postulated to consist of several different types, including sustained attention, or vigilance; divided attention; and selective (focused) attention.[221] Sustained attention is defined as a continuous allocation of processing resources for the detection of rare events. Deficits in sustained attention typically occur toward the end of a long test session. Divided attention occurs when an animal has to respond differently to varied stimuli, often involving different sensory channels within the same test session, which requires optimal allocation of processing resources. Selective attention occurs when an animal has to focus resources on a restricted number of sensory channels, while ignoring the rest.

The 5-choice serial reaction time task (5-CSRTT), recently reviewed by Robbins,[221] was developed as a rat version of the continuous performance test (CPT), which is used in clinical settings to measure attentional deficits in ADHD and schizophrenia. Briefly, in this test, the animal has to watch for the occurrence of a brief (e.g., 0.5 s) target stimulus (a light) to appear in one of five holes and then perform a nose-poke into the hole that contained it. Correct responses are reinforced by the presentation of food pellets in a magazine at the rear of the chamber, and incorrect responses are punished by a brief time-out (darkness). Several types of errors are possible during performance of the task, including errors of commission, which are incorrect responses; errors of omission, which are failures to respond during the allotted time limit (e.g., 5 s limited hold); and premature responses, which are responses that occur after the initiation of the trial but prior to the presentation of the stimulus (i.e., anticipatory responses). These latter deficits are hypothesized to occur when inhibitory control of highly pre-potent responses has been lost and are considered to be an indication of impulsivity.[222] Perseveration of responding can also occur, which represents an additional type of inhibitory deficit and is considered to be a form of compulsive, rather than impulsive behavior.[221] Following extensive training, performance generally reaches high levels (e.g. >80% accuracy; <15% omissions), with improvements in accuracy still detectable in "normal" animals. Experimental manipulations such as changing the intensity, the duration, or the frequency of the visual stimuli can also be used to alter the difficulty of the task. Thus, the basic 5-CSRTT task can serve as a measure for efficacy versus sustained attentional deficits, as well as response inhibition deficits, a type of "executive function." The 5-CSRTT assay is also being used successfully with mice.[223]

Another task, the lateralized reaction time task (LRTT), which is similar to the 5-CSRTT, but which measures visuospatial divided attention and motor initiation is also being used by several groups.[224] In this task animals initiate the presentation of a visual target stimulus, which is presented in one of only two possible spatial locations and then make a response toward the location of the target, requiring both sustained and divided attention.

Over the past several decades many studies have been performed to pharmacologically characterize the 5-CSRTT using both systemically and intracerebrally administered drugs. In addition, the effects of central manipulations such as neurochemical lesions on various aspects of attentional control have been studied. The reader is referred to Robbins[221] for a thorough review of the findings.

Since similar tests can be performed in humans, it is expected that this assay may provide translational information regarding the clinical potential of novel ADHD drugs. However, although psychomotor stimulants such as D-amphetamine are known to enhance performance in sustained attention tasks in humans, this has proven difficult to observe in the rat 5-CSRTT task,[225] since they do not appear to reliably improve accuracy in the model. However, several studies have observed evidence for improved accuracy with psychomotor stimulants. In a study that used both fixed intertrial intervals (ITI's) and variable ITI's,[226] D-amphetamine and methylphenidate did produce an increase in accuracy, as well as reduced response latency and decreased anticipatory responding (regardless of the ITI used). In another study that used "poor-performer" rats, MPH was shown to increase the accuracy of the poor-performing rats, but had no effect in the normal rats.[227]

A thorough review of the pharmacology of attentional tests in rodents and humans would be extremely helpful toward establishing the predictive validity of the preclinical models, but it is speculated that novel agents that improve performance in these tasks in rodents would be worthy of consideration for clinical evaluation.

Assessment of Impulsivity

Impulsivity plays a role in several psychiatric disorders including ADHD, mania, and substance abuse disorders. In ADHD, impulse control deficits are evident in a variety of experimental tasks including the continuous performance test and the stop signal reaction time test.[228,229] A review article by Evenden[222] has comprehensively described the concept of impulsivity, along with the behavioral approaches that have been used to study it. Impulsivity is broadly defined as "actions without foresight" that are "poorly conceived, prematurely expressed, unduly risky, or inappropriate to the situation, and that often result in undesirable outcomes." Impulse control or behavioral inhibition can be described as an active inhibitory mechanism that modulates the desire for primary reinforcers, and is supported by a large literature on the neural basis of the different types of behavioral inhibition.[230]

By focusing on different aspects of impulsive behavior, several behavioral paradigms have been developed to measure impulsivity in humans, as well as in animals.[231] These paradigms can be broadly divided into two categories: those measuring motoric impulsivity (impulsive action) and those measuring impulsive decision-making (impulsive choice).[vi]

Several tasks that measure motoric impulsivity are available for preclinical and clinical use. In the go/no-go task, the subject must make a particular response when the "go" signal is presented and must refrain from making the response when the "no-go" signal is presented, either prior to the "go" signal or concurrently with it. The stop signal reaction time (SSRT) task is similar except that the "Stop" signal occurs after the presentation of the "go" signal, making it harder for the subject to inhibit their behavior. As mentioned above, the 5-CSRTT task can also be used to measure aspects of motoric impulsivity (i.e., premature or anticipatory responding).

Impulsive choice involves decision-making processes rather than motoric inhibition, and in this case there is no "pre-potent" response that is present and then inhibited.[231] The delay-discounting task, which measures "tolerance to the delay of gratification" is the most commonly used task of this type, and can also be used preclinically as well as clinically in the form of operant tasks or questionnaire-based tests. The impulsive choice in these tests is the choice of a smaller reward that is available immediately over a larger award that is delayed. Much less work has been done with these impulsivity models than with, for example, the 5-CSRTT task, but their development and pharmacological characterization will be an important body of work for the ADHD field.

[vi] Please refer to Williams *et al.*, Current concepts in the classification, treatment and modeling of pathological gambling and other impulse control disorders, Volume 3, *Reward Deficits Disorders*, for further discussion and description of models of impulsivity.

THE NEED TO DEVELOP PRECLINICAL COGNITION ASSAYS IN ANIMAL SPECIES

The most challenging aspect of preclinical model or assay development is attempting to create tools to predict clinical outcomes that are either not well defined or may have poor behavioral correlates in animal species, as is the case with executive dysfunction in ADHD. One of the most prominent neuropsychological theories of ADHD postulates that ADHD symptomology stems from a primary deficit in EF,[73] (see above), which has been defined as neurocognitive processes that maintain an appropriate problem-solving set to attain a later goal.[232] These fundamental cognitive processes include the abilities to inhibit inappropriate behaviors and thoughts (i.e., impulse control); to regulate attention and action; to plan, initiate and monitor one's actions; and to coordinate goal-directed actions.[233] Neuropsychological and imaging studies indicate that there are both structural and functional insufficiencies in PFC circuitry in ADHD patients and that they contribute significantly to the observed EF deficits. A recent meta-analysis of 83 studies of EF in ADHD found that there were EF dysfunctions across all domains tested, including measures of response inhibition, vigilance, verbal and spatial working memory, set-shifting, and planning.[41] It was concluded that ADHD is associated with weaknesses in several key EF domains. However, since the magnitude of the group difference on EF measures was much smaller than the group difference in other ADHD symptoms, together with the estimate that fewer than half of the children with ADHD exhibit significant impairment on any specific EF task,[120] it was concluded that EF deficits are significantly associated with ADHD but are not the single necessary and sufficient cause of the disorder in all individuals.

However, the presence of cognitive dysfunction is particularly common in adolescents and adults with ADHD, with over 90% of adults seeking treatment manifesting cognitive dysfunction.[81] In addition, stimulants are viewed as being effective versus the hyperactivity and attentional symptoms of ADHD but typically do not adequately address the additional cognitive symptoms.[81] Thus, the cognitive deficits observed in the disorder, are still only poorly controlled and are a major contributor to poor functional outcome in ADHD patients. Therefore, the cognitive deficits manifested in ADHD patients represent a major unmet medical need and is a major focus of preclinical experimentation in both industry and academia.[vii]

Despite the clinical efforts that are ongoing, cognitive deficits that are observed in ADHD patients are not well defined and the field would greatly benefit from a comprehensive analysis similar to the one conducted by the measurement and treatment research to improve cognition in schizophrenia (MATRICS) initiative, which was begun in 2003, to study the cognitive deficits in schizophrenia (see website for details: http://www.matrics.ucla.edu[viii]). This effort, by combining the efforts of academic, governmental, and industrial scientists made significant advances in defining the cognitive

---

[vii] See Lindner *et al.*, Development, optimization and use of preclinical behavioral models to maximize the productivity of drug discovery for Alzheimer's disease, for further discussion and description of procedures commonly used to assess cognitive function in rodents and non-human primates.

[viii] See also Jones *et al.*, Developing new drugs for schizophrenia: from animals to the clinic, in Volume 1, *Psychiatric Disorders*, for further discussion of MATRICS and other initiatives.

deficits in schizophrenia, classifying them into seven different but overlapping cognitive domains. This in turn, helped to identify the preclinical and clinical cognition models/batteries that should be used to evaluate the potential utility of novel compounds. Therefore, to increase confidence in clinical success it is proposed that the cognitive domains affected in ADHD be systematically identified and characterized such that preclinical behavioral batteries addressing these domains can be assembled and used for profiling new compounds. Much work has already been done in this area, but individual labs working on ADHD have not systematically set up the various models that are available and have not thoroughly characterized those pharmacologically using similar experimental conditions. In addition, reported findings have not been systematically replicated by independent laboratories. Therefore, at this time, the predictive validity of the preclinical cognition models for ADHD remains largely unestablished and a considerable effort will be required to build a preclinical database that will ultimately serve to direct compounds toward clinical development.[ix]

Aside from the attention and impulsivity models mentioned above, the conclusions from the recent meta-analysis of EF studies[41] suggest that there are several cognitive domains that can be investigated using preclinical models, including spatial working memory and set-shifting. Although verbal working memory and planning were also concluded to be dysfunctional in ADHD, these domains cannot be adequately assessed in animal models. Spatial working memory, however, has been well studied in rodents and non-human primates and attentional set-shifting models that mimic the behavioral flexibility required by the Wisconsin Card-Sorting test in humans have also been developed and are in use preclinically.[234-236] Comprehensive reviews of the pharmacology of these models would also be extremely useful in evaluating their predictive validities with respect to identifying novel compounds for clinical investigation. Ultimately, however, the predictive utility of preclinical models can only be achieved via retrospective feedback from clinical studies.

TRANSLATIONAL BIOMARKERS IN ADHD DRUG DEVELOPMENT

Use of Biomarkers in the Drug Development of ADHD Compounds

Biomarkers have become key components of the drug development of new compounds for many therapeutic areas including ADHD. Based on the biomarkers definitions working group,[237] biomarkers are defined as "a characteristic that is objectively measured and evaluated as an indicator of normal biological processes, pathogenic processes, or pharmacologic responses to a therapeutic intervention." Under this broad definition, a variety of outcomes may be considered as biomarkers and used in the development of compounds in ADHD. Results from biomarker studies are used to help the selection of viable drug candidates, set go/no-go decision criteria, increase confidence that compounds show adequate pharmacology, bridge the response from animal to human, and help in

---

[ix] For a comprehensive and critical review of impaired cognition in various neurologic and psychiatric disorders, and issues arising from the clinical assessment of candidate drugs being developed for their treatment, see Schneider, Issues in design and conduct of clinical trials for cognitive-enhancing drugs, in Volume 2, *Neurologic Disorders*.

the selection of an adequate therapeutic dose range. Coupled with exposure–response analysis, the use of biomarkers can have a tremendous impact on the efficiency and cost-effectiveness of developing new drug candidates and allow better predictions of doses and dosing regimen. Although not covered herein, biomarkers may also be used for assessment of safety endpoints as defined by a compound's toxicity profile.

Depending on the mechanism of action, different biomarkers are selected based on the intended use (fit-for-purpose). Results are used in the proper context to determine that the new ADHD compound achieves a pharmacologically active target, reaches its site of action, and shows proof of mechanism or proof of pharmacology. An ideal biomarker can be defined by its ability to fulfill the following criteria.

Evidence of Compound Activity or Proof of Mechanism: One of the primary selection criteria for a mechanistic biomarker is that the observed responses confirm the drug hits its intended target and exhibits desired pharmacodynamic activity and specificity for the intended ligand.

Measure of Central Activity: The biomarker of choice needs to reflect activation of the target receptor at the site of action, which in the case of ADHD is most likely to be found in the central brain compartment. Some examples include changes in CSF monoamines or quantitative electroencephalogram (EEG) spectral power responses.

Translatability: An ideal biomarker for early drug development would establish a direct link between preclinical and clinical studies. In short, the same biomarker endpoint that is measured in preclinical species should also be measurable in humans. Furthermore, the target exposure triggering a response in preclinical species can be directly translated into a target exposure in human. However, with drugs with precedented mechanisms, scaling based on a response that is not directly translatable has been very successful.

PK/PD Relationship: The specificity of a biomarker response can often be garnered by appropriate exposure–response relationships. The usefulness of a biomarker is maximal when a time course of response can be characterized, in contrast to a biomarker that provides an all-or-none type of response. The relationship between exposure and response can be used to establish a target concentration and thus predict doses likely to be effective in humans. Rather than dose, this corrects for differences in pharmacokinetics between the preclinical species under study and humans. From that relationship, the dose that is needed to maintain a target concentration over the dosing interval can be identified. With compounds that share the same mechanism of action of marketed drugs or are developed as backup compounds, the target exposure is typically defined by benchmarking against the positive control or the lead compound. The availability of a positive control provides opportunity for better estimate of likelihood of success, selection of relevant doses, and optimization of study design and thus allows more rapid development.

Relationship to Outcome: In addition to the concept of translatability between preclinical and clinical studies, a further step is required to link biomarker response to clinical outcome. Understanding of the link between the exposure providing biomarker response and therapeutic effect (e.g., changes in an ADHD symptom severity scale) can be used to establish early signs of efficacy and is critical to quantify the risk of making development decisions based on the biomarker response.

The use of biomarkers as part of the drug development continuum for a new ADHD compound is illustrated in Figure 10.1. Although the scheme presented

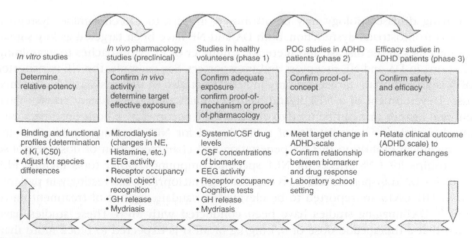

Figure 10.1   The use of biomarkers in the development of a new ADHD compound

simplifies the drug development process, types of biomarkers that can be obtained at each step are provided as well as the main objective relative to biomarker use. The type of biomarker is dependent on the mechanism of action and what is known about the pharmacological properties. The order is loosely based on the classification proposed by Danhof.[238] Most activities are related to the translatability of biomarkers between preclinical and early clinical studies. However, for compounds whose mechanisms have been precedented, information is available over the full development cycle including demonstration of efficacy (e.g., as determined by changes in ADHD symptom severity scales).

Types of Biomarkers Used in Early Drug Development

Drug Concentrations

Regardless of mechanism of action, the exposure observed following oral dosing of a new compound must match and exceed the target exposure set by preclinical studies at a dose that is considered well tolerated. Achievement of a target exposure (expressed as free fraction) and ability to maintain the exposure over a dosing interval is the lowest requirement for a new compound. As a surrogate for drug concentrations at the target site, studies have been conducted in which CSF is sampled and drug concentrations are measured in this matrix to estimate brain exposure levels. This can be accomplished as part of the initial Phase I study in healthy volunteers to confirm that the drug penetrates the CNS. However, this assumes an oversimplification of the brain as the site of action,[239] and its usefulness is considered limited.

Positron Emission Tomography/Receptor Occupancy

Positron emission tomography (PET) studies have been used successfully to measure receptor occupancy over a dose range in humans and results correlated with therapeutic benefit. Indeed, PET ligands have been key tools not only in determining receptor occupancy of individual compounds, but also in understanding the underlying pathophysiology of disease. In ADHD, there is compelling evidence to suggest that underlying disease etiology may be attributed, in part, to catecholamine dysregulation and frontostriatal dysfunction. Both DA and NE have been targeted as key signaling molecules in the disease and there are a number of PET approaches to examining alterations in DA and NE receptors and transporters. For example, the NE transporter (NET) is an important target not only in ADHD but also in depression and substance abuse. Development of a NET ligand has been challenging, but recent studies have identified ligands that can be used to evaluate NET occupancy in both preclinical and clinical models.[240,241] Availability of a PET ligand for NET binding would allow for the preclinical evaluation of CNS penetration and characterization of dose–response relationships for CNS effects for NET specific compounds. Other tools include PET ligands for DA transporters and D_2 receptors (e.g., raclopride). Interestingly, in patients with ADHD DATs are reported to be elevated in caudate regions of treatment naive brain.[242] DAT-imaging studies have been conducted with MPH. These studies have shown that a therapeutic dose of 0.5 mg/kg of MPH is expected to block more than 60% of DAT.[243] In that study, large intersubject variability was observed in the increase in extracellular DA for a similar level of DA blockade, potentially explaining the large subject variability in response to MPH observed between patients.

In summary, PET biomarker endpoints can be used not only to understand the underlying etiology of disease but also to further understand the degree of binding of novel compounds which in turn can be used to select appropriate exposure-dose ranges. Although the use of PET as a primary biomarker can be attractive, the difficulty associated with developing a suitable ligand, the additional regulatory requirements, the limited number of research centers available to conduct these studies and the relatively long time required to complete, can limit its usefulness as part of a development program. In addition, compounds that exhibit multiple receptor pharmacology would require multiple markers for PET imaging. Nevertheless, there are few approaches that can determine the true human Ki and exposure issues as elegantly as PET.

Quantitative Electroencephalogram

Quantitative electroencephalogram (qEEG) fulfills many of the criteria of an ideal biomarker. Measurements are non-invasive, changes in EEG signal represent changes at the site of action, and results are amenable to exposure–response analysis preclinically and in humans. This technique has been used successfully to extrapolate effect from animals to human with other CNS indications.[244] Children with ADHD exhibit abnormalities in specific frequency bands including alternations in beta, a spectral band known to be associated with alertness and increases in other spectral frequencies within frontotemporal regions.[245] Most of the studies using quantitative EEG have focused upon responses following treatment with MPH.[246-249] Typical endpoints focus upon alterations in the theta/beta ratios in frontal and parietal brain regions suggesting qEEG may have some utility as a means to establish centrally mediated pharmacodynamic activity in patients. However, to date, qEEG has not proved robust in predicting individual treatment response. Further study is merited.

EEG using evoked response models has proved to be slightly more sensitive. In evoked response potential models, a cognitive task is typically included and EEG responses recorded during performance of the task. Oddball auditory tasks, continuous performance tasks, and attention tasks such as the Stroop interference test (a measure of the ability to inhibit automatic responses) are often performed. Although a number of studies have reported pharmacodynamic responses in ERP endpoints following stimulant treatment, test and re-test is often an issue with these endpoints and the specificity of the response requires additional work. Despite the variability, EEG endpoints can be used in preclinical models and possess translatable utility. Thus work continues on EEG biomarker endpoints as tools for ADHD drug development.

Functional Magnetic Resonance Imaging

The use of functional magnetic resonance imaging as a tool to aid in understanding ADHD has recently been reviewed.[111] For the most part, fMRI has been employed further to elucidate the behavioral and cognitive deficits associated with the disease rather than specific pharmacological responses or as a tool to predict clinical benefit. fMRI can be performed in awake animals and humans, but considerable methodology work is required to prove utility as a tool for early decisions in the clinic.

Cerebrospinal Fluid Endpoints

Although a few reports have described alterations in CSF monoamines in patients with ADHD, such studies are rare as collection of CSF in pediatric patients is still considered to be invasive. Nevertheless, abnormalities in homovanillic acid levels have been reported and that baseline levels correlate with clinical benefit of stimulant treatment.[250] In current drug development, most CSF measures are used to assess pharmacodynamic activity associated with specific mechanistic activity of compounds rather than as predictors of clinically efficacious responses.

Neuroendocrine Data

Alteration of noradrenergic tone increases circulating levels of hypothalamic-pituitary-adrenal hormones including adrenocorticotropin (ACTH), growth hormone and cortisol following acute administration.[x] Specifically, NE induces the release of corticotrophic releasing hormone from the hypothalamic paraventricular nucleus which in turn regulates both ACTH and cortisol levels. Stimulation of adrenergic α_2 receptors (either through direct stimulation of hypothalamic median eminence neurons or indirect stimulation of somatotrophs) are thought to underlie increases in growth hormone release. Although neuroendocrine endpoints have been important tools to understand phenotypic traits associated with psychoaffective disorders, pediatric populations do exhibit gender specific responses.[251,252] In addition, neuroendocrine endpoints like GH exhibit cyclical and diurnal levels of expression.[253,254] Nevertheless, basal morning levels are relatively stable thus allowing a suitable 3–4 h window to assess changes with drug administration in subjects. Extensive endogenous variability of neuroendocrine endpoints to assess ADHD disease state can be problematic. Despite significant variability, neuroendocrine endpoints remain important mechanistic biomarker tools for specific types of pharmacology.

---

[x] For further discussion of effects of stress and changes in the hypothalamic-pituitary-adrenal axis in other behavioral disorders, please refer to Cryan *et al.*, Developing more efficacious antidepressant medications: improving and aligning preclinical detection and clinical assessment tools, Large *et al.*, Developing therapeutics for bipolar disorder: from animal models to the clinic, Steckler *et al.*, Developing novel anxiolytics: improving preclinical detection and clinical assessment; in this volume.

An example of the utility of neuroendocrine endpoints involves use as a mechanistic endpoint to establish pharmacology. For example, NRIs such as atomoxetine can stimulate the release of salivary cortisol[253] and reboxetine (Edronax®) can stimulate growth hormone (GH) following a single dose administration.[255] Compounds with direct α_2-adrenoceptor agonist activity such as guanfacine and clonidine have also been shown to induce a GH response following a single dose of guanfacine or clonidine in adults and pediatric patients[256,257] Increases in neuroendocrine endpoints are translational and GH changes have also been measured in rats following administration of clonidine.[258,259] Alterations with neuroendocrine endpoints have also been demonstrated with several compounds including tricyclic antidepressants (desipramine and imipramine), in addition to the NRIs reboxetine and atomoxetine[255,260] (unpublished observations). While many of the compounds described above have shown some utility in the treatment of ADHD, they in and of themselves are not predictive of efficacy. Rather, neuroendocrine endpoints reflect monoaminergic tone and are useful mechanistic markers of centrally mediated pharmacodynamic activity.

Physiologic Measures

Sympathetic endpoints have also proved useful in assessing noradrenergic tone. Although innervation of the iris is complex and involves different pathways, mydriasis – defined as an increase in pupillary diameter – has been used as a biomarker of NRI activity. Indeed, venlafaxine (Effexor®), a dual 5-HT/NE reuptake inhibitor and reboxetine, a more selective NRI, both increase resting pupil diameter in humans.[261-264,286] These changes are thought to be centrally mediated. As part of their first-in-human study, Pereira et al.[287] included measurement of pupillary light reflex following administration of LY2124275, a second-generation NRI. Results showed exposure-related increases in pupillary diameter and decreases in constriction rates. Thus, pupillary responses, specifically mydriasis, can be used to assess pharmacodynamic activity and establish proof of pharmacology.

Other physiologic measures such as salivary flow offer distinct advantages as a central biomarker of α_2-adrenoreceptor agonist activity. The response is amenable to exposure-response modeling and methodology can be easily implemented as part of a Phase I study. Although no data are available following the administration of guanfacine, decreases in salivary flow have been measured following administration of clonidine.[265-269]

Disease- or Outcome-Based Biomarkers

The main characteristics of ADHD are inattention, hyperactivity, and impulsivity. New treatments aim to improve these behavioral symptoms but also ameliorate cognitive disfunction. Numerous studies have been conducted to investigate the cognitive effects of stimulants and other compounds using different tests (reaction time, memory, learning, vigilance, etc.) with varying results. This topic has been elegantly summarized by Pietrzak et al. with regard to the effects of immediate-release MPH on cognitive function in ADHD patients.[270] The effects of a new drug on different domains of cognitive function are important to understand a drug's characteristics. However, their use for decision-making in clinical development is limited. Several batteries of test are available and can be used in early Phase I studies (e.g., CogState Ltd).[271] However, improvements in these endpoints are difficult to detect in a healthy population with no known impairment, limiting their usefulness as part of an early development program.[xi]

Small studies using laboratory classroom setting have been used successfully to evaluate the effect of different formulations of stimulants in children with ADHD.[272–275]. These studies used a crossover study design to evaluate the time course of response in relation to the pharmacokinetic profiles of new extended-release formulations of different stimulants (discussed in detail in below). Although not a biomarker *per se*, results can be extended to efficacy in the general ADHD population.

Overall, the use of biomarkers can greatly enhance a drug development program. The selection of an ideal biomarker varies greatly depending on the mechanism of action. To establish such milestones as proof of mechanism, proof of pharmacology, or proof that the drug reaches its site of action, different methods may be employed. The challenge is greater when developing a compound with a new mechanism of action since the uncertainty in terms of defining the target is large considering that no prior information is available in the clinic.

CHALLENGES IN CLINICAL DEVELOPMENT

As is the case for many neurologic and psychiatric indications, the clinical development program of a drug for ADHD must confront the unknown validity of its preclinical and translational models. This problem is particularly acute for ADHD, because the approved treatments for ADHD (psychostimulants and atomoxetine) were developed only after there was clinical evidence of their potential efficacy in humans, rather than being developed from a drug discovery program that was informed by a deep neurobiological understanding of the disease. Indeed, the preclinical models of ADHD have been, in large part, reverse-engineered from the knowledge that psychostimulants are a clinically efficacious treatment. The early clinical program for a new treatment for ADHD is discussed here, in this light.

A second challenge that rather uniquely confronts ADHD is that the majority of the known patient population is pediatric, and an extensive program of clinical studies must be conducted in this age range. It is often assumed, that the pathophysiology of ADHD is similar in children and in adults, and that efficacy of a drug for ADHD will not differ in children versus adults. In fact, this assumption is untested, and we discuss below both general issues related to pediatric drug development and the specific issue of possible differences between adults and children.

[xi] Please see Schneider, Issues in design and conduct of clinical trials for cognitive-enhancing drugs, in Volume 2, *Neurologic Disorders* for further discussion regarding testing of compounds with cognitive-enhancing potential.

Early Clinical Development for ADHD

The clinical development program of a new chemical entity for the treatment of ADHD must be initiated in adult volunteers, rather than in pediatric patients, as discussed below.

The availability of an "outcome biomarker" would greatly facilitate such a clinical program, but no such biomarker is available presently. In its absence, it still may be possible to obtain useful pharmacodynamic information in a "first-in-human" study by inclusion of simple drug effect questionnaires rating subjective effects such as sedation, euphoria, and dizziness. Neurocognitive endpoints, such as those reviewed above, could also be evaluated in early clinical studies, but their value as biomarkers for efficacy in ADHD is not established. PK-PD modeling can then be undertaken to characterize the exposure–response relationship for these effects, and this information (taken with preclinical predictions of the efficacious concentration range and the adverse event profile) can then be used in setting the dose to be tested in initial proof of concept (POC) studies in patients with ADHD.

Intermediate between a functional outcome biomarker and a full proof of concept endpoint is the approach of seeking an "early signal of efficacy (ESOE)." One experimental paradigm that has been used repeatedly in drug development for ADHD, and which may be useful as an ESOE, is the "laboratory school" or "analog classroom" model.[273,276] In this model, the effects of ADHD treatments are assessed in a controlled classroom setting, using both observational measures of behavior, as well as academic performance measures (e.g., timed tests of arithmetic). Assessments are made repeatedly throughout a single day, allowing the collection of data for PK-PD modeling. These studies generally require a sample size of about 50 subjects, and often feature a crossover design, allowing the comparison of multiple doses of a single agent, or of multiple different agents and placebo. Only a handful of centers across the United States have both facilities for and experience in conducting this type of study.

Virtually all of the development programs for approved psychostimulant medications included analog classroom studies, usually during Phase II or Phase III, and these studies would seem appropriate to be considered for use even earlier in development, if a drug is hypothesized to have an effect in the healthy volunteer population. The analog classroom model would lend itself easily to the inclusion of neuropsychological and cognitive measures as well. While this type of study has typically been conducted with pediatric patients, it has also been adapted for use with adult subjects, as a "simulated workplace" paradigm.[277] The possibility that new compounds for ADHD would have positive effects on cognition and behavior in healthy volunteers leads to the possibility that "analog classroom" or "simulated workplace" studies might be useful in Phase I of clinical development, rather than being restricted to later phases.

The typical early Phase II program for ADHD drug development has used small-scale, short-duration crossover studies designed to provide initial proof of differentiation from placebo.[184] The subjects in these studies typically had symptoms of at least moderate severity and had been carefully screened for comorbid conditions such as depression, anxiety, or substance abuse, which were exclusionary. The primary endpoint is typically the change from baseline in ADHD symptoms as measured by total score on an investigator-rated global scale, such as the ADHD-rating scale.[278] In addition, efficacy may also have been evaluated using a responder analysis (defined as ⩾30% improvement from baseline in total ADHD-RS score).

Timing of Pediatric Studies: Ethical and Regulatory Issues

In the typical course of drug development, pediatric trials are planned and performed only after extensive testing and approval in adults, if ever. For ADHD however, commercial imperatives require that any new drug be tested and shown safe and efficacious in children as part of its core development program. Moreover, new European regulations require the submission of a "Pediatric Investigational Plan" prior to entering Phase II in adults (although the plan may request a deferral of pediatric studies).[279] At what point then, should pediatric studies in ADHD begin?

FDA guidance document E11, "Clinical Investigation of Medicinal Products in the Pediatric Population," provides general guidelines on the appropriate timing of pediatric studies in the development of new chemical entities (NCEs). Among the central criteria identified in this document are the prevalence and severity of the disease under study, the availability of alternative treatments, and the chemical novelty of the compound under development. In the case of ADHD, prevalence is high, but the availability of already approved treatments that are both safe and effective, and the fact that ADHD is not life threatening, weighs in favor of deferring pediatric studies until there is a reasonable indication of safety and potential efficacy in adults who are administered the new compound. Recent precedent with atomoxetine and modafinil also supports the deferral of pediatric studies in ADHD until a substantial body of adult data is available. Atomoxetine had been studied in a substantial number of adults as a treatment for depression,[280] and modafinil[281] had been studied and approved for the treatment of adults with narcolepsy, before pediatric studies in ADHD were conducted. Other compounds initially evaluated in adult patients with ADHD include the nicotinic agonist ABT-418[282] and most recently the ampakine allosteric modulator CX717.[283]

One approach to the timing of pediatric studies in the development program is depicted in Figure 10.2. This figure illustrates the need to establish a database of safety and tolerability, as well as initial POC, in adults, prior to the initiation of any pediatric clinical study. Appropriate preclinical studies of developmental toxicology clearly must precede dosing in children, and it would be at the development sponsor's discretion whether to invest in these animal studies prior to establishing adult POC.

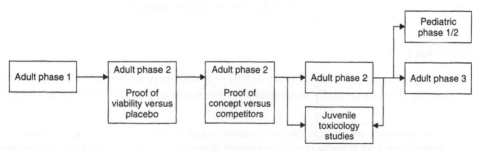

Figure 10.2 Staged clinical development of pharmaceutical agents for juvenile populations

For a compound showing good safety and tolerability in adults, it may be possible to advance to pediatric dosing after a few hundred adults have been exposed to the drug.[xii]

Differential Efficacy in Children Versus Adults

This adult-first approach to POC in ADHD is based on the implicit assumption that the underlying neurobiology and clinical response to treatment is comparable across the lifespan, despite the fact that ADHD symptom presentation changes over development. In fact, available data suggest that treatment response in adults is not always comparable to that observed in children and adolescents. For example, the treatment effect size typically observed in adult trials with atomoxetine (approximately 0.4) is substantially less than that observed in pediatric trials with atomoxetine (approximately 0.7).[284] Various explanations related to comorbidity and other factors have been offered, but by contrast, a recent review of psychostimulant use in adults with ADHD showed that they are associated with a "robust clinical response that is highly consistent with that observed in pediatric studies using equipotent daily doses."[285] Taken together, these results indicate that the treatment effect observed in an adult POC study may not be predictive of the true effect size which may be obtained in future clinical trials in children and adolescents. Achieving proof of concept in children, after establishing it in adults, is further complicated by the use of different efficacy endpoints, or of differential validity of efficacy endpoints, in children versus adults.

What could account for differences in treatment response between adults and younger age groups? One possibility is that children and adults with ADHD have differential neurobiology (e.g., there could be developmental differences in the relative density of neurotransmitter receptor subtypes). The issue of differential treatment effects could arise in at least two other scenarios. First, future drug development efforts could be developmentally targeted. That is, they might target neurobiological processes that are more relevant to one age group than another (e.g., myelination). Second, a treatment might be targeted to address symptoms that are more common in one age group than another (e.g., hyperactivity). If the clinical development plan for a new compound requires proof of concept in adults before advancing to studies of children, then it is possible that a compound with poor efficacy in adults could be discontinued despite having unrecognized benefits in children. Translational models should ideally, therefore, be evaluated for their validity in both children and adults, and the possibility of differential validity must be recognized and accounted for. This will be a notable challenge for ADHD and for any other condition in which developmental processes may distinguish adults and children with the disease.

SUMMARY

As discussed throughout this chapter, ADHD is a relatively common disorder in children causing developmentally inappropriate symptoms of inattention, impulsivity, and

---

[xii] For further discussion regarding regulatory guidelines regarding testing candidate drugs for potential abuse liability, please refer to Rocha *et al.*, Development of medications for heroin and cocaine addiction and regulatory aspects of abuse liability testing, in Volume 3, *Reward Deficit Disorders*.

hyperactivity of which inattention and impulsivity often persist into adulthood. Left untreated ADHD can result in significant impairment including poor academic performance, lower incomes, greater marital problems, social maladaptation, and a higher risk for injuries. Though treatment options exist, a significant unmet medical need continues. This continued need is driven by many factors including a lack of understanding and acceptance of the disorder within the general population and the inability of current medications to fully treat the disorder in all patients including core symptoms and cognitive impairments. In both cases, a greater understanding of the biological etiology of ADHD would improve our ability to identify and treat this medical population. While significant advancements have been made in identifying genetic and neurological risk factors, as yet no biological diagnostic tool exists. As such, the search for novel, more effective medications relies heavily on assays in animal models, which are proposed to mimic symptoms found in ADHD. Since no animal model has been found that can reliably model the full disorder most preclinical drug discovery efforts rely on these assays to establish proof of mechanism while determining proof of concept (i.e., proving that the new drug target is effective in treating ADHD) in a clinical setting and using translatable biomarkers to bridge the gap. As novel mechanisms are tested in the clinic it will be important to re-evaluate them in a systematic and comprehensive manner in current animal models to better define their utility in predicting clinical outcomes in ADHD patients. Only through these means can more accurate models be identified which can ultimately help to better understand the disorder and more quickly bring effective medications to patients in need.

ACKNOWLEDGEMENTS

The authors would like to thank Betty Pettersen, Gregg Cappon, and Vamsi Bollu for their helpful insights and comments during the development of this chapter.

REFERENCES

1. NIH Consensus Statement on ADHD (2000). National Institutes of Health Consensus Development Conference Statement: Diagnosis and treatment of attention-deficit/hyperactivity disorder (ADHD). *J Am Acad Child Adolesc Psychiatry*, 39(2):182–193.
2. Polanczyk, G., de Lima, M.S., Horta, B.L., Biederman, J., and Rohde, L.A. (2007). The worldwide prevalence of ADHD: A systematic review and metaregression analysis. *Am J Psychiatry*, 164(6):942–948.
3. Skounti, M., Philalithis, A., and Galanakis, E. (2007). Variations in prevalence of attention deficit hyperactivity disorder worldwide. *Eur J Pediatr*, 166(2):117–123.
4. Adewuya, A.O. and Famuyiwa, O.O. (2007). Attention deficit hyperactivity disorder among Nigerian primary school children: Prevalence and co-morbid conditions. *Eur Child Adolesc Psychiatry*, 16(1):10–15.
5. Meyer, A. and Sagvolden, T. (2006). Fine motor skills in South African children with symptoms of ADHD: Influence of subtype, gender, age, and hand dominance. *Behav Brain Funct*, 2:33.

6. Fayyad, J., De Graaf, R., Kessler, R., Alonso, J., Angermeyer, M., Demyttenaere, K. *et al.* (2007). Cross-national prevalence and correlates of adult attention-deficit hyperactivity disorder. *Br J Psychiatry*, 190:402–409.

7. Kessler, R.C., Adler, L., Ames, M., Barkley, R.A., Birnbaum, H., Greenberg, P. *et al.* (2005). The prevalence and effects of adult attention deficit/hyperactivity disorder on work performance in a nationally representative sample of workers. *J Occup Environ Med*, 47(6):565–572.

8. Gaub, M. and Carlson, C.L. (1997). Gender differences in ADHD: A meta-analysis and critical review. *J Am Acad Child Adolesc Psychiatry*, 36(8):1036–1045.

9. Smalley, S.L., McGough, J.J., Moilanen, I.K., Loo, S.K., Taanila, A., Ebeling, H. *et al.* (2007). Prevalence and psychiatric comorbidity of attention-deficit/hyperactivity disorder in an adolescent Finnish population. *J Am Acad Child Adolesc Psychiatry*, 46(12):1575–1583.

10. Goldman, L.S., Genel, M., Bezman, R.J., and Slanetz, P.J. (1998). Diagnosis and treatment of attention-deficit/hyperactivity disorder in children and adolescents. Council on Scientific Affairs, American Medical Association. *JAMA*, 279(14):1100–1107.

11. American Psychiatric Association (2000). *Diagnostic and Statistical Manual of the Mental Disorders (4th Edn, Text Revision, DSM-IV-RT)*. American Psychiatric Association, Washington, DC.

12. Palmer, E.D. and Finger, S. (2001). An early description of ADHD (Inattention Subtype): Dr. Alexander Crichton and the 'Mental Restlessness' (1798). *Child Psychol Psychiatry Rev*, 6:66–73.

13. Hoffman, H. (1845). *The Story of Fidgety Phillip*. In Struwelpeter Menu, 19th Century German Stories: VCU Department of Foreign Languages.

14. Still, G.F. (1902). Some abnormal psychical conditions in children. *Lancet*, 1:1008–1012.

15. Still, G.F. (1902). Some abnormal psychical conditions in children. *Lancet*, 1:1077–1082.

16. Still, G.F. (1902). Some abnormal psychical conditions in children. *Lancet*, 1:1163–1168.

17. Volkmar, F. (2005). Toward understanding the basis of ADHD. *Am J Psychiatry*, 162(6):1043–1044.

18. Klein, C., Wendling, K., Huettner, P., Ruder, H., and Peper, M. (2006). Intra-subject variability in attention-deficit hyperactivity disorder. *Biol Psychiatry*, 60(10):1088–1097.

19. Castellanos, F.X., Sonuga-Barke, E.J., Scheres, A., Di Martino, A., Hyde, C., and Walters, J.R. (2005). Varieties of attention-deficit/hyperactivity disorder-related intra-individual variability. *Biol Psychiatry*, 57(11):1416–1423.

20. Castellanos, F.X. and Tannock, R. (2002). Neuroscience of attention-deficit/hyperactivity disorder: The search for endophenotypes. *Nat Rev Neurosci*, 3(8):617–628.

21. Russell, V.A. (2007). Neurobiology of animal models of attention-deficit hyperactivity disorder. *J Neurosci Methods*, 161(2):185–198.

22. Lahey, B.B., Applegate, B., McBurnett, K., Biederman, J., Greenhill, L., Hynd, G.W. *et al.* (1994). DSM-IV field trials for attention deficit hyperactivity disorder in children and adolescents. *Am J Psychiatry*, 151(11):1673–1685.

23. Lubke, G.H., Muthen, B., Moilanen, I.K., McGough, J.J., Loo, S.K., Swanson, J.M. *et al.* (2007). Subtypes versus severity differences in attention-deficit/hyperactivity disorder in the Northern Finnish Birth Cohort. *J Am Acad Child Adolesc Psychiatry*, 46(12):1584–1593.

24. Rasmussen, E.R., Neuman, R.J., Heath, A.C., Levy, F., Hay, D.A., and Todd, R.D. (2002). Replication of the latent class structure of attention-deficit/hyperactivity disorder (ADHD) subtypes in a sample of Australian twins. *J Child Psychol Psychiatry*, 43(8):1018–1028.

25. Althoff, R.R., Copelan, W.E., Stanger, C., Derks, E.M., Todd, R.D., Neuman, R.J. *et al.* (2006). The latent class structure of ADHD is stable across informants. *Twin Res Hum Genet*, 9(4):507–522.

26. Hardy, K.K., Kollins, S.H., Murray, D.W., Riddle, M.A., Greenhill, L., Cunningham, C. *et al.* (2007). Factor structure of parent- and teacher-rated attention-deficit/hyperactivity disorder

symptoms in the preschoolers with attention-deficit/hyperactivity disorder treatment study (PATS). *J Child Adolesc Psychopharmacol*, 17(5):621–634.

27. McGough, J.J. and Barkley, R.A. (2004). Diagnostic controversies in adult attention deficit hyperactivity disorder. *Am J Psychiatry*, 161(11):1948–1956.

28. Biederman, J., Mick, E., and Faraone, S.V. (2000). Age-dependent decline of symptoms of attention deficit hyperactivity disorder: Impact of remission definition and symptom type. *Am J Psychiatry*, 157(5):816–818.

29. Larsson, H., Lichtenstein, P., and Larsson, J.O. (2006). Genetic contributions to the development of ADHD subtypes from childhood to adolescence. *J Am Acad Child Adolesc Psychiatry*, 45(8):973–981.

30. Diamantopoulou, S., Rydell, A.M., Thorell, L.B., and Bohlin, G. (2007). Impact of executive functioning and symptoms of attention deficit hyperactivity disorder on children's peer relations and school performance. *Dev Neuropsychol*, 32(1):521–542.

31. Fuchs, L., Fuchs, D., Compton, D., Powell, S., Seethaler, P., Capizzi, A. *et al.* (2006). The cognitive correlates of third-grade skills in arithmetic, algorithmic computation and arithmetic word problems. *J Educ Psychol*, 98(1):29–43.

32. Rabiner, D. and Coie, J.D. (2000). Early attention problems and children's reading achievement: A longitudinal investigation. The Conduct Problems Prevention Research Group. *J Am Acad Child Adolesc Psychiatry*, 39(7):859–867.

33. Rodriguez, A., Jarvelin, M.R., Obel, C., Taanila, A., Miettunen, J., Moilanen, I. *et al.* (2007). Do inattention and hyperactivity symptoms equal scholastic impairment? Evidence from three European cohorts. *BMC Public Health*, 7(1):327.

34. Burke, J.D., Loeber, R., White, H.R., Stouthamer-Loeber, M., and Pardini, D.A. (2007). Inattention as a key predictor of tobacco use in adolescence. *J Abnorm Psychol*, 116(2):249–259.

35. Rodriguez, D., Tercyak, K.P., and Audrain-McGovern, J. (2007). Effects of inattention and hyperactivity/impulsivity symptoms on development of nicotine dependence from mid adolescence to young adulthood. *J Pediatr Psychol* (in press).

36. Gardner, T.W., Dishion, T.J., and Posner, M.I. (2006). Attention and adolescent tobacco use: A potential self-regulatory dynamic underlying nicotine addiction. *Addict Behav*, 31(3):531–536.

37. Friedman, N.P., Haberstick, B.C., Willcutt, E.G., Miyake, A., Young, S.E., Corley, R.P. *et al.* (2007). Greater attention problems during childhood predict poorer executive functioning in late adolescence. *Psychol Sci*, 18(10):893–900.

38. Martel, M., Nikolas, M., and Nigg, J.T. (2007). Executive function in adolescents with ADHD. *J Am Acad Child Adolesc Psychiatry*, 46(11):1437–1444.

39. Martinussen, R., Hayden, J., Hogg-Johnson, S., and Tannock, R. (2005). A meta-analysis of working memory impairments in children with attention-deficit/hyperactivity disorder. *J Am Acad Child Adolesc Psychiatry*, 44(4):377–384.

40. Thorell, L.B. (2007). Do delay aversion and executive function deficits make distinct contributions to the functional impact of ADHD symptoms? A study of early academic skill deficits. *J Child Psychol Psychiatry*, 48(11):1061–1070.

41. Willcutt, E.G., Doyle, A.E., Nigg, J.T., Faraone, S.V., and Pennington, B.F. (2005). Validity of the executive function theory of attention-deficit/hyperactivity disorder: A meta-analytic review. *Biol Psychiatry*, 57(11):1336–1346.

42. Massetti, G.M., Lahey, B.B., Pelham, W.E., Loney, J., Ehrhardt, A., Lee, S.S., *et al.* (2008). Academic achievement over 8 years among children who met modified criteria for attention-deficit/hyperactivity disorder at 4–6 years of age. *J Abnorm Child Psychol*, 36(3):399–410.

43. Toplak, M.E. and Tannock, R. (2005). Time perception: Modality and duration effects in attention-deficit/hyperactivity disorder (ADHD). *J Abnorm Child Psychol*, 33(5): 639–654.

44. Abikoff, H.B., Jensen, P.S., Arnold, L.L., Hoza, B., Hechtman, L., Pollack, S. *et al.* (2002). Observed classroom behavior of children with ADHD: Relationship to gender and comorbidity. *J Abnorm Child Psychol*, 30(4):349–359.

45. Bauermeister, J.J., Shrout, P.E., Chavez, L., Rubio-Stipec, M., Ramirez, R., Padilla, L. *et al.* (2007). ADHD and gender: Are risks and sequela of ADHD the same for boys and girls?. *J Child Psychol Psychiatry*, 48(8):831–839.

46. Biederman, J., Kwon, A., Aleardi, M., Chouinard, V.A., Marino, T., Cole, H. *et al.* (2005). Absence of gender effects on attention deficit hyperactivity disorder: Findings in nonreferred subjects. *Am J Psychiatry*, 162(6):1083–1089.

47. Graetz, B.W., Sawyer, M.G., and Baghurst, P. (2005). Gender differences among children with DSM-IV ADHD in Australia. *J Am Acad Child Adolesc Psychiatry*, 44(2):159–168.

48. Derks, E.M., Hudziak, J.J., and Boomsma, D.I. (2007). Why more boys than girls with ADHD receive treatment: A study of Dutch twins. *Twin Res Hum Genet*, 10(5):765–770.

49. Busch, B., Biederman, J., Cohen, L.G., Sayer, J.M., Monuteaux, M.C., Mick, E. *et al.* (2002). Correlates of ADHD among children in pediatric and psychiatric clinics. *Psychiatr Serv*, 53(9):1103–1111.

50. Sprafkin, J., Gadow, K.D., Weiss, M.D., Schneider, J., and Nolan, E.E. (2007). Psychiatric comorbidity in ADHD symptom subtypes in clinic and community adults. *J Atten Disord*, 11(2):114–124.

51. Kessler, R.C., Adler, L., Barkley, R., Biederman, J., Conners, C.K., Demler, O. *et al.* (2006). The prevalence and correlates of adult ADHD in the United States: Results from the National Comorbidity Survey Replication. *Am J Psychiatry*, 163(4):716–723.

52. Biederman, J. (2004). Impact of comorbidity in adults with attention-deficit/hyperactivity disorder. *J Clin Psychiatry*, 65(Suppl 3):3–7.

53. Faraone, S.V. and Biederman, J. (2005). What is the prevalence of adult ADHD? Results of a population screen of 966 adults. *J Atten Disord*, 9(2):384–391.

54. Barkley, R.A. (2004). Driving impairments in teens and adults with attention-deficit/hyperactivity disorder. *Psychiatr Clin North Am*, 27(2):233–260.

55. Harpin, V.A. (2005). The effect of ADHD on the life of an individual, their family, and community from preschool to adult life. *Arch Dis Child*, 90(Suppl 1):i2–i7.

56. Brehaut, J.C., Miller, A., Raina, P., and McGrail, K.M. (2003). Childhood behavior disorders and injuries among children and youth: A population-based study. *Pediatrics*, 111(2):262–269.

57. Rowe, R., Maughan, B., and Goodman, R. (2004). Childhood psychiatric disorder and unintentional injury: Findings from a national cohort study. *J Pediatr Psychol*, 29(2):119–130.

58. Barbaresi, W.J., Katusic, S.K., Colligan, R.C., Weaver, A.L., and Jacobsen, S.J. (2007). Long-term school outcomes for children with attention-deficit/hyperactivity disorder: A population-based perspective. *J Dev Behav Pediatr*, 28(4):265–273.

59. Currie, J. and Stabile, M. (2006). Child mental health, human capital accumulation: The case of ADHD. *J Health Econ*, 25(6):1094–1118.

60. Biederman, J., Monuteaux, M.C., Mick, E., Spencer, T., Wilens, T.E., Silva, J.M. *et al.* (2006). Young adult outcome of attention deficit hyperactivity disorder: A controlled 10-year follow-up study. *Psychol Med*, 36(2):167–179.

61. Barkley, R.A., Fischer, M., Smallish, L., and Fletcher, K. (2006). Young adult outcome of hyperactive children: Adaptive functioning in major life activities. *J Am Acad Child Adolesc Psychiatry*, 45(2):192–202.

62. Birnbaum, H.G., Kessler, R.C., Lowe, S.W., Secnik, K., Greenberg, P.E., Leong, S.A. *et al.* (2005). Costs of attention deficit-hyperactivity disorder (ADHD) in the US: Excess costs of persons with ADHD and their family members in 2000. *Curr Med Res Opin*, 21(2):195–206.

63. De Ridder, A. and De Graeve, D. (2006). Healthcare use, social burden and costs of children with and without ADHD in Flanders, Belgium. *Clin Drug Investig*, 26(2):75–90.

64. King, S., Griffin, S., Hodges, Z., Weatherly, H., Asseburg, C., Richardson, G., *et al.* (2006). A systematic review and economic model of the effectiveness and cost-effectiveness of methylphenidate, dexamfetamine and atomoxetine for the treatment of attention deficit hyperactivity disorder in children and adolescents. *Health Technol Assess* 10(23): iii-iv, xiii-146.

65. Pelham, W.E., Foster, E.M., and Robb, J.A. (2007). The economic impact of attention-deficit/hyperactivity disorder in children and adolescents. *Ambul Pediatr*, 7(1 Suppl):121-131.

66. Baughman, F.A., Jr (2001). Questioning the treatment for ADHD. *Science*, 291(5504):595.

67. Diller, L. (1998). *Running on Ritalin: A physician reflects on children, society, and performance in a pill*. Bantam Books, New York.

68. Faraone, S.V. (2005). The scientific foundation for understanding attention-deficit/hyperactivity disorder as a valid psychiatric disorder. *Eur Child Adolesc Psychiatry*, 14(1):1-10.

69. Rohde, L.A., Szobot, C., Polanczyk, G., Schmitz, M., Martins, S., and Tramontina, S. (2005). Attention-deficit/hyperactivity disorder in a diverse culture: Do research and clinical findings support the notion of a cultural construct for the disorder? *Biol Psychiatry*, 57(11):1436-1441.

70. Douglas, V.I. (1972). Stop, look, and listen: The problem of sustained attention and impulse control in hyperactive and normal children. *Can J Behav Sci*, 4:259-282.

71. Mattes, J.A. (1980). The role of frontal lobe dysfunction in childhood hyperkinesis. *Compr Psychiatry*, 21(5):358-369.

72. Pennington, B.F. and Ozonoff, S. (1996). Executive functions and developmental psychopathology. *J Child Psychol Psychiatry*, 37(1):51-87.

73. Barkley, R.A. (1997). Behavioral inhibition, sustained attention, and executive functions: Constructing a unifying theory of ADHD. *Psychol Bull*, 121(1):65-94.

74. Swanson, J.M., Kinsbourne, M., Nigg, J., Lanphear, B., Stefanatos, G.A., Volkow, N. *et al.* (2007). Etiologic subtypes of attention-deficit/hyperactivity disorder: Brain imaging, molecular genetic and environmental factors and the dopamine hypothesis. *Neuropsychol Rev*, 17(1):39-59.

75. Wender, P. (1971). *Minimal brain dysfunction in children*. Wiley-Liss, New York.

76. Sagvolden, T., Johansen, E.B., Aase, H., and Russell, V.A. (2005) A dynamic developmental theory of attention-deficit/hyperactivity disorder (ADHD) predominantly hyperactive/impulsive and combined subtypes. *Behav Brain Sci* 28(3):397-419 discussion 419-368.

77. Gainetdinov, R.R., Wetsel, W.C., Jones, S.R., Levin, E.D., Jaber, M., and Caron, M.G. (1999). Role of serotonin in the paradoxical calming effect of psychostimulants on hyperactivity. *Science*, 283(5400):397-401.

78. Oades, R.D. (2007). Role of the serotonin system in ADHD: Treatment implications. *Expert Rev Neurother*, 7(10):1357-1374.

79. Arnsten, A.F. (2006). Fundamentals of attention-deficit/hyperactivity disorder: Circuits and pathways. *J Clin Psychiatry*, 67(Suppl 8):7-12.

80. Zametkin, A.J. and Rapoport, J.L. (1987). Neurobiology of attention deficit disorder with hyperactivity: Where have we come in 50 years? *J Am Acad Child Adolesc Psychiatry*, 26(5):676-686.

81. Wilens, T.E. and Decker, M.W. (2007). Neuronal nicotinic receptor agonists for the treatment of attention-deficit/hyperactivity disorder: Focus on cognition. *Biochem Pharmacol*, 74:1212-1223.

82. Perlov, E., Philipsen, A., Hesslinger, B., Buechert, M., Ahrendts, J., Feige, B., Bubl, E., Hennig, J., Ebert, D., and van Eslt Tebartz, L. (2007). Reduced cingulate glutamate/glutamine-to-creatinine ratios in adult patients with attention deficit/hyperactivit disorder: A magnet resonance spectroscopy study. *J Psychiatric Res*, 41:934-941.

83. Russell, V.A., Sagvolden, T., and Johansen, E.B. (2005). Animal models of attention-deficit hyperactivity disorder. *Behav Brain Funct* (epub);1:9.

84. Faraone, S.V., Perlis, R.H., Doyle, A.E., Smoller, J.W., Goralnick, J.J., Holmgren, M.A. *et al.* (2005). Molecular genetics of attention-deficit/hyperactivity disorder. *Biol Psychiatry*, 57(11):1313-1323.

85. Faraone, S.V. and Khan, S.A. (2006). Candidate gene studies of attention-deficit/hyperactivity disorder. *J Clin Psychiatry*, 67(Suppl 8):13-20.

86. Dorval, K.M., Wigg, K.G., Crosbie, J., Tannock, R., Kennedy, J.L., Ickowicz, A. *et al.* (2007). Association of the glutamate receptor subunit gene GRIN2B with attention-deficit/hyperactivity disorder. *Genes Brain Behav*, 6(5):444-452.

87. Friedel, S., Saar, K., Sauer, S., Dempfle, A., Walitza, S., Renner, T. *et al.* (2007). Association and linkage of allelic variants of the dopamine transporter gene in ADHD. *Mol Psychiatry*, 12(10):923-933.

88. Ogdie, M.N., Macphie, I.L., Minassian, S.L., Yang, M., Fisher, S.E., Francks, C. *et al.* (2003). A genomewide scan for attention-deficit/hyperactivity disorder in an extended sample: Suggestive linkage on 17p11. *Am J Hum Genet*, 72(5):1268-1279.

89. Muir, T. and Zegarac, M. (2001). Societal costs of exposure to toxic substances: Economic and health costs of four case studies that are candidates for environmental causation. *Environ Health Perspect*, 109(Suppl 6):885-903.

90. Slotkin, T.A. (2004). Cholinergic systems in brain development and disruption by neurotoxicants: Nicotine, environmental tobacco smoke, organophosphates. *Toxicol Appl Pharmacol*, 198(2):132-151.

91. Slotkin, T.A., Ryde, I.T., Tate, C.A., and Seidler, F.J. (2007). Lasting effects of nicotine treatment and withdrawal on serotonergic systems and cell signaling in rat brain regions: Separate or sequential exposure during fetal development and adulthood. *Brain Res Bull*, 73(4-6):259-272.

92. Liang, K., Poytress, B.S., Chen, Y., Leslie, F.M., Weinberger, N.M., and Metherate, R. (2006). Neonatal nicotine exposure impairs nicotinic enhancement of central auditory processing and auditory learning in adult rats. *Eur J Neurosci*, 24(3):857-866.

93. Langley, K., Holmans, P.A., van den Bree, M.B., and Thapar, A. (2007). Effects of low birth weight, maternal smoking in pregnancy and social class on the phenotypic manifestation of Attention Deficit Hyperactivity Disorder and associated antisocial behaviour: Investigation in a clinical sample. *BMC Psychiatry*, 7:26.

94. Schmitz, M., Denardin, D., Laufer Silva, T., Pianca, T., Hutz, M.H., Faraone, S. *et al.* (2006). Smoking during pregnancy and attention-deficit/hyperactivity disorder, predominantly inattentive type: A case-control study. *J Am Acad Child Adolesc Psychiatry*, 45(11):1338-1345.

95. Kharrazi, M., DeLorenze, G.N., Kaufman, F.L., Eskenazi, B., Bernert, J.T., Jr, Graham, S. *et al.* (2004). Environmental tobacco smoke and pregnancy outcome. *Epidemiology*, 15(6):660-670.

96. Lahti, J., Raikkonen, K., Kajantie, E., Heinonen, K., Pesonen, A.K., Jarvenpaa, A.L. *et al.* (2006). Small body size at birth and behavioural symptoms of ADHD in children aged five to six years. *J Child Psychol Psychiatry*, 47(11):1167-1174.

97. Ward, C., Lewis, S., and Coleman, T. (2007). Prevalence of maternal smoking and environmental tobacco smoke exposure during pregnancy and impact on birth weight: Retrospective study using Millennium Cohort. *BMC Public Health*, 7:81.

98. Jacobsen, L.K., Picciotto, M.R., Heath, C.J., Frost, S.J., Tsou, K.A., Dwan, R.A. *et al.* (2007). Prenatal and adolescent exposure to tobacco smoke modulates the development of white matter microstructure. *J Neurosci*, 27(49):13491-13498.

99. Fried, P.A., Watkinson, B., and Siegel, L.S. (1997). Reading and language in 9- to 12-year olds prenatally exposed to cigarettes and marijuana. *Neurotoxicol Teratol*, 19(3):171-183.

100. Yolton, K., Dietrich, K., Auinger, P., Lanphear, B.P., and Hornung, R. (2005). Exposure to environmental tobacco smoke and cognitive abilities among U.S. children and adolescents. *Environ Health Perspect*, 113(1):98–103.

101. Kahn, R.S., Khoury, J., Nichols, W.C., and Lamphear, B.P. (2003). Role of dopamine transporter genotype and maternal prenatal smoking in childhood hyperactive-impulsive, inattentive, and oppositional behaviors. *J Pediatr*, 143(1):104–110.

102. Neuman, R.J., Lobos, E., Reich, W., Henderson, C.A., Sun, L.W., and Todd, R.D. (2007). Prenatal smoking exposure and dopaminergic genotypes interact to cause a severe ADHD subtype. *Biol Psychiatry*, 61(12):1320–1328.

103. Todd, R.D. and Neuman, R.J. (2007). Gene-environment interactions in the development of combined type ADHD: Evidence for a synapse-based model. *Am J Med Genet B Neuropsychiatr Genet*, 144(8):971–975.

104. Valera, E.M., Faraone, S.V., Murray, K.E., and Seidman, L.J. (2007). Meta-analysis of structural imaging findings in attention-deficit/hyperactivity disorder. *Biol Psychiatry*, 61(12):1361–1369.

105. Castellanos, F.X., Lee, P.P., Sharp, W., Jeffries, N.O., Greenstein, D.K., Clasen, L.S. *et al.* (2002). Developmental trajectories of brain volume abnormalities in children and adolescents with attention-deficit/hyperactivity disorder. *JAMA*, 288(14):1740–1748.

106. Shaw, P., Eckstrand, K., Sharp, W., Blumenthal, J., Lerch, J.P., Greenstein, D. *et al.* (2007). Attention-deficit/hyperactivity disorder is characterized by a delay in cortical maturation. *Proc Natl Acad Sci USA*, 104(49):19649–19654.

107. Shaw, P., Lerch, J., Greenstein, D., Sharp, W., Clasen, L., Evans, A. *et al.* (2006). Longitudinal mapping of cortical thickness and clinical outcome in children and adolescents with attention-deficit/hyperactivity disorder. *Arch Gen Psychiatry*, 63(5):540–549.

108. Bonelli, R.M. and Cummings, J.L. (2007). Frontal-subcortical circuitry and behavior. *Dialogues Clin Neurosci*, 9(2):141–151.

109. Doyle, A.E. (2006). Executive functions in attention-deficit/hyperactivity disorder. *J Clin Psychiatry*, 67(Suppl 8):21–26.

110. Dickstein, S.G., Bannon, K., Xavier Castellanos, F., and Milham, M.P. (2006). The neural correlates of attention deficit hyperactivity disorder: An ALE meta-analysis. *J Child Psychol Psychiatry*, 47(10):1051–1062.

111. Paloyelis, Y., Mehta, M.A., Kuntsi, J., and Asherson, P. (2007). Functional MRI in ADHD: A systematic literature review. *Expert Rev Neurother*, 7(10):1337–1356.

112. Konrad, K., Neufang, S., Hanisch, C., Fink, G.R., and Herpertz-Dahlmann, B. (2006). Dysfunctional attentional networks in children with attention deficit/hyperactivity disorder: Evidence from an event-related functional magnetic resonance imaging study. *Biol Psychiatry*, 59(7):643–651.

113. Ashtari, M., Kumra, S., Bhaskar, S.L., Clarke, T., Thaden, E., Cervellione, K.L. *et al.* (2005). Attention-deficit/hyperactivity disorder: A preliminary diffusion tensor imaging study. *Biol Psychiatry*, 57(5):448–455.

114. Casey, B.J., Epstein, J.N., Buhle, J., Liston, C., Davidson, M.C., Tonev, S.T. *et al.* (2007). Frontostriatal connectivity and its role in cognitive control in parent-child dyads with ADHD. *Am J Psychiatry*, 164(11):1729–1736.

115. Durston, S., Huslhoff Pol, H.E., Schnack, H.G., Buitelaar, J.K., Steenhuis, M.P., Minderaa, R.B., Kahn, R.S., and van Engeland, H. (2004). Magnetic resonance imaging of boys with attention-deficit/hyperactivity disorder and their unaffected siblings. *J Am Acad Child Adolesc Psychiatry*, 43(3):332–340.

116. Castellanos, F.X., Margulies, D.S., Kelly, C., Uddin, L.Q., Ghaffari, M., Kirsch, A., *et al.* (2008). Cingulate-precuneus interactions: A new locus of dysfunction in adult attention-deficit/hyperactivity disorder. *Biol Psychiatry*, 63(3):332–337.

117. Fransson, P. (2006). How default is the default mode of brain function? Further evidence from intrinsic BOLD signal fluctuations. *Neuropsychologia*, 44(14):2836–2845.

118. Greicius, M.D. and Menon, V. (2004). Default-mode activity during a passive sensory task: Uncoupled from deactivation but impacting activation. *J Cogn Neurosci*, 16(9):1484–1492.

119. Clare Kelly, A.M., Uddin, L.Q., Biswal, B.B., Castellanos, F.X., and Milham, M.P. (2008). Competition between functional brain networks mediates behavioral variability. *Neuroimage*, 39(1):527–537.

120. Nigg, J.T., Willcutt, E.G., Doyle, A.E., and Sonuga-Barke, E.J. (2005). Causal heterogeneity in attention-deficit/hyperactivity disorder: Do we need neuropsychologically impaired subtypes? *Biol Psychiatry*, 57(11):1224–1230.

121. Doyle, A.E., Biederman, J., Seidman, L.J., Weber, W., and Faraone, S.V. (2000). Diagnostic efficiency of neuropsychological test scores for discriminating boys with and without attention deficit-hyperactivity disorder. *J Consult Clin Psychol*, 68(3):477–488.

122. Toplak, M.E., Jain, U., and Tannock, R. (2005). Executive and motivational processes in adolescents with Attention-Deficit-Hyperactivity Disorder (ADHD). *Behav Brain Funct*, 1(1):8.

123. Doyle, A.E., Faraone, S.V., Seidman, L.J., Willcutt, E.G., Nigg, J.T., Waldman, I.D. *et al.* (2005). Are endophenotypes based on measures of executive functions useful for molecular genetic studies of ADHD?. *J Child Psychol Psychiatry*, 46(7):774–803.

124. Waldman, I.D. (2005). Statistical approaches to complex phenotypes: Evaluating neuropsychological endophenotypes for attention-deficit/hyperactivity disorder. *Biol Psychiatry*, 57(11):1347–1356.

125. Gottesman, I.I. and Gould, T.D. (2003). The endophenotype concept in psychiatry: Etymology and strategic intentions. *Am J Psychiatry*, 160(4):636–645.

126. Gould, T.D. and Gottesman, I.I. (2006). Psychiatric endophenotypes and the development of valid animal models. *Genes Brain Behav*, 5(2):113–119.

127. Crosbie, J., Perseuse, D., Barr, C.L., and Schachar, R.J. (2008). Validating psychiatric endophenotypes: Inhibitory control and attention deficit hyperactivity disorder. *Neurosci Biobehav Rev*, 32:40–55.

128. Nigg, J.T., Blaskey, L.G., Stawicki, J.A., and Sachek, J. (2004). Evaluating the endophenotype model of ADHD neuropsychological deficit: Results for parents and siblings of children with ADHD combined and inattentive subtypes. *J Abnorm Psychol*, 113(4):614–625.

129. Schachar, R.J., Crosbie, J., Barr, C.L., Ornstein, T.J., Kennedy, J., Malone, M. *et al.* (2005). Inhibition of motor responses in siblings concordant and discordant for attention deficit hyperactivity disorder. *Am J Psychiatry*, 162(6):1076–1082.

130. Waldman, I.D., Nigg, J.T., Gizer, I.R., Park, L., Rappley, M.D., and Friderici, K. (2006). The adrenergic receptor alpha-2 A gene (ADRA2A) and neuropsychological executive functions as putative endophenotypes for childhood ADHD. *Cogn Affect Behav Neurosci*, 6(1): 18–30.

131. Slaats-Willemse, D., Swaab-Barneveld, H., de Sonneville, L., van der Meulen, E., and Buitelaar, J. (2003). Deficient response inhibition as a cognitive endophenotype of ADHD. *J Am Acad Child Adolesc Psychiatry*, 42(10):1242–1248.

132. Anstey, K.J., Dear, K., Christensen, H., and Jorm, A.F. (2005). Biomarkers, health, lifestyle, and demographic variables as correlates of reaction time performance in early, middle, and late adulthood. *Q J Exp Psychol A*, 58(1):5–21.

133. MacDonald, S.W., Hultsch, D.F., and Dixon, R.A. (2003). Performance variability is related to change in cognition: Evidence from the Victoria Longitudinal Study. *Psychol Aging*, 18(3):510–523.

134. Williams, B.R., Strauss, E.H., Hultsch, D.F., Hunter, M.A., and Tannock, R. (2007). Reaction time performance in adolescents with attention deficit/hyperactivity disorder: Evidence

of inconsistency in the fast and slow portions of the RT distribution. *J Clin Exp Neuropsychol*, 29(3):277–289.

135. Johnson, K.A., Robertson, I.H., Kelly, S.P., Silk, T.J., Barry, E., Daibhis, A. *et al.* (2007). Dissociation in performance of children with ADHD and high-functioning autism on a task of sustained attention. *Neuropsychologia*, 45(10):2234–2245.

136. Kuntsi, J., McLoughlin, G., and Asherson, P. (2006). Attention deficit hyperactivity disorder. *Neuromolecular Med*, 8(4):461–484.

137. Walhovd, K.B. and Fjell, A.M. (2007). White matter volume predicts reaction time instability. *Neuropsychologia*, 45(10):2277–2284.

138. Anstey, M., Mack, H.A., Christensen, H., Li, S.C., Reglade-Meslin, C., Maller, J., Kumar, R., Dear, K., Easteal, S., and Sachdev, P. (2007). Corpus callosum size, reaction time speed and variability in mild cognitive disorders and in a normative sample. *Neuropsychologia*, 45(8):1911–1920.

139. van Beijsterveldt, C.E. and van Baal, G.C. (2002). Twin and family studies of the human electroencephalogram: A review and a meta-analysis. *Biol Psychol*, 61(1–2):111–138.

140. Hall, M.H., Schulze, K., Pijsdijke, F., Picchioni, M., Ettinger, U., Bramon, E., Freedman, R., Murray, R.M., and Sham, P. (2006). Heritability and reliability of P300, P50 and duration mismatch negativity. *Behav Genet*, 36(6):845–857.

141. Carmelli, D., Swan, G.E., DeCarli, C., and Reed, T. (2002). Quantitative genetic modeling of regional brain volumes and cognitive performance in older male twins. *Biol Psychol*, 61(1–2):139–155.

142. Thompson, P.M., Cannon, T.D., Narr, K.L., van Erp, T. *et al.* (2001). Genetic influences on brain structure. *Nat Neurosci*, 4(12):1253–1258.

143. van't Ent, D., Lehn, H., Derks, E.M., Hudziak, J.J., Van Strien, N.M., Veltman, D.J., De Geus, E. J., Todd, R.D., and Boomsma, D.I. (2007). A structural MRI study in monozygotic twins concordant or discordant for attention/hyperactivity problems: Evidence for genetic and environmental heterogeneity in the developing brain. *Neuroimag*, 35(3):1004–1020.

144. Posthuma, D., de Geus, E.J., Neale, M.C., Hulshoff Pol, H.E., Baare, W.E.C., Kahn, R.S. *et al.* (2000). Multivariate genetic analysis of brain structure in an extended twin design. *Behav Genet*, 30(4):311–319.

145. Dickerson, B.C., Fenstermacher, E., Salat, D.H., Wolk, D.A., Maguire, R.P., Desikan, R. *et al.* (2008). Detection of cortical thickness correlates of cognitive performance: Reliability across MRI scan sessions, scanners, and field strengths. *Neuroimage*, 39(1): 10–18.

146. Lasky-Su, J., Lange, C., Biederman, J., Tsuang, M., Doyle, A.E., Smoller, J.W., *et al.* (2008). Family-based association analysis of a statistically derived quantitative traits for ADHD reveal an association in DRD4 with inattentive symptoms in ADHD individuals. *Am J Med Genet B Neuropsychiatr Genet*, 147:100–106.

147. Syed, Z., Dudbridge, F., and Kent, L. (2007). An investigation of the neurotrophic factor genes GDNF, NGF, and NT3 in susceptibility to ADHD. *Am J Med Genet B Neuropsychiatr Genet*, 144(3):375–378.

148. Kent, L., Green, E., Hawi, Z., Kirley, A. *et al.* (2005). Association of the paternally transmitted copy of common Valine allele of the Val66Met polymorphism of the brain-derived neurotrophic factor (BDNF) gene with susceptibility to ADHD. *Molecular Psychiatry*, 10(10):939–943.

149. Tsai, S.J. (2007). Attention-deficit hyperactivity disorder may be associated with decreased central brain-derived neurotrophic factor activity: Clinical and therapeutic implications. *Med Hypotheses*, 68(4):896–899.

150. Xu, X., Mill, J., Zhou, K., Brookes, K., Chen, C.K., and Asherson, P. (2007). Family-based association study between brain-derived neurotrophic factor gene polymorphisms and

attention deficit hyperactivity disorder in UK and Taiwanese samples. *Am J Med Genet B Neuropsychiatr Genet*, 144(1):83–86.

151. Staller, J.A. and Faraone, S.V. (2007). Targeting the dopamine system in the treatment of attention-deficit/hyperactivity disorder. *Expert Rev Neurother*, 7(4):351–362.

152. Kroutil, L.A., Van Brunt, D.L., Herman-Stahl, M.A., Heller, D.C., Bray, R.M., and Penne, M.A. (2006). Nonmedical use of prescription stimulants in the United States. *Drug Alcohol Depend*, 84(2):135–143.

153. Novak, S., Kroutil, L.A., Williams, R.L., and Van Brunt, D.L. (2007). The nonmedical use of prescription ADHD medications: Results from a national Internet panel. *Subst Abuse Treat Prev Policy*, 2(1):32.

154. Wilens, T.E., Faraone, S.V., Biederman, J., and Gunawardene, S. (2003). Does stimulant therapy of attention-deficit/hyperactivity disorder beget later substance abuse? A meta-analytic review of the literature. *Pediatrics*, 111(1):179–185.

155. Swanson, J.M., Elliott, G.R., Greenhill, L.L., Wigal, T., Arnold, L.E., Vitiello, B. *et al.* (2007). Effects of stimulant medication on growth rates across 3 years in the MTA follow-up. *J Am Acad Child Adolesc Psychiatry*, 46(8):1015–1027.

156. Charach, A., Ickowicz, A., and Schachar, R. (2004). Stimulant treatment over five years: Adherence, effectiveness, adverse effects. *J Am Acad Child Adolesc Psychiatry*, 43(5):559–567.

157. Darredeau, C., Barrett, S.P., Jardin, B., and Pihl, R.O. (2007). Patterns, predictors of medication compliance, diversion, misuse in adult prescribed methylphenidate users. *Hum Psychopharmacol*, 22(8):529–536.

158. Miller, A.R., Brehaut, J.C., Raina, P., McGrail, K.M., and Armstrong, R.W. (2004). Use of medical services by methylphenidate-treated children in the general population. *Ambul Pediatr*, 4(2):174–180.

159. Safren, S.A., Duran, P., Yovel, I., Perlman, C.A., and Sprich, S. (2007). Medication adherence in psychopharmacologically treated adults with ADHD. *J Atten Disord*, 10(3):257–260.

160. Kemner, J.E. and Lage, M.J. (2006). Effect of methylphenidate formulation on treatment patterns and use of emergency room services. *Am J Health Syst Pharm*, 63(4):317–322.

161. Olfson, M., Marcus, S.C., Zhang, H.F., and Wan, G.J. (2007). Continuity in methylphenidate treatment of adults with attention-deficit/hyperactivity disorder. *J Manag Care Pharm*, 13(7):570–577.

162. Cheng, J.Y., Chen, R.Y., Ko, J.S., and Ng, E.M. (2007). Efficacy and safety of atomoxetine for attention-deficit/hyperactivity disorder in children and adolescents-meta-analysis and meta-regression analysis. *Psychopharmacology (Berl)*, 194(2):197–209.

163. Spencer, T.J., Kratochvil, C.J., Sangal, R.B., Saylor, K.E., Bailey, C.E., Dunn, D.W. *et al.* (2007). Effects of Atomoxetine on Growth in Children with Attention-Deficit/Hyperactivity Disorder Following up to Five Years of Treatment. *J Child Adolesc Psychopharmacol*, 17(5):689–700.

164. Chronis, A.M., Jones, H.A., and Raggi, V.L. (2006). Evidence-based psychosocial treatments for children, adolescents with attention-deficit/hyperactivity disorder. *Clin Psychol Rev*, 26(4):486–502.

165. Klingberg, T., Fernell, E., Olesen, P.J., Johnson, M., Gustafsson, P., Dahlstrom, K. *et al.* (2005). Computerized training of working memory in children with ADHD-a randomized, controlled trial. *J Am Acad Child Adolesc Psychiatry*, 44(2):177–186.

166. Shalev, L., Tsal, Y., and Mevorach, C. (2007). Computerized progressive attentional training (CPAT) program: Effective direct intervention for children with ADHD. *Child Neuropsychol*, 13(4):382–388.

167. Toplak, M.E., Connors, L., Shuster, J., Knezevic, B., and Parks, S. (2008). Review of cognitive, cognitive-behavioral, and neural-based interventions for Attention-Deficit/Hyperactivity Disorder (ADHD). *Clin Psychol Rev*, 28(5):801–823.

168. Faraone, S.V., Biederman, J., Spencer, T.J., and Aleardi, M. (2006). Comparing the efficacy of medications for ADHD using meta-analysis. *MedGenMed*, 8(4):4.
169. Majewicz-Hefley, A. and Carlson, J.S. (2007). A meta-analysis of combined treatments for children diagnosed with ADHD. *J Atten Disord*, 10(3):239–250.
170. Crenshaw, T.M., Kavale, K.A., Forness, S.R., and Reeve, R.E. (1990). Attention deficit hyperactivity disorder and the efficacy of stimulant medication: A meta-analysis. *Advances LearningBehav Disabilities*, 1:135–165.
171. Bradley, C. (1937). The behavior of children receiving benzedrine. *Am J Psychiatry*, 94(3):577–585.
172. Brown, W.A. (1998). Images in psychiatry. *Am J Psychiatry*, 155:7.
173. Shetty, T. and Chase, T.N. (1976). Central monoamines and hyperkinase of childhood. *Neurology*, 26:1000–1002.
174. Zametkin, A.J., Karoum, F., Linnoila, M., Rapoport, J.L., Brown, G.L., Chuang, L.W., and Wyatt, R.J. (1985). Stimulants, urinary catecholamines, and indoleamines in hyperactivity. A comparison of methylphenidate and dextroamphetamine. *Arch Gen Psychiatry*, 42:251–255.
175. Zametkin, A., Papoport, J.L., Murphy, D.L., Linnoila, M., Karoum, F., Potter, W.Z., and Ismond, D. (1985). Treatment of hyperactive children with monoamine oxidase inhibitors. II. Plasma and urinary monoamine findings after treatment. *Arch Gen Psychiatry*, 42:969–973.
176. Elia, J., Borcherding, B.G., Potter, W.Z., Mefford, I.N., Rapoport, J.L., and Keysor, C.S. (1990). Stimulant drug treatment of hyperactivity: Biochemical correlates. *Clin Pharmacol Ther*, 48:57–66.
177. Kuczenski, R. and Segal, D.S. (2001). Locomotor effects of acute, repeated threshold doses of amphetamine, methylphenidate: Relative roles of dopamine, norepinephrine. *J Pharmacol Exp Ther*, 296(3):876–883.
178. Berridge, C.W., Devilbiss, D.M., Andrzejewski, M.E., Arnsten, A.F., Kelley, A.E., Schmeichel, B. *et al.* (2006). Methylphenidate preferentially increases catecholamine neurotransmission within the prefrontal cortex at low doses that enhance cognitive function. *Biol Psychiatry*, 60(10):1111–1120.
179. Brozoski, T.J., Brown, R.M., Rosvold, H.E., and Goldman, P.S. (1979). Cognitive deficit caused by regional depletion of dopamine in prefrontal cortex of rhesus monkey. *Science*, 205(4409):929–932.
180. Arnsten, A.F. and Dudley, A.G. (2005). Methylphenidate improves prefrontal cortical cognitive function through alpha2 adrenoceptor and dopamine D1 receptor actions: Relevance to therapeutic effects in Attention Deficit Hyperactivity Disorder. *Behav Brain Funct*, 1(1):2.
181. Ramos, B.P. and Arnsten, A.F. (2007). Adrenergic pharmacology and cognition: Focus on the prefrontal cortex. *Pharmacol Ther*, 113(3):523–536.
182. Winsberg, B.G., Bialer, I., Kupietz, S., and Tobias, J. (1972). Effects of imipramine and dextroamphetamine on behavior of neuropsychiatrically impaired children. *Am J Psychiatry*, 128(11):1425–1431.
183. Wilens, T.E., Biederman, J., Prince, J., Spencer, T.J., Faraone, S.V., Warburton, R., Schleifer, D., Harding, M., Linehan, C., and Geller, D. (1996). Six-week, double-blind, placebo-controlled study of desipramine for adult attention deficit hyperactivity disorder. *Am J Psychiatry*, 153(9):1147–1153.
184. Spencer, T., Biederman, J., Wilens, T. *et al.* (1998). Effectiveness and tolerabilitiy of tomoxetine in adults with attention deficit hyperactivity disorder. *Am J Psychiatry*, 155:693–695.
185. Bymaster, F.P., Katner, J.S., Nelson, D.L., Hemrick-Luecke, S.K., Threlkeld, P.G., Heiligenstein, J.H., Morin, S.M., Gehlert, D.R., and Perry, K.W. (2002). Atomoxetine increases extracellular levels of norepinephrine and dopamine in prefrontal cortex of rat: A potential

mechanism for efficacy in attention deficit/hyperactivity disorder. *Neuropsychopharmacology*, 27(5):699-711.

186. Connor, D.F., Fletcher, K.E., and Swanson, J.M. (1999). A meta-analysis of clonidine for symptoms of attention-deficit hyperactivity disorder. *J Am Acad Child Adolesc Psychiatry*, 38(12):1551-1559.

187. Arnsten, A.F. and Goldman-Rakic, P.S. (1990). Analysis of alpha-2 adrenergic agonist effects on the delayed nonmatch-to-sample performance of aged rhesus monkeys. *Neurobiol Aging*, 11(6):583-590.

188. Arnsten, A.F., Steere, J.C., Jentsch, D.J., and Li, B.M. (1998). Noradrenergic influences on prefrontal cortical cognitive function: Opposing actions at postjunctional alpha 1 versus alpha 2-adrenergic receptors. *Adv Pharmacol*, 42:764-767.

189. Wilens, T.E. (2006). Mechanism of action of agents used in attention-deficit/hyperactivity disorder. *J Clin Psychiatry*, 67(Suppl 8):32-38.

190. Weisler, R.H. (2007). Emerging drugs for attention-deficit/hyperactivity disorder. *Expert Opin Emerg Drugs*, 12(3):423-434.

191. Davids, E., Zhang, K., Tarazi, F.I., and Baldessarini, R.J. (2003). Animal models of attention-deficit hyperactivity disorder. *Brain Res*, 42(1):1-21.

192. Sagvolden, T., Russell, V.A., Aase, H., Johansen, E.B., and Farshbaf, M. (2005). Rodent models of attention-deficit hyperactivity disorder. *Biol Psychiatry*, 57(11):1239-1247.

193. Sagvolden, T. (1998). Behavioural validation of the spontaneously hypertensive rat (SHR) as an animal model of attention deficit/hyperactivity disorder (AD/HD). *Neurosci Biobehav Res*, 24:31-39.

194. Johansen, E.B., Sagvolden, T., and Kvande, G. (2005). Effects of delayed reinforcers on the behavior of an animal model of attention-deficit/hyperactivity disorder (ADHD). *Behav Brain Res*, 162(1):47-61.

195. Knardahl, S. and Sagvolden, T. (1979). Open-field behavior of spontaneously hypertensive rats. *Behav Neural Biol*, 27(2):187-200.

196. Myers, M.M., Musty, R.E., and Hendley, E.D. (1982). Attenuation of hyperactivity in the spontaneously hypertensive rat by amphetamine. *Behav Neural Biol*, 34:42-54.

197. Sagvolden, T., Metzger, M.A., Schiorbeck, H.K., Rugland, A.-L., Spinnangr, I., and Sagvolden, G. (1992). The spontaneously hypertensive rat (SHR) as an animal model of childhood hyperactivity (ADHD): Changed reactivity to reinforcers and to psychomotor stimulants. *Behav Neural Biol*, 58:103-112.

198. Bull, E., Reavill, C., Hagan, J.J., Overend, P., and Jones, D.N.C. (2000). Evaluation of the spontaneously hyperactive rat as a model of attention deficit hyperactivity disorder: Acquisition and performance of the DRL-60s test. *Behav Brain Res*, 109:27-35.

199. Sagvolden, T., Pettersen, M.B., and Larsen, M.C. (1993). Spontaneously hypertensive rats (SHR) as a putative animal model of childhood hyperkinesis: SHR behavior compared to four other rat strains. *Physiol Behav*, 54:1047-1055.

200. van den Bergh, F.S., Bloemarts, E., Chan, J.S., Groenink, L., Olivier, B., and Oosting, R.S. (2006). Spontaneously hypertensive rats do not predict symptoms of attention-deficit hyperactivity disorder. *Pharmacol Biochem Behav*, 83(3):380-390.

201. Barr, C.L., Feng, Y., Wigg, K., Bloom, S., Roberts, W., Malone, M., Achachar, R., Tannock, R., and Kennedy, J.L. (2000). Identification of DNA variants in the SNAP-25 gene and linkage study of these polymorphisms and attention-deficit hyperactivity disorder. *Mol Psychiatry*, 5(4):405-409.

202. Hess, E.J., Jinnah, H.A., Kozak, C.A., and Wilson, M.C. (1992). Spontaneous locomotor hyperactivity in a mouse mutant with a deletion including the Snap gene on chromosome 2. *J Neurosci*, 12(7):2865-2874.

203. Heyser, C.J., Wilson, M.C., and Gold, L.H. (1995). Coloboma hyperactive mutant exhibits delayed neurobehavioral developmental milestones. *Brain Res Dev Brain Res*, 89(2):264–269.

204. Hess, E.J., Collins, K.A., and Wilson, M.C. (1996). Mouse model of hyperkinesis implicates SNAP-25 in behavioral regulation. *J Neurosci*, 16(9):3104–3111.

205. Bruno, K.J., Freet, C.S., Twining, R.C., Egami, K., Grigson, P.S., and Hess, E.J. (2007). Abnormal latent inhibition and impulsivity in coloboma mice, a model of ADHD. *Neurobiol Dis*, 25(1):206–216.

206. Jones, S.R., Gainetdinov, R.R., Jaber, M., Giros, B., Wightman, R.M., and Caron, M.G. (1998). Profound neuronal plasticity in response to inactivation of the dopamine transporter. *Proc Natl Acad Sci USA*, 95(7):4029–4034.

207. Zhuang, X., Oosting, R.S., Jones, S.R., Gainetdinov, R.R., Miller, G.W., Caron, M.G., and Hen, R. (2001). Hyperactivity and impaired response inhibition in hyperdopaminergic mice. *Proc Natl Acad Sci USA*, 98:1982–1987.

208. Luthman, J., Lindqvist, E., Young, D., and Cowburn, R. (1990). Neonatal dopamine lesion in the rat results in enhanced adenylate cyclase activity without altering dopamine receptor binding or dopamine- and adenosine 3':5'-monophosphate-regulated phosphoprotein (DARPP-32) immunoreactivity. *Exp Brain Res*, 83(1):85–95.

209. Kostrzewa, R.M., Kostrzewa, J.P., Kostrzewa, R.A., Nowak, P., and Brus, R. (2007). Pharmacological models of ADHD. *J Neural Transm*; Nov 12; [Epub ahead of print].

210. van der Kooij, M.A. and Glennon, J.C. (2007). Animal models concerning the role of dopamine in attention-deficit hyperactivity disorder. *Neurosci Biobehav Rev*, 31:597–618.

211. Cada, A.M., Gray, E.P., and Ferguson, S.A. (2000). Minimal behavioral effects from developmental cerebellar stunting in young rats induced by postnatal treatment with alpha-difluoromethylornithine. *Neurotoxicol Teratol*, 22(3):415–420.

212. Ferguson, S.A., Cada, A.M., Gray, E.P., and Paule, M.G. (2001). No alterations in the performance of two interval timing operant tasks after alpha-difluoromethylornithine (DFMO)-induced cerebellar stunting. *Behav Brain Res*, 126(1–2):135–146.

213. Shaywitz, B.A., Klopper, J.H., Yager, R.D., and Gordon, J.W. (1976). Paradoxical response to amphetamine in developing rats treated with 6-hydroxydopamine. *Nature*, 261(5556): 153–155.

214. Luthman, J., Fredriksson, A., Lewander, T., Jonsson, G., and Archer, T. (1989). Effects of amphetamine and methylphenidate on hyperactivity produced by neonatal 6- hydroxydopamine treatment. *Psychopharmacology (Berl)*, 99:241–250.

215. Moran-Gates, T., Zhang, K., Baldessarini, R.J., and Tarazi, F.I. (2005). Atomoxetine blocks motor hyperactivity in neonatal 6- hydroxydopamine-lesioned rats: Implications for treatment of attention-deficit hyperactivity disorder. *Int J Neurophsychopharmacol*, 8(3):439–444.

216. Archer, T., Danysz, W., Fredriksson, A., Jonsson, G., Luthman, J., Sundstrom, E., and Teiling, A. (1988). Neonatal 6-hydroxydopamine-induced dopamine depletions: Motor activity and performance in maze leaning. *Pharmacol Biochem Behav*, 31:357–364.

217. Stancheva, S., Papazova, M., Alova, L., and Lazarova-Bakarova, M. (1993). Impairment of learning and memory in shuttle box-trained rats neonatally injected with 6-hydroxydopamine. Effects of nootropic drugs. *Acta Physiol Pharmacol Bulg*, 19(3):77–82.

218. Speiser, Z., Shved, A., and Gitter, S. (1983). Effect of propranolol treatment in pregnant rats on motor activity and avoidance learning of the offspring. *Psychopharmacology (Berl)*, 79(2–3):148–154.

219. Dell'Anna, M.E., Calzolari, S., Molinari, M., Iuvone, L., and Calimici, R. (1991). Neonatal anoxia induces trnsitory hyperactivity, permanent spatial memory deficits and CA1 cell density reduction in developing rats. *Behav Brain Res*, 45:125–134.

220. Gramatté, T. and Schmidt, J. (1986). The effect of early postnatal hypoxia on the effectiveness of drugs influencing motor behaviour in adult rats. *Biomed Biochim Acta*, 45(8):1069–1074.

221. Robbins, T.W. (2002). The 5-choice serial reaction time task: Behavioral pharmacology and functional neurochemistry. *Psychopharmacology (Berl)*, 163(3–4):362–380.

222. Evenden, J.L. (1999). Varieties of impulsivity. *Psychopharmacology (Berl)*, 146:348–361.

223. Patel, S., Stolerman, I.P., Asherson, P., and Sluyter, F. (2006). Attentional performance of C57Bl/6 and DBA/2 mice in the 5-choice serial reation time task. *Beh Brain Res*, 170:197–203.

224. Jentsch, J.D. (2005). Impaired visuospatial divided attention in the spontaneously hypertensive rat. *Beh Brain Res*, 157:323–330.

225. Cole, B.J. and Robbins, T.W. (1989). Effects of 6-hydroxydopamine lesions of the nucleus accumbens septi on performance of a 5-choice serial reaction time task in rats: Implications for theories of selective attention and arousal. *Behav Brain Res*, 33:165–179.

226. Bizarro, L., Patel, S., Murtagh, C., and Stolerman, I.P. (2004). Differential effects of psychomotor stimulants on attentional performance in rats: Nicotine, amphetamine, caffeine and methylphenidate. *Behav Pharmacol*, 15(3):195–206.

227. Puumala, T., Ruotsalainen, S., Jakala, P., Kovisto, E., Riekkinenen, P., and Sirvio, J. (1996). Behavioral and pharmacological studies on the validation of a new animal model for attentional deficit hyperactivity disorder. *Neurobiol Learn Mem*, 66:198–211.

228. Solanto, M.V. (1998). Neuropsychopharmacological mechanisms of stimulant drug action in attention-deficit hyperactivity disorder: A review and integration. *Beh Brain Res*, 94(1):127–152.

229. Solanto, M.V. (2002). Dopamine dysfunction in AD/HD: Integrating clinical and basic neuroscience research. *Behav Brain Res*, 130(1–2):65–71.

230. Nigg, J. (2000). On inhibition/disinhibition in developmental psychopathology: Views from cognitive and personality psychology and a working inhibition taxonomy. *Psychol Bull*, 126(2):220–246.

231. Winstanley, C.A., Eagle, D.M., and Robbins, T.W. (2006). Behavioral models of impulsivity in relation to ADHD: Translation between clinical and preclinical studies. *Clin Psychol Rev*, 26:379–395.

232. Welsh, M.C. and Pennington, B.F. (1988). Assessing frontal lobe functioning in children: Views from developmental psychology. *Devel Neuropsychol*, 4(3):199–230.

233. Arnsten, A.F.T. and Li, B.M. (2005). Neurobiology of executive functions: Catecholamine influences on prefrontal cortical functions. *Biol Psychiatry*, 57:1377–1384.

234. Roberts, A.C. (1996). Comparison of cognitive function in human and non-human primates. *Brain Res Cogn Brain Res*, 3(3–4):319–327.

235. Birrell, J.M. and Brown, V.J. (2000). Medial frontal cortex mediates perceptual attentional set shifting in the rat. *J Neurosci*, 20:4320–4324.

236. Chudasama, Y. and Robbins, T.W. (2006). Functions of frontostriatal systems in cognition: Comparative neuropsychopharmacological studies in rats, monkeys and humans. *Biol Psychol*, 73(1):19–38.

237. Biomarkers Definitions Working Group. (2001). Biomarkers and surrogate endpoints: Preferred definitions and conceptual framework. *Clin Pharmacol Ther*, 69(3):89–95.

238. Danhof, M., Alvan, G., Dahl, S.G., Kuhlmann, J., and Paintaud, G. (2005). Mechanism-based pharmacokinetic-pharmacodynamic modeling – A new classification of biomarkers. *Pharmaceutical Res*, 22(9):1432–1437.

239. De Lange, E.C.M. and Danhof, M. (2002). Considerations in the use of cerebrospinal fluid pharmacokinetics to predict brain target concentrations in the clinical setting: Implications of the barriers between blood and brain. *Clin Pharmacokin*, 41(10):691–703.

240. Lin, K.-S., Ding, J., and Logan, Y.-S. (2006). PET imaging of norephinephrine transporters. *Curr Pharmaceut Design*, 12:3831–3845.

241. Schou, M., Pike, V.W. *et al.* (2007). Development of radioligands for imaging of brain norepinephrine transporters in vivo with positron emission tomography. *Curr Top Med Chem*, 7(18):1806–1816.

242. Spencer, T.J., Biederman, J. *et al.* (2007). Further evidence of dopamine transporter dysregulation in ADHD: A controlled PET imaging study using altropane. *Biol Psychiatry*, 62(9):1059–1061.

243. Volkow, N.D., Wang, G.-J., Fowler, J.S., and Ding, Y.-S. (2005). Imaging the effects of methylphenidate on brain dopamine: New model on its therapeutic actions for attention-deficit/hyperactivity disorder. *Bio Psychiatry*, 57:1410–1415.

244. Danhof, M. (2002). Electroencephalography parameters as biomarkers: Extrapolation from laboratory animals to humans. *Methods Find Exp Clin Pharmacol*, 24(Suppl. D):63–64.

245. Clarke, A.R., Barry, R.J. *et al.* (2007). Coherence in children with Attention-Deficit/Hyperactivity Disorder and excess beta activity in their EEG. *Clin Neurophysiol*, 118(7):1472–1479.

246. Clarke, A.R., Barry, R.J. *et al.* (2005). Effects of methylphenidate on EEG coherence in attention-deficit/hyperactivity disorder. *Int J Psychophysiol*, 58(1):4–11.

247. Rowe, D.L., Robinson, P.A. *et al.* (2005). Stimulant drug action in attention deficit hyperactivity disorder (ADHD): Inference of neurophysiological mechanisms via quantitative modeling. *Clin Neurophysiol*, 116(2):324–335.

248. Pliszka, S.R. (2007). Pharmacologic treatment of attention-deficit/hyperactivity disorder: Efficacy, safety and mechanisms of action. *Neuropsychol Rev*, 17(1):61–72.

249. Pliszka, S.R., Liotti, M. *et al.* (2007). Electrophysiological effects of stimulant treatment on inhibitory control in children with attention-deficit/hyperactivity disorder. *J Child Adolesc Psychopharmacology (Berl)*, 17(3):356–366.

250. Castellanos, F.X., Elia, J., Kruesi, M.J., Marsh, W.L., Gulotta, C.S., Potter, W.Z., Ritchie, G.F., Hamburger, S.D., and Rapoport, J.L. (1996). Cerebrospinal fluid homovanillic acid predicts behavioral response to stimulants in 45 boys with attention deficit/hyperactivity disorder. *Neuropsychopharmacology*, 14(2):125–137.

251. Hatzinger, M., Brand, S. *et al.* (2007). Hypothalamic-pituitary-adrenocortical (HPA) activity in kindergarten children: Importance of gender and associations with behavioral/emotional difficulties. *J Psychiatr Res*, 41(10):861–870.

252. Sondeijker, S., Ferdinand, F.E.R.F. *et al.* (2007). Disruptive behaviors and HPA-axis activity in young adolescent boys and girls from the general population. *J Psychiatr Res*, 41(7):570–578.

253. Charmandari, E., Pincus, S.M., Matthews, D.R., Dennison, E., Fall, C.H.D., and Hindmarsh, P.C. (2001). Joint growth hormone and cortisol spontaneous secretion is more asynchronous in older females than in their male counterparts. *J Clin Endocrinol Metabol*, 86:3393–3399.

254. Müller, U., Clark, L., Lam, M.L., Moore, R.M., Murphy, C.L., Richmond, N.K., Sandhu, R.S., Wilkins, I.A., Menon, D.K., Sahakian, B.J. *et al.* (2005). Lack of effects of guanfacine on executive memory functions in healthy male volunteers. *Psychopharmacology*, 182:205–213.

255. Schüle, C., Baghai, R., Schmidbauer, S., Bidlingmaier, M., Strasburger, C.J., and Laakmann, G. (2004). Reboxetine acutely stimulates cortisol, ACTH, growth hormone and prolactin secretion in healthy male subjects. *Psychoendocrinol*, 29:185–200.

256. Halperin, J.M., Newcorn, J.H., McKay, K.E., Siever, L.J., and Sharma, V. (2003). Growth hormone response to guanfacine in boys with attention deficit hyperactivity disorder: A preliminary study. *J Child Adolesc Psychopharmacol*, 13:283–294.

257. Balldin, J., Berggren, U., Eriksson, E., Lindstedt, G., and Sundkler, A. (1993). Guanfacine as an alpha-2-agonist inducer of growth hormone secretion – a comparison with clonidine. *Psychopharmacology (Berl)*, 18:45–55.

258. Durand, D., Martin, J.B., and Brazeau, P. (1977). Evidence for a role of α-adrenergic mechanisms in the regulations of episodic growth hormone secretion in the rat. *Endocrinology*, 100:7228.

259. Krulich, L., Mayfield, M.A., Steele, M.K., McMillan, B.A., McCann, S.M., and Koenig, J.I. (1982). Differential effects of pharmacological manipulations of central alpha1- and alpha2-adrenergic receptors on the secretion of thyrotropin and growth hormone in male rats. *Endocrinology*, 110:792.

260. Laarkmann, G., Schoen, H.W., Blaschke, D., and Wittmann, M. (1985). Dose-dependent growth hormone, prolactin and cortisol stimulation after i.v. administration of desimipramine in human subjects. *Psychoneuroendocrin*, 1:83–93.

261. Szabadi, E., Bradshaw, C.M., Boston, P.F., and Langley, R.W. (1998). The human pharmacology of reboxetine. *Human Psychopharmacol*, 13:S3–S12.

262. Bitsios, P., Szabadi, E., and Bradshaw, C.M. (1999). Comparison of the effects of venlafaxine, paroxetine and desipramine on the pupillary light reflex in man. *Psychopharmacology (Berl)*, 143:286–292.

263. Phillips, M.A., Szabadi, E., and Bradshaw, C.M. (2000). Comparison of the effects of clonidine and yohimbine on spontaneous pupillary fluctuations in healthy human volunteers. *Psychopharmacology (Berl)*, 150:85–89.

264. Siepmann, T., Ziemssen, T. *et al.* (2007). The effects of venlafaxine on autonomic functions in healthy volunteers. *J Clin Psychopharmacol*, 27(6):687–691.

265. Dollery, C.T., Davies, D.S., Draffan, G.H., Dargie, H.J., Dean, C.R., Reid, J.L., Clare, R.A., and Murray, S. (1976). Clinical pharmacology and pharmacokinetics of clonidine. *Clin Pharmacol Ther*, 19(1):11–17.

266. Warren, J.B., Dollery, C.T., Fuller, R.W., Williams, V.X., and Gertz, B.J. (1989). Assessment of MK-912, an α2-adrenoceptor antagonist, with use of intravenous clonidine. *Clin Pharmacol Ther*, 46:103–109.

267. Warren, J.B., Dollery, C.T., Sciberras, D., and Goldberg, M.R. (1991). Assessment of MK-467, a peripheral α2-adrenergic receptor antagonist, with intravenous clonidine. *Clin Pharmacol Ther*, 50:71–77.

268. Porchet, H.C., Piletta, P., and Dayer, P. (1992). Pharmacokinetic-pharmacodynamic modelling of the effects of clonidine on pain threshold, blood pressure, and salivary flow. *Eur J Clin Pharmacol*, 42:655–662.

269. Phillips, M.A., Bitsios, P., Szabadi, E., and Bradshaw, C.M. (2000). Comparison of the antidepressants reboxetine, fluvoxamine and amitriptyline upon spontaneous pupillary fluctuations in healthy human volunteers. *Psychopharmacology (Berl)*, 149:72–76.

270. Pietrzak, R.H., Mollica, C.M., Maruff, P., and Snyder, P.J. (2006). Cognitive effects of immediate-relaease methylphenidate in children with attention/hyperactivity disorder. *Neurosc Biobehavior Rev*, 30:1225–1245.

271. Collie, A., Darekar, A., Weissgerber, G., Toh, M.K., Snyder, P.J., Maruff, P., and Huggins, J.P. (2007). Cognitive testing in early-phase clinical trials: Development of a rapid computerized test battery and application in a simulated Phase 1 study. *Contemp Clin Trials*, 28:391–400.

272. Greenhill, L.L., Swanson, J.M., Steinhoff, K., Freid, J., Posner, K., Lerner, M., Wigal, S., Clausen, S.B., Zhang, Y., and Tullock, S. (2003). A pharmacokinetic/pharmacodynamic study comparing a single morning dose of Adderall to twice-daily dosing in children with ADHD. *J Am Acad Child Adolesc Psychiatry*, 42(10):1234–1241.

273. Swanson, S.B. Wigal, T. Wigal, E. Sonuga-Barke, L.L. Greenhill, J. Biederman, S. Kollins, A. Stehli Nguyen, H.H. DeCory, S.J., Hirshe Dirksen, S.J., and Hatch COMACS Study Group. (2004).

A comparison of once-daily extended-release methylphenidate formulations in children with attention-deficit/hyperactivity disorder in the laboratory school (The Comacs Study). *Pediatrics,* 113:206–216.

274. Lyseng-Williamson, K.A. and Keating, G.M. (2002). Extended-release methylphenidate (Ritalin LA). *Drugs,* 62(15):2251–2259.

275. Quinn, D., Wigal, S., Swason, J., Hirsch, S., Ottolini, Y., Dariani, M., Roffman, M., Zeldis, J., and Cooper, T. (2004). Comparative pharmacodynamics, plasma concentrations of d-threo-methylphenidate hydrochloride after single doses of d-threo-methylphenidate hydrochloride, d,l-threo-methylphenidate hydrochloride in a double-blind, placebo-controlled, cross-over laboratory school study in children with attention-deficit/hyperactivity disorder. *J Am Acad Child Adolesc Psychiatry,* 43(11):1422–1429.

276. Wigal, S.B., McGough, J.J., McCracken, J.T. *et al.* (2005). A laboratory school comparison of mixed amphetamine slats extended release (Adderall XR) and atomoxetine (Strattera) in school-aged children with Attention Deficit/Hyperactivity Disorder. *Journal of Attention Disorders,* 9:275–289.

277. Biederman, J., Mick, E., Fried, R. *et al.* (2005). A simulated workplace experience for non-medicated adults with and without ADHD. *Psychiatr Serv,* 56:1617–1620.

278. Adler L.A., Faraone S.V., Spencer T.J., *et al.* (2007). The reliability and validity of self and investigator ratings of ADHD in adults. *J Atten Disorders,* Nov 19 [epub ahead of print].

279. Regulation (EC) No 1901/2006 of the European Parliament and of the Council of 12 December 2006 on medicinal products for paediatric use and amending Regulation (EEC) No 1768/92, Directive 2001/20/EC, Directive 2001/83/EC and Regulation (EC) No 726/2004. *Official Journal of the European Union.* 2006 December 27:378/1–19.

280. Preti, A. (2002). Tomoxetine. *Curr Opin Investig Drugs,* 3:272–277.

281. Ballon, J.S. and Feifel, D. (2006). A systematic review of modafinil: Potential clinical uses and mechanisms of action. *J Clin Psychiatry,* 67:554–566.

282. Wilens, T.E., Biederman, J., Spencer, T.J., *et al.* (1999). A pilot controlled clinical trial of ABT-418, a cholinergic agonist, in the treatment of adults with Attention Deficit Hyperactivity disorder. *Am J Psychiatry* 156-1931-1937.

283. Adler, L.A., Stein, M., and Mansbach, H. (2006). *Treatment of adult ADHD with the novel ampakine CX717.* Presented at the American Academy of Child and Adolescent Psychiatry, San Diego.

284. Michelson, D., Adler, L., Spencer, T. *et al.* (2003). Atomoxetine in adults with ADHD:Two randomized, placebo-controlled studies. *Biolog Psychiatry,* 53:112–120.

285. Spencer, T., Biederman, J., and Wilens, T. (2004). Stimulant treatment of adult attention deficity/hyperactivity disorder. *Psychiatr Clin N Am,* 27:361–372.

286. Theofilopoulos, N., McDade, G., Szabadi, E. *et al.* (1995). Effects of reboxetine and desipramine on the kinetics of the pupillary light reflex. *Brit J Clin Pharmacol,* 39:251–255.

287. Pereira, A., Ledent, E., Bervoets, L. *et al.* (2006). Pupillary light reflex effect of a new selective norepinephrine reuptake inhibitor assessed during the first human dose study. *Clin Pharmacol Ther,* 79(2):Suppl 44.

Preclinical Animal Models of Autistic Spectrum Disorders (ASD)

Jennifer A. Bartz[1], Larry J. Young[2], Eric Hollander[1], Joseph D. Buxbaum[1] and Robert H. Ring[3]

[1]Department of Psychiatry, Mount Sinai School of Medicine, New York, NY, USA
[2]Department of Psychiatry and Behavioral Sciences, Center for Behavioral Neuroscience, Yerkes National Primate Research Center, Emory University School of Medicine, Atlanta, GA, USA
[3]Wyeth Research, Discovery Neuroscience, Depression and Anxiety Disorders, Princeton, NJ, USA

Animal and Translational Models for CNS Drug Discovery,
Vol. 1 of 3: Psychiatric Disorders
Robert McArthur and Franco Borsini (eds), Academic Press, 2008

353

INTRODUCTION

Autism spectrum disorders (ASD) is a term used to describe the spectrum of pervasive developmental disorders (PDD) recognized by the *Diagnostic and Statistical Manual of Mental Disorders* (DSM-IV-TR),[i] and includes autistic disorder, Asperger's disorder, and PDD-not otherwise specified (PDD-NOS).[ii] These neurodevelopmental disabilities are characterized by impairments in three core areas of development: reciprocal social interaction, verbal and non-verbal communication or stereotyped behavior, and restricted interests and activities. In general, impairments occur prior to 3 years of age (although that onset is only required for a diagnosis of autism and Asperger's disorder) and tend to be lifelong.

Numerous epidemiological studies have revealed a substantial increase in the prevalence rates of ASD in the United States over the past 20 years.[1] This trend toward

---

[i] Please refer to the *Diagnostic and Statistical Manual of Mental Disorders, Fourth Edition-Text Revision* (DSM-IV-TR), or *The International Statistical Classification of Diseases and Related Health Problems 10th Revision*, published by the American Psychiatric Association and the World Health Organization, respectively, for current diagnostic criteria manuals in use.

[ii] Although Childhood Disintegrative Disorder and Rett's Disorder are included in the autism spectrum disorders, they will not be the focus of the present chapter because of their distinctive presentation and symptomatology (1).

an epidemic was highlighted by results of a recent multi-site collaborative study conducted by the US Centers for Disease Control, which placed estimates of ASD prevalence across the United States at 6.7 per 1000 children aged 8 years old.[2] Although the increase in prevalence may simply reflect improvements in disease education, widening of diagnostic criteria, and increased clinical surveillance, the changes will undoubtedly translate into increased burdens on social, educational, and medical systems, and indicate that ASD is a growing and significant public health concern. Despite improvements in diagnosis and education, treatment options for ASD have been limited by a relative lack of drug discovery efforts aimed specifically at developing, and not simply re-labeling, pharmacotherapies for child and adult patients. This stands in stark contrast to other neuropsychiatric disorders (e.g., anxiety disorders, mood disorders, schizophrenia, and bipolar disorder) where substantial investments have been made.[iii] Indeed, to date, only risperidone (Risperdal®) has been approved by the US Food and Drug Administration (FDA) for the treatment of irritability associated with autism; no drugs have yet been approved for the treatment of autism *per se*.

The limited availability and efficacy of treatments for ASD highlights the need for improved understanding of disease etiology. Critical to the success of this endeavor will be the development of behavioral assays and animal models of ASD that can provide researchers with experimental systems that enable investigation into specific mechanisms underlying the pathophysiology of ASD. Moreover, assays and models are essential in providing pharmaceutical researchers with the means to translate scientific discovery into the successful development of novel therapeutics for the treatment of ASD.

In this chapter, we examine the clinical phenomenology of ASD, moving from historical perspectives on the disorder to modern diagnostic criteria, design of clinical trials, and current pharmacological treatments. Building off this background, we review efforts to define endophenotypes and uncover the genetic risk factors behind ASD. We then turn to a discussion on the preclinical modeling of ASD in animals, focusing on assays that are being used for phenotypic assessment of behaviors relevant to the three core ASD domains, and review several animal models of ASD. Particular focus is placed on the validation criteria that each model has met, which demonstrates its utility for both basic and applied neurobiological research. Given the profound need for new treatment options for ASD, we end with a discussion on translational roles animal models play in drug discovery research, emphasizing the issues and challenges associated with adapting current behavioral assays and animal models of ASD to the demands of a high-throughput environment.

CLINICAL PHENOMENOLOGY OF ASD

A primary goal driving the development of any animal model of human disease is to provide an experimental system that allows researchers to make accurate predictions

---

[iii] Please refer to Joel *et al.*, Animal models of obsessive-compulsive disorder: From bench to bedside via endophenotypes and biomarkers, in this volume, or Williams *et al.*, Current concepts in the classification, treatment and modeling of pathological gambling and other impulse control disorders, in Volume 3, *Reward Deficit Disorders* for further discussion of the treatment of disorders such as ASD, OCD and impulse control-disorders through opportunistic re-labeling of drugs for other disorders. See also Heidbreder, Impulse and reward deficit disorders: Drug discovery and development, in Volume 3, *Reward Deficit Disorders* for discussion of how these disorders may be modeled.

about the disease in humans. Consequently, it is essential that the process of developing and validating animal models for ASD begin with, and be guided by, an understanding of the measures that objectively characterize the clinical phenomenology for these disorders. As we discuss in the following section, the clinical picture (diagnostic criteria, clinical instruments, treatment options) of autism and ASD has evolved considerably over the past 60 years, and researchers today have the means to engage in meaningful efforts to develop models that provide accurate predictions about the human disease condition.

Historical Origins

Autism was first recognized by Leo Kanner and Hans Asperger, who separately published accounts of the disorder in 1943 and 1944, respectively.[3,4] Although both accounts were written independently of one another, as Frith[3] noted, they both emphasized autistic children's inability to establish normal peer relationships and their desire for sameness. Specifically, Kanner's observations focused on "autistic aloneness" (i.e., an "inability to relate themselves in the ordinary way to people and situations" and a general preference for interacting with objects over people), desire for sameness, and discrete areas of ability. Asperger also emphasized the child's difficulty integrating socially with others. Finally, both emphasized the peculiar communication styles of these children, as well as movement stereotypies.

Diagnostic Criteria and Core Symptom Domains of ASD

Today, experts have come to a consensus on the specific criteria required for a diagnosis of autism and related spectrum disorders (i.e., ASD). These have been captured in the *Diagnostic and Statistical Manual of Mental Disorders* (DSM),[5] which instructs clinicians that individuals must present with abnormalities in all three of the following symptom domains to meet a diagnosis of autistic disorder: (1) qualitative impairments in social interaction, (2) qualitative impairments in communication, and (3) restricted repetitive and stereotyped patterns of behavior, interests, and activities. A minimum of two items from the first domain must be endorsed, while at least one item from the latter two domains must be endorsed, calling attention to the prominence of impaired social interactions in ASD. In addition, because autistic disorder is a developmental disorder, the delayed or abnormal functioning must occur prior to 3 years of age (in at least one symptom domain). Asperger's disorder is marked by impairments in the social and restricted and repetitive behaviors and interests domains, but a diagnosis of Asperger's disorder does not require specific language disruption (although individuals may show language abnormalities, especially more subtle abnormalities like overly formal speech). Finally, a diagnosis of PDD-NOS is given when an individual shows impairments in the social domain and either the communication or repetitive and restrictive behaviors and interests domains; in addition, the requirement for symptom onset prior to 3 years of age is not required for a diagnosis of PDD-NOS. The World Health Organization's *International Classification of Diseases* (ICD) provides a similar diagnostic scheme.

Domain 1: Impairments in Social Functioning

The first domain concerns impairments in social functioning, which can vary widely between individuals but, according to the DSM, are generally "gross and sustained."

Specifically, individuals with ASD often fail to use standard non-verbal behaviors to regulate social interactions with others. For example, they tend to avoid direct eye contact with others, have a limited range of affective expression (or do not direct their affective expressions to others) and have difficulty coordinating gesture (descriptive, conventional, instrumental, informational, or emphatic) with speech to aid in social communication. Individuals with ASD also have difficulty developing age-appropriate peer relationships; younger children often show little interest in same-age peers, and older children (and adults) – who may be more motivated to form peer relationships – often lack the social skills to facilitate this goal. Failure to share enjoyment, interests, and achievements with others is also a hallmark of ASD, as well as a lack of social and/or emotional reciprocity. More generally, individuals with ASD have difficulty engaging in two-way interactions; however, the precise quality of this deficit varies across individuals and varies within individuals across situations. For example, Wing and Gould[6] identified three distinct styles of impairments that can undermine social interactions: aloof, passive, and odd. Finally, as noted by Kanner, awareness of and/or interest in others are often impaired, which can undermine the individual's ability to be empathic.

Although not typically used to establish a diagnosis, research has found evidence for specific social cognitive deficits in individuals with ASD. For example, individuals with ASD have difficulty recognizing faces,[7-9] and also have difficulty processing the affective states of others, both in terms of recognizing facial displays of emotions[10,11] and affective speech comprehension.[10,12] fMRI studies of face processing and facial expression identification also support social processing deficits in ASD.[13,14] It is likely that these deficits in social cognition contribute, in part, to the more general social functioning deficits described earlier, including deficits in social and emotional reciprocity, and the failure to share enjoyment and empathize with others.

Domain 2: Impairments in Verbal and Non-verbal Communication

The second domain reflects impairments in verbal and non-verbal communication. Specifically, ASD can be associated with delayed development of spoken language, with some individuals never achieving this milestone. Spoken language, if developed, tends to be stereotyped, repetitive, and/or idiosyncratic, and pitch, intonation, volume, rhythm, and/or rate are often abnormal. Moreover, the ability to initiate or sustain conversation with others can be limited, resulting in a relatively one-sided interaction with little "give-and-take." The pragmatic use of language may also be impaired, as evidenced by an inability to understand humor, irony, or implied meaning. Similarly, as noted, the use of non-verbal behaviors to regulate social interactions with others can be impaired, either occurring less than would be expected, or exaggerated and not well-integrated into conversation. Moreover, if there is an absence of spoken language, this is not typically supplemented by the use of non-verbal behaviors (gesture, eye contact) to aid in communication. Finally, make-believe and/or imitative play can be impaired; if it occurs at all, play and/or imitation often have a mechanical quality and lack variety and spontaneity.

Domain 3: Restricted and Repetitive Behaviors and/or Interests

The third symptom domain concerns restricted and repetitive behaviors and/or interests. Individuals with ASD often have intense preoccupations that can be abnormal in their intensity but not content (e.g., dinosaurs), or can be abnormal in content (e.g., metal objects or street signs); these preoccupations can be so encompassing that they seriously interfere with the individual's social functioning or other activities. Preoccupation with parts of objects (e.g., repetitive spinning of wheels on a toy car) and repetitive behavior directed at objects (e.g., lining up toys in the same way over and over) are also characteristic. Rigid adherence to often non-functional routines and rituals as well as a desire for sameness and extreme distress in response to trivial changes (e.g., moving the couch in the living room) are also hallmarks of ASD. This symptom domain can also manifest itself in stereotyped and repetitive motor mannerisms, typically involving the hands (e.g., clapping and finger flipping) or the whole body (e.g., rocking). Finally, attachment to unusual objects (e.g., a lead pipe) is observed in individuals with ASD.

Associated ASD Symptom Domains

In addition to the three core symptom domains, a number of symptoms are associated with ASD. In particular, anxiety, hyperactivity, short attention span, irritability, mood instability, aggression, self-injurious behavior, and poor impulse control are associated with this disorder. Aggressive and irritable symptoms are common in children,[15] and as many as a quarter of adults with an ASD diagnosis have a history of irritability.[16] Moreover, mania-like symptoms including irritability, psychomotor agitation, excessive involvement with pleasurable activities with little regard for the behavioral consequences, labile mood, and grandiosity are seen in higher functioning individuals with ASD.[17] Although not core ASD characteristics, these symptoms are problematic as they are often severe enough to disrupt family life significantly and affect developmental and educational progress.[18] In addition, hyper- and hyposensitivity to the sound, sight, smell, taste, or touch of certain stimuli is also associated with ASD. This sensitivity can be paradoxical, for example, a child may be thrown into a tantrum in response to the phone ringing but barely notice a fire alarm. Finally, a diagnosis of mental retardation often accompanies a diagnosis of autism (but not Asperger's disorder since it is listed as an exclusionary criterion for Asperger's).

Clinical Measurements of ASD

Diagnostic Instruments

Although a psychiatric evaluation can be used to determine whether or not an individual meets DSM criteria, the gold standard for diagnosing autism and related spectrum disorders consists of two standardized assessments: the Autism Diagnostic Observation Schedule-Generic (ADOS-G),[19,20] a semi-structured behavioral assessment that combines unstructured conversation with structured activities and interview questions to probe for social and communicative behavior; and the Autism Diagnostic Interview-Revised (ADI-R),[21] an extensive, semi-structured psychiatric interview in which the patient's parent or guardian is asked to report on the patient's behaviors and development during the fourth and fifth years of childhood. The ADI-R yields scores for the three core ASD symptom domains: Qualitative Abnormalities in Reciprocal Social Interaction, Qualitative Abnormalities in Communication, and Restricted, Repetitive, and Stereotyped Patterns of Behavior.

In addition, instruments have been developed to identify broader dimensions of behaviors associated with ASD, or the "broader phenotype." In particular, the Social Responsiveness Scale (SRS),[22] the Children's Communication Checklist (CCC),[23] and the Social Communication Questionnaire (SCQ)[24,25] are examples of such instruments. These instruments do not yield scores on the three core domains specified by the DSM and ICD, so they cannot be used to establish diagnosis; however, as Volkmar *et al.*[26] noted, when used in conjunction with the DSM or ICD, these instruments allow for the assessment of a wider range of behavior associated with ASD and thus have the potential to shed light on etiological heterogeneity.

ASD Outcome Measures

To date, the predominant (but by no means the only) outcome measures that have been used in treatment studies of ASD are the Aberrant Behavior Checklist (ABC),[27,28] Clinical Global Impressions Scale-Improvement (CGI-I),[29] and Yale-Brown Obsessive-Compulsive Scale (YBOCS).[30,31] In addition, the Vineland Adaptive Behavior Scale[32] and the SRS have recently been used, but on a very limited basis. It is noteworthy that these outcome measures are based on third party reports of problematic behaviors; and, although useful, are limited by the fact that they do not tap the underlying processes or specific skills that contribute to the quality of the individual's social and communicative functioning. The CGI and YBOCS are administered and rated by a clinician and the ABC and SRS are questionnaire or checklist style instruments that are completed by the caregiver (or sometimes others with knowledge about the person in question). The Vineland includes both a clinician-administered survey interview (semi-structure style) and parent report checklist. Below is a brief description of these instruments.

The CGI-I, which is used as an outcome measure in clinical trials for a number of psychiatric disorders, employs a 7-point scale to determine the individual's improvement in response to treatment and has been successfully used as an outcome measure in numerous psychopharmacology trials in ASD including the Research Units of Pediatric Psychopharmacology (RUPP) trial of risperidone in children with ASD.[15] As noted, the CGI is a clinician-rated instrument; scores are based on all available data including direct observation, other assessment scales, and patient report to inform clinical judgment. The CGI-I can also be tailored to target specific symptom domains such as the social domain.

The YBOCS is also a clinician-administered instrument measuring the time spent, distress, interference, resistance, and control in relation to obsessions and compulsions based on a 5-point scale. This scale, which has excellent reliability and validity, is the gold standard to measure treatment outcomes in clinical trials for obsessive-compulsive disorder (OCD) and has been adapted to assess changes in repetitive behaviors in autism and ASD.[33,34] In addition, the Yale-Brown Obsessive-Compulsive Checklist assesses past and present occurrences of different symptom patterns, including aggressive, contamination, sexual, religious, magical, somatic and symmetry obsessions as well as cleaning/washing, checking, repeating, counting, ordering/arranging, and hoarding/saving compulsions.

The ABC is a 58-item parent-rated instrument consisting of 5 subscales measuring irritability, social withdrawal, stereotypic behavior, hyperactivity, and inappropriate speech. Parents/guardians are asked to report the extent to which each item is problematic on a scale ranging from 0 (not a problem) to 3 (severe problem).

The Vineland Adaptive Behavior Scale is a survey interview conducted by clinicians with parents/guardians and/or teachers to measure the level of an individual's personal and social skills required for everyday living. The Vineland taps five domains of adaptive behavior: communication (receptive, expressive, written); daily living skills (personal, domestic, community); socialization (personal relationships, play and leisure time, coping skills), motor skills (fine, gross); and maladaptive behavior (internalizing, externalizing, other). In addition, as noted, there is a parent/caregiver rating form.

Finally, the SRS,[22] which was mentioned above as an instrument to assess the broader dimension of behaviors associated with ASD, has also been used to measure treatment response in individuals ages 4–18 years of age. The SRS is a caregiver/educator rating scale of social behaviors specific to ASD, including social awareness, social information processing, and social motivation and yields a quantitative score that has been useful in detecting milder social impairments in endophenotyping studies of family members of individuals with ASD.

Current Pharmacological Treatment Strategies

The most valuable type of validity for animal models of any disorder is achieved by demonstrating that a pharmacological agent that shows efficacy in humans produces a measurable and relevant effect in an animal model of that disease. This enables researchers to make predictions about the potential of novel mechanisms of action to deliver efficacy in the clinic. Achieving this predictive validity during the development of an animal model requires comprehensive understanding of current pharmacological strategies used for the targeted disease. Clinically efficacious classes of compounds, or mechanisms of action, also provide important insights into the molecular pathways, neurotransmitter systems, or specific neural circuits implicated in the pathophysiology underlying symptom domains of the disorder under study, which, in turn, can be exploited as guidance for future drug development.

To date, there are relatively few well-designed, placebo-controlled, empirical studies of pharmacological agents in the treatment of ASD symptoms despite the fact that such treatments are common in clinical practice. Moreover, many of the studies that have been conducted have serious limitations, including small subject numbers and poorly characterized populations.[iv] Below, we review the major findings to date for studies on the use of monoamine reuptake inhibitors (selective serotonin reuptake inhibitors [SSRIs] and selective norepinephrine reuptake inhibitors), antipsychotics, anticonvulsants and mood stabilizers; we conclude this section by highlighting some novel pharmacological approaches that may have therapeutic value in the treatment of autism and by outlining unmet needs in this area.

Serotonin Reuptake Inhibitors

Selective serotonin reuptake inhibitors may be especially useful in treating stereotyped motor behaviors, adherence to routines and rituals, and intense preoccupations that

---

[iv] Please refer to McEvoy and Freudenreich, Issues in the design and conductance of clinical trials, in this Volume for a discussion of the consequences of small subject numbers and poorly characterized patient populations on clinical trail outcome.

can characterize ASD. In addition, they may be effective in treating anxiety – a relatively common associated symptom. Rationale for the use of SSRIs in ASD comes from the relative success they have had in treating symptoms of OCD; although not all OCD patients respond to SSRIs, they are generally considered the first-line of pharmacological treatment in this disorder.[35] In particular, it is thought that the obsessions (persistent, intrusive thoughts) and compulsions (repetitive, ritualized behaviors that the individual feels compelled to perform) in OCD are akin to the repetitive behaviors and restricted interests in ASD, and that both may be driven by a strong desire for sameness and order.[36] This relationship receives some support from genetic studies in which rare mutations are proposed to produce ASD and/or OCD.[37,38] Additional rationale for the use of SSRIs in ASD comes from observations of elevated peripheral serotonin levels in autism.[37,39]

There are several reports investigating SSRIs (fluoxetine [Prozac®], fluvoxamine [Luvox®], paroxetine [Seroxat®, Paxil®], citalopram [Celexa®], escitalopram [Lexapro®], and sertraline [Zoloft®]) in the treatment of ASD symptoms; these range from individual case reports, to retrospective chart reviews, to open-label clinical trials, to double-blind, placebo-controlled clinical trials. As noted, many of these investigations have methodological limitations, including small samples, and sample heterogeneity (in terms of age, disability level, psychiatric comorbidity, and the use of concomitant medications); nonetheless, collectively they suggest that SSRIs have the potential to reduce repetitive and ritualistic behaviors, improve global functioning, and may improve aspects of communication and social relatedness. The following review provides highlights from this research (interested readers are referred to Schapiro *et al.*[36] for a more detailed analysis[v]). One retrospective chart review and three open-label trials found beneficial outcomes following treatment with fluoxetine in individuals with autism or ASD; specifically, the retrospective review found reductions in irritability, stereotypy, inappropriate speech, and lethargy (as assessed by the ABC) following fluoxetine treatment,[38] and the open-label trials found improvements in overall clinical severity of illness and perseverative and compulsive behaviors (as assessed by the CGI),[40] mood, social interaction and language,[41] and social interaction and communication, repetitive and other problem behaviors, and overall functioning.[42] Finally, Hollander and colleagues report results from two placebo-controlled trials of fluoxetine in the treatment of autism and ASD. Specifically, Buchsbaum *et al.*[43] report improvements on the CGI for half the ASD patients in the study and improvements on the obsessions subscale of the YBOCS for all ASD patients in the study. Hollander *et al.*[44] investigated low-dose liquid fluoxetine in children and adolescents with autism and found significant reductions in repetitive behaviors (as assessed by the YBOCS), and improvements on the CGI-I.

In contrast to fluoxetine, studies investigating fluvoxamine in ASD are mixed. One placebo-controlled, double-blind study showed that fluvoxamine reduced repetitive thoughts and behaviors in adults with autistic disorder[34]; however, these beneficial effects were not replicated in a separate placebo-controlled, double-blind study of child and adolescent subjects with ASD.[45] With respect to citalopram and escitalopram, a retrospective chart review suggests that citalopram may be efficacious in treating

---

[v] Please refer also to Joel *et al.*, Animal models of obsessive-compulsive disorder: From bench to bedside via endophenotypes and biomarkers, in this volume.

symptoms associated with ASD,[46] and an open-label trial of escitalopram showed significant improvements on global functioning (assessed by CGI) and irritability (assessed by the ABC-Community Version) in patients with ASD.[47]

To date, only open-label studies have been conducted to investigate the efficacy of sertraline in ASD. Preliminary results show improvements in self-injurious behavior and aggression in mentally retarded adults, five of whom were diagnosed with autistic disorder[48]; another study found improvements on the CGI and decreased aggression (but not social or language improvements) in adults with ASD[49]; and a case series reported significant improvements in behavior symptoms in eight of nine children with autistic disorder.[50]

Finally, dual serotonin norepinephrine reuptake inhibitors (SNRIs), which enhance norepinephrine and serotonin neurotransmission, may have therapeutic value in treating ASD symptoms. In a retrospective open-label designed study, Hollander *et al.*[51] showed that low doses of venlafaxine (Effexor®) improved repetitive behaviors and restricted interests in children and young adults with ASD.

Typical and Atypical Neuroleptics

Much of the early pharmacological work in autism and related spectrum disorders focused on neuroleptics, and although these agents were shown to improvement stereotyped and other problematic behaviors and to increase engagement, as Campbell and colleagues[52] have shown, significant side effects (including sedation, withdrawal, and tardive dyskinesia) seriously limit their usefulness. More recently, these drugs have been replaced by atypical neuroleptics, which have been used to treat self-injury, agitation, stereotyped movements, and behavior problems in autism.[53] The most extensively studied neuroleptic is risperidone, which is currently the only US FDA approved medication for the treatment of irritability associated with autism in children.

Anticonvulsants and Mood Stabilizers

As noted, although atypical neuroleptics are used for the treatment of irritability and impulsive aggression in autism, concerns about weight gain and metabolic syndrome have prompted the continued search for treatments for these symptoms, and mood-stabilizing anticonvulsants may be a viable alternative. The potential value of mood-stabilizing anticonvulsants is further reinforced by the fact that a large minority of individuals with autism or ASD have comorbid epilepsy or sub-threshold epilepsy. In addition, further support for the potential value of mood-stabilizing anticonvulsants in autism comes from observations of comorbid affective disorders characterized by mania-like symptoms in individuals with autism.[17]

To date, valproate (Depakote®), lamotrigine (Lamictal®), levetiracetam (Keppra®), and carbamazepine (Tegretol®) have been investigated in the context of autism. In particular, Hollander *et al.*[54] conducted an open-label trial of valproate in ASD and found significant improvements in repetitive behaviors, social relatedness, aggression, and mood lability. Moreover, a follow-up double-blind, placebo-controlled pilot study of valproate in ASD also found significant improvements in repetitive behaviors.[55] Evidence for the potential value of lamotrigine was obtained from a large open-label study of children with epilepsy, a subset of whom had autism; eight of the thirteen children with autism showed improvements in attention, eye contact, irritability, and emotional lability.[56] However, a subsequent double-blind placebo-controlled trial of children with autistic disorder found no evidence for improvements in such symptoms following lamotrigine treatment,[57] although the large placebo response in this study may have been a factor. One open-label study of levetiracetam in boys with ASD showed significant improvements in hyperactivity, impulsivity, mood lability, and aggression,[58] although the therapeutic effects of levetiracetam in ASD were not replicated in a preliminary trial conducted by Wasserman *et al.*[59] Finally, although widely used in clinical practice, to our knowledge, no studies have investigated the efficacy of carbamazepine in autism.

Novel Pharmacological Approaches

With the exception of the repetitive behaviors domain, the pharmacological agents reviewed above do not target core symptom domains of autism; rather, most target such associated symptoms as irritability, aggression, and mood lability. Yet it is widely acknowledged that deficits in social behavior are the defining feature of ASD, and pharmacological treatments that target this domain are sorely needed. In addition, agents that target communication, as well as general cognition and executive functioning skills are also needed, as deficits in these areas can seriously impair an individual's ability to function, even those who are relatively "high-functioning." With this in mind, researchers are beginning to explore novel pharmacological approaches that target the social and communication symptom domains, as well as cognition/executive functioning. In this regard, glutamatergic agents and, possibly, the peptide oxytocin (OT) may hold promise.

Rationale for the use of glutamatergic agents in the treatment of ASD comes from studies showing activation of the glutamatergic system in autism[60-62] (the reader is referred to reference[63] for a detailed review of this literature), as well as genetic studies implicating neuroligin and neurexins, involved in glutamatergic synaptogenesis, and other glutamatergic genes in ASD (see below and reference[64]). Fragile X syndrome and tuberous sclerosis, both of which often present with ASD symptoms, demonstrate altered glutamatergic signaling. A double-blind, placebo-controlled pilot study of D-cycloserine showed significant improvements on the CGI and social withdrawal subscale of the ABC in children with autism.[65] A case study found that dextromethorphan resulted in improvements in problem behaviors associated with autism[66]; however, a follow-up mixed group/single-case, double-blind, placebo-controlled trial found no group differences between dextromethorphan and placebo in the treatment of problem behaviors and core symptoms of autism, although three of the eight participants who showed a behavioral profile consistent with attention-deficit hyperactivity disorder responded positively to dextromethorphan.[67] Finally, memantine (Namenda®), which has received approval from the FDA to treat memory loss in Alzheimer's disease, may be useful in targeting cognitive/executive functioning in ASD.[63] To date, no controlled studies have investigated the therapeutic potential of memantine in ASD; however, a few open label trials have yielded promising results.[190-192] The Mount Sinai group is currently leading a Cure Autism Now/Autism Speaks funded multi-site controlled clinical trial to investigate its therapeutic potential in this population.

Finally, as we address in detail at the end of this chapter, oxytocin, a nine-amino acid peptide hormone that acts as a neuromodulator in the brain, may hold promise for treating social/social-communicative deficits in ASD. Studies with rodents and non-human primates have shown that oxytocin, and the structurally similar peptide vasopressin, are involved in the regulation of affiliative behaviors including sexual behavior, mother–infant and adult–adult pair-bond formation, separation distress, and other aspects of social affiliation and social cognition. Moreover, four recent studies suggest that oxytocin may play an important role in human social behavior.[64,68-70] Oxytocin has also been implicated in repetitive behaviors, for example, the central administration of oxytocin has been shown to induce a variety of stereotyped behaviors including stretching, repetitive grooming, startle, and squeaking in mice,[71-74] grooming in rats,[71,75] and wing-flapping in chicks.[76] Over the years, a number of researchers have suggested that dysregulated oxytocin may be implicated in autism and related spectrum disorders given that deficits in social interaction and repetitive behaviors are core features of ASD, and that oxytocin is involved in the regulation of affiliative and repetitive behaviors.[76-84] As we discuss at the end of this chapter, efforts are now underway to investigate the therapeutic potential of oxytocin in the treatment of core ASD symptoms.

Unmet Needs

In summary, the above review suggests that a number of pharmacological agents hold promise for treating isolated symptoms of autism. In particular, SSRIs and SNRIs may be of value in treating repetitive behaviors, intense preoccupations and resistance to change, as well as associated anxiety. Neuroleptics and, in particular, the atypical neuroleptic risperidone, has been effective in treating irritability associated with autism. Anticonvulsants may be helpful in addressing repetitive behaviors, irritability, impulsivity, mood lability, and aggression. Similarly, mood stabilizers such as lithium may hold value in treating mood instability, but well-controlled clinical studies are needed. What is clear from the above review is that most of the pharmacological treatments target associated symptoms of ASD and that there is an absence of pharmacological treatments that target two of the three core symptom domains of ASD – that is, the social and communicative deficits. What is also clear from the above review is that most of the pharmacological treatments that are currently used to treat symptoms of ASD are based on their utility in the treatment of other psychiatric disorders (e.g., schizophrenia, OCD, attention-deficit hyperactivity disorder, depression, and anxiety), and that there has been very little deliberate drug development in this area.

TRANSLATIONAL RESEARCH IN ASD: ENDOPHENOTYPES AND GENETIC RISK FACTORS

One of the main goals of translational ASD research is to develop pharmacological interventions to treat the symptoms of ASD. This goal cannot be accomplished without animal models with face, construct, and predictive validity. Unfortunately, there is no single animal model that recapitulates all of the core symptoms of ASD. Further complicating the development of animal models is the fact that ASD is a heterogeneous disorder, perhaps involving dozens of genetic risk factors. One strategy for developing animal models with face and construct validity is to model the individual endophenotypes or risk factors. But in assessing the validity of animal models, one must be aware of the underlying neurobiological and genetic correlates of the disorder. Here we discuss briefly the known neurobiological endophenotypes and genetics risk factors of ASD.

ASD Endophenotypes

A number of morphometric and neuropathological studies have revealed brain abnormalities in ASD. A recent meta-analysis of brain size based on magnetic resonance imaging (MRI) and postmortem brain weight revealed that brain size in ASD is slightly reduced at birth, dramatically increased within the first year of life, but then plateaus so that by adulthood the majority of cases were within normal range.[85] One MRI study revealed that at 2–3 years of age, ASD boys had more cerebral (18%) and cerebellar (39%) white matter, and more cerebral cortical gray matter (12%) than normal.[86] In contrast, cerebellar vermi are reduced in ASD compared to normal.[86,87] Postmortem microscopic analyses have revealed cellular abnormalities in ASD including decreased numbers of Purkinje cells in the cerebellum, brainstem and olivary dysplasia,[88] and decreased cell number and increased cell-packing density in several limbic structures.[89]

Functional magnetic resonance imaging (fMRI) studies have revealed abnormalities in brain activation patterns that accompany the social and cognitive deficits found in ASD. For example, the deficits in social perception and emotional engagement are associated with reduced activity in the amygdala.[13,90,91] Individuals with ASD display deficits in individual face recognition as well as extracting emotional information from faces. This deficit is accompanied by a reduction in activation of the fusiform face area (FFA) during face perception tasks.[13,14] In fact, autistic subjects show hyperactivation in other cortical regions during these tasks compared to normal controls, indicating that some aspects of face perception are being performed in alternate cortical structures.[13]

Genetic Risk Factors for ASD

Heritability studies suggest that ASD is one of the most heritable of all psychiatric disorders, yet the underlying genetic basis of ASD remains elusive. Twin studies reveal 60–90% concordance rate among monozygotic twins, whereas 0–10% among dizygotic twins, depending on the phenotypic definitions.[92] This heritability pattern suggests that multiple genes, perhaps in the dozens, are involved in the etiology of ASD. Genetic analysis of ASD is further complicated by the fact that ASD is a heterogeneous disorder, with multiple genetic paths leading to the various points of the ASD diagnosis spectrum. Nevertheless, several genome-wide linkage and association studies have identified multiple chromosomal loci as risk factors for ASD, with chromosomal regions 2q, 7q, 17q, and 16p yielding the most common positive results.[93] Over 30 candidate genes have been reported as potential risk factors for ASD.[93] These candidate genes include genes involved in synaptogenesis (neurexins, neuroligins), brain development (EN2, HOXA1, RELN), language (FOXP2), and social behavior (oxytocin receptor [OXTR] and vasopressin receptor [AVPR1A]) (see reference[93] for a comprehensive listing). Perhaps the strongest case for a single gene contributing to idiopathic ASD is that of the neuroligins (NLGN). Neuroligins interact with neurexins transsynaptically and are thought to play an important role in synapse formation and maintenance.[94] Loss-of-function mutations in NLGN3 and NLGN4 have been reported in affected siblings with ASD[95] as well as in a large pedigree where NLGN4 mutations were associated with ASDs and/or mental retardation.[96] However, it should be noted that these are apparently rare mutation causes of ASD since no mutations in these genes have been reported in other ASD populations.[97,98]

Rett syndrome and Fragile X syndrome are examples of monogenic neurodevelopmental disorders that present with autistic behavioral phenotypes. Rett syndrome results from the mosaic expression of mutant copies of the X-linked methyl CpG-binding protein 2 gene (*MeCP2*) in females. MeCP2 functions as a DNA methylase and is thought to play an important role in gene regulation.[99] Fragile X syndrome results from an expansion of a trinucleotide repeat in the 5′ untranslated region of the *FMR1* gene that prevents expression of the encoded protein, FMRP.[100] FMRP plays an important role in regulating translation, including at the synapse, by inhibiting protein translation.[96] Since Rett and Fragile X syndromes arise from known mutations of single genes, these disorders are particularly amenable for study using transgenic mouse models and provide an excellent examples of how animal models can be informative in the development of pharmacological treatment strategies for neurodevelopmental disorders.[vi]

Elucidating the behavioral and neurobiological endophenotypes and genetic risk factors of ASD is only the first step toward drug development for the treatment of ASD. Animal models are essential for understanding the fundamental neurobiology regulating the behavioral endophenotype and how these systems are affected by genetic risk factors. This knowledge will serve as the foundation for the development of candidate pharmacological interventions.

PRECLINICAL MODELING OF ASD IN ANIMALS: BEHAVIORAL ASSAYS AND ASD MODELS

Animal models of ASD are clearly essential for the development of biologically based pharmacological therapies for the treatment of ASD. However, ASD is a uniquely human disorder, and there is no one animal model that captures all of the core features of ASD. However, animal models can provide insights into the neural mechanisms regulating behaviors relevant to ASD and to the contribution of genetic risk factors associated with ASD. Ultimately, animal models should prove useful in identifying candidate targets for pharmacological interventions for ASD. In this section, we will discuss the behavioral assays and animal models that have been developed for preclinical investigation of ASD.

Before proceeding, it is important to note a working distinction between "assays" and "models" of ASD used in this review. Assays should be regarded as tests or procedures developed to provide investigators with the means to observe and measure

---

[vi] For further discussion of genetic models of learning disabilities, the reader is invited to refer to Shilyansky *et al.*, Molecular and cellular mechanisms of learning disabilities: a focus on Neurofibromatosis type I, in Volume 2, *Neurologic Disorders*.

a specific phenotype (usually behavior) in an animal, which is thought to be related to a particular symptom or symptom domain observed in ASD patients (e.g., duration of olfactory investigation in the social recognition paradigm as an etholog of social recognition deficits in ASD). Behavioral assays can be used to examine and measure the impact of genotype (e.g., mutation, knockout, strain), pharmacological intervention (e.g., drug, toxic compound), or other experimental manipulations (e.g., lesion, infection) on a relevant phenotype. By comparison, animal "models" are paradigms that have been developed to recapitulate an aspect of human pathophysiology or endophenotype, which results in a phenotype that is reminiscent of the human condition. As discussed below, the appropriateness of an assay or model for use in preclinical research is dependent on the type and degree of validity (e.g., face, construct, predictive) they have demonstrated or achieved during development.[vii]

Behavioral Assays Used to Measure ASD-like Symptoms in Animals

In this age of genomics and transgenic technology, the mouse has become the premier species to model perhaps all heritable psychiatric disorders. Consequently, considerable effort has been devoted to develop behavioral testing paradigms in mice that are relevant to ASD. The goal is to design paradigms with face validity for the behavioral phenotype found in ASD, although it is unclear whether these paradigms in mice will have construct or predictive validity. For example, Crawley and colleagues have proposed a battery of behavioral tests to model the social deficits and repetitive, restrictive behavior in ASD.[101,102] While each of these tests may be informative, they must be interpreted in the context of a complete battery of assays that examine motor behavior, sensory processing, and emotionality.[viii]

Although ASD features communication deficits and increased repetitive and restricted behaviors, assay development in the preclinical ASD research field has largely focused on rodent paradigms that model phenotypic parameters of social interaction and cognition. This bias towards social behavior in part reflects the fact that mice are highly social animals; however, it also reflects commonalities in symptomatic overlap with social aspects of other neuropsychiatric conditions such as schizophrenia, bipolar and anxiety disorders in particular, many of the assays used to model social interaction and cognition deficits of ASD in animals were originally developed for research on these disorders. Unless otherwise noted, all assays discussed have been developed as paradigms of rodent (mouse or rat) behavior.

[vii] For further and detailed discussions regarding criteria of validity, the reader is invited to refer to discussions by Steckler *et al.*, Developing novel anxiolytics: improving preclinical detection and clinical assessment; Joel *et al.*, Animal models of obsessive-compulsive disorder: from bench to bedside via endophenotypes and biomarkers, Large *et al.*, Developing therapeutics for bipolar disorder: from animal models to the clinic in this volume; Lindner *et al.*, Development, optimization and use of preclinical behavioral models to maximize the productivity of drug discovery for Alzheimer's Disease in Volume 2, *Neurologic Disorders*; Koob, The role of animal models in reward deficit disorders: views from academia, Markou *et al.*, Contribution of animal models and preclinical human studies to medication development for nicotine dependence, in Volume 3, *Reward Deficits Disorders*.

[viii] Please refer to Large *et al.*, Developing therapeutics for bipolar disorder (BPD): From animal models to the clinic, in this Volume for further discussion of the development of test batteries needed to characterize disorders with multiple behavioral components.

Assays Modeling Social Interaction and Cognition

Crawley and colleagues proposed a social investigation task to quantify social interest and motivation,[101,102] a core feature of the social deficits in ASD. This task is performed in a three-chambered arena. In one chamber, a novel mouse is placed within a wire cage to restrict its movement. An empty wire cage is placed in the third chamber to control for the novelty of the cage. The experimental animal is placed in the center chamber and allowed to move freely through all chambers. The time spent in and entries into each chamber and the time spent sniffing each wire cage is quantified. Most mouse strains spend most of the time near the novel stimulus mouse. The second phase of this test involves a social novelty task. A new novel stimulus animal is placed in the empty wire cage, while the original stimulus mouse remains. Again, the time in each cage and investigating each wire cage is quantified. Most strains will spend more time investigating the novel mouse cage.

As noted, individuals with ASD exhibit deficits in face recognition and in the ability to infer emotional information from faces; they also show specific neurobiological alterations when processing faces. Similar deficits can be measured in rodents using the social recognition task, which measures the ability to recognize another rodent over time and disruptions in the neural processing of social cues. In this task, the experimental mouse is exposed to the same novel mouse in four successive 1 min pairings with a 10 min inter-trial interval.[103] In a fifth trial, the experimental mouse is exposed to a new novel female. During each pairing the time, that the experimental mouse spends investigating the stimulus animal is recorded. Typically, mice will habituate to the familiar mouse on later trials and spend less time in olfactory investigation, but return to initial levels of investigation in the fifth trial. Mice with impaired social recognition will fail to habituate to the familiar mouse. Control experiments using cotton balls scented with non-social scents can be used to determine whether the deficits are selective for social learning.

Social play behavior is a distinct form of social interaction that occurs across ontogeny in mammalian species.[104] In humans and rodents, play behaviors are believed to be critical in the establishment of stable social relationships.[105] Individuals with ASD tend to be less interested in other children and are often unresponsive to the approaches of other children. They are also often reluctant to engage in play activities with their peers, and when they do, their play typically lacks a true interactive, cooperative quality.[19] Play behavior can be modeled in rodents using a variety of phenotypic measurements, thus offering investigators with the potential for assaying a key behavioral deficit observed in ASD. One common measurement of play behavior is pinning, which is observationally defined as an animal lying down with its dorsal surface in contact with test cage while another animal is found standing over it.[106] Pinning behavior was used as a primary behavioral assay in the validation of an amygdala lesion model of ASD in rats.[107] In that study, deficits in pinning behavior observed in juvenile rats helped reveal age-dependent effects of amygdala lesions on social behavior, emphasizing the importance of the amygdala in the development of social behaviors, and providing specific behavioral evidence supporting the face validity of early life amygdala lesioning as an animal model of social interaction deficits in ASD.[107] Behavioral assays of social play were also used in the original validation studies for the neonatal Borna disease virus

(BDV) infection model of ASD.[108] Neonatal BDV infection produces significant changes to normal (uninfected) patterns of social behavior in infected rats, including reduced social interaction in the open field and decreased aggression toward the intruders in the resident-intruder assay.[109] Viral infections (e.g., rubella virus, herpes simplex virus, cytomegalovirus, and human immunodeficiency virus) have long been implicated in the etiology of ASD.[110] BDV infection also produces changes in play behaviors, including pinning and play solicitation.[108] These examples illustrate the relevance of play behaviors as measurements of social interaction, and the important role behavioral assays based on play behavior can have in validating models of ASD.

Social interaction deficits in ASD are also evident in the way children with ASD relate to parents and caregivers (e.g., diminished responsiveness to parents/caregivers, failure to share enjoyment with parents/caregivers, etc.). Measuring ultrasonic vocalizations (USVs) produced by neonatal rodent pups, which have been removed from their dam, is frequently used as an assay to measure separation-induced anxiety, but in the context of animal models of ASD, it has been used to examine social attachment. The basic paradigm involves a cage equipped to capture and record sound emitted at ultrasonic frequencies (typically in a 20–100 kHz range). Recording of USVs is made in sequence at intervals that capture changes in the vocalization of neonates when dam is present with her pup(s), followed by USVs that follow the removal of the dam from her pup(s), and ending with an interval when the dam has been returned to her pup(s). Variations can include recording from litters or single pups. The USV assay has been used to reveal and measure deficits in attachment behavior for several animal models of ASD including oxytocin (−/−) mice, rat 5-methoxytryptamin model, and μ-opioid receptor (−/−) mice.[111-113]

Nest-building is a home cage activity shared by all members of the home cage; although this activity primarily functions to provide an area for members of the group to sleep and huddle,[114] it is principally considered to be an index of social behavior.[115] When provided with suitable material mice of both sexes build nests and are typically found lying in the nest during the daytime; this helps to provide shelter, camouflage the mice from predators, enhance thermoregulation, and facilitates reproduction.[116] By introducing a usable piece of nesting material (usually a small amount of pressed cotton), an investigator can score whether test subjects are able to build a nest, how the location of a nest changes within the cage over time, and the position of the subject during periods of rest with respect to the position of the nest.[116] When gross abnormalities in motor behavior and non-related stereotypies can be excluded, these parameters of nesting behavior provide a readout of home cage behavior. This paradigm has been used to reveal and characterize deficits in nest-building behavior in several animal models of neuropsychiatric disorders featuring deficits in social behavior,[117,118] including the *Dvl* (−/−) mouse model of ASD.[119]

Arakawa *et al.* has proposed using the semi-naturalistic environment of a visible burrow system (VBS) as a behavioral assay for modeling deficits in social behavior observed in ASD.[120] When mixed sex groups of mice or rats are housed in the VBS, social hierarchies are formed between animals, which are characterized by individual differences in offensive and defensive behavior.[121,122] The VBS features a cage environment that closely resembles the conditions in which rodents live in a natural setting, and creates a paradigm where investigators can observe a variety of agonistic social behaviors expressed during the formation of a colony.[123] The process of familiarization that occurs between conspecifics during colony formation is integral to the establishment of these hierarchies and can be objectively observed over time using various behavioral assessments of social interaction. In the VBS paradigm described by Arakawa, social behaviors (e.g., huddle, being alone, allogrooming, self-grooming, approach to the front or the back of the approached animal, flight, chasing, following, and mounting) of C57/Bl6 mice were observed over a 15-day test period, and the frequency of each behavior was scored in 10 min intervals.[120] Results from this study identified huddling and approach from the front as the most stable social behaviors expressed across the different phases of colony formation. As animals become more familiar with one another, investigatory activity decreases between conspecifics, while passive body contact increases.[124] This is consistent with previous reports suggesting that C57BL/6 mice express more huddling behavior with a novel animal compared to other strains of mice (BALB/cJ and FVB/NJ), which cannot be attributed to an adaptive thermoregulatory behavior alone.[125] The VBS paradigm may be particularly well suited for assessing phenotypic differences in social interaction that occur between animals in a group, which has face validity for assessing deficits in social interaction and cognition that present themselves in a group setting.

Assays Modeling Restricted and Repetitive Behaviors

Restrictive behavior and adherence to routine can also be assayed in mice using tasks involving reversal learning. For example, in the Morris water maze, mice are trained to locate a hidden platform submerged in a circular pool of opaque water. Over several trials, mice with intact spatial learning and memory will quickly swim to the hidden platform. In the final probe trial, the platform is moved and the mice typically circle over the location where the platform was previously located. In the final phase, the platform is placed in a new location.[ix] Delay or deficient acquisition during the reversal phase could serve as a measure of cognitive rigidity in ASD.[101] Reversal learning in the T-maze task can be another measure of cognitive rigidity. Mice are trained to enter one arm of the maze to receive a food reward. Once the mouse has learned this task, the food reward is moved to the other arm, requiring the mouse to reverse its pattern of exploration to obtain the food.

As examples of some of the behavioral variance in the above tasks in inbred strains of mice, useful to define trait loci in the murine genome, there have been several recent studies looking at different strains of inbred mice and assessing the degree to which there were differences in behavioral tasks that were relevant to ASD. In a large study conducted by the laboratory of Dr. Crawley, 10 inbred strains were characterized in assays of sociability, preference for social novelty, and reversal learning.[107] In social behaviors, the mice were monitored to see whether they would prefer initially to interact with a novel mouse or to explore an empty quadrant, and 6 of the 10 strains

---

[ix] Please refer to Lindner et al., Development, optimization and use of preclinical behavioral models to maximize the productivity of drug discovery for Alzheimer's Disease, or Wagner et al., Huntington Disease in Volume 2, *Neurologic Disorders*, for further discussion of the Morris water maze and other procedures used to assess cognitive abilities in rodents.

of mice tested spent more time in the side of the apparatus with the novel mouse. In a follow-up experiment, the mice were given the opportunity of choosing between spending time with a known mouse or with a novel mouse. Again most strains showed preference for social novelty, spending more time with the novel mouse. The authors looked at anxiety-like behaviors using the elevated plus maze, and identified high levels of anxiety in some strains, which may contribute to lower levels of social approach. These authors also looked at reversal learning, and some strains failed to show a quadrant preference in a reversal probe trial. Interestingly, over all strains, the BTBR T+tf/J showed deficits both in social behaviors (without heightened anxiety as a potential cause) as well as in reversal learning, and thus represents a model with deficits similar to those seen in ASDs. Conversely, the FVB/NJ strain showed high levels of sociability and appropriate reversal learning in these studies.

In a similar study, another group looked at social behaviors and again found that BTBR showed very low levels of social behaviors while the FVB/NJ strain showed very high levels of social behaviors.[118,119] In the first paradigm, a mouse was placed in a cage and allowed to explore freely for 15 min; after the end of the 15 min, a second mouse was added to the cage and behaviors were monitored for 20 min (a resident-intruder challenge). In the second paradigm, both mice were added at the same time and social interactions were monitored (which resulted in less aggression than the more familiar resident-intruder paradigm). In both paradigms, FVB/NJ showed high levels of social behavior and BTBR T+tf/J displayed low levels of social behavior.

Animal Models of ASD

The complexity of the human makes it impossible for any one animal model to recapitulate all aspects of ASD. Models with face validity should display behavioral similarity with the characteristics of ASD and models with construct validity should share common neurobiological mechanisms. One strategy for developing models of ASD with face validity is to target individual endophenotypes associated with ASD (e.g., social cognition and motivation, communication, or repetitive and restrictive behaviors). However, the degree of construct validity in these models is often difficult to assess, and models with face validity, but not construct validity will not be useful in the pursuit of treatments for ASD. Models with construct validity are based on known underlying neurobiological mechanisms or candidate genes for ASD.

Neuropeptides and Models of Social Interaction and Cognition

The neuropeptides oxytocin and arginine vasopressin (AVP) have been implicated in the regulation of a wide range of affiliative behaviors including parental nurturing, mother–infant bonding, and social attachments in a variety of species. OT and OT receptor knockout mice have been used to examine the role of this neuropeptide system in regulating the social brain and may represent models of ASD with face, construct and perhaps predictive validity. When mouse pups are separated from their nest and mother, they emit ultrasonic distress vocalizations. However, OT and OT receptor knockout pups emit significantly fewer isolation distress calls than their wildtype littermates, suggesting that social isolation may not be aversive to the mutants.[112,126] This is supported by the results of a reunion task in which 10-day-old pups are separated from their mother by a divider with small holes that allow the pups to freely enter the chamber with the mother, but do not allow the mother to reunite with the pup. In this task, after one learning trial, wildtype pups quickly reunited with their mother, while OT knockout pups did not, despite similar locomotor activity (L.J.Young, unpublished data). Maternal nurturing behavior is moderately disrupted in OT knock-outs and severely impaired in OT receptor knockouts.[126,127] In addition, OT knockout males display complete social amnesia in the social recognition test, despite a normal ability to recognize familiar non-social scents.[103] The deficit in social recognition is completely rescued with an infusion of OT prior to, but not after the initial exposure, suggesting that the deficit lies in the processing of social stimuli.[128] Fos activation studies revealed that although wildtype and knockout mice display similar levels of neuronal activation in the olfactory bulb in an initial 2 min social exposure, OT knock-out males display decreased amygdala activation. Rather, OT knockout males exhibited abnormally elevated levels of Fos activation in the cortex and hippocampus following a social exposure, suggesting that OT knockout mice use alternate neural pathways in processing social information. Finally, a single infusion of OT into the amygdala, but not the olfactory bulb rescued the recognition abilities. There are intriguing parallels between the deficits in social recognition in OT knockout mouse model and altered face recognition and perception in ASD. In particular, as previously mentioned, ASD subjects display decreased amygdala activation during face perception tasks, but elevated activation in other cortical areas.[13]

Voles represent another animal model that has provided insights in the neuropeptidergic regulation of social cognition.[78,129] Vole species vary tremendously with respect to their social behavior. Prairie voles are highly social and socially monogamous. In contrast, montane and meadow voles are relatively asocial (socially aloof), and do not form adult–adult attachments. OT and AVP play central roles in facilitating social bond formation between adult prairie voles.[130] Specifically, OT interacts with the dopamine in the nucleus accumbens to facilitate social attachments in females, while AVP acts in the ventral pallidum to facilitate social attachments in males. Interestingly, prairie voles have high densities of OT receptors in the nucleus accumbens and vasopressin V1a receptors in the ventral pallidum, while montane and meadow voles do not.[130]

The species differences in V1a receptor expression is thought to be a major contributor to species differences in male social behavior patterns, since altering receptor expression patterns in the meadow vole brain leads to the development of social attachments.[131] Even within prairie voles, there is considerable individual variation in both V1a receptor expression patterns in the brain, and in the expression of social behavior. In fact, polymorphisms in a highly repetitive microsatellite DNA sequence located in the promoter of the gene encoding the V1a receptor (*avpr1a*) are associated with both variation in receptor expression, and social behavior in male prairie voles.[132] These studies in voles have led investigators to examine whether similar polymorphisms in microsatellites in the human *AVPR1a* may be associated with ASD. Indeed, three independent studies have reported modest associations between polymorphisms in the *AVPR1a* and ASD, with one study suggesting that these polymorphisms mediate variation in social skills in ASD.[133-135] These studies suggest that while variations in *AVPR1a* are not a major genetic risk factor for ASD, they may contribute additively to other genetic factors, and may contribute to the core social cognitive deficits found in some cases of ASD. These studies illustrate that investigations into the neural and genetic mechanism underlying normal social cognitive functions in animal models, related to the social endophenotype in ASD, can lead to potential targets for pharmacological intervention in ASD.

Foxp2 (–/–) Mice as a Model of Communication Deficits in ASD

The behavioral endophenotype of ASD that is perhaps the most difficult to model in animals is the impairment in language communication. One interesting exception involved mutants of *foxp2*. Mutations in *FOXP2* have been reported in a family in which half of the members have severe speech and language impairments.[136] *FOXP2* is located on 7q31 which has been implicated in autism linkage studies. Interestingly, *FOXP2* is expressed at high levels in brain regions involved in birdsong learning in finches and canaries, and its expression varies seasonally with song production, suggesting a conserved role for this gene in vocal communication in birds and man.[137,138] Furthermore, heterozygous *foxp2* knockout mice display severely reduce USVs when separated from the mother.[139] Subsequent gene associations analyses have failed to implicate *FOXP2* mutations in idiopathic ASD, however a significant proportion of individuals with alterations at the *FOXP2* locus meet criteria for ASD,[124] and the *foxp2* knockout model provides a tool to understand the genetics of language development and its possible relationship to other ASD endophenotypes.[140]

Models of Repetitive and Restrictive Behaviors in ASD

As mentioned above, "higher order" repetitive behavior, such as insistence on sameness, can be examined using reversal learning in the Morris water maze and T-maze. In addition to the differences across mouse strains discussed above, animal models of repetitive and restrictive behaviors in ASD generally fall into three categories: repetitive behavior induced by brain insults, repetitive behavior induced by pharmacological agents, and repetitive behavior induced by restricted environments or experience.[141] Various knockout mouse models of ASD display stereotypies including excessive grooming, repetitive forepaw movements or tail chasing.[141] One particularly informative model of repetitive and restrictive behavior is the deer mouse (*Peromyscus maniculatus*). When raised in standard laboratory cages, deer mice display repetitive hind limb jumping and backward somersaulting. However, when raised in larger, more complex environments, substantially fewer individuals display this behavior. Lewis and colleagues have used this environmental influence and individual variation to explore the neurobiological correlates of this stereotypy.[141] In this model, stereotypies are reduced with intrastriatal D_1 dopamine receptor antagonist or NMDA selective antagonist. The stereotypies are associated with an imbalance in the direct and indirect cortico-basal ganglia pathways. This and other models of repetitive and restrictive behaviors may be useful for identifying potential pharmacological targets for reducing repetitive and restrictive behavior in ASD.[x]

---

[x] For further discussion of the deer mouse as a model of repetitive behaviors, please refer to Joel *et al.*, Animal models of obsessive-compulsive disorder: From bench to bedside via endophenotypes and biomarkers, in this volume.

Models Based on Candidate ASD Genes

Using techniques like gene targeting by homologous recombination, researchers have been able to develop more precise animal models of human disease including ASD. The development of animal models that manipulate the expression of genes implicated in ASD enable investigators with the means to evaluate the contribution of these candidate genes to disease pathogenesis, and to explore the neurobiological mechanisms underlying genotype–phenotype relationships. The models discussed below were developed to investigate the contributions of genes implicated in ASD by linkage or association studies, such that the models would have construct validity, and offer translational opportunities for deeper exploration of pathophysiology.

Engrailed 2 (En2) Knockout Mouse

EN2 is a homeobox transcription factor gene that has been identified as an ASD susceptibility gene in several studies.[142,143] In fact, some risk assessment calculations suggest that the risk allele contributes to as many as 40% of ASD cases in the general population.[142] In mice, *En2* expression is primarily restricted to the cerebellum during nervous system development. Consistent with this, *En2* knockout mice display cerebellar hypoplasia, a reduction in the number of Purkinje neurons in the cerebellum, and foliation defects, all of which parallel features observed in ASD (although neuropathological analyses in ASD have been severely hampered by limited samples, inconsistent processing, and diagnostic concerns). *En2* knockout mice also display several behavioral abnormalities consistent with ASD.[144] Juvenile males display a reduction in play behavior, social investigation and allogrooming compared to wildtypes. The differences in social behavior are reduced in adults; however, adult knockout males display increased levels of autogrooming (repetitive) behavior. Deficits in spatial learning and memory tasks were detected in *En2* knockout mice as well. Thus the *En2* knockout mouse model displays both face (social behavior disruption) and construct (cerebellar defects, genetic risk factor) validity. However, the model does not presently suggest potential pharmacological interventions to reverse these deficits.

Neuroligin (Nlgn) Knockout Mice

Neuroligins play a critical role in synaptogenesis and synapse maintenance through their transynaptic interactions with neurexins. Loss-of-function mutations in NLGN3 and NLGN4 have been found in affected siblings with ASD and these genes have been proposed to cause rare monogenic forms of autism.[145-147] Neurexins, the binding partners for neuroligins, have also recently been implicated as ASD susceptibility genes,[148] highlighting the significance of synapse formation and maintenance in the etiology of ASD. A knockout mouse approach has been employed to study the role of neuroligins in synapse formation and function. Neuroligin 1,2,3 triple knockouts displayed an altered balance of glutamatergic and GABAergic neurotransmission, but a normal number of synapses. The altered neurotransmission was associated with altered synaptic protein distribution, rather than a decrease in synapse number. Thus neuroligins are required for the proper maintenance and function of the synapse rather than formation. This model provides an example of how animal models are useful for determining the cellular function of genes implicated in ASD etiology.

Phosphatase and Tensin Homolog on Chromosome Ten (PTEN) Mutant Mice

Phosphatase and tensin homolog on chromosome ten (*PTEN*) is a tumor suppressor gene and important negative regulator of PI3K intracellular signaling processes, which in the central nervous system are important for mediating neuronal migration and neurite extension.[149] Recently, a transgenic mouse line has been generated in which *Pten* expression is cleverly deleted in restricted populations of neurons in the cerebral cortex (layers III–V) and dentate gyrus (granular layer and polymorphic layer) of the hippocampus.[150,151] These Pten mutant mice have a deregulated PI3K pathway in neurons isolated from the cortex and hippocampus and display deficits in a wide range of social interaction and learning assays including social interaction/learning, nest-building, social preference test, and caged social interaction.[151] These deficits in social interaction and social learning are reminiscent of those observed in ASD, which suggest these animals have good face validity as a model of symptoms in the ASD social domain. Interestingly, *Pten* mutant mice also exhibit neuroanatomical abnormalities that are hallmarked by a phenotype of progressive macrocephaly.[152] This offers additional face, and perhaps construct, validity to the model, as increased brain volume has been reported in ASD patients.[153] Moreover, a screen of 88 individuals with apparently idiopathic ASD with macrocephaly identified one individual with a *de novo* PTEN mutation.[154]

Animal Models of Monogenic Disorders with ASD Phenotypes

Fragile X Syndrome and the mGluR Theory

The behavioral phenotype of *Fmr1* knockout mice is generally consistent with the human Fragile X phenotype. *Fmr1* knockouts display increased locomotor activity, reduced habituation to an open field, increased susceptibility to audiogenic seizure, and low levels of social interaction.[155,156] *Fmr1* knockout mice also have dendritic abnormalities similar to those found in humans. Interestingly, *Fmr1* knockout mice exhibit enhanced metabotropic glutamate receptor (mGluR)-dependent long-term depression (LTD). mGluR-dependent LTD requires the translation of pre-existing mRNAs at the synapse. Bear and colleagues have proposed that the exaggerated LTD seen in *Fmr1* knockout mice is due to the absence of the FMRP, which functions to put a brake on this translation.[96] The exaggerated LTD could alter synaptic development during critical periods of synaptogenesis, resulting in altered neuronal connections and behavioral phenotype. If the mGluR theory of Fragile X syndrome is correct, then mGluR antagonists may actually prove to be a viable pharmacological treatment strategy for Fragile X syndrome.[96] However, it is important to note that it is unclear if other forms of ASD involve the same underlying mechanisms, which is an important limitation in animal models of monogenic disorders.

Some insights into the molecular pathophysiology of Fragile X syndrome were recently afforded by studies showing that the p21-activated kinase associates with FMRP, and further those abnormalities in dendritic spines and long-term potentiation (LTP), as well as behavioral deficits in locomotor activity, stereotypy, anxiety, and trace fear conditioning are all ameliorated in *Fmr1* knockouts when PAK is inhibited.[157]

It is of interest to point out that the *Fmr1* knockout mouse model is one of only two animal models of ASD that has achieved criteria for predictive validity.[158] Ventura *et al.*

demonstrated that amphetamine improved performance in a novel object recognition task, thus reversing the cognitive impairments observed in these animals.[159] Increases in prefrontal release of dopamine were also observed with amphetamine in these animals. Although more commonly used to treat symptoms of hyperactivity, drugs that enhance dopaminergic activity (e.g., amphetamine, methylphenidate) in the CNS have been reported to be efficacious in treating cognitive impairments in patients with ASD.

Rett Syndrome and Phenotype Reversibility in Mice

Mecp2 knockout mice have been used as a model for Rett's syndrome and display altered motor function, gait, balance, and reduction in social interaction.[160] In addition, *Mecp2* knockout mice display reduced LTP in hippocampal neurons. Recently a mouse model of Rett syndrome was created in which the endogenous *Mecp2* gene was silenced by the insertion of a *lox-stop* cassette, but could be reactivated conditionally by deleting the cassette using Cre recombination. Mutants with the cassette in place developed typical symptoms of *Mecp2* knockouts, including altered gait and a reduction of LTP. Remarkably, however, if the cassette was deleted in symptomatic animals, resulting in expression of *Mecp2*, both the behavioral deficits and the reduction in LTP were rescued.[161] This remarkable finding does not suggest an immediate therapeutic intervention for Rett syndrome, but does demonstrate that the neurobiological deficits associated with this disorder may be reversible.

ANIMAL MODELS OF ASD IN DRUG DISCOVERY RESEARCH

Translational Roles for Animal Models in ASD Drug Research

Translational research is often referred to as a two-way street that seeks to translate scientific discoveries arising from the laboratory into clinical applications in one direction, while novel insights into disease pathogenesis made in the clinic work in the other direction to shape basic research at the bench. Animal models play a critical role in this endeavor, serving as experimental platforms for a variety of translational objectives for preclinical drug research including new target identification, preclinical validation of candidate targets or mechanisms, biomarker discovery, and the prioritization of experimental therapeutics. In this section, we discuss the translational roles for animal models in achieving preclinical research goals for ASD.

New Target Identification

The identification and validation of new targets for therapeutic drug development is the lifeblood of the pharmaceutical industry, which aims to provide patients with continual improvements in treatment options for human disease. The current of lack of approved pharmacological treatments for ASD discussed earlier illustrates the enormous unmet medical needs facing this patient population. It also emphasizes the need to increase focus on translational research aimed at identifying and validating targets for new ASD drug development.

In combination with a variety of discovery-based techniques such as gene expression profiling, global proteomic or metabolomic analysis, and quantitative trait locus

(QTL) mapping, animal models of disease offer excellent platforms for studies focused on new target identification. Experimental strategies using these types of approaches have been widely used to identify and implicate novel targets in animal models of other neuropsychiatric disorders, including schizophrenia,[162] depression,[163] and anxiety disorders.[164] Published reports indicate comparatively fewer studies that have been undertaken in animal models of ASD. Several representative examples of how new target identification studies have been successfully performed in animal models of ASD are discussed below.

Several new target identification studies have focused on the *Fmr1*(−/−) mouse model of Fragile X and ASD behavioral phenotypes discussed earlier. In the first example, researchers used the *Fmr1*(−/−) mice experimentally to address a key hypothesis aimed at explaining the mechanism through which mutations in the *FMR* gene lead to cognitive deficits in humans. This hypothesis proposes that mutations in *FMRP*, which functions as a RNA-binding protein, result in altered patterns of translation for mRNAs normally associated with FMRP-mRNP complexes.[165] Using a combination of immunoprecipitation and microarray analysis, researchers were able to capture and identify mRNAs (ligands) that were physically associated with the FMRP-mRNP complex in adult wild type brains, and compare these mRNA profiles with those obtained from *Fmr1*(−/−) mice.[166] Comparative analysis of these two profiles revealed a compendium of mRNAs whose translation is potentially altered in *Fmr1*(−/−) mice, thus providing novel insights into the potential molecular mechanisms underlying the phenotypes observed in this model. In a separate study using *Fmr1*(−/−) mice and a combination of microarray-based expression profiling and *in situ* hybridization, researchers identified microtubule-associated protein 2 and amyloid beta precursor protein as targets of interest for future.[167]

Other examples include models and assays of ASD not previously discussed here, but that offer good perspectives on how new target identification studies can be executed using animal models of ASD. Repetitive beam breaks in an open field is a measurement of repetitive behavior in rodents and has been proposed as a behavioral assay that offers a phenotypic measurement of the repetitive behaviors observed in ASD.[115] Using subcongenic strains of mice developed from a parental B6.129-Il10−/− knockout/congenic strain, researchers mapped a QTL interval on chromosome 1 (*Reb1*) that governs repetitive beam breaks in the open field.[168] This suggested that a gene(s) localized to this region of the genome might participate in the neurobiological mechanisms underlying the differences in repetitive behaviors observed in these mice. Combining this QTL analysis with differential gene expression profiling in amygdala tissue, researchers were able to identify two candidate genes for *Reb1*, the peptidylglycine alpha-amidating monooxygenase *Pam* and the (serine/threonine kinase *Stk25*) QTL.

Smith-Lemli-Opitz syndrome is a neurodevelopmental disorder that is caused by mutations in the gene encoding 7-dehydrocholesterol reductase (*DHCR7*), which plays an important role in normal cholesterol synthesis.[169] In children, Smith-Lemli-Opitz syndrome results in a spectrum of behavioral symptoms characteristic of ASD.[170] *Dhcr7* knockout mice (*Dhcr7*−/−) feature abnormalities in the development and functioning of the central serotonergic system, which have also been reported in patients with ASD.[171] Using a combination of microarray-based global gene expression profiling and immunohistochemical approaches, researchers were able to identify numerous gene products (mRNAs) that differed in expression between ($Dbcr7-/-$) and wild type, each of which can be considered new targets of interest for future investigation.[172] Each of these examples represents a new target discovery project that demonstrates how animal models of ASD can be used to identify specific molecular targets, but for each example, separate investigation is required to examine its potential as a new drug discovery target.

New Target Validation

Once a target of interest (e.g., enzyme, channel, receptor) has been identified, regardless of how it was discovered, evidence must then be obtained that will help establish a rationale supporting its therapeutic potential as a drug discovery target. Generally, the experimental process through which this preclinical proof-of-concept is obtained is often referred to as "target validation." This would be distinct from the proof-of-concept achieved by demonstrating efficacy for a target, or novel mechanism of action, in the clinic. The evidence supporting preclinical proof-of-concept usually involves demonstrating that an experimental agent (e.g., drug, mutation, transgene, siRNA), which can selectively modulate the function of the target, produces a measurable change in a biological function relevant to the targeted disease. In the context of ASD drug discovery, target validation could involve the significant reversal of deficits in social interaction, social cognition, repetitive behavior, or any other relevant phenotype, in an animal model of ASD that has established strong face or construct validity.

Biomarker Discovery

A biomarker is generally defined as an objective biological measurement (e.g., protein, metabolic product, fMRI image) that serves as an indicator of normal or pathogenic biological processes, or responses (e.g., efficacy, safety) to a therapeutic agent. In a clinical setting, biomarkers offer the potential for categorizing subsets of patients in a more reliable and consistent manner, predicting prognosis and response to treatment, and possibly assisting with early detection of illness in high-risk patients. Not surprisingly, modern paradigms of drug discovery research require developing research strategies for the identification of biomarker(s) as an essential component to the programmatic efforts for a given drug target or targeted therapeutic indication.[173] Although many current biomarker discovery efforts are driven by clinical studies, researchers have increasingly turned to animal models as translational platforms for biomarker discovery and characterization.

In contrast to human studies, very little biomarker research has been reported using animal models of ASD. An excellent example illustrating that this can be done successfully is exemplified in a study featuring the combined proteomic and transcriptomic (microarray) profiling of CD1 mice that were selectively bred for either high-anxiety-related behavior (HAB-M) or low-anxiety-related behavior (LAB-M).[174] In this study, researchers identified glyoxalase-I as a protein marker of extremes in trait anxiety, which now has potential as a biomarker of the anxiety in humans. This same type of discovery strategy could quite easily be used to identify biomarkers that correlate with extremes in phenotypes (e.g., social interaction, repetitive behaviors) related to ASD. In comparison to other strains of inbred mice, Balb/c mice are a good example of strain-based extremes in ASD-related phenotypes, and could serve as a platform for ASD research.[175] Balb/c mice exhibit low sociability, increased prevalence of anxiety and aggressive behaviors, large brain size, underdevelopment of the corpus callosum, and reduced levels of brain serotonin synthesis, all phenotypes similar to those observed in human ASD patients. Extreme behavioral phenotypes in animal models have also been developed based on selective breeding, transgenesis, targeted neuroanatomical lesion, or pharmacological challenge. Future efforts around the development and validation of new animal models of ASD should include considerations for use as platforms in translational research to identify biomarkers.

Evidence-based Identification and Prioritization of Candidate Therapeutics

Once a drug target has been identified and sufficient validation has been achieved to initiate chemistry efforts to discovery and development of novel compounds, animal models serve an essential role in the evaluation and prioritization of compounds in the development process. Animal models of ASD could also be used preclinically to investigate whether a drug(s), approved for another related indication, might have potential utility for treating specific symptoms of ASD. For instance, if evidence can be generated preclinically that a drug approved for a non-related indication, which would not *a priori* be expected to be efficacious for the treatment of social deficits in Rett's syndrome, strongly reverses social deficits or relevant changes in LTP in $Mecp2(-/-)$ mice, this may provide a rationale to investigate its utility as a therapeutic for Rett's in humans.

Oxytocin: An Example of an Animal Model Driven Drug Intervention for ASD

There is now considerable evidence that OT modulates aspects of social behavior and social cognition in animals. As discussed in detail above, OT is involved in the processing of social stimuli in mice and modulates social motivation. In voles, OT plays a role in the formation of social bonds. Additionally, as noted, there is preliminary evidence showing that OT is involved in social information processing in humans. Specifically, studies show that OT infusion enhances interpersonal trust,[176] decreases amygdala activation while viewing socially threatening stimuli[68] and, particularly relevant to ASD, enhances the ability to read social signals from subtle facial expressions.[70] Indeed, given that OT has been implicated in the regulation of affiliative behaviors – as well as repetitive behaviors – and that deficits in social behavior and repetitive behaviors are core ASD symptoms, a number of researchers have suggested that oxytocin may be implicated in autism and related spectrum disorders.[76-84]

In support of this idea, research has found decreased plasma OT in children with autism compared to age-matched controls.[177] A second study also found evidence for dysregulated OT in adults with ASD; however, this study found higher OT plasma levels in the ASD group compared to controls.[178] Genetic studies also support a role of OT in ASD. Linkage analysis implicated the region of chromosome 3 in which OXTR is found as a susceptibility locus for ASD.[179] This study was reinforced by a study of Han Chinese family trios, which showed evidence of association of two single nucleotide polymorphisms (SNPs) in the oxytocin receptor with ASD.[180] This latter-finding has now been replicated by an independent group: Jacob *et al.* looked at these two polymorphisms in 57 Caucasian autism trios, and observed a significant association with one of them and autism, despite of the modest scale of the study.[181] Finally, in recent careful analyses of copy number variation (CNV) in 121 unrelated subjects with ASD, a microdeletion encompassing the oxytocin receptor gene was identified.[182] The affected child and the mother both carried the deletion; the child had a diagnosis of autism, while the mother was diagnosed with psychological symptoms including possible OCD and phobias.

Based on the extensive work in animals and the findings showing altered plasma OT levels in ASD, Hollander and colleagues have been interested in the potential therapeutic value of OT in treating core ASD symptoms.[82-84] In a double-blind, placebo-controlled, cross-over investigation, Hollander *et al.* administered a synthetic form of OT (Pitocin) (or placebo) via intravenous infusion to 15 adults with ASD over a 4h period; each participant was randomly assigned to receive OT and placebo challenges on separate occasions (administration order was counter-balanced). Results showed a significant reduction in repetitive behaviors following OT administration compared to placebo.[82] In addition, OT also facilitated participants' ability to identify emotions in speech intonation – a key deficit shared by many individuals with ASD.[84] Interestingly, though, the effect of OT on social information processing was a function of time and *administration order*. Whereas those who received placebo 1st tended to revert to baseline after a delay (of approximately 2 weeks), those who received oxytocin 1st retained the ability to accurately assign emotional significance to speech intonation. This finding is consistent with studies showing that low doses of OT facilitate social recognition in rodents,[183] and with the aforementioned studies showing that a single ICV injection of OT can rescue social memory acquisition in mice with social memory deficits produced in OT knockout mice.[184]

Although these preliminary findings are encouraging, there are obstacles that must be overcome before OT can be considered a viable treatment for core ASD symptoms. In particular, it is unclear whether OT administered peripherally efficiently passes the blood-brain barrier and, if so, in what quantities. In addition, intravenous administration is highly impractical for a drug that is to be given on a daily basis. Intranasal administration, which is currently only available in Europe, would be one way to overcome these obstacles because this administration modality has been shown to penetrate into cerebrospinal fluid[185] and is more practical and user-friendly for patients. Indeed, Hollander's group is conducting a pilot study to investigate intranasal OT in the treatment of core ASD symptoms and preliminary findings from this investigation are promising.[186]

Model Development and Validation: Issues, Needs, and Challenges

Lack of ASD Animal Models with Predictive Validity

The ability to make predictions about whether or not a novel mechanism of action, or experimental drug, is likely to have relevant clinical effects in humans based on effects in preclinical animal models is an integral part of the path pharmaceutical companies take toward the discovery and development of novel therapeutics. Although pharmaceutical researchers share interest in developing and using animal models with face and construct validity, it is an expectation that models with predictive validity will serve as the primary platforms driving new target discovery/validation, test compound screening, and decision-making around the prioritization of therapeutic compounds for clinical development. This is particularly true in CNS drug development, where pharmaceutical companies strive to mitigate the recognized risks of lower probabilities (7%) that CNS drugs entering clinical development will succeed in gaining approval to enter the marketplace, when compared to other therapeutic areas (15%).[187] Thus, the drug discovery process for behavioral disorders places a premium on the use of animal models that have achieved predictive validity as part of their development.

The ability to achieve predictive validity for models of ASD has been complicated historically by the absence of approved phamacotherapies for the treatment of symptoms in ASD. This is emphasized by the fact that, to date, only two models of ASD have successfully achieved the criterion for predictive validity, using compounds that were not developed specifically for ASD.[158] Moreover, the atypical antipsychotic risperidone (Risperdal®), which has now been approved for the treatment of irritability associated with autism in children and adolescents, may have clinical utility that is too narrow to serve as an appropriate reference compound for animal models needing to achieve criterion of predictive validity in other symptom domains of ASD. This creates a quagmire as the current lack of available treatment options may, in part, be linked to the limited or inadequate predictive validity of current animal models of ASD, which, subsequently, hinders the development of novel therapeutics for ASD.[xi]

Therefore, in the absence of approved drugs for ASD, it is recommended that future efforts focus on the development of animal models of ASD that place a greater emphasis on achieving predictive validity using drugs that, although not officially labeled for use in treating ASD, are widely used to manage specific symptoms of the disorder. A summary of these drugs was described in detail earlier.

Balancing Validity and Reliability with Demands of a High-Throughput Environment

Selecting behavioral assays and/or animal models for use in supporting a drug discovery and development program presents numerous challenges. Most of these challenges, however, are not unique to the targeted therapeutic area of ASD; rather they represent general considerations, which highlight the often profound differences in demand and expectation that exist between different research environments. For instance, the need to accommodate throughput in pharmaceutical industry can be much larger in scale than most academic or government researchers are accustomed to, consequently, this places limitations on the types of behavioral assays and animal

---

[xi] Pharmacological isomorphism, or the amelioration of abnormal behaviors present in the animal model by clinically effective drugs, is an important, but not necessarily sufficient criterion for the establishment of the predictive validity of that behavioral model of a disorder. Please refer to Please refer to Steckler *et al.*, Developing novel anxiolytics: improving preclinical detection and clinical assessment, Joel *et al.*, Animal models of obsessive-compulsive disorder: From bench to bedside via endophenotypes and biomarkers, in this volume, or to Lindner *et al.*, Development, optimization and use of preclinical behavioral models to maximize the productivity of drug discovery for Alzheimer's Disease, in Volume 2, *Neurological Disorders* for further discussion of the strengths and limitations of pharmacological isomorphism in establishing model validity.

models that can be used. Meeting these demands, without compromising model validity and/or validity, is a crucial challenge in selecting which models will most successfully serve in a behavioral screen for ASD or any neuropsychiatric disorder. Here we discuss some of the challenges facing the development and adaptation of animal models for use with behavioral screening in a drug discovery environment.

Although many animal models may offer good validity as disease models, the maintenance of colonies sufficient in size to support the demands of a high-throughput environment may be limited by a variety of issues. Running a behavioral screen can require large cohorts of animals, many of which may differ greatly in their health and reproductive fitness. This can be particularly true with genetically modified animals. Strain, transgene, knockout or knockin effects on the health and reproductive fitness can vary widely for animals, limiting availability. For instance, if a particular strain or genetically modified animal does not breed well, requires cumbersome or complicated mating protocols, or suffers from lethality that limits their use to a narrow developmental window, the ability to maintain colonies of sufficient size to support the demands of a behavioral screen can be time-consuming (slow) and resource intensive.

Reliability is an important criterion for evaluating the utility of any animal model. It is particularly true for models that will be used in the context of a drug discovery operation, where the screening of large numbers of test compounds leaves little room for inconsistency or instability in the measurable outcomes of a given model.[xii]

Behavioral pharmacology groups working in drug discovery and development divisions are required to use animal models to screen large numbers of compounds for prioritization, etc. It is often surprising, but male animals are used more routinely in behavioral panels than females, owing to convenience of use and avoidance of the complications and physiological challenges associated with controlling the estrus cycle in females. This specific issue may raise concerns over the use of animal models to screen novel therapeutic compounds for psychiatric disorders such as depression, where epidemiology studies clearly show a bias towards females; however, operational bias towards using male animals may be an advantage for autism, where males are roughly four times more likely to have the disorder.

Reaching Consensus on Gold Standards in Assays and Models of ASD

As discussed in detail, there are numerous behavioral assays and animal models relevant to ASD, which demonstrate potential for use in drug discovery research. Moreover, on the basic conceptual aspects behind designing a battery of animal models for the evaluation of behavioral phenotypes relevant to ASD have been thoroughly discussed.[101,102] However, experts in the field still have not reached a consensus regarding which assays or models are the most relevant to ASD, and its symptom domains. Establishing a consensus on which assays and models represent gold standards within the field would be an important first step in recruiting pharmaceutical companies into a focused

---

[xii] For further discussion regarding the demands placed upon behavioral pharmacologists developing and working with animal models of behavioral disorders within the context of pharmaceutical drug discovery environments, please refer to Lindner *et al.*, Development, optimization and use of preclinical behavioral models to maximize the productivity of drug discovery for Alzheimer's Disease, in Volume 2, *Neurological Disorders*.

effort to discovery and developing novel therapeutics for ASD. Moving forward, it is critical that collaborative effort be made amongst academic, clinical, government, and pharmaceutical research to establish a consensus on which animal models should be consider as the gold standard(s) in the field.

SUMMARY AND FUTURE DIRECTIONS

Autism spectrum disorders are a class of neurodevelopmental disorders defined by social deficits, a lack of verbal and non-verbal communication skills, and rigid, repetitive, stereotyped behavior patterns and/or restricted interests. In addition to these three core symptom domains, ASD is often accompanied by a number of associated features (e.g., mental retardation, seizures, anxiety, and self-injury), ADHD-like symptoms, and affective instability. ASD impairments are generally gross and sustained, with onset typically prior to 3 years of age (usually by 18 months) and lasting throughout the individual's lifespan. Needless to say, the typical outcome for individuals with ASD is not promising, and studies indicate that even those with the best profiles (e.g., average to superior IQs) are often unemployed, underemployed, have difficulty living independently, and face persistent social isolation.[188] Given that ASD is a life-long disorder, it places a tremendous burden on caregivers; moreover, the special educational (e.g., occupational therapy, speech, special instruction) and medical needs required by individuals with ASD place a significant load on society as a whole. Indeed, it is estimated that the cost of caring for individuals with autism over their lifetime is $35 billion per year; however, this may be an underestimate because many expenses, for example alternative therapies, are paid for out-of-pocket by families and are difficult to measure.[189]

To date, relatively small efforts have been made to develop pharmacological treatments that target core ASD symptom domains. Indeed, most of the drug development in this area has been based on adopting treatments that have been successful in other psychiatric disorders like schizophrenia, OCD, attention-deficit hyperactivity disorder, depression, and anxiety; as a result, most available treatments target associated symptoms of ASD, rather than the core symptoms that are unique to the disorder. Pharmacological treatments that target social and communicative deficits of ASD are sorely needed. In addition, drugs that target neurocognitive deficits are needed. Although not a core feature of ASD, these deficits afflict a large majority of the ASD population (even the so-called "high-functioning" individuals), and significantly undermine their ability to function on a daily basis (e.g., independent self-care) and meet their true potential (e.g., although intellectually able, many individuals with ASD fail to complete school and cannot hold down a job because the lack the required organizational skills).

On the clinical side, more work is needed to develop adequate outcome measures. The majority of outcome measures typically used in clinical trials are based on third party reports of problematic behaviors. Although useful, they do not tap the underlying processes or specific skills that contribute to the quality of the individual's social and communicative functioning. Understanding these skills and processes are important because, presumably, they are at the heart of the problematic behavior. In addition, adequate surrogate outcome measures that reflect changes in key systems in response to treatment (e.g., fMRI, evoked potentials, prepulse inhibition) are needed. Tracking surrogate markers is important because the effects of a drug may not immediately translate to observable behavior but may contribute to behavioral changes down the road. The identification of surrogate markers may also shed light on the biological factors implicated in the target disruptive behavior as well as the underlying therapeutic mechanisms of a particular drug. Finally, a better understanding of the mediators and moderators of treatment response is needed. While this is important for many disorders, it is especially important for ASD because ASD is such a heterogeneous disorder, not only in terms of symptom presentation, but also with respect to etiology (i.e., it is generally thought that autism and related spectrum disorders have multiple causes resulting from interactions between numerous genetic and environmental factors). The incorporation of genetics, endophenotypic measures, and functional imaging into treatment trials will be instrumental to this goal as these techniques can shed light on the relevant genes and brain systems involved in treatment response.

In conclusion, because of the relatively unique features of ASD, and because of the heterogeneity of these disorders, drug development in this area may especially benefit from approaches that draw upon preclinical work with animal models to develop novel treatment studies that integrate genetics, endophenotyping, and functional imaging to understand better the mediators and moderators of treatment response. Although progress is being made, future success in this area will require more close collaboration between clinical investigators, who can identify the relevant disease phenomena and unmet needs, and preclinical investigators, who can identify novel targets that can be moved into clinical trials. In addition, a key component of this effort will be to develop consortiums to rapidly screen promising target compounds that have been developed in animal models. Indeed, such a treatment network was recently established in by Cure Autism Now/Autism Speaks and holds promise for innovative drug development.

REFERENCES

1. Yeargin-Allsopp, M., Rice, C., Karapurkar, T., Doernberg, N., Boyle, C., and Murphy, C. (2003). Prevalence of autism in a US metropolitan area. *JAMA*, 289(1):49–55.
2. CDC. (2007). Prevalence of Autism Spectrum Disorders – Autism and Developmental Disabilities Monitoring Network, 14 Sites, United States, 2002. *Surveillance Summaries, MMWR*, 56(SS-1):12–27.
3. Asperger, H. (1991). Die autistischen psychopathen im Kindesalter, Archiv fur Psychiatrie und Nervenkrankheiten, 117:76–136. In: Frith, U. (ed.) Autism and *Asperger Syndrome*. Cambridge, UK: Cambridge University Press; pp. 37–92.
4. Kanner, L. (1943). Autistic disturbances of affective contact. *Nervous Child*, 2:217–250.
5. American Psychiatric Association. (2000). *Diagnostic and statistical manual of mental disorders*, 4th edition. American Psychiatric Association, Washington, DC.
6. Wing, L. and Gould, J. (1979). Severe impairments of social interaction, associated abnormalities in children: Epidemiology, classification. *J Autism Dev Disord*, 9(1):11–29.
7. Szatmari, P., Tuff, L., Finlayson, M.A., and Bartolucci, G. (1990). Asperger's syndrome and autism: Neurocognitive aspects. *J Am Acad Child Adolesc Psychiatry*, 29(1):130–136.
8. Davies, S., Bishop, D., Manstead, A.S., and Tantam, D. (1994). Face perception in children with autism and Asperger's syndrome. *J Child Psychol Psychiatry*, 35(6):1033–1057.

9. Barton, J.J. (2003). Disorders of face perception and recognition. *Neurol Clin*, 21(2):521–548.

10. Hobson, R.P., Ouston, J., and Lee, A. (1988). Emotion recognition in autism: Coordinating faces and voices. *Psychol Med*, 18(4):911–923.

11. Tantam, D., Monaghan, L., Nicholson, H., and Stirling, J. (1989). Autistic children's ability to interpret faces: A research note. *J Child Psychol Psychiatry*, 30(4):623–630.

12. Rutherford, M.D., Baron-Cohen, S., and Wheelwright, S. (2002). Reading the mind in the voice: A study with normal adults and adults with Asperger syndrome and high functioning autism. *J Autism Dev Disord*, 32(3):189–194.

13. Pierce, K., Muller, R.A., Ambrose, J., Allen, G., and Courchesne, E. (2001). Face processing occurs outside the fusiform 'face area' in autism: Evidence from functional MRI. *Brain*, 124(Pt 10):2059–2073.

14. Schultz, R.T., Gauthier, I., Klin, A., Fulbright, R.K., Anderson, A.W., Volkmar, F. *et al.* (2000). Abnormal ventral temporal cortical activity during face discrimination among individuals with autism and Asperger syndrome. *Arch Gen Psychiatry*, 57(4):331–340.

15. Arnold, L.E., Vitiello, B., McDougle, C., Scahill, L., Shah, B., Gonzalez, N.M. *et al.* (2003). Parent-defined target symptoms respond to risperidone in RUPP autism study: Customer approach to clinical trials. *J Am Acad Child Adolesc Psychiatry*, 42(12):1443–1450.

16. Allen, D.A., Steinberg, M., Dunn, M., Fein, D., Feinstein, C., Waterhouse, L. *et al.* (2001). Autistic disorder versus other pervasive developmental disorders in young children: Same or different? *Eur Child Adolesc Psychiatry*, 10(1):67–78.

17. Towbin, K.E., Pradella, A., Gorrindo, T., Pine, D.S., and Leibenluft, E. (2005). Autism spectrum traits in children with mood and anxiety disorders. *J Child Adolesc Psychopharmacol*, 15(3):452–464.

18. Research Units on Pediatric Psychopharmacology Autism Network. (2005). Risperidone treatment of autistic disorder: Longer-term benefits and blinded discontinuation after 6 months. *Am J Psychiatry*, 162(7):1361–1369.

19. Lord, C., Risi, S., Lambrecht, L., Cook, E.H., Jr, Leventhal, B.L., DiLavore, P.C. *et al.* (2000). The autism diagnostic observation schedule-generic: A standard measure of social and communication deficits associated with the spectrum of autism. *J Autism Dev Disord*, 30(3):205–223.

20. Lord, C., Rutter, M., and DiLavre, P.C. (1998). *Autism Diagnostic Observational Schedule-Generic (ADOS-G)*. Psychological Corporation, San Antonio, TX.

21. Rutter, M., Lord, C., and LeCouteur, A. (1994). *Autism Diagnostic Interview-Revised (ADI-R)*, 3rd edition. Department of Psychiatry, University of Chicago, Illinois.

22. Constantino, J.N. (2002). *The Social Responsiveness Scale*. Western Psychological Services, Los Angeles.

23. Bishop, D.V.M. (1998). Development of the children's communication checklist: A method for assessing qualitative aspects of communicative impairments in children. *J Child Psychol Psychiatry*, 39:879–891.

24. Berument, S.K., Rutter, M., Lord, C., Pickles, A., and Bailey, A. (1999). Autism screening questionnaire: Diagnostic validity. *Br J Psychiatry*, 175:444–451.

25. Rutter, M., Bailey, A., Lord, C., and Berument, S.K. (2003). *Social Communication Questionnaire*. Western Psychological Services, Los Angeles, CA.

26. Volkmar, F.R., Lord, C., Bailey, A., Schultz, R.T., and Klin, A. (2004). Autism and pervasive developmental disorders. *J Child Psychol Psychiatry*, 45(1):135–170.

27. Aman, M.G., Richmond, G., Stewart, A.W., Bell, J.C., and Kissel, R.C. (1987). The aberrant behavior checklist: Factor structure and the effect of subject variables in American and New Zealand facilities. *Am J Ment Defic*, 91(6):570–578.

28. Aman, M.G. and Singh, N.N. (1986). *Manual for the Aberrant Behavior Checklist*. Slosson Educational Publications, East Aurora, NY.

29. Connors, C.K. and Barkley, R.A. (1985). Clinical Global Impresion Scale (CGI). *Psychopharmacol Bull*, 21:809–843.
30. Goodman, W.K., Price, L.H., Rasmussen, S.A., Mazure, C., Fleischmann, R.L., Hill, C.L. *et al.* (1989). The Yale-Brown Obsessive Compulsive Scale. I. Development, use, and reliability. *Arch Gen Psychiatry*, 46(11):1006–1011.
31. Goodman, W.K., Price, L.H., Rasmussen, S.A., Mazure, C., Delgado, P., Heninger, G.R. *et al.* (1989). The Yale-Brown Obsessive Compulsive Scale. II. Validity. *Arch Gen Psychiatry*, 46(11):1012–1016.
32. Sparrow, S.S., Balla, D.A., and Cichetti, D.V. (1984). *Vineland Adaptive Behavior Scale*. American Guidance Service, Circle Pines, MN.
33. McDougle, C.J., Kresch, L.E., Goodman, W.K., Naylor, S.T., Volkmar, F.R., Cohen, D.J. *et al.* (1995). A case-controlled study of repetitive thoughts and behavior in adults with autistic disorder and obsessive-compulsive disorder. *Am J Psychiatry*, 152(5):772–777.
34. McDougle, C.J., Naylor, S.T., Cohen, D.J., Volkmar, F.R., Heninger, G.R., and Price, L.H. (1996). A double-blind, placebo-controlled study of fluvoxamine in adults with autistic disorder. *Arch Gen Psychiatry*, 53(11):1001–1008.
35. Kaplan, A. and Hollander, E. (2003). A review of pharmacologic treatments for obsessive-compulsive disorder. *Psychiatric Services*, 54:1111–1118.
36. Schapiro, M.L., Wasserman, S., and Hollander, E. (2007). Treatment of autism with selective serotonin reuptake inhibitors and other antidepressants. In Hollander, E. and Anagnostou, E. (eds.), *Clinical Manual for the Treatment of Autism*. American Psychiatric Publishing, Inc., Washington, DC.
37. Cook, E.H. and Leventhal, B.L. (1996). The serotonin system in autism. *Curr Opin Pediatr*, 8(4):348–354.
38. Fatemi, S.H., Realmuto, G.M., Khan, L., and Thuras, P. (1998). Fluoxetine in treatment of adolescent patients with autism: A longitudinal open trial. *J Autism Dev Disord*, 28(4):303–307.
39. Schain, R.J. and Freedman, D.X. (1961). Studies on 5-hydroxyindole metabolism in autistic and other mentally retarded children. *J Pediatr*, 58:315–320.
40. Cook, E.H., Jr, Rowlett, R., Jaselskis, C., and Leventhal, B.L. (1992). Fluoxetine treatment of children and adults with autistic disorder and mental retardation. *J Am Acad Child Adolesc Psychiatry*, 31(4):739–745.
41. DeLong, G.R., Teague, L.A., and McSwain Kamran, M. (1998). Effects of fluoxetine treatment in young children with idiopathic autism. *Dev Med Child Neurol*, 40(8):551–562.
42. DeLong, G.R., Ritch, C.R., and Burch, S. (2002). Fluoxetine response in children with autistic spectrum disorders: Correlation with familial major affective disorder and intellectual achievement. *Dev Med Child Neurol*, 44(10):652–659.
43. Buchsbaum, M.S., Hollander, E., Haznedar, M.M., Tang, C., Spiegel-Cohen, J., Wei, T.C. *et al.* (2001). Effect of fluoxetine on regional cerebral metabolism in autistic spectrum disorders: A pilot study. *Int J Neuropsychopharmacol*, 4(2):119–125.
44. Hollander, E., Phillips, A., Chaplin, W., Zagursky, K., Novotny, S., Wasserman, S. *et al.* (2005). A placebo controlled crossover trial of liquid fluoxetine on repetitive behaviors in childhood and adolescent autism. *Neuropsychopharmacology*, 30(3):582–589.
45. McDougle, C.J., Kresch, L.E., and Posey, D.J. (2000). Repetitive thoughts and behavior in pervasive developmental disorders: Treatment with serotonin reuptake inhibitors. *J Autism Dev Disord*, 30(5):427–435.
46. Namerow, L.B., Thomas, P., Bostic, J.Q., Prince, J., and Monuteaux, M.C. (2003). Use of citalopram in pervasive developmental disorders. *J Dev Behav Pediatr*, 24(2):104–108.
47. Owley, T., Walton, L., Salt, J., Guter, S.J., Jr, Winnega, M., Leventhal, B.L. *et al.* (2005). An open-label trial of escitalopram in pervasive developmental disorders. *J Am Acad Child Adolesc Psychiatry*, 44(4):343–348.

48. Hellings, J.A., Kelley, L.A., Gabrielli, W.F., Kilgore, E., and Shah, P. (1996). Sertraline response in adults with mental retardation and autistic disorder. *J Clin Psychiatry*, 57(8):333–336.

49. McDougle, C.J., Brodkin, E.S., Naylor, S.T., Carlson, D.C., Cohen, D.J., and Price, L.H. (1998). Sertraline in adults with pervasive developmental disorders: A prospective open-label investigation. *J Clin Psychopharmacol*, 18(1):62–66.

50. Steingard, R.J., Zimnitzky, B., DeMaso, D.R., Bauman, M.L., and Bucci, J.P. (1997). Sertraline treatment of transition-associated anxiety and agitation in children with autistic disorder. *J Child Adolesc Psychopharmacol*, 7(1):9–15.

51. Hollander, E., Kaplan, A., Cartwright, C., and Reichman, D. (2000). Venlafaxine in children, adolescents, and young adults with autism spectrum disorders: An open retrospective clinical report. *J Child Neurol*, 15(2):132–135.

52. Campbell, M., Armenteros, J.L., Malone, R.P., Adams, P.B., Eisenberg, Z.W., and Overall, J.E. (1997). Neuroleptic-related dyskinesias in autistic children: A prospective, longitudinal study. *J Am Acad Child Adolesc Psychiatry*, 36(6):835–843.

53. McDougle, C.J., Scahill, L., McCracken, J.T., Aman, M.G., Tierney, E., Arnold, L.E. *et al.* (2000). Research Units on Pediatric Psychopharmacology (RUPP) Autism Network. Background and rationale for an initial controlled study of risperidone. *Child Adolesc Psychiatr Clin N Am*, 9(1):201–224.

54. Hollander, E., Dolgoff-Kaspar, R., Cartwright, C., Rawitt, R., and Novotny, S. (2001). An open trial of divalproex sodium in autism spectrum disorders. *J Clin Psychiatry*, 62(7):530–534.

55. Hollander, E., Soorya, L., Wasserman, S., Esposito, K., Chaplin, W., and Anagnostou, E. (2006). Divalproex sodium vs. placebo in the treatment of repetitive behaviours in autism spectrum disorder, *Int J Neuropsychopharmacol*, 9(2):209–213.

56. Uvebrant, P. and Bauziene, R. (1994). Intractable epilepsy in children. The efficacy of lamotrigine treatment, including non-seizure-related benefits. *Neuropediatrics*, 25(6):284–289.

57. Belsito, K.M., Law, P.A., Kirk, K.S., Landa, R.J., and Zimmerman, A.W. (2001). Lamotrigine therapy for autistic disorder: A randomized, double-blind, placebo-controlled trial. *J Autism Dev Disord*, 31(2):175–181.

58. Rugino, T.A. and Samsock, T.C. (2002). Levetiracetam in autistic children: An open-label study. *J Dev Behav Pediatr*, 23(4):225–230.

59. Wasserman, S., Iyengar, R., Chaplin, W.F., Watner, D., Waldoks, S.E., Anagnostou, E. *et al.* (2006). Levetiracetam versus placebo in childhood and adolescent autism: A double-blind placebo-controlled study. *Int Clin Psychopharmacol*, 21(6):363–367.

60. Aldred, S., Moore, K.M., Fitzgerald, M., and Waring, R.H. (2003). Plasma amino acid levels in children with autism and their families. *J Autism Dev Disord*, 33(1):93–97.

61. Rolf, L.H., Haarmann, F.Y., Grotemeyer, K.H., and Kehrer, H. (1993). Serotonin and amino acid content in platelets of autistic children. *Acta Psychiatr Scand*, 87(5):312–316.

62. Moreno-Fuenmayor, H., Borjas, L., Arrieta, A., Valera, V., and Socorro-Candanoza, L. (1996). Plasma excitatory amino acids in autism. *Invest Clin*, 37(2):113–128.

63. Anagnostou, E., Collins, G., and Hollander, E. (2007). Promising new avenues of treatment and future directions for patients with autism. In Hollander, E. and Anagnostou, E. (eds.), *Clinical Manual for the Treatment of Autism*. American Psychiatric Publishing, Inc., Washington, DC.

64. Kosfeld, M., Heinrichs, M., Zak, P.J., Fischbacher, U., and Fehr, E. (2005). Oxytocin increases trust in humans. *Nature*, 435(7042):673–676.

65. Posey, D.J., Kem, D.L., Swiezy, N.B., Sweeten, T.L., Wiegand, R.E., and McDougle, C.J. (2004). A pilot study of D-cycloserine in subjects with autistic disorder. *Am J Psychiatry*, 161(11):2115–2117.

66. Woodard, C., Groden, J., Goodwin, M., Shanower, C., and Bianco, J. (2005). The treatment of the behavioral sequelae of autism with dextromethorphan: A case report. *J Autism Dev Disord*, 35(4):515–518.

67. Woodard, C., Groden, J., Goodwin, M., and Bodfish, J. (2007). A placebo double-blind pilot study of dextromethorphan for problematic behaviors in children with autism. *Autism*, 11(1):29–41.

68. Kirsch, P., Esslinger, C., Chen, Q., Mier, D., Lis, S., Siddhanti, S. *et al.* (2005). Oxytocin modulates neural circuitry for social cognition and fear in humans. *J Neurosci*, 25(49):11489–11493.

69. Domes, G., Heinrichs, M., Glascher, J., Buchel, C., Braus, D.F., and Herpertz, S.C. (2007). Oxytocin attenuates amygdala responses to emotional faces regardless of valence, *Biol Psychiatry*, 62(10):1187–1190.

70. Domes, G., Heinrichs, M., Michel, A., Berger, C., and Herpertz, S.C. (2007). Oxytocin improves "mind-reading" in humans. *Biol Psychiatry*, 61(6):731–733.

71. Drago, F., Pedersen, C.A., Caldwell, J.D., and Prange, A.J., Jr (1986). Oxytocin potently enhances novelty-induced grooming behavior in the rat. *Brain Res*, 368(2):287–295.

72. Insel, T.R. and Winslow, J.T. (1991). Central administration of oxytocin modulates the infant rat's response to social isolation. *Eur J Pharmacol*, 203(1):149–152.

73. Meisenberg, G. and Simmons, W.H. (1983). Centrally mediated effects of neurohypophyseal hormones. *Neurosci Biobehav Rev*, 7(2):263–280.

74. Nelson, E. and Alberts, J.R. (1997). Oxytocin-induced paw sucking in infant rats. *Ann N Y Acad Sci*, 807:543–545.

75. Van Wimersma Greidanus, T.B., Kroodsma, J.M., Pot, M.L., Stevens, M., and Maigret, C. (1990). Neurohypophyseal hormones and excessive grooming behaviour. *Eur J Pharmacol*, 187(1):1–8.

76. Panksepp, J. (1992). Oxytocin effects on emotional processes: Separation distress, social bonding, and relationships to psychiatric disorders. *Ann N Y Acad Sci*, 652:243–252.

77. Insel, T.R., O'Brien, D.J., and Leckman, J.F. (1999). Oxytocin, vasopressin, and autism: Is there a connection? *Biol Psychiatry*, 45(2):145–157.

78. Lim, M.M., Bielsky, I.F., and Young, L.J. (2005 Apr-). Neuropeptides and the social brain: Potential rodent models of autism. *Int J Dev Neurosci*, 23(2-3):235–243.

79. McCarthy, M.M. and Altemus, M. (1997). Central nervous system actions of oxytocin and modulation of behavior in humans. *Mol Med Today*, 3(6):269–275.

80. Modahl, C., Fein, D., Waterhouse, L., and Newton, N. (1992). Does oxytocin deficiency mediate social deficits in autism? *J Autism Dev Disord*, 22(3):449–451.

81. Waterhouse, L., Fein, D., and Modahl, C. (1996). Neurofunctional mechanisms in autism. *Psychol Rev*, 103(3):457–489.

82. Hollander, E., Novotny, S., Hanratty, M., Yaffe, R., DeCaria, C.M., Aronowitz, B.R. *et al.* (2003). Oxytocin infusion reduces repetitive behaviors in adults with autistic and Asperger's disorders. *Neuropsychopharmacology*, 28(1):193–198.

83. Bartz, J.A. and Hollander, E. (2006). The neuroscience of affiliation: Forging links between basic and clinical research on neuropeptides and social behavior. *Horm Behav*, 50(4):518–528.

84. Hollander, E., Bartz, J., Chaplin, W., Phillips, A., Sumner, J., Soorya, L. *et al.* (2007). Oxytocin increases retention of social cognition in autism. *Biol Psychiatry*, 61(4):498–503.

85. Redcay, E. and Courchesne, E. (2005). When is the brain enlarged in autism? A meta-analysis of all brain size reports. *Biol Psychiatry*, 58(1):1–9.

86. Courchesne, E., Karns, C.M., Davis, H.R., Ziccardi, R., Carper, R.A., Tigue, Z.D. *et al.* (2001). Unusual brain growth patterns in early life in patients with autistic disorder: An MRI study. *Neurology*, 57(2):245–254.

87. Kaufmann, W.E., Cooper, K.L., Mostofsky, S.H., Capone, G.T., Kates, W.R., Newschaffer, C.J. *et al.* (2003). Specificity of cerebellar vermian abnormalities in autism: A quantitative magnetic resonance imaging study. *J Child Neurol*, 18(7):463–470.

88. Bailey, A., Luthert, P., Dean, A., Harding, B., Janota, I., Montgomery, M. *et al.* (1998). A clinicopathological study of autism. *Brain*, 121(Pt 5):889–905.

89. Bauman, M.L. and Kemper, T.L. (2005). Neuroanatomic observations of the brain in autism: A review and future directions. *Int J Dev Neurosci*, 23(2-3):183-187.

90. Baron-Cohen, S., Ring, H.A., Wheelwright, S., Bullmore, E.T., Brammer, M.J., Simmons, A. *et al.* (1999). Social intelligence in the normal and autistic brain: An fMRI study. *Eur J Neurosci*, 11(6):1891-1898.

91. Critchley, H.D., Daly, E.M., Bullmore, E.T., Williams, S.C., Van Amelsvoort, T., Robertson, D. M. *et al.* (2000). The functional neuroanatomy of social behaviour: Changes in cerebral blood flow when people with autistic disorder process facial expressions. *Brain*, 123(Pt 11):2203-2212.

92. Bailey, A., Le Couteur, A., Gottesman, I., Bolton, P., Simonoff, E., Yuzda, E. *et al.* (1995). Autism as a strongly genetic disorder: Evidence from a British twin study. *Psychol Med*, 25(1):63-77.

93. Yang, M.S. and Gill, M. (2007). A review of gene linkage, association and expression studies in autism and an assessment of convergent evidence. *Int J Dev Neurosci*, 25(2):69-85.

94. Varoqueaux, F., Aramuni, G., Rawson, R.L., Mohrmann, R., Missler, M., Gottmann, K. *et al.* (2006). Neuroligins determine synapse maturation and function. *Neuron*, 51(6):741-754.

95. Jamain, S., Quach, H., Betancur, C., Rastam, M., Colineaux, C., Gillberg, I.C. *et al.* (2003). Mutations of the X-linked genes encoding neuroligins NLGN3 and NLGN4 are associated with autism. *Nat Genet*, 34(1):27-29.

96. Bear, M.F., Huber, K.M., and Warren, S.T. (2004). The mGluR theory of fragile X mental retardation. *Trends Neurosci*, 27(7):370-377.

97. Blasi, F., Bacchelli, E., Pesaresi, G., Carone, S., Bailey, A.J., and Maestrini, E. (2006). Absence of coding mutations in the X-linked genes neuroligin 3 and neuroligin 4 in individuals with autism from the IMGSAC collection. *Am J Med Genet B Neuropsychiatr Genet*, 141(3):220-221.

98. Gauthier, J., Bonnel, A., St-Onge, J., Karemera, L., Laurent, S., Mottron, L. *et al.* (2005). NLGN3/NLGN4 gene mutations are not responsible for autism in the Quebec population. *Am J Med Genet B Neuropsychiatr Genet*, 132(1):74-75.

99. Amir, R.E., Van den Veyver, I.B., Wan, M., Tran, C.Q., Francke, U., and Zoghbi, H.Y. (1999). Rett syndrome is caused by mutations in X-linked MECP2, encoding methyl-CpG-binding protein 2. *Nat Genet*, 23(2):185-188.

100. O'Donnell, W.T. and Warren, S.T. (2002). A decade of molecular studies of fragile X syndrome. *Annu Rev Neurosci*, 25:315-338.

101. Moy, S.S., Nadler, J.J., Magnuson, T.R., and Crawley, J.N. (2006). Mouse models of autism spectrum disorders: The challenge for behavioral genetics. *Am J Med Genet C Semin Med Genet*, 142(1):40-51.

102. Moy, S.S., Nadler, J.J., Young, N.B., Perez, A., Holloway, L.P., Barbaro, R.P. *et al.* (2007). Mouse behavioral tasks relevant to autism: Phenotypes of 10 inbred strains. *Behav Brain Res*, 176(1):4-20.

103. Ferguson, J.N., Young, L.J., Hearn, E.F., Insel, T.R., and Winslow, J.T. (2000). Social amnesia in mice lacking the oxytocin gene. *Nat Genet*, 25:284-288.

104. Vanderschuren, L.J., Niesink, R.J., and Van Ree, J.M. (1997). The neurobiology of social play behavior in rats. *Neurosci Biobehav Rev*, 21(3):309-326.

105. Panksepp, J. (1981). The ontogeny of play in rats. *Dev Psychobiol*, 14(4):327-332.

106. Vanderschuren, L.J., Spruijt, B.M., Hol, T., Niesink, R.J., and Van Ree, J.M. (1995). Sequential analysis of social play behavior in juvenile rats: Effects of morphine. *Behav Brain Res*, 72(1-2):89-95.

107. Wolterink, G., Daenen, L.E., Dubbeldam, S., Gerrits, M.A., van Rijn, R., Kruse, C.G. *et al.* (2001). Early amygdala damage in the rat as a model for neurodevelopmental psychopathological disorders. *Eur Neuropsychopharmacol*, 11(1):51-59.

108. Pletnikov, M.V., Moran, T.H., and Carbone, K.M. (2002). Borna disease virus infection of the neonatal rat: Developmental brain injury model of autism spectrum disorders. *Front Biosci*, 7:d593–d607.

109. Lancaster, K., Dietz, D.M., Moran, T.H., and Pletnikov, M.V. (2007). Abnormal social behaviors in young and adult rats neonatally infected with Borna disease virus. *Behav Brain Res*, 176(1):141–148.

110. Ciaranello, A.L. and Ciaranello, R.D. (1995). The neurobiology of infantile autism. *Annu Rev Neurosci*, 18:101–128.

111. Moles, A., Kieffer, B.L., and D'Amato, F.R. (2004). Deficit in attachment behavior in mice lacking the mu-opioid receptor gene. *Science*, 304(5679):1983–1986.

112. Winslow, J.T., Hearn, E.F., Ferguson, J., Young, L.J., Matzuk, M.M., and Insel, T.R. (2000). Infant vocalization, adult aggression, and fear behavior of an oxytocin null mutant mouse. *Horm Behav*, 37:145–155.

113. Kahne, D., Tudorica, A., Borella, A., Shapiro, L., Johnstone, F., Huang, W. et al. (2002). Behavioral and magnetic resonance spectroscopic studies in the rat hyperserotonemic model of autism. *Physiol Behav*, 75(3):403–410.

114. Schneider, C.W. and Chenoweth, M.B. (1970). Effects of hallucinogenic and other drugs on the nest-building behaviour of mice. *Nature*, 225(5239):1262–1263.

115. Crawley, J.N. (2004). Designing mouse behavioral tasks relevant to autistic-like behaviors. *Ment Retard Dev Disabil Res Rev*, 10(4):248–258.

116. Deacon, R.M. (2006). Assessing nest building in mice. *Nat Protoc*, 1(3):1117–1119.

117. Ballard, T.M., Pauly-Evers, M., Higgins, G.A., Ouagazzal, A.M., Mutel, V., Borroni, E. et al. (2002). Severe impairment of NMDA receptor function in mice carrying targeted point mutations in the glycine binding site results in drug-resistant nonhabituating hyperactivity. *J Neurosci*, 22(15):6713–6723.

118. Keisala, T., Minasyan, A., Jarvelin, U., Wang, J., Hamalainen, T., Kalueff, A.V. et al. (2007). Aberrant nest building and prolactin secretion in vitamin D receptor mutant mice. *J Steroid Biochem Mol Biol*, 104(3–5):269–273.

119. Lijam, N., Paylor, R., McDonald, M.P., Crawley, J.N., Deng, C.X., Herrup, K. et al. (1997). Social interaction and sensorimotor gating abnormalities in mice lacking Dvl1. *Cell*, 90(5):895–905.

120. Arakawa, H., Blanchard, D.C., and Blanchard, R.J. (2007). Colony formation of C57BL/6J mice in visible burrow system: Identification of eusocial behaviors in a background strain for genetic animal models of autism. *Behav Brain Res*, 176(1):27–39.

121. Blanchard, D.C., Cholvanich, P., Blanchard, R.J., Clow, D.W., Hammer, R.P., Jr, Rowlett, J.K. et al. (1991). Serotonin, but not dopamine, metabolites are increased in selected brain regions of subordinate male rats in a colony environment. *Brain Res*, 568(1–2):61–66.

122. Blanchard, R.J., McKittrick, C.R., and Blanchard, D.C. (2001). Animal models of social stress: Effects on behavior and brain neurochemical systems. *Physiol Behav*, 73(3):261–271.

123. Blanchard, R.J., Fukunaga, K., Blanchard, D.C., and Kelley, M.J. (1975). Conspecific aggression in the laboratory rat. *J Comp Physiol Psychol*, 89(10):1204–1209.

124. Kareem, A.M. (1983). Effect of increasing periods of familiarity on social interactions between male sibling mice. *Anim Behav*, 31:919–926.

125. Mondragon, R., Mayagoitia, L., Lopez-Lujan, A., and Diaz, J.L. (1987). Social structure features in three inbred strains of mice, C57Bl/6J, Balb/cj, and NIH: A comparative study. *Behav Neural Biol*, 47(3):384–391.

126. Takayanagi, Y., Yoshida, M., Bielsky, I.F., Ross, H.R., Kawamata, M., Onaka, T. et al. (2006). Pervasive social deficits but normal parturition in oxytocin receptor-deficient mice. *Proc Natl Acad Sci USA*, 102:16096–16101.

127. Pedersen, C.A., Vadlamudi, S.V., Boccia, M.L., and Amico, J.A. (2006). Maternal behavior deficits in nulliparous oxytocin knockout mice. *Genes Brain Behav*, 5(3): 274–281.

128. Ferguson, J.N., Aldag, J.M., Insel, T.R., and Young, L.J. (2001). Oxytocin in the medial amygdala is essential for social recognition in the mouse. *J Neuroscience*, 21:8278–8285.

129. Lim, M.M. and Young, L.J. (2006). Neuropeptidergic regulation of affiliative behavior and social bonding in animals. *Horm Behav*, 50(4):506–517.

130. Young, L.J. and Wang, Z. (2004). The neurobiology of pair bonding. *Nat Neurosci*, 7(10):1048–1054.

131. Lim, M.M., Wang, Z., Olazábal, D.E., Ren, X., Terwilliger, E.F., and Young, L.J. (2004). Enhanced partner preference in promiscuous species by manipulating the expression of a single gene. *Nature*, 429:754–757.

132. Hammock, E.A.D. and Young, L.J. (2005). Microsatellite instability generates diversity in brain and sociobehavioral traits. *Science*, 308:1630–1634.

133. Kim, S., Young, L.J., Gonen, D., Veenstra-VanderWeele, J., Courchesne, R., Courchesne, E. *et al.* (2001). Transmission disequilibrium testing of arginine vasopressin receptor 1A (AVPR1A) polymorphisms in autism. *Mol Psychiatry*, 7:503–507.

134. Wassink, T.H., Piven, J., Vieland, V.J., Pietila, J., Goedken, R.J., Folstein, S.E., *et al.* (2004). Examination of AVPR1a as an autism susceptibility gene. *Mol Psychiat*, ePub.

135. Yirmiya, N., Rosenberg, C., Levi, S., Salomon, S., Shulman, C., Nemanov, L. *et al.* (2006). Association between the arginine vasopressin 1a receptor (AVPR1a) gene and autism in a family-based study: Mediation by socialization skills. *Mol Psychiatry*, 11(5):488–494.

136. Lai, C.S., Fisher, S.E., Hurst, J.A., Vargha-Khadem, F., and Monaco, A.P. (2001). A forkhead-domain gene is mutated in a severe speech and language disorder. *Nature*, 413(6855):519–523.

137. Haesler, S., Wada, K., Nshdejan, A., Morrisey, E.E., Lints, T., Jarvis, E.D. *et al.* (2004). FoxP2 expression in avian vocal learners and non-learners. *J Neurosci*, 24(13):3164–3175.

138. Teramitsu, I., Kudo, L.C., London, S.E., Geschwind, D.H., and White, S.A. (2004). Parallel FoxP1 and FoxP2 expression in songbird and human brain predicts functional interaction. *J Neurosci*, 24(13):3152–3163.

139. Shu, W., Cho, J.Y., Jiang, Y., Zhang, M., Weisz, D., Elder, G.A. *et al.* (2005). Altered ultrasonic vocalization in mice with a disruption in the Foxp2 gene. *Proc Natl Acad Sci USA*, 102(27):9643–9648.

140. Gauthier, J., Joober, R., Mottron, L., Laurent, S., Fuchs, M., De Kimpe, V. *et al.* (2003). Mutation screening of FOXP2 in individuals diagnosed with autistic disorder. *Am J Med Genet A*, 118(2):172–175.

141. Lewis, M.H., Tanimura, Y., Lee, L.W., and Bodfish, J.W. (2007). Animal models of restricted repetitive behavior in autism. *Behav Brain Res*, 176(1):66–74.

142. Benayed, R., Gharani, N., Rossman, I., Mancuso, V., Lazar, G., Kamdar, S. *et al.* (2005). Support for the homeobox transcription factor gene ENGRAILED 2 as an autism spectrum disorder susceptibility locus. *Am J Hum Genet*, 77(5):851–868.

143. Gharani, N., Benayed, R., Mancuso, V., Brzustowicz, L.M., and Millonig, J.H. (2004). Association of the homeobox transcription factor, ENGRAILED 2, 3, with autism spectrum disorder. *Mol Psychiatry*, 9(5):474–484.

144. Cheh, M.A., Millonig, J.H., Roselli, L.M., Ming, X., Jacobsen, E., Kamdar, S. *et al.* (2006). En2 knockout mice display neurobehavioral and neurochemical alterations relevant to autism spectrum disorder. *Brain Res*, 1116(1):166–176.

145. Chih, B., Afridi, S.K., Clark, L., and Scheiffele, P. (2004). Disorder-associated mutations lead to functional inactivation of neuroligins. *Hum Mol Genet*, 13(14):1471–1477.

146. Comoletti, D., De Jaco, A., Jennings, L.L., Flynn, R.E., Gaietta, G., Tsigelny, I. *et al.* (2004). The Arg451Cys-neuroligin-3 mutation associated with autism reveals a defect in protein processing. *J Neurosci*, 24(20):4889–4893.

147. Laumonnier, F., Bonnet-Brilhault, F., Gomot, M., Blanc, R., David, A., Moizard, M.P. *et al.* (2004). X-linked mental retardation and autism are associated with a mutation in the NLGN4 gene, a member of the neuroligin family. *Am J Hum Genet*, 74(3):552–557.

148. Szatmari, P., Paterson, A.D., Zwaigenbaum, L., Roberts, W., Brian, J., Liu, X.Q. *et al.* (2007). Mapping autism risk loci using genetic linkage and chromosomal rearrangements. *Nat Genet*, 39(3):319–328.

149. Penn, H.E. (2006). Neurobiological correlates of autism: A review of recent research. *Child Neuropsychol*, 12(1):57–79.

150. Kwon, C.H., Zhou, J., Li, Y., Kim, K.W., Hensley, L.L., Baker, S.J. *et al.* (2006). Neuron-specific enolase-cre mouse line with cre activity in specific neuronal populations. *Genesis*, 44(3):130–135.

151. Kwon, C.H., Luikart, B.W., Powell, C.M., Zhou, J., Matheny, S.A., Zhang, W. *et al.* (2006). Pten regulates neuronal arborization and social interaction in mice. *Neuron*, 50(3):377–388.

152. Kwon, C.H., Zhu, X., Zhang, J., Knoop, L.L., Tharp, R., Smeyne, R.J. *et al.* (2001). Pten regulates neuronal soma size: A mouse model of Lhermitte-Duclos disease. *Nat Genet*, 29(4):404–411.

153. Fombonne, E., Roge, B., Claverie, J., Courty, S., and Fremolle, J. (1999). Microcephaly and macrocephaly in autism. *J Autism Dev Disord*, 29(2):113–119.

154. Buxbaum, J.D., Cai, G., Chaste, P., Nygren, G., Goldsmith, J., Reichert, J. *et al.* (2007). Mutation screening of the PTEN gene in patients with autism spectrum disorders and macrocephaly. *Am J Med Genet B Neuropsychiatr Genet*, 144(4):484–491.

155. Mineur, Y.S., Huynh, L.X., and Crusio, W.E. (2006). Social behavior deficits in the Fmr1 mutant mouse. *Behav Brain Res*, 168(1):172–175.

156. Spencer, C.M., Alekseyenko, O., Serysheva, E., Yuva-Paylor, L.A., and Paylor, R. (2005). Altered anxiety-related and social behaviors in the Fmr1 knockout mouse model of fragile X syndrome. *Genes Brain Behav*, 4(7):420–430.

157. Hayashi, M.L., Rao, B.S., Seo, J.S., Choi, H.S., Dolan, B.M., Choi, S.Y. *et al.* (2007). Inhibition of p21-activated kinase rescues symptoms of fragile X syndrome in mice. *Proc Natl Acad Sci USA*, 104(27):11489–11494.

158. Belzung, C., Leman, S., Vourc'h, P., and Andres, C. (2005). Rodent models for autism: A critical review. *Drug Discov Today Dis Models*, 2(2):93–101.

159. Ventura, R., Pascucci, T., Catania, M.V., Musumeci, S.A., and Puglisi-Allegra, S. (2004). Object recognition impairment in Fmr1 knockout mice is reversed by amphetamine: Involvement of dopamine in the medial prefrontal cortex. *Behav Pharmacol*, 15(5–6):433–442.

160. Zoghbi, H.Y. (2005). MeCP2 dysfunction in humans and mice. *J Child Neurol*, 20(9):736–740.

161. Guy, J., Gan, J., Selfridge, J., Cobb, S., and Bird, A. (2007). Reversal of neurological defects in a mouse model of Rett syndrome. *Science*, 315(5815):1143–1147.

162. Klink, R., Boksa, P., and Joober, R. (2003). Pharmacogenomics and animal models of schizophrenia. *Drug Dev Res*, 60(2):95–103.

163. Crowley, J.J. and Lucki, I. (2005). Opportunities to discover genes regulating depression and antidepressant response from rodent behavioral genetics. *Curr Pharm Des*, 11(2):157–169.

164. Uys, J.D., Stein, D.J., and Daniels, W.M. (2006). Neuroproteomics: Relevance to anxiety disorders. *Curr Psychiatry Rep*, 8(4):286–290.

165. Jin, P. and Warren, S.T. (2000). Understanding the molecular basis of fragile X syndrome. *Hum Mol Genet*, 9(6):901–908.

166. Brown, V., Jin, P., Ceman, S., Darnell, J.C., O'Donnell, W.T., Tenenbaum, S.A. *et al.* (2001). Microarray identification of FMRP-associated brain mRNAs and altered mRNA translational profiles in fragile X syndrome. *Cell*, 107(4):477–487.

167. D'Agata, V., Warren, S.T., Zhao, W., Torre, E.R., Alkon, D.L., and Cavallaro, S. (2002). Gene expression profiles in a transgenic animal model of fragile X syndrome. *Neurobiol Dis*, 10(3):211–218.

168. de Ledesma, A.M., Desai, A.N., Bolivar, V.J., Symula, D.J., and Flaherty, L. (2006). Two new behavioral QTLs, Emo4 and Reb1, map to mouse Chromosome 1: Congenic strains and candidate gene identification studies. *Mamm Genome*, 17(2):111–118.

169. Irons, M., Elias, E.R., Salen, G., Tint, G.S., and Batta, A.K. (1993). Defective cholesterol biosynthesis in Smith-Lemli-Opitz syndrome. *Lancet*, 341(8857):1414.

170. Sikora, D.M., Pettit-Kekel, K., Penfield, J., Merkens, L.S., and Steiner, R.D. (2006). The near universal presence of autism spectrum disorders in children with Smith-Lemli-Opitz syndrome. *Am J Med Genet A*, 140(14):1511–1518.

171. Waage-Baudet, H., Lauder, J.M., Dehart, D.B., Kluckman, K., Hiller, S., Tint, G.S. *et al.* (2003). Abnormal serotonergic development in a mouse model for the Smith-Lemli-Opitz syndrome: Implications for autism. *Int J Dev Neurosci*, 21(8):451–459.

172. Waage-Baudet, H., Dunty, W.C., Jr, Dehart, D.B., Hiller, S., and Sulik, K.K. (2005). Immunohistochemical and microarray analyses of a mouse model for the smith-lemli-opitz syndrome. *Dev Neurosci*, 27(6):378–396.

173. Colburn, W.A. (2003). Biomarkers in drug discovery and development: From target identification through drug marketing. *J Clin Pharmacol*, 43(4):329–341.

174. Kromer, S.A., Kessler, M.S., Milfay, D., Birg, I.N., Bunck, M., Czibere, L. *et al.* (2005). Identification of glyoxalase-I as a protein marker in a mouse model of extremes in trait anxiety. *J Neurosci*, 25(17):4375–4384.

175. Brodkin, E.S. (2007). BALB/c mice: Low sociability and other phenotypes that may be relevant to autism. *Behav Brain Res*, 176(1):53–65.

176. Kosfeld, M., Heinrichs, M., Zak, P.J., Fischbacher, U., and Fehr, E. (2005). Oxytocin increases trust in humans. *Nature*, 435:673–676.

177. Modahl, C., Green, L., Fein, D., Morris, M., Waterhouse, L., Feinstein, C. *et al.* (1998). Plasma oxytocin levels in autistic children. *Biol Psychiatry*, 43(4):270–277.

178. Jansen, L.M., Gispen-de Wied, C.C., Wiegant, V.M., Westenberg, H.G., Lahuis, B.E., and van Engeland, H. (2006). Autonomic and neuroendocrine responses to a psychosocial stressor in adults with autistic spectrum disorder. *J Autism Dev Disord*, 36(7):891–899.

179. Ylisaukko-oja, T., Alarcon, M., Cantor, R.M., Auranen, M., Vanhala, R., Kempas, E. *et al.* (2006). Search for autism loci by combined analysis of Autism Genetic Resource Exchange and Finnish families. *Ann Neurol*, 59(1):145–155.

180. Wu, S., Jia, M., Ruan, Y., Liu, J., Guo, Y., Shuang, M. *et al.* (2005). Positive association of the oxytocin receptor gene (OXTR) with autism in the Chinese Han population. *Biol Psychiatry*, 58(1):74–77.

181. Jacob, S., Brune, C.W., Carter, C.S., Leventhal, B.L., Lord, C., and Cook, E.H., Jr (2007). Association of the oxytocin receptor gene (OXTR) in Caucasian children and adolescents with autism. *Neurosci Lett*, 417(1):6–9.

182. Sebat, J., Lakshmi, B., Malhotra, D., Troge, J., Lese-Martin, C., Walsh, T. *et al.* (2007). Strong association of de novo copy number mutations with autism. *Science*, 316(5823): 445–449.

183. Popik, P., Vetulani, J., and van Ree, J.M. (1992). Low doses of oxytocin facilitate social recognition in rats. *Psychopharmacology (Berl)*, 106(1):71–74.

184. Ferguson, J.N., Aldag, J.M., Insel, T.R., and Young, L.J. (2001). Oxytocin in the medial amygdala is essential for social recognition in the mouse. *J Neurosci*, 21(20):8278–8285.

185. Born, J., Lange, T., Kern, W., McGregor, G.P., Bickel, U., and Fehm, H.L. (2002). Sniffing neuropeptides: A transnasal approach to the human brain. *Nat Neurosci*, 5(6):514–516.

186. Bartz, J., Anagnostou, E., Fan, J., and Hollander, E. (2006). Oxytocin and experimental therapeutics in autism spectrum disorders. *Neuropsychopharmacology*, 31:S1–S9.

187. Pangalos, M.N., Schechter, L.E., and Hurko, O. (2007). Drug development for CNS disorders: Strategies for balancing risk and reducing attrition. *Nat Rev Drug Discov*, 6(7):521–532.

188. Howlin, P. (2003). Outcome in high-functioning adults with autism with and without early language delays: Implications for the differentiation between autism and Asperger syndrome. *J Autism Dev Disord*, 33(1):3–13.

189. Ganz, M.L. (2006). The Costs of Autism. In Moldin, S.O. and Rubenstein, J.L.R. (eds.), *Understanding Autism: From Basic Neuroscience to Treatment*. CRC Press: New York, NY, pp. 475–498.

190. Chez, M.G., Burton, Q., Dowling, T., Chang, M., Khanna, P., and Kramer, C. (2007). Memantine as adjunctive therapy in children diagnosed with autistic spectrum disorders: an observation of initial clinical response and maintenance tolerability. *J Child Neurol*, 22(5):574–579.

191. Niederhofer, H. (2007). Glutamate antagonists seem to be slightly effective in psychopharmacologic treatment of autism. *J Clin Psychopharmacol*, 27(3):317–318.

192. Erickson, C.A., Posey, D.J., Stigler, K.A., Mullett, J., Katschke, A.R., and McDougle, C.J. (2007). A retrospective study of memantine in children and adolescents with pervasive developmental disorders. *Psychopharmacology (Berl)*, 191(1):141–147.

Translational Models of Sleep and Sleep Disorders

Scott M. Doran[1], Thomas Wessel[2], Thomas S. Kilduff[3], Fred Turek[4] and John J. Renger[1]

[1]Merck Research Laboratories, West Point, PA 19486, USA
[2]Sepracor, 84 Waterford Drive, 3-North, Marlborough, MA 01752, USA
[3]SRI International, Biosciences Division, 333 Ravenswood Avenue, Menlo Park, CA 94025, USA
[4]Center for Sleep and Circadian Biology, Northwestern University, Evanston, IL 60208, USA

Animal and Translational Models for CNS Drug Discovery,
Vol. 1 of 3: Psychiatric Disorders
Robert McArthur and Franco Borsini (eds), Academic Press, 2008

INTRODUCTION

Sleep disorders are an international health concern and pose elevated risk factors for the development of other medical and psychiatric disorders including depression, obesity, and cardiovascular disease. The American Sleep Disorders Association Diagnostic Steering Committee has identified 89 classifiable sleep and circadian disorders, including those resulting from primary psychiatric disorders.[1] Sleep disorders have enormous socioeconomic impact based on the combined cost of the three most prevalent sleep disorders: insomnia, sleep-related breathing disorders, and excessive daytime sleepiness (EDS).[2] In the United States, for example, sleep problems extract about USD 15 billion a year in direct medical costs from the economy, and potentially another USD 150 billion yearly has been estimated in lost productivity.[3] These figures may be an underestimate as sleep disorders are under-diagnosed and under-treated.

In the general population, at least 30% complain of sleep difficulties and around 10% suffer daytime consequences. Insomnia, for example, has an estimated prevalence between 9% and 50% in the general adult population in Europe and the United States, depending on the insomnia definition used in different studies.[4] The 1-year prevalence estimates of insomnia symptoms vary according to the survey, with rates of 10–40% reported in the general population and rates as high as 66% in primary care and psychiatric settings.[5-9]

The costs associated with sleep disorders are difficult to estimate because of the frequent comorbidities (see below). Nevertheless, using insomnia as an example, there are substantial direct (e.g., medical care or self-treatment) and indirect (e.g., loss of productivity) costs associated with this sleep disorder. Insomnia-related morbidity and mortality, and property damage resulting from accidents make sleep disorders a significant public health issue.[3,10-14] The increased number of medical consultations, medication use, number of medical tests performed, number of hospitalization days, and emergency visits calculated in population-based studies[15,16] contribute to approximately USD 14 billion direct costs associated with insomnia in the United States.[4] However, indirect costs are considerably higher, estimated to exceed USD 75 billion in 1994.[13] As evaluated in non-managerial personnel, the cost of absenteeism alone – which is significantly more prevalent in individuals with insomnia than in good sleepers[17] – has been estimated to be approximately USD 143 million per day or more than USD 57 billion per year.[4]

In view of the serious consequences of the condition, it is surprising that sleep disorders such as insomnia remain under-diagnosed and under-treated.[18,19] Although approximately half the patients in primary care have sleep difficulties, such problems are often not discussed with physicians and, thus, insomnia symptoms frequently go undetected by healthcare professionals (cf., Ref. 20). In two surveys, general practice physicians were unaware of severe insomnia in 60–64% of the cases,[8,21] and it appears that physicians were not aware of the high rate of psychopathology and substance abuse among these patients. Constraints on time for the office visit may contribute to the failure to discuss sleep problems, but the reasons for under-recognition of chronic insomnia and its under-treatment can be traced in part to inadequate knowledge of sleep medicine.[22] Health professionals also have concerns about the safety and efficacy of pharmacologic treatments for sleep disorders, due in part to the relatively small amount of information on long-term efficacy of treatments for insomnia, the effects on comorbid disorders, and the potential improvements in daytime functioning possible with appropriate treatment.

CLINICAL DESCRIPTION OF PREVALENT SLEEP DISORDERS
Insomnia

Insomnia is a heterogeneous disorder of reduced sleep quality, duration, or efficiency. Diagnostic criteria proposed in the DSM-IV[23] and in ICD-10[24] defines insomnia as a problem either initiating or maintaining sleep during the night or recurrent early morning awakenings. Insomnia is diagnosed for problems persisting for at least 1 month and leading to patient complaints of diminished sleep quality or non-restorative sleep. In addition, the DSM-IV requires patients to report daytime impairment or distress as a diagnostic criterion. Typical daytime consequences of insomnia include complaints of fatigue, decreased psychomotor performance, inattentiveness and memory impairment, or dysphoria. Additionally, patients with insomnia have greater work absenteeism, more visits to the healthcare system, and an increased incidence of developing depression.[5,25-27]

Individuals with insomnia have higher rates of medical illnesses than people without sleep problems, with 53% of adults with serious insomnia reporting two or more health problems[28] and more frequent use of medical services.[6] For example, one study in Italy found that insomniacs have significantly more medical encounters ($p < 0.0001$), more laboratory tests ($p < 0.0001$), and more prescriptions filled

($p < 0.0001$) than non-insomniacs.[29] Greater sleep disturbance severity is correlated with a worse outcome and increased pain severity among those patients who experience pain[30] and a worse outcome in a number of other medical illnesses, including increased risk of mortality among institutionalized elderly individuals, greater disability among stroke patients, and increased risk of mortality among patients with cardiovascular disease.[31,32]

Insomnia is often comorbid with other conditions, including psychiatric disorders, chronic medical conditions and drug or substance consumption/abuse.[i] Chronic medical conditions associated with insomnia include chronic pain syndromes, coronary heart disease, asthma, gastrointestinal disorders, vascular disorders, chronic fatigue, and endocrine and metabolic disorders.[33] Certain medications including stimulants, steroids, antihypertensives, or antidepressants have been reported to precipitate insomnia.[34] Comorbidity with psychiatric disorders is common, and it is estimated that 40% or more of the adults suffering from insomnia have a diagnosable psychiatric disorder.[6,35] Depression, generalized anxiety disorder, attention-deficit/hyperactivity disorder, and schizophrenia are all frequently comorbid with insomnia. One European epidemiological study documented the presence of significant insomnia in 71% of patients with dementia, 69% of depressive disorder, 61% of anxiety disorder, and 32% of alcoholism patients.[36] Overall, insomnia is thought to be more strongly associated with depression than with any other medical disorder in the primary care setting.[37] Insomnia may also be the presenting complaint when it is caused by an underlying sleep disorder such as sleep apnea, or by restless leg syndrome/periodic limb movements during sleep.

Sleep Apnea

Sleep apnea is known to interfere with optimal sleep and to cause next-day mental impairments and long-term physiologic sequelae.[38] Several risk factors contribute to sleep apnea including age, obesity, and narrowing of the upper airway, so a diagnosis of sleep apnea requires nocturnal respiratory and sleep monitoring. Sleep apnea manifests as obstructive or centrally mediated breathing cessation leading to repetitive arousals from sleep and cyclic episodes of hypoxia. Between 2% and 5% of adults suffer clinical sleep apnea on a regular basis,[38,39] although transient sleep apnea can occur following administration of alcohol or sedatives. Obstructive (but not central) sleep apnea originates from a simple mechanism: upper airway muscle relaxation blocks airflow to interfere with normal respiration during sleep. However, the long-term consequences of sleep apnea are not simple, because sleep apnea is known to impair cognition, mood, and daytime performance[40]; it correlates with heart

---

[i]Changes in sleep, mood, and cognition are common themes throughout this series. For further discussion, the reader is invited to see, among others, Millan, The discovery and development of pharmacotherapy for psychiatric disorders: a critical survey of animal and translational models, and perspectives for their improvement or Cryan *et al.*, Developing more efficacious antidepressant medications: Improving and aligning preclinical detection and clinical assessment tools in this volume, Merchant *et al.*, Animal models of Parkinson's Disease to aid drug discovery and development, in Volume 2, *Neurological Disorders*, or Little *et al.*, Pharmacotherapy of alcohol dependence: improving translation from the bench to the clinic, in Volume 3, *Reward Deficit Disorders*.

disease and hypertension,[41,42] and it affects blood glucose regulation and insulin resistance.[43-45]

Narcolepsy

Narcolepsy is an under-diagnosed, chronic neurological and heritable disorder that is characterized by a disturbance of sleep/wake state control, intermittent cataplexy, and rapid eye movement (REM) sleep intrusions into the day of otherwise healthy people. Patients can present with a confusing mix of symptoms in which sleep intrudes into wakefulness and vice versa. The classic tetrad of clinical features of daytime sleepiness, hypnagogic hallucinations, sleep paralysis, and cataplexy do not usually occur simultaneously at the onset of their disease,[46,47] but usually evolve as the disease manifests itself, most frequently during the second decade of life.[48] The diagnosis of narcolepsy should be considered even in patients with sleepiness alone, as only about one-third of patients will have all four of the classical symptoms. In an epidemiologic survey of closely to 19000 participants in five European countries (United Kingdom, Germany, Italy, Portugal, and Spain), narcolepsy was found to affect 47 individuals/100000 inhabitants.[49] While the etiology of narcolepsy remains elusive, subsequent neuroepidemiologic studies point to possible environmental exposures before the age of onset in genetically susceptible individuals (reviewed in Ref. 50).

Narcolepsy is related to the degeneration of hypocretin (orexin) neurons in the brain.[51,52] The reason for hypocretin cell loss is still unexplained.[53] Notwithstanding, the degree of hypocretin deficiency appears to parallel the severity of clinical symptoms in patients with narcolepsy and the decreased levels of hypocretin can be measured in the (cerebrospinal fluid) CSF patients with narcolepsy.[54] Mignot and colleagues, for example, report that humans with CSF orexin levels less than 110ng/L typically have severe narcolepsy with cataplexy.[55] Narcolepsy following diencephalic stroke is also associated with low orexin levels.[56] With one exception,[52] (humans with narcolepsy do not have not genetic abnormalities in the hypocretin system but narcolepsy is highly associated with specific human haplotypes of the HLA allele DQB1*0602.[57][ii] On the other hand, animals with genetic mutations in the hypocretin pathway manifest cataplexy, sleepiness, and sleep disruption.[60,61]

Excessive Daytime Sleepiness

Differential diagnosis of EDS covers a broad range of central nervous system (CNS) disorders, including obstructive sleep apnea (the major cause of daytime sleepiness, especially in males), insufficient sleep, residual effects from hypnotic agents, chronic fatigue syndrome, chronic demyelinating diseases, degenerative processes, or space-occupying lesions in the brain, such as hypothalamic tumors, and chronic toxic-metabolic encephalopathies.

[ii]Hypocretin/orexin pathophysiology is discussed in detail below because natural mutations in the hypocretin system offer a unique window into the genetics of sleep/wake control. Additionally, hypocretin and sleep control are now linked with metabolic disorders[58,59] helping to refine our understanding of the mechanisms by which hypothalamic control is maintained over multiple homeostatic systems.

SLEEP NEUROBIOLOGY

Understanding the neural control of sleep and wakefulness has largely paralleled the history of neuroscience discovery as a whole. As new tools and methodologies became available to research, sleep scientists have been quick to take advantage of those techniques and apply them to common, replicable experimental paradigms related to sleep. This section provides an overview of the classical techniques used to measure sleep, while subsequent sections of this chapter describe progress from relatively crude methods of brain transection and lesion studies to more complicated methods including gene cloning and the production of transgenic models. Approaches in this section are largely historical, illustrating insights, and principles that have emerged as research has progressed.

Sleep and its Measurement

Immobility and Posture

Observational studies were initially used to study sleep across species. A stereotypical sleep posture is a widely accepted criterion for identification of sleep or "sleep-like" states across organisms. Immobility in the shark, recumbence of the horse, stillness of the zebra fish, and drooped antennae of the honeybee reliably differentiate sleep from wake across diverse species.[62-65] As laboratory techniques improved and focused on the nuances of the immobility during sleep, the skeletal muscles were found to produce small bursts of motion during sleep. The use of electromyography (EMG) to measure muscle tone changes was introduced by Max[66] who reported that nocturnal patterns of hand and arm activity in deaf-mute patients were regular and occurred in cycles during sleep. These muscle cycles were rhythmic, mimicking the newly discovered cyclic nocturnal patterns of electroencephalographic (EEG) amplitude and frequency oscillations during sleep.[67,68] Both muscle and EEG cycles were immediately thought to reflect nocturnal information processing, because hand and arm movements are a primary means of communication for deaf-mute patients.

Cyclic patterns of physiologic activity during sleep challenged theories of sleep and wake as discontinuous, orthogonal mind-brain-body states. Instead, muscle tone, and later EEG, eye movements and body temperature were all found to exhibit gradual transitions both between and within states of arousal suggesting "curvilinear phases for both wakefulness and sleep."[69] The measurement of these curvilinear processes was extended not only to measurement of the EEG and EMG, but also to other circadian phenomena such as locomotion, temperature, and sleep-related eye movements.

Electroencephalogram

Richard Caton[70] initiated the recording of brain electrical activity by placing electrodes on the exposed cortex. In 1929, Hans Berger demonstrated that recording brain- (and not muscle-) derived electrical signals from the intact skull was possible.[71] Six years later, using scalp EEG electrodes, Loomis and his associates described cyclic patterns of amplitude fluctuations during sleep that were modifiable by external cues.[67,68] These descriptions of transient EEG waves during sleep included time-dependent rhythmical changes in frequency (e.g., alpha [8–12 Hz] and theta [4 Hz and

8 Hz] rhythms) that correlated with states of arousal and sleep and laid the foundation of the electrophysiological study of sleep.

Nocturnal cycles of increasing EEG amplitude (e.g., slow wave activity, SWA; for definitions of various physiologic terms used in sleep research, refer Table 12.1), reduced EEG frequency, and runs of transient waves were eventually examined in sufficient detail to suggest that sleep was not a unitary state.[72] Intermittent EEG patterns resembling those observed in awake, subjects were also observed during sleep when the subject was immobile and otherwise non-responsive. The combination of periodic electrooculogram (EOG) activity during sleep with total EMG immobility and EEG activation led to the description of REM sleep. Subsequently, other physiological features such as decreased body temperature and heart rate variability were described to characterize REM sleep more fully.[73,74] These physiological concomitants of sleep are found in nearly all mammals and their disruption may lead to sleep disorders such as the parasomnias.[75,76]

Sleep and wake patterns are identified or "scored" by visually or algorithmically evaluating changes in amplitude and frequency of concurrent scalp EEG, skeletal EMG, and orbital EOG signals, together referred to as polysomnographic (PSG) recordings. Sleep/wake "states" are assessed by classifying sections of these recordings (4 s, 10 s, or 30 s "epochs") as waking, slow wave sleep (SWS) or REM sleep by summing the relative contributions from fast, slow, and transiently expressed frequencies within these physiologic signals for each epoch. SWA is the canonical EEG feature of brain activity within sleep because SWA is easily extracted from EEG recordings using Fast Fourier transformation (FFT) analysis to quantify spectral "power."[77][iii]

Computerized analyses of spectral power within the EEG are used to quantify time- and space-coherent oscillating bands such that hours of EEG recordings (a complex, non-stationary signal) can be quickly parsed, averaged, and compared as a series of small series of values. How the EEG "responds" (in general) to drug effects, the nature of the recording environment, time spent awake, or circadian phase in humans and laboratory animals remains a challenging question because there are so many degrees of freedom in the EEG signal. SWA descriptions support a "two process model" of sleep regulation designed to explain timing and intensity of sleep across the circadian day.[78] According to the two-process model, the homeostatic sleep-related "Process S" is a physiologic phenomenon that interacts with the circadian system ("Process C") to time the daily occurrence of sleep and wakefulness.

Localization of Sleep/Wake Brain Regions

Early investigations of the neurobiology underlying sleep/wake processes were conducted in the 1930s when Bremer[79] demonstrated that brainstem transections at low medullary levels (encephale isolé) allowed cats to undergo normal sleep/wake cycles while transections at the junction of the pons and midbrain (cerveau isolé) produced

---

[iii] The use of EEG has and is being used as a translational research tool for drug discovery in many therapeutic indications aside from sleep. Please refer to Millan, The discovery and development of pharmacotherapy for psychiatric disorders: a critical survey of animal and translational models, and perspectives for their improvement, in this volume for a discussion of the use of EEG and other imaging techniques in psychiatric drug discovery.

Table 12.1 Definition of sleep-related terms used to describe the structure of sleep and its disorders

Terms/Synonyms	Definition	Physiologic source
Sleep structure Sleep architecture	The patterned recurrence of sleep/wake stages across a day or a sleep period. Sleep/wake and NREM/REM alternation cycles.	Interactions between the hypothalamus, cortex, and brainstem work to modify global neurotransmitter levels to change brain cell firing from an environmentally responsive mode to an internally generated tendency towards neuronal burst firing
Rapid eye movement (REM) Paradoxical sleep	Brief periods of sleep that include rapid eye movements, polkiothermy, and skeletal atonia	REM normally arises after periods of NREM sleep but not immediately after periods of wake. Brainstem mechanisms of unknown source shift global CNS neurotransmission from a largely monoaminergic state to a highly cholinergic state
Non-rapid eye movement (NREM) Sleep stages 1–4	Sleep not accompanied by rapid eye movements. Typically 75% of all sleep and occurring in cycles that culminate with REM sleep bouts	Arousal state of non-wake and non-REM sleep. Includes light and deep sleep. Appears to result from hyperpolarization of the thalamus by retraction of activating neurotransmission from the brainstem.
Slow wave activity (SWA) Delta activity Sleep stages 3 and 4 Slow wave sleep (SWS)	Low frequency (0.5–4 Hz) EEG waves	Slow oscillations in the cortex interacting with burst firing in the thalamus
Spectral power	Extracted value from Fast Fourier Transformation used to compare EEG amplitude and zero crossing duration	Extracellular ion flow around pyramidal cells in the cortex produce aligned magnetic dipoles that are detected by surface electrodes. Signals are recorded across time while spectral power eliminates time factor during data reduction
Sleep fragmentation Sleep disruption	Changes in arousal state from sleep to wake	Shifts in arousal state sufficient to change EEG and EMG signals towards wake-like signals.

chronically drowsy cats. Bremer concluded that the reduction in cerebral "tone" (i.e., the loss of wakefulness) following cerveau isolé resulted from interruption of ascending sensory inputs. This "passive deafferentation" theory of sleep as a default process predicted that sleep would occur during periods of decreasing environmental demand. In the late 1940s, Moruzzi and Magoun[80] specified the role of the ascending brainstem reticular activating system (ARAS) showing how electrical stimulation of the ARAS, even after severing ascending sensory pathways, produced desynchronized (wakeful) EEG signals in the cerebral cortex. These observations led to the concept that tonic activity in the reticular formation, rather than input from sensory pathways as Bremer proposed, was sufficient to produce an activated, wakeful cortex.

In the late 1950s, Batini *et al.* evolved the mid-pontine pretrigeminal preparation that transected the brainstem at the pontine level rostral to the trigeminal nerve. This animal was constantly awake (insomniac), leading to the conclusion that input from a sleep "center" in the lower brainstem had been interrupted by the transection.[81] These results led to the idea that sleep must be an active process with a "center" in the lower pons or medulla that inhibits a wakefulness "center" in the rostral pons. Although these results were transformative for the field of sleep research, Hess had proposed the concept that sleep was an active state of the brain requiring activation of a sleep "center" in the 1920s.[82] In any case, 50 years later, the localization of the sleep "center" in the lower brainstem remains unknown, although "sleep active" neurons have been reported in the nucleus tractus solitarius.[83]

After World War I, a worldwide influenza epidemic occurred from which an estimated 25–40 million fatalities resulted. One variant of this disease caused chronic insomnia in patients from whom post-mortem brain studies revealed extensive cell loss in the anterior hypothalamus and the adjacent basal forebrain (BF). Based on observations of these patients, von Economo suggested the existence of distinct centers in the brain regulating wakefulness and sleep with the posterior hypothalamus proposed to maintain wakefulness while the anterior hypothalamic/BF region was important for sleep induction.[84] Subsequently, Nauta demonstrated that lesions of the anterior hypothalamus severely disrupted sleep and wakefulness,[85] providing direct experimental evidence for this region as involved in the regulation of sleep. In the 1960s, Sterman, McGinty and others found that lesions of the pre-optic/BF region resulted in a decrease of sleep,[86] whereas stimulation of the median pre-optic hypothalamus facilitated sleep onset with a very short latency.[87] It should be noted that the pre-optic/BF region also plays an important role in the regulation of several autonomic functions, particularly body temperature regulation, and that ambient temperature strongly influences sleep.

Results from both diencephalic and brainstem studies supported these regions as critical for sleep expression. Lesion studies specific to the posterior lateral hypothalamus (PLH) were found to increase sleep in rats,[85] cats,[88] and in monkeys.[89] Despite these intriguing results, little attention was focused on the posterior hypothalamus until it was recognized the histaminergic (HA) cells were exclusive to this region, specifically found in the tuberomammillary nuclei (TMN).[90] Antihistamines are known soporifics and HA-containing TMN cell bodies project to the cortex. Injections of the $GABA_A$ receptor agonist muscimol into the posterior hypothalamus-induced long-lasting hypersomnia and suppressed REM sleep whereas injections directed toward the ventral posterolateral hypothalamus increased both non-REM (NREM) and REM sleep.[91] Such effects contrasted sharply with injections into the pre-optic and anterior hypothalamus that resulted in insomnia. The suprachiasmatic nuclei (SCN), an important circadian cell group in the rostral hypothalamus, does not seem to play a direct role in the regulation of sleep amounts, but sleep/wake rhythms are disrupted by bilateral SCN lesions.[92,93] SCN lesions flatten the expression distribution of sleep and wakefulness across the 24h period,[94-96] lending support to the hypothesis that posterior hypothalamus neurons maintain wake while sleep results from functional blockade of a posterior hypothalamic waking center.

The Hypocretin/Orexin System

Although the role of the hypocretins as signaling peptides was formally described early in 1998,[97,98] localization of the cell bodies expressing the hypocretin (Hcrt) peptides and descriptions of their efferent projections was first reported at the 1997 *Society for Neuroscience* meeting.[99,100] Cell bodies expressing this gene were restricted to an area of the hypothalamus centered around the perifornical nucleus (PFH). The Hcrt peptides were found to bind to cell lines expressing orphan G-protein-coupled receptors.[98] Hcrt neurons are restricted to the tuberal region of the hypothalamus, specifically, the PFH and the dorsal and lateral hypothalamus. Hcrt projection neurons widely distribute in the brain[101-105] and spinal cord[106] with densest extra-hypothalamic projections to the locus coeruleus (LC).[101,107,108] Other projection sites include the cerebral cortex, olfactory bulb, hippocampus, amygdala, septum, diagonal band of Broca (DBB), bed nucleus of the stria terminalis, thalamus, midbrain, brainstem, and spinal cord.

Afferent control of the Hcrt neurons is of great interest and two noteworthy articles[109,110] have contributed the majority of our knowledge on this aspect to date. Sakurai and collaborators[109] created a transgenic mouse with enhanced green fluorescent protein (EGFP) and described afferents from the amygdala, BF cholinergic neurons, GABAergic neurons in the pre-optic area (POA), and serotonergic neurons in the median/paramedian raphé nuclei. Surprisingly, although cholinergic neurons in the BF had reciprocal connections with Hcrt cells, the monoamine-containing groups that are innervated by the Hcrt neurons did not.

The Hcrt peptides have uniformly been reported as excitatory by either eliciting depolarization and/or increased spike frequency in many regions and cell types within the CNS. Of particular interest are findings that Hcrt directly excites cellular systems involved in waking and arousal. An excitatory effect of Hcrt has been reported in the LC,[107,108,111] the dorsal raphé nucleus DRN,[112,113] the TMN,[114-116] the lateral dorsal tegmentum (LDT),[117,118] the cholinergic BF,[119] and both dopaminergic (DA) and non-DA neurons in the ventral tegmentum area (VTA),[120,121] among many other regions.

Widespread Hcrt projections suggest the Hcrt system subserves multiple physiologic functions. In addition to feeding regulation, the Hcrt system has been implicated in neuroendocrine,[122-126] cardiovascular,[127,128] water balance,[129] and gastrointestinal[130] control.

Two landmark articles[131,132] indicated that dysfunction of the Hcrt system can result in the sleep disorder narcolepsy. Narcolepsy is characterized by EDS, episodes of muscle weakness (cataplexy) triggered by emotional stimulation, and abnormalities of REM sleep. A genetic component of this disorder has been established in both humans and dogs. In narcoleptic dogs, the canarc-1 gene, transmitted in Doberman pinschers and Labrador retrievers as an autosomal recessive trait with full penetrance, was identified as a deletion mutation in the hcrtr2 gene, resulting in a truncated, non-functional protein.[131,132] In a remarkable convergence, Hcrt null mutant mice were found to exhibit periods of "behavioral arrest" that strongly resemble the cataplectic attacks and sleep onset REM periods characteristic of narcolepsy.[131] These mice also have altered sleep architecture with increased REM and NREM sleep, short-latency REM periods, and decreased sleep bout lengths, primarily during the dark (active) period (for further discussion regarding sleep architecture see below).

Since publication of these articles, several other animal models of narcolepsy have been produced. In Hcrt/ataxin-3 mice, Hcrt cells begin to degenerate within 4 weeks after birth to produce a phenotype strikingly similar to human narcolepsy including behavioral arrests, premature entry into REM sleep, poorly consolidated sleep patterns, and late-onset obesity.[133] A rat model of Hcrt cell degeneration has been produced by conjugating the Hcrt2 peptide to the ribosome-inactivating protein saporin and injection of the conjugate into the PLH.[134] These rats have increased SWS (particularly in the dark phase of an light-dark [LD] cycle), REM sleep, and sleep onset REM sleep periods.[134,135] Hcrtr2 null mutant mice have a syndrome distinct from Hcrt null mutant mice,[136] implying a greater role for Hcrtr1 in narcolepsy than previously appreciated. Since narcolepsy is characterized by both EDS and abnormal REM sleep, dysfunction of the Hcrt system in narcoleptic dogs, mice, and humans suggests that this system plays an important role in both waking and REM sleep regulation.

We (TK) proposed a model (illustrated in Figure 12.1) whereby Hcrt cells are involved in both normal arousal state control and the EDS of narcolepsy.[137] During waking, Hcrt cells might promote arousal through excitation of "wake-active" monoaminergic populations in the TMN, LC, and DRN. Hcrt cells could also promote EEG desynchronization via excitatory inputs onto cholinergic cell groups of the BF and the pons (LdT, PPT). During NREM sleep, reduced Hcrt cell activity, perhaps due to release of GABA[138] from the POA,[139] would decrease excitation to monoaminergic and cholinergic groups thereby facilitating cortical synchronization. During REM sleep, excitatory input from Hcrt cells onto cholinergic cells would facilitate cortical desynchronization, but excitatory effects onto the monoaminergic cell groups might be blocked by presynaptic inhibition,[140] since GABA levels are high in both the LC[141] and DRN[138] during REM. Absence of excitatory input from Hcrt cells could result in net excitation of "REM on" groups in the LdT and PPT through disinhibition. The suggestion that Hcrt cells activated "Wake on/REM on" brain areas was controversial but was initially supported by observations of increased Hcrt1 release during REM.[142] An alternative hypothesis proposed that activity of the Hcrt system was not related to wakefulness *per se* but was related, more specifically, to activation of the somatomotor system.[143] Indeed, subsequent studies characterized the discharge pattern of presumptive Hcrt

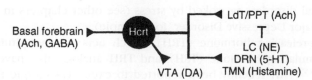

Figure 12.1   Model illustrating major connections from the Hcrt cells to some of the brain regions implicated in arousal state control. See Kilduff and Peyron[137] for full explanation of model

cells as highest during wakefulness, particularly active wakefulness involving exploratory behavior[144,145] but silent during REM sleep.

Other Neurochemicals Involved in Sleep/Wake Control

The emphasis in the foregoing sections has been on "systems neurobiology," that is, the role of defined and localized neurotransmitter systems and their putative roles in sleep/wake control. While such a neural systems description has produce fundamental insights into the control of sleep and wakefulness, an equally impressive literature exists on sleep substances and their contributions to behavioral state control. Fortunately, the "sparks vs. soup" approaches are highly complementary research strategies and valuable insights to sleep/wake expression will arise from both approaches. In fact, the most provocative and potentially fruitful areas are likely to result from the interaction between these two approaches, as illustrated below in the cases of adenosine and Prostaglandin D_2.

A number of lymphokines (e.g., interleukin-1, tumor necrosis factor alpha), inflammatory molecules, and growth factors have been shown to promote NREM sleep and have been the subject of many excellent reviews.[146,147] Since these molecules are not stored intracellularly, or solely released by neurons, they are generally not considered neurotransmitters *per se* but clearly have biological activity in the CNS. Specific immune molecules, such as interleukin-6, promote NREM sleep and are elevated in sleep disorders with EDS as a symptom. Although it is likely that alterations in sleep during infection are mediated by immune molecules, the extent to which such mechanisms play a role in the regulation of "normal" sleep and wakefulness remains uncertain.

Similarly, a number of peptides have been implicated in sleep/wake control but, since most neuropeptides do not cross the blood-brain barrier, peptidergic control of sleep/wake has only been tested in animals. Peptides associated with activation of the hypothalamo-pituitary adrenal (HPA) axis that have been reported to have wake-promoting activity include corticotrophin-releasing factor (CRF)[148,149] and adrenocorticotropic hormone (ACTH)[150]; an effect that is not surprising given the nature of stress on behavior when the HPA axis is involved. As indicated above, hypocretin/orexin also has wake-promoting activity,[108,151] and we recently suggested an alerting component of the stress response might be mediated by CRF activation of CRF receptor-1 on Hcrt cells.[152] In contrast to the wake-promoting activity of ACTH, another pro-opiomelanocortin (POMC)-derived peptide, α-melanocyte stimulating hormone (α-MSH), has a sleep-promoting effect as does corticotropin-like intermediate lobe peptide (CLIP).[153] Hypothalamic protein signaling leading to wake promotion via stress responses is consistent with other models that link sleep pattern changes with a variety of behavioral disorders provoked by stress (see other chapters in this volume on "Anxiety and Major Depressive Disorder" for example).

Thyrotropin-releasing hormone (TRH), which acts on the pituitary to release thyrotropin-stimulating hormone (TSH), and TRH analogs also have wake-promoting activity.[154,155] TRH recently been reported to excite GABAergic thalamic perigeniculate and thalamocortical neurons,[156] suggesting that TRH is an intrinsic regulator of thalamocortical network activity related to EEG desynchronization. However, in a clinical study,[157] TRH exerted a "weak" effect on the sleep EEG as evidenced by a slight decrease in sleep efficiency and a trend toward wakefulness during the night. The authors suggested that TRH may contribute to the sleep disturbance seen in depressed patients.

Neuropeptide Y (NPY) has long been known to be a potent inducer of feeding when administered intracerebroventricularly (ICV). Effects of NPY on sleep in rodents have been somewhat contradictory, perhaps due to the different times of day various studies were conducted. An early study relied on qualitative (visual) EEG assessment in three strains of rats to report (depending on the rat strain used) either (1) behavioral signs of sedation but a reduction of synchronized EEG activity, (2) increased synchronized EEG activity, or (3) increased EEG desynchronization-indicating an awakening effect of the peptide.[158] High doses of NPY administered during the day have been reported to have little effect on sleep onset latency or NREM sleep quantity but reduced spectral power across all EEG frequencies.[159] More recently, both ICV and lateral hypothalamic injections of NPY administered early in the wake period transiently suppressed NREM and REM sleep during the first hour after the injection (corresponding to the period when food intake is increased) while inducing changes in EEG SWA.[160] In humans, intravenous NPY has been reported to reduce sleep latency in young men,[161] older men, and older women.[162]

Melatonin is produced by the pineal gland during the night in both diurnal and nocturnal species. Specific receptors for melatonin are found in the cortex, SCN, and hypothalamic regions involved in thermoregulation. Exogenous melatonin is a popular hypnotic available in both physiological (0.03 mg) and pharmacological (1–10 mg) doses. Physiologic doses can help in sleep onset processes when sleep initiation is attempted at abnormal times such as occurs following travel across time zones,[163,164] especially when combined with appropriately timed light exposure.[165,166] Melatonin helps synchronize circadian rhythms in totally blind individuals.[167]

Melanin-concentrating hormone (MCH) is a peptide that is coextensive, but not co-localized, with the Hcrt neuronal population and MCH has profound effects on both SWS and REM sleep, in particular when administered ICV.[168] Additionally, the Fos protein is expressed in MCH neurons during recovery from REM sleep deprivation.[168,169] Other peptides with REM-promoting activity include prolactin,[170,171] vasoactive intestinal polypeptide (VIP)[171,172] and pituitary adenylate cyclase activating polypeptide (PACAP).[171-175] Both peripheral[176] and ICV[177] infusion of insulin increases SWS in rats. These effects could be related to postprandial sleepiness. Insulin also stimulates insulin-like growth factor-1 (IGF-1) receptors, although the molar doses of IGF-1 needed to promote sleep are much lower than that of insulin.[178]

Several of the peptides described above (MCH, insulin, melatonin) also influence feeding patterns. The link between feeding and sleep includes descriptions of putative increases in wakefulness during periods when food is available, if the food source of interest is only transiently available (see Ref. 179 for a review). Whether food-seeking and sleep interact via sleep or circadian rhythm signals remains a matter of study. Conversely, metabolic alterations, in the form of insufficient or excessive feeding, are also known to alter normal sleep patterns to produce interesting animal models to explore the link between sleep and metabolism.

Sleep Homeostasis and the Timing of Sleep and Wakefulness

Sleep is traditionally considered a homeostatic physiological process because longer periods of wakefulness increase our need to sleep, the duration of recovery sleep (RS), and EEG features thought to be unique to sleep, SWA in the EEG. SWA (traditionally, 0.5–4 Hz) occurs spontaneously during sleep in all species and increases in magnitude during periods of wakefulness such that its expression is greatest during the first part of every sleep period.[180] Recently, evidence for sleep as an allostatic process[181] has come from chronic partial sleep loss studies that have established that lost sleep is not fully recovered as sleep duration, and SWA do not exceed baseline levels after chronic partial restriction in humans[182,183] or rats.[184] iv Acute, total sleep loss clearly produces immediate, homeostatic-like responses in sleep expression.[185-189] However, chronically disturbed sleep, like that of clinical sleep disorders, does not adhere to descriptions of homeostasis. Instead, chronic sleep disruptions might unbalance homeostatic sleep responses sufficiently to cause persistent imbalances in sleep expression. McEwen suggested that chronic partial sleep loss evokes allostatic responses in physiologic mediators outside the sleep system itself and that poor, or restricted, sleep may be responsible for disrupting activity in physiologic mediators of global processes including metabolism, parasympathetic tone, glycogen levels, and pro-inflammatory cytokines. The unbalanced physiologic control that results from poor sleep might explain the observed relationships between sleep and diseases of allostatic overload such as hypertension, diabetes, anxiety, and depression.[190]

A variation of the two-process model discussed above, the "opponent process" model, emerged to explain how sleep and circadian phase interact after lesions of the central circadian pacemaker, the SCN.[191] The opponent process model suggested that, at certain times of day, unidentified SCN "alerting signals" oppose the physiologic accumulation of the homeostatic need to sleep. Considerable research has since focused on SCN efferent projections as potentially involved in Process S, including the ventral lateral pre-optic (VLPO) area.[192] In contrast, other regions such as Hcrt cells[193] and LC[194] are suggested to drive wakefulness. The neurochemical basis of "alerting" signals theoretically emanating from the SCN remain unknown, but it is noteworthy that CSF Hcrt1 levels increase as waking duration increases in both rats[195] and squirrel monkeys.[196] CSF Hcrt1 levels are amplified by increased activity of animals, but a correlation exists such that Hcrt1 appears to be tracking physiology to maintain wakefulness.

ANIMAL MODELS OF SLEEP

The validity of animal models for any clinical disorder is established, among other criteria, by a precise understanding of the physiologic mechanisms underlying that disorder, that is, construct validity.[197] v The physiological mechanisms responsible for

---

iv For further discussion regarding allostatic models, please refer to Koob, The role of animal models in reward deficit disorders: views from academia, in Volume 3, *Reward Deficits*.

v For further and detailed discussions regarding criteria of validity, the reader is invited to refer to discussions by Steckler *et al.*, Developing novel anxiolytics: improving preclinical detection and clinical insomnia, sleep apnea, and EDS are not fully understood but genetic research has been essential to help dissect not only sleep disorders, but also increasingly the physiology underlying normal sleep as well. For example, genetic manipulation of the Hcrt system has furthered our understanding of the sleep disorder narcolepsy as discussed above. Other models of normal and disturbed sleep rely upon the combination of sleep research methodology, molecular biology, and molecular genetics.

One *caveat* in the choice of animal model for studies of normal sleep or sleep disorders is the fact that adult human sleep tends to be consolidated into a single bout that occurs during the night. Exceptions to this general rule occur in cultures in which the siesta is common and in occupations in which 24 h staffing is necessary such as aboard ship. Despite these limitations, when one considers the characteristics of sleep shared by humans and animals including a stereotypical recumbent posture, elevated arousal threshold, reversibility to the waking state, circadian organization, and homeostatic regulation, it is evident that the similarities outweigh the differences and the underlying neurobiological mechanisms are likely to be similar as well.

Cats

Cats were originally the most popular animal species for natural sleep and contributed to key neurological discoveries, including isolation of the brain areas responsible for maintaining sleep, wake, or behavioral responsiveness as described above (for a review see Refs. 198, 199). At the time Loomis *et al.* described use of EEG in humans, Bremer began his series of experiments evaluating cat EEG as part of his transection studies. The first demonstration of REM sleep in animals was found in cats,[200] and cats provided the first set of animal EEG sleep patterns against which other laboratory animal species would later be compared. Cats remain a key species for studying sleep behavior[201-209] and an experimental species in which to examine the neurophysiology of sleep-related corticothalamic activity (see Refs. 210, 211), hypothalamic/POA initiation of sleep, and the relationship between sleep and body temperature control.[86,212,213] Nevertheless, cats have limitations for sleep studies as they have environmentally dependent sleep/wake patterns, weak circadian organization of sleep, and are difficult to train in behavioral tasks relevant for sleep research today.

Rats

Rat sleep was defined using EEG to indicate arousal state for the first time when Swisher[214] confirmed that laboratory rats produced similar cycles of inactive (non-REM) and "activated" (REM) sleep as that seen by Jouvet and others in cats. Clear differences between rat and cat EEG/ EMG signals were soon reported as cats showed

---

assessment, Joel *et al.*, Animal models of obsessive-compulsive disorder: from bench to bedside via endophenotypes and biomarkers, in this volume; Lindner *et al.*, Development, optimization and use of preclinical behavioral models to maximize the productivity of drug discovery for Alzheimer's Disease, Merchant *et al.*, Animal models of Parkinson's Disease to aid drug discovery and development, in Volume 2, *Neurologic Disorders*; Koob, The role of animal models in reward deficit disorders: views from academia, Markou *et al.*, Contribution of animal models and preclinical human studies to medication development for nicotine dependence, in Volume 3, *Reward Deficits Disorders*.

full immobility and atonia during paradoxical sleep but rats produced more variable patterns of motor inactivity during REM sleep, including less pronounced spiking EEG patterns than typically recorded in cat EEG. The architecture of sleep differs between cats and rats. Cats spend about 15% of their day in REM sleep while experiencing individual REM periods of about 6 min each that recur in cycles about every 20–30 min.[207,208] Rats also experience about 15% of their day in REM sleep but the bouts range from 0.5 to 1.5 min and recur about once every 10 min during sleep. Rats spend about 50% of a 24 h period in NREM sleep, comprised of 3–7 min bouts interspersed with 3–6 min wakefulness bouts.[215-220] Depending on their age and health status, adult humans spend from 15 to 25% of a sleep period in REM sleep in bouts of 10 to 30 min in duration, with 80 to 120 min between REM periods in healthy individuals.[221]

Today, rats are the preferred species for pharmaceutical research due to ease of handling, resilience to EEG and EMG recording methods, relative uniformity of sleep patterns within strains (but see below), and general utility in pharmacokinetic and safety assessment studies. However, strain differences have been reported, and one should be aware of them when choosing a particular strain for screening and evaluating compounds during the drug discovery process.[vi] Tang and Sanford, for example,[215,222] reported differences in baseline wake and NREM sleep in four different rat strains (Fischer 344, Lewis, Wistars, and Sprague-Dawley) overall and as a function of diurnal ratio (amount in light versus amount in darkness). Baseline REM sleep percentages are not reported to vary significantly across strains but REM sleep responses to simple stressors (e.g., cage changes) do vary by strain. Stress differences were expected based on known differences in rat strain responses to stress and well-established stress–learning–sleep relationships across species. Clearly, not all rat strains have similar sleep or sleep responses to stressors, even for normal behavioral testing (such as open field-testing). Furthermore, individual differences in sleep patterns of Wistar rats following testing and re-testing can be seen.[222]

Rats, like humans, respond to sleep-promoting ("soporific") compounds by increasing total sleep time and, typically, non-REM sleep.[223] Sleep latency is difficult to measure in rats, which have extremely short-sleep cycles and few periods of continuous wakefulness. Rat sleep is better characterized by evaluating the amount of each sleep state as a function of time of day versus vehicle dosing. Sleep/wake architecture-modifying effects of experimental or standard compounds can be evaluated by comparing the number of entries and duration of a given sleep/wake state as a function of time of day. Rat sleep architecture is best measured using chronic dosing in crossover designs to allow (1) comparison with acute dosing, (2) testing for withdrawal or rebound effects after dosing discontinuation, (3) comparison of early versus delayed responses to dosing, and (4) consideration of individual animal differences. As with humans, chronic zolpidem dosing in rats results in reduced REM sleep, increased delta

---

[vi]Please refer to Millan, The discovery and development of pharmacotherapy for psychiatric disorders: a critical survey of animal and translational models, and perspectives for their improvement, Steckler *et al.*, Developing novel anxiolytics: improving preclinical detection and clinical assessment, in this volume; Hunter, animal and translational models of neurological disorders: an industrial perspective, in Volume 2, *Neurologic Disorders*, or Markou *et al.*, Contribution of animal models and preclinical human studies to medication development for nicotine dependence, in Volume 3, *Reward Deficit Disorders*, for further discussion of the drug discovery process.

sleep and fewer wake episodes during peak exposure.[223] Additionally, post-zolpidem rebound insomnia on the first vehicle day after 7 days zolpidem dosing was seen by the significant decrease in SWA and an increase in light sleep for the first hour of the sleep period on the first vehicle day. Unexpectedly, re-initiating chronic zolpidem dosing after a washout week following the first period of chronic dosing revealed an increase in the zolpidem sleep response. This was interpreted as sensitization of sleep to zolpidem, not due to the short half-life compound, but due to plasticity of the underlying sleep physiology mechanisms.

Ease of use, laboratory resilience, and the ability to train rats on sleep-relevant behavioral tasks (including attention, memory, and learning) make rats the most common animal species for pharmaceutical sleep research. Rat responses to sleep-modifying compounds in terms of sleep and EEG pattern changes are predictive of similar changes in humans. For example, zolpidem causes dose-dependent increases in high frequency (β) EEG activity (in the range of 15–50 Hz) during wake, an effect that is counter to normal EEG patterns sleep onset, but an effect explained as a compensatory response to sedative effects of activation of α_1 subunit-containing GABA$_A$ receptors[224] High frequency EEG effects in rodents appear selective to activation of the α_1 subunit of the GABA$_A$ receptor as barbiturates do not produce this effect either in rats[224] or in humans.[225] Furthermore, increased β frequency EEG spectral power following zolpidem administration has been correlated with plasma levels in rats[226] and in humans.[227] Inter-species correlation of EEG to plasma effects (a pharmacodynamic/pharmacokinetic [PK/PD] relationship) is thus a very powerful tool to understand CNS effects of novel compounds and mechanisms of action.[vii] For example, examination of the effects of gaboxadol (THIP), a selective extrasynaptic GABA$_A$ receptor agonist with functional selectivity for the $\delta4$ subunit-containing GABA$_A$ receptors, on rat EEG spectral activity during sleep established a correlation with both monkey and human EEG spectral activity after the same doses of THIP (see Figure 12.2).

Monkeys

Due to shared evolutionary ancestry, non-human primates (NHP) are likely the optimal translational species to study sleep, cognition, and other behaviors.[228,229] Studies investigating changes in primate brain activity during wake and sleep originally focused on deep brain structures complementing the early systems localization work pioneered in cats (above). Adey *et al.*[230] were among the first to document chimpanzee sleep while recording from surface and intracortical EEG electrodes. They reported a number of EEG signals, and brain areas of sleep-dependent activation that were different

---

[vii] For further discussion on the importance of PK/PD relationships in animal and human responses to drugs, please refer to Millan, The discovery and development of pharmacotherapy for psychiatric disorders: a critical survey of animal and translational models, and perspectives for their improvement, Cryan *et al.*, Developing more efficacious antidepressant medications: Improving and aligning preclinical detection and clinical assessment tools, Large *et al.*, Developing therapeutics for bipolar disorder: from animal models to the clinic, in this volume, Merchant *et al.*, Animal models of Parkinson's Disease to aid drug discovery and development, in Volume 2, *Neurological Disorders*, or Markou *et al.*, Contribution of animal models and preclinical human studies to medication development for nicotine dependence, in Volume 3, *Reward Deficit Disorders*.

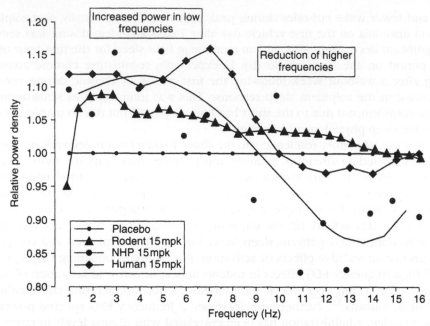

Figure 12.2 Non-REM spectral profile of gaboxadol (THIP) across species

from cats but more closely resembling humans.[231-234] Subsequently, sleep has been studied in detail in various NHP species including African Greens,[228,235] squirrel monkeys,[236,237] baboons,[238-241] rhesus,[242-244] and marmosets.[245] A survey of monkey sleep literature determined chimpanzee daily activity and sleep patterns to be most similar to humans, but that rhesus monkeys are better suited to sleep studies based on their diurnal activity cycles, sleep architecture, and ease of laboratory handling.[228]

The chimpanzee sleep studies of Adey and colleagues, primarily sponsored by NASA in the 1960s, produced the first telemetric biological data collection devices amenable to recording sleep in animals without requiring them to be tethered by recording wires.[246] Telemetric recording was critical for investigating monkey sleep because monkeys rarely adapt to tethered wire attachments and to being chair-restrained to allow skin penetrating electrodes to remain in place. All early non-human primate sleep studies recorded monkey sleep in chair-restrained animals even up to 24 h of continuous recording. This may be a reason for the variability in sleep patterns and responses to pharmacological treatment in these early studies. Crofts and associates[245] reviewed several studies to find squirrel monkey sleep reported to be 54.8% of a 24 h day in one study[247] while another study found 82.4% of the monkey day dedicated to sleep.[236] These differences are most likely the result of experimental differences in recording environment, with additional sources of variability from sleep scoring, socialization, and stress. Today, telemetry-based monkey sleep recording is essential to allow minimally disturbed, unrestrained animals to provide crucial data exploring the pharmacophysiology of sleep and circadian rhythms, EEG patterns and concurrent behavior, and the effects of aging versus health.

Crofts *et al.*[245] addressed both individual differences and recording stability across time for marmoset sleep in animals recorded telemetrically. Crofts reported high intra-subject stability along with high test/re-test reliability in home-cage recorded animals. Several NHP species show sleep/wake patterns roughly similar to human sleep. Human sleep occurs in a single major sleep bout at night, 15–20% REM sleep, and a pre-dominance of light sleep.[221] NHP have intra-sleep cycles shorter than human intra-sleep cycles of 90–100 min.[248] Overall sleep patterns, individual sleep pattern stability, similar brain structure, similar EEG and body temperature patterns, and very similar behavioral repertoire make monkeys the best animal species to study sleep and wakefulness for translational studies. Very few studies compare sleep effects of known sleep or wake-promoting agents between NHPs and humans using EEG as a direct measure of sleep. More typically, monkey studies have included simple behavioral observation of chair-restrained primates after dosing (cf., Refs. 244, 249, 250).

Non-human primates are diurnal and have similar circadian patterns of SCN projection and pineal gland activity as humans. Thus, they are an excellent choice for evaluating sleep effects of circadian phase-modifying compounds like melatonin. Zhdanova *et al.*[251] reviewed the animal melatonin literature across multiple species to find oral doses of melatonin that caused rats, cats, and monkeys to fall asleep more quickly, but sleep architecture responses differed across species. Differences in the response to melatonin may arise because melatonin may provide a different sleep signal to nocturnal versus diurnal animals. Zhdanova and colleagues evaluated the effects of melatonin in three monkey species (*Macaca nemestrina*, *M. mulatta*, and *M. fascicularis*) using both acute and chronic (4 weeks) dosing regimes.[252] Only the 5 µg/kg oral dose of melatonin produced earlier sleep onset without altering sleep offset times or sleep efficiency. However, high doses (40–320 µg/kg) increased nocturnal activity, as indicated by an increase in sleep fragmentation, an effect observed previously in human subjects treated with high doses of melatonin.[253]

The sleep effects of ramelteon, a selective melatonin receptor 1/2 agonist, versus zolpidem, a short-acting non-benzodiazepine GABA$_A$ positive modulator, were measured in unrestrained crab-eating macaques.[254] Significant decreases in sleep latency with increased sleep duration were seen in otherwise normal animals with sleep effects of ramelteon (0.3 mg/kg) exceeding the effects of orally dosed melatonin (0.3–1 mg/kg) or zolpidem (up to 100 mg/kg). Quantitative EEG (qEEG) parameters during sleep following administration of ramelteon and melatonin were not different from that recorded during baseline sleep but zolpidem (30 mg/kg) indicated a reduction in slow wave qEEG activity during NREM sleep. qEEG effects were directly translated to human sleep studies finding the same qualitative changes in sleep and EEG SWA patterns.[255,256]

Aged Animals

Effects of age on normal sleep and response to sleep deprivation are well documented and are consistent between species. Rats, cats, dogs, monkeys, mice, humans, and now even invertebrate species (for reviews see Refs. 257–263) tend to have more disrupted day/night sleep pattern distributions as animals age. Increasing age is related to decreased NREM and REM sleep, decreased overall sleep quantity, increased sleep fragmentation, and reduced restorative effects of sleep in all species studied. Multi-day

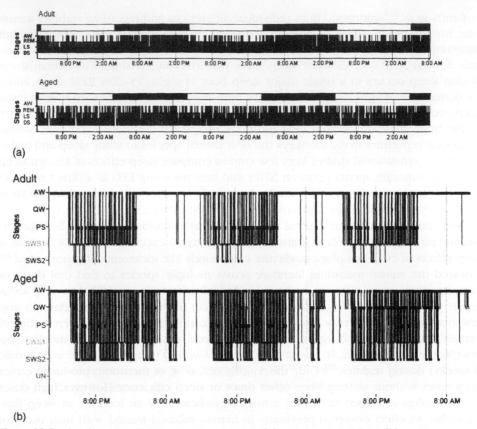

Figure 12.3 Aged versus adult sleep patterns in rats (a) and rhesus monkeys (b)

sleep patterns comparing aged rats and aged rhesus monkeys with their younger conspecifics show the characteristic re-distribution of sleep into the wake period, increased state shifts, and reductions in non-REM and REM sleep (see Figure 12.3). Sleep deprivation in aged humans and aged rhesus results in reduced RS[264] (Doran unpublished observations) but sleep deprivation-related performance impairments are not as severe in older versus younger subjects.[265-267]

Many hypotheses exist to explain the effects of aging on sleep including reduced homeostatic sleep drive,[268] reduced circadian promotion of wakefulness,[269,270] and age-modified circadian/homeostatic interactions.[271] Ancoli-Israel, however, has proposed that age alone does not impair sleep-medical and psychological problems impair sleep.[272] When medication and medical condition-related sleep disorders are accounted for, very few sleep pattern differences can be found between healthy adults and people of advanced age. Furthermore, little or no evidence is available finding cell death or abnormalities in the neurophysiologic systems responsible for sleep with increasing age.[273,274] The effects of aging on sleep remain a reliable behavioral phenotype even though the neurologic mechanisms by which aging changes sleep remain elusive. Murillo-Rodriguez and colleagues reported higher adenosine levels are required to activate adenosine A1 receptors in aged animals, suggesting this receptor might lose potency as a function of age.[220] Whatever the mechanism, aged animals provide a natural model for impaired sleep because health, sleep, and behavioral effects are consistent across species, and all three parameters depend on intact CNS activity.

Sleep Deprivation

Manaceine[275] was the first to document total sleep deprivation experiments in animals when she reported that puppies kept awake for 3–4 days would die and younger animals suffered mortality sooner. Manaceine noted decreases in body temperature of 4–5°C and an average of 15% reduction in body weight at death. Pierón (1913) (as reported in Ref. 69 and Kleitman[276]) followed up these studies to confirm the lethal consequences of sleep loss in puppies and to characterize post-mortem brains and spinal cords from surviving and non-surviving dogs. Neither study reported morphologic effects of sleep loss on brain tissue, but both noted reductions in red blood cell counts preceding coma, convulsions, and death that occurred during sleep deprivation. In a seminal series of studies, Rechtschaffen and colleagues[277-281] confirmed that sleep deprivation was fatal in rats. Greater experimental control was introduced into these studies by adapting the revolving cage technique first described by Bast *et al.*[282] to keep cats walking to stay awake. Rechtschaffen used the animals' own EEG patterns to trigger a moving platform and, to dissociate continuous wakefulness effects from accumulating effects of enforced locomotion, yoked-control animals were placed on the same moving platform that was controlled by the experimental animal's EEG. Rechtschaffen's studies were influential in shifting the focus of sleep deprivation studies from cats to rats. Today, most studies using environmental and pharmacologic manipulations to produce sleep deprivation and to measure the consequent effects use rodents as experimental subjects.

Impairments following sleep deprivation procedures in rats and monkeys are models for the daytime performance decrements known to accompany narcolepsy, sleep apnea, and insomnia. As described above, distinct differences between acute and chronic sleep deprivation emerge when evaluating immediate recovery versus long-term adaptive sleep patterns. Acute sleep deprivation in rhesus monkeys has been used to test the efficacy of wake-promoting compounds to improve cognition[229] and sleep fragmentation imposed on rats decreases selective and executive attention.[283,284] Chronic sleep restriction decreases total leukocytes and lymphocyte counts while increasing circulating levels of IgM in rats, effects that should increase susceptibility to infections.[285] Acute total sleep deprivation studies alter HPA axis activity but one study found stress responses in general (increases in corticosterone and ACTH) were not elevated early in chronic sleep restriction. Additionally, novel stressor effects on HPA responses were suppressed.[286] These results data suggest that chronic sleep loss does not produce a stress response alone but does impair the ability to muster a transient stress response to novel stimuli. Chronic animal sleep restriction studies more closely the chronic sleep problems suffered by human patients but most published studies focus on acute sleep deprivation when examining drug effects on overcoming the cognitive or stress effects of sleep loss.

Translational sleep deprivation studies between animals and humans use Rechtschaffen's strategy of timing wake-promoting interventions using each experimental subject's own EEG patterns. Both animal and human studies find that *acute total* sleep deprivation causes degraded mental performance,[187,229,287] altered immunological cell functioning,[288-291] susceptibility to disease, and an increased drive to sleep.[292] Daytime consequences of *chronic partial* sleep restriction in animals and humans include cumulative cognitive, mood, and immuno-functioning impairments.[293-299] In all species tested, acute total sleep deprivation increases circulating levels of "stress" corticotropin-releasing factor, plasma ACTH and corticosterone and progesterone while reducing testosterone.[300] The use of sleep deprivation approaches in translational studies will be of particular benefit to understanding of the therapeutic role of "restorative sleep" on the effects of stress on mood, cognition and immune responses.

INSOMNIA

Primary insomnia can occur as episodes of acute insomnia lasting 2 or 3 weeks, transient insomnia lasting less than a week, or chronic insomnia, which can last for periods of at least 1 month up to years. Acute and transient insomnia may occur in anyone at certain times, for example, in association with emotional or physical discomfort,[301] or sleeping at a time that is inconsistent with the daily biological rhythm, for example, "jet lag."[302] Chronic insomnia may follow episodes of acute or transient insomnia and factors such as worrying or having unreasonable expectation of sleep duration may contribute to persistence. Each of these insomnia sub-types has been modeled in animals using stress events to provoke transient insomnia such as the "cage change" model first reported by Michaud and colleagues.[303] Chronic insomnia has been modeled in rats via the administration of caffeine,[304] or by housing animals in cages with widely spaced wire floors suspended over water.[305-307] While these models do not purport to alter the neurological mechanisms driving insomnia, they do promote disturbed sleep either transiently (for about 2h after a cage change) or chronically (up to 12h after caffeine administration). Pharmacologic improvements of sleep patterns under experimentally disruptive conditions are considered supporting evidence for the likelihood of efficacy in humans with insomnia.

Pharmacological Models of Insomnia

Several strategies have been attempted to model the sleep disruption patterns known to define human insomnia. The earliest of these strategies used pharmacologic induction of wakefulness in the sleep phase of the circadian cycle. The disruption of sleep by caffeine intake in both humans[308-311] and rat[307,312] has prompted the proposal of acute caffeine ingestion as a translatable model of insomnia. Paterson and associates used caffeine to induce sleep onset effects and then reversed the sleep onset delays with the established sedative-hypnotics zolpidem and trazodone.[304] This pharmacologic insomnia animal model provides a well-controlled and an easily manipulated procedure from which reversal of induced wakefulness may indicate therapeutic potential for sleep induction. However, there are complications and construct weaknesses using this model to select potential sleep therapeutics. Specifically, compounds with strong sedative hypnotic efficacy rather than those able to enhance or promote normal sleep patterns will show stronger effects in a caffeine-induced model of insomnia. Furthermore, stimulants have a time course of effect that will, in most cases, have a short onset to action followed by subsequent clearance. This type of pharmacodynamic effect mimics sleep onset insomnia or "early" insomnia, thereby favoring compounds with strong sedating effects that emerge soon after administration. Additional concerns with this pharmacological model, as a general principle, include identifying compounds that are good at reversing stimulant mechanisms *per se*, but perhaps not ideal for restoring "normal" or "restorative" sleep in insomniacs. The relevance of the temporal interaction and dose–response relationship of drugs identified using this model to clinical response in insomniacs is unclear. Furthermore, the reversal of an acute administration caffeine does not necessarily predict the effect of chronic administration of a novel pharmacological treatment of insomnia in humans.

Noise Disruption Model of Insomnia

Contention exists as to whether human sleepers can adapt to, or remain persistently disturbed by constant noise during the sleep period (for a review see Ref. 313). Intermittent bursts of noise clearly cause momentary periods of wake but the effect of chronic noise on long-term sleep patterns is reported by some to produce chronic sleep disruption[314] while others claim humans habituate to chronic noise.[315,316] Basner and colleagues[317] recently conducted the first chronic (nine nights) human study under tightly controlled laboratory conditions assessing aircraft noise levels on EEG-defined sleep parameters. They reported that small, transient arousals were present at low noise levels (45 dBA) while only high noise (65 dBA) was able to cause awakenings, as traditionally scored using clinical sleep measures. Lower noise levels caused small interruptions in sleep continuity known to disrupt next-day human functioning.[318,319] Sleep arousals were too brief to be scored as stage changes or as classic arousals, but still sufficient to disrupt sleep stage continuity.

Rats subjected to airport noise modified to the higher frequencies within the rat hearing range produced both acute[218] and chronic[219] sleep pattern changes. Rats chronically subjected to adapted airport noise showed significant and cumulative increases in wake and reductions in both slow wave and REM sleep. Subsequently, Rabat *et al.*[320] showed that this procedure impaired long-term spatial memory, with variation in the memory effect positively correlating with daily variation in SWS bouts and cumulative SWS amounts across the 9 days of noise exposure. Rabat's procedure appears to model insomnia and insomnia-impaired sleep and cognition more successfully than other procedures that use white noise of continuous frequencies[321] through its use of randomized and discontinuous noise patterns adapted to the rat's hearing that were naturally disruptive.

Environmental noise models have been used to induce short-term "insomnia" in healthy human subjects in several studies examining the sleep maintenance effects of sleep-promoting compounds. Saletu[322,323] and others have documented that simulated traffic noise in sleep laboratories is effective at producing an increase in the number of awakenings and the amount of Stage 1 sleep. In contrast, white noise in sleep laboratories appears to be more effective at reducing sleep latency, but only in some patients.[324] This comparison of findings across studies lends support to the idea that inconsistent, sporadic noise rather than constant noise provides a translational animal to human sleep model. In human studies that did use simulated traffic noise cinolazepam (Gerodorm®), zolpidem, zaleplon, and rameleton were found to decrease the number of awakenings due to environmental noise in human subjects. In one study comparing effects of lormetazepam (Noctamid®, 2 mg) to zolpidem (10 mg) during traffic noise exposure, both compounds increased total sleep time when compared to placebo and both compounds reduced the amount of light (Stage 2) sleep.[325] Lormetazepam, but not zolpidem, reduced noise-related arousals by 20%. Overall, disruptive environmental noise appears to be a good translational model for testing the effect of sleep maintenance compounds in both animals and good sleeping humans but is not useful for testing sleep latency. Furthermore, noise models can be used chronically in both animals and humans to document long-term changes in sleep architecture.

Behavioral Stress Model of Insomnia

Stress is still considered the primary precipitating factor leading to clinical insomnia. The mechanisms by which stress contributes to persistent insomnia remain unclear, although the principles of allostatic sleep modification have the most circumstantial support. Stress effects on rodent sleep were recently reviewed by Pawlyk *et al.*[326] comparing sleep effects across stress methods and strains. Stress intensity, estimated by measuring plasma cortisol or epinephrine levels after the stressor, tends to increase sleep at low levels and to decrease sleep at high levels. Stress modality appears crucial to the sleep response (see Ref. 327–331). For example, when conditioned stress is used, sleep effects are more persistent and resistant to extinction.[332-334] Re-exposure to stress cues re-establishes altered sleep patterns observed initially during conditioning to the stressor. REM sleep decreases are the most consistent stress-sleep effect recorded after conditioned stress, but decreases in total sleep are common during stressed animal's next sleep period.

Stress-related sleep disruptions in rodents are generally consistent with the altered sleep quantity and continuity indicative of insomnia. However, the recurrence of insomnia following periods of stress common to human insomnia experiences is not consistently reported for rodents given fearful cues sometime after fear conditioning.[333,335] Acute rodent stress procedures model acute reductions in total sleep and REM sleep time, suggesting rodent sleep responses to stress are a better model of stress disorders generally rather than primary insomnia. Cage change manipulations combined with novel object presentation and social stressors produce transient sleep loss from which rodents soon recover.[215,216] Unfortunately, the sleep effects of cage change and open field stressors are quite variable between rat and mice strains, suggesting very subtle differences in neurophysiology may be responsible for translating wakeful stress experiences into acute or chronic sleep changes.[viii]

[viii]Please refer to Cryan *et al.*, Developing more efficacious antidepressant medications: Improving and aligning preclinical detection and clinical assessment tools, in this volume, or Koob, The role of animal models in reward deficit disorders: views from academia, in Volume 3, *Reward Deficit Disorders* for further discussion of the use of random and continuous environmental stress to model behavioral disorders, including sleep.

SLEEP APNEA

Recently, natural animal models for sleep apnea have been explored (the English bulldog) and symptom induction models (chronic intermittent hypoxia) have been developed. Chronic sleep fragmentation with enforced awakenings of rats and monkeys has been developed as a model to evoke the daytime stress and cognitive consequences of sleepiness due to sleep apnea.

Airway Obstruction

English bulldogs of a certain age have spontaneous sleep apnea becoming more severe during REM sleep with weight gain and age, paralleling the human condition. Hendricks *et al.*[336] provided the first laboratory report of disrupted nocturnal breathing and sleep patterns in the English bulldog (i.e., breathing lapses, blood oxygen desaturation, nocturnal arousals, and daytime hypersomnolence). Like humans, nocturnal breathing is worse during REM sleep in these animals since the upper airways constrict and upper airway control is reduced. Similar to humans with sleep apnea, the bulldog has upper airway muscle edema and fibrosis as well.[337] Few efforts have been made to attempt pharmacologic reversal of Bulldog sleep apnea, but some reductions in apnea, but not reversals, of the concurrent sleep fragmentation were seen when apneic bulldogs were given the serotonin 5-HT$_3$ receptor antagonist ondansetron.[338]

Rats fed a chronically high-fat diet have only been reported to show one feature of sleep apnea, central respiratory pauses, while other features (sleep disruption and increased nocturnal apnea) did not develop.[339] Central apnea pauses induced by the high-fat diet were prevented with co-administration of metformin (Fortamet®/Glucophage®), suggesting insulin dysregulation is part of a positive feedback between obesity and sleep apnea in humans. Obese Zucker rats evaluated for naturally occurring sleep apnea have smaller airways than non-obese members of the same strain, but no evidence has emerged finding obese rats express apnea during sleep (see Refs. 340,341).

Philip *et al.*[342] has reported an induced obstructive airway model of sleep apnea using collagen injections into the upper airway of cynomologus monkeys (*M. fascicularis*). Monkeys injected with collagen have obstructed nocturnal breathing but no differences in daytime respiration. Monkey sleep apnea reduced total sleep time, reduced time in all sleep states, and increased sleep fragmentation. Sleep in these monkeys was recorded in restraint chairs. During wake, breathing patterns were reported to be normal. Injected collagen is absorbed by the body in about 3–6 months so this is a reversible model of sleep apnea, a useful feature for an animal model of sleep apnea because apnea can be reversed in humans that achieve weight loss, undergo surgery, or adhere to continuous positive airway pressure (CPAP) treatment.[343]

Intermittent Hypoxia

Because sleep apnea causes both blood oxygen desaturation and intermittent awakenings, these two symptoms have been experimentally imposed on animals both separately and together to understand better how sleep apnea interferes with animal models of cognition, cardiovascular physiology, and energy metabolism. Cyclic desaturations accompany apneic episodes in patients because breath holding decreases blood oxygen content. Cyclic blood oxygen desaturations are produced during rodent sleep by rapidly modulating the gas fraction of an animal's living environment. Gozal et al.[40] has standardized the rodent intermittent hypoxia (IH) model cycling ambient oxygen content from normal concentration (21%) to restricted (10%) once every 60–90 s to simulate the deoxygenation pattern experienced by patients with sleep apnea.

In rats, consequences of IH include cognitive impairments, selective neuronal degeneration, gliosis, changes in brain neurochemistry, and increased inflammatory processes among other collateral damage (reviewed in Refs. 344–346). Daily rhythms of blood glucose and corticosterone were reversed and pancreatic β cell proliferation increased significantly in mice exposed to sleep-period IH. Mouse glucose and β cell responses to IH were exacerbated by glucose infusion-further supporting the idea that sleep apnea contributes directly to diabetes and obesity.[347,348] Sleep apnea is a chronic disease and chronic IH in rodents causes long-term, set-point modifying, changes in a variety of physiologic systems including carotid body sensitivity,[349] hypertension and tyrosine hydroxylase activity in various brain areas.[350] As in the case of sleep deprivation, chronic, rather than acute, animal IH studies provide the more predictive strategy for human disease. Veasey et al.[351] found long-term IH resulted in sleep architecture impairments and oxidative damage to wake-promoting neurons in the mouse forebrain. She suggests persistent sleepiness resulting from human sleep apnea might partially result from cumulative neuronal damage of wake-control neurons due to persistent, intermittent hypoxia during sleep. Additionally, other studies inducing long-term IH in rodents have reported apoptosis in frontal and hippocampal cortex.[40,352,353] These and other studies are establishing a close link between intermittent hypoxia and cognitive impairments related to sleep apnea.

Sleep Fragmentation

A model of the sleep fragmentation that occurs as a consequence of the repeated brief arousals that characterize sleep apnea has recently been described.[295] This procedure forces rats to undergo 30 interruptions of sleep per hour by a cage floor programmed to move at 0.02 m/s in cycles of 30 s "on" followed by 90 s "off." This procedure reduces sleep quality (shorter sleep bout durations) for both non-REM and REM sleep and increased sleepiness, that is, the latency to fall asleep when permitted. In fact, rats may adapt to chronic sleep patterns with long-term fragmentation as they produce near-baseline levels of non-REM sleep although REM sleep was reduced by intermittent platform movements. Compared to sleep state control, experimental animals, but not yoked controls, showed increased forebrain adenosine levels; a proposed neural mechanism for controlling sleep and sleepiness. Sleep fragmented rats showed impairments of attentional performance[284] and decreases in hippocampal long-term potentiation (LTP) measured ex vivo after sleep fragmentation.[354]

Enforced locomotion in rats appears to produce the expected sleep and cognitive effects known to occur in humans who experience sleep fragmentation without concurrent sleep loss [reviewed in Ref. 319). Sleep fragmentation by repetitive arousals is not unique to sleep apnea so animal models of enforced sleep fragmentation (as opposed to cumulative sleep deprivation) generalizes to other medical and psychiatric disorders defined by frequent, brief arousals from sleep as part of a given disease such as restless legs syndrome.[355,356] Furthermore, intermittent hypoxia procedures using young animals found even more striking results[344,352,357] including hyperactivity and cortical response findings, suggesting a link between childhood sleep apnea and attention-deficit problems.

SLEEP AND METABOLIC DISORDERS

Studies by Rechtschaffen, Bergmann and colleagues revealed that chronic total sleep deprivation over a 2-week period (and longer) leads to hyperphagia, increased energy expenditure (i.e., weight loss), initial hyperthermia followed by hypothermia, elevated sympathetic tone (increased norepinephrine levels and adrenal hypertrophy) and an increased thyroid hormone turnover.[278] More recent studies report that long-term sleep deprivation leads to a decrease in the putative satiety hormone, leptin, as well as reduced serum levels of growth hormone, prolactin, and insulin-like growth factor.[358] Similarly, during a 20-day period of selected REM sleep deprivation, rats developed hyperphagia, increased metabolic rate (i.e., elevated uncoupling protein-1 expression in brown adipose tissue), and decreased leptin levels accompanied by upregulated mRNA expression of NPY, an orexigenic neuropeptide, and downregulated mRNA expression of POMC, an anorectic neuropeptide, in the hypothalamus.[359,360] Decreased leptin and increased ghrelin levels in the serum have been observed in association with increased feeding following just a 5-h period of sleep deprivation.[361]

Effects of Metabolism on Sleep/Wake Cycle

While sleep deprivation studies have made it clear that sleep is important in maintaining energy balance and normal metabolic function; studies in genetic and experimental animal models have revealed that metabolic pathways reciprocally interact to influence sleep/wake regulation. An important neuropeptide link between the sleep/wake and energy balance regulatory systems was the discovery that hypocretin peptides are involved in sleep/wake regulation (see above). Narcoleptic patients are reported to have an elevated body mass index (BMI),[362] and energy expenditure problems in Hcrt-deficient mice may be related to disruption of their sleep/wake patterns.[363] Therefore, Hcrt appears to play an important role in the co-regulation of sleep and energy metabolism as it may be involved in coordinating periods of sleep, food consumption, and energy storage.

Recent clinical and epidemiological studies in humans linking short sleep with obesity, diabetes and the metabolic syndrome[364,365] renewed interest in animal models focused on genetic, cellular, and physiological mechanisms by which loss of sleep can impact metabolic function. Sleep loss effects on metabolic function led to developing animal models addressing the reverse question: what are the effects of altered metabolism on sleep/wake patterns? A majority of neuroendocrine changes that occur in response to sleep loss are similar in humans and animals, so animal models may be valuable for exploring mechanistic links and common physiological/molecular components between sleep regulatory and energy metabolism regulating systems.

Animal Models Linking Sleep to Obesity

Mice fed a high-fat diet show interactions between the sleep/wake and metabolic regulatory systems with diet-induced obese mice expressing more NREM sleep time and increased sleep fragmentation. Conversely, food deprivation in rats results in decreased sleep time.[366,367] Recent studies with *ob/ob* leptin-deficient mouse found that these obese mice sleep more, have severely fragmented sleep/wake patterns, and disrupted circadian distribution of REM sleep time and NREM SWA.[368] Thus, many of the primary neuropeptides and neurotransmitters involved in the regulation of energy homeostasis also mediate sleep/wake states, suggesting mechanistic overlap between metabolic and sleep/wake regulatory systems. A common thread in animal models of obesity (whether genetic or diet-induced) is that total sleep time is increased; however, sleep is less consolidated as evidenced by frequent arousals from sleep during the normal sleep period and increased sleep during the normal wake period.

Many consequences of sleep loss are consistent between human and animal studies including: (1) increased food intake and appetite, (2) decreased leptin and increased ghrelin levels, (3) activation of the sympathetic nervous system, (4) elevation of corticosterone levels, (5) alterations in glucose utilization, and (6) an increase in cardiovascular risk factors. However, there is one major difference between sleep loss studies in humans and in animal models for sleep loss: while chronic total sleep loss in animals leads to a negative energy balance and loss of weight, short-sleep time in humans has been associated with weight gain and or increased BMI. It has been suggested that these differences in weight response between humans and rodents may involve methodological issues, rather than actual physiological differences in response to sleep loss.[369] While almost all animal studies have involved long-term total sleep deprivation (or total REM deprivation), the human clinical and epidemiological studies have involved chronic partial sleep loss.[369] A second methodological difference is that partial chronic sleep loss studies in a clinical setting are usually carried out in sedentary volunteers under bed-rest conditions, while current procedures for depriving animals of sleep for an extended period of time require some degree of forced locomotor activity or physical manipulation of the animal to keep it awake. A third methodological difference in rodent and controlled human chronic sleep loss studies is that, in human studies, nutrient intake is usually controlled by giving control and experimental subjects meals with identical caloric intake or by using constant glucose infusion. Therefore, these experiments do not assess *ad lib* food intake and body weight changes, as has been the case in animal sleep deprivation studies.

VACCINES

One study used telemetry-based primate EEG sleep recording during drug administration[370] to evaluate the effects of common vaccines on marmoset sleep and cognition. Vaccine administration immediately increased the amount of NREM sleep and chronically reduced REM sleep. Vaccine effects on rat sleep also find increased NREM sleep immediately after vaccination[371] but no changes in REM sleep. While no similar studies have been run in humans, two different studies in humans document how sleep disruption immediately after vaccination with hepatitis A antigen[372] or influenza vaccine[373] resulted in significantly reduced long-term antibody titer response. Together, these results suggest strong translatability of immune system-related sleep responses across species. As described above, lymphokines and inflammatory molecules interact with sleep even to the level of influencing local cortical synchronization.[374,375] The sleep response and relationships within the sleep-metabolism-immunology triad is an intersection of interests that deserves more research based on the many intriguing links including obvious (sickness requires sleep to heal) and less obvious (bacterial enterotransmission during sleep deprivation)[294,358] evidence of necessary co-incident activity.

GENETIC ASPECTS OF HUMAN AND ANIMAL SLEEP

Natural polymorphisms link sleep behavior and gene loci in cases such as the rare disease Fatal Familial Insomnia (FFI). FFI is linked to a GAC to AAC mutation (codon 178) on the PRNP gene locus of human chromosome 20 showing Mendelian inheritance with autosomal dominant frequency.[376] Interestingly, Gambetti *et al.*[377] found a prion mutation can lead to either Creutzfeldt–Jakob Disease (CJD) or to FFI if another polymorphism is present at codon 129 (valine for CJD or methionine for FFI). In those cases where FFI does occur, the disease involves the loss of neurons in the anterior and dorsomedial thalamic nuclei,[378] pointing to the importance of the thalamus in sleep. Destruction of these thalamic nuclei can explain the hallmark loss of SWS and resulting insomnia in FFI. It remains to be understood whether these prion proteins have a normal physiological function in sleep or if their accumulation in specific regions has the effect on sleep in FFI.[379]

As mentioned earlier, narcolepsy is another example of human genetic sleep disorder. This disease is highly sporadic and its phenotypic expression tends to be variable. Studies in narcoleptic dog and mouse models that had implicated the Hcrt system as a likely cause of narcolepsy were supported when Hcrt levels in narcoleptic humans were found to be undetectable in CSF from seven of nine narcoleptic patients.[51] In subsequent post-mortem analyses, prepro-hcrt mRNA was undetectable in two narcoleptic brains, although mRNA for MCH was readily detectable in both controls and narcoleptics.[52] Immunohistochemistry showed an 85–95% reduction in the number of Hcrt-containing cells in narcoleptic brains with no evident change in the number of MCH cells.[380] These studies suggest that degeneration of the Hcrt cells may be the cause of human narcolepsy. Increased staining for glial fibrillary acid protein in the PFH suggests that Hcrt cells degenerate in narcolepsy, possibly by an autoimmune mechanism.[380] Interestingly, the molecular basis of the human narcolepsy remains elusive because mutations in the orexin/hypocretin prepro-peptide, or the two Hcrt-receptors, have not been found in the majority of narcolepsy patients.[381] Demonstration of a narcoleptic phenotype in both spontaneously and engineered orexin ligand or orexin receptor mutants strongly implicates Hcrt signaling deficiency as the root cause of narcolepsy in rodent and canine models as well as human narcolepsy patients.

There is now a good deal of evidence from different species, including flies, rodents and humans, for characteristics or traits of the sleep/wake cycle being under at least some degree of genetic control. Very little is known about which specific genes or molecular networks producing differential sleep/wake expression between individuals or within individual interacting with environmental factors. Three general approaches have been used to uncover genetic control of sleep/wake traits. One approach has been to alter the sleep/wake state of the animal (e.g., sleep deprivation) and determine changes in gene expression in response to the altered state. A second approach has been to look for genetic variation (either natural or induced) in sleep/wake traits with the ultimate objective being to uncover the genes and gene networks underlying the variation. A third approach has been to look at the effects of altered "candidate genes" on sleep/wake traits.

Changes in Sleep State Alter Changes in Gene Expression

One way to link a putative sleep function or trait to a specific gene is to alter that function/trait and determine which genes are altered. Widespread changes in gene expression have been documented within the brain in conjunction with changes in behavioral states.[382-386] The expression of a number of genes is upregulated during RS after SD.[384-387] In studies of the cerebral cortex of spontaneous wake, sleep-deprived and sleeping rats, 10% of transcripts change their expression from day to night, about half of these genes owe their expression changes to the sleep/wake state and were independent of time of day.[382] In general, gene expression data support the hypothesis that sleep is involved in protein synthesis and neural plasticity, but also suggested a novel role for sleep in membrane trafficking and maintenance. Gene expression studies involving different brain regions in mice and rats following acute or chronic sleep deprivation indicate sleep loss triggers generalized inflammatory and stress responses in the brain.[278,358] Ubiquity of sleep loss effects on neural function is exemplified by the finding that transcripts with higher expression during wakefulness versus sleep belong to different functional categories in fruit flies. Interestingly, in some cases, state-dependent fly gene categories overlap with genes identified as varying with wake and sleep in the rat.[360]

While gene expression studies have identified hundreds of genes to be associated with sleep/wake state or sleep loss, such studies are, by their nature, correlative and linkage between a sleep function or trait and a specific gene needs to be supported by more direct genetic approaches. While such linkages have been found to some genetic regions, as discussed in the next section, very few specific genes have actually been linked to specific defined sleep/wake traits or EEG characteristics.

Evidence for Genetic Control of Sleep/Wake Traits

While environmental factors clearly have a major impact on the sleep/wake cycle and individual characteristics of the sleep/wake states (e.g., sleep deprivation leads to an increase in NREM sleep and SWA), there is evidence for a substantial role of genetic factors in contributing to the expression of a number of sleep/wake phenotypes. To date, three species have provided support for the genetic control of sleep and wake traits: fruit flies, laboratory mice, and humans. Interestingly, evidence supporting genetic control of sleep/wake traits in these species comes from diverse approaches.

Fruit Flies

Drosophila has been a model organism for studying formal properties and genetic control of circadian rhythms for over half a century[388,389] but only in the last decade have fruit flies been used to elucidate genetic components of sleep regulation.[390-392] Recent recognition that fruit flies share fundamental features of mammalian sleep, even if they do not have the equivalent of EEG activity, has enabled fly geneticists to use tools available to screen for specific mutations associated with sleep/wake traits. Because sleep in thousands of individual flies can be monitored rapidly and economically, it is possible to set up a reverse genetics screen and search for flies with genetically controlled differences in the amount of sleep or the response to sleep deprivation.[392,393] Similarly, given the thousands of lines of flies with known genetic deletions or disruptions, forward genetics can screen for sleep/wake patterns in known genes. Surprisingly, although a number of mutant lines showing altered traits such as short sleep or no sleep rebound after sleep deprivation in flies have been identified, few specific genes have been linked to the altered traits in flies.[393] One exception is the "Shaker" mutant fly detected in a screen of 9000 mutant lines and found to sleep only one-third the amount of wild-type flies.[394] The altered sleep phenotype is due to the mutation in a voltage-dependent potassium channel. Given the broad range of effects of this channel on overall neural cellular function, its role in normal sleep physiology remains unclear.

Inbred Mice

A few groups have attempted to perform high-throughput mutagenesis screening studies for sleep/wake mutants in mice using markers for adult EEG/EMG states (e.g., just EMG in pups or highly sensitive motion detectors[395]). Inbred mouse strains have provided some of the strongest evidence for the genetic control of sleep and for linking specific genomic regions to sleep/wake traits.[396] Valatx and colleagues, in the 1970s, established that various sleep/wake traits associated with REM sleep differed between strains and were inherited in specific patterns when hybrids were produced.[397] A few groups have attempted to isolate genes associated with specific sleep/wake traits by crossing two inbred strains to create F_2 mice and then inbreeding these F_2 mice to create recombinant inbred strains.[396] This approach has led to the identification of a handful of genomic regions (Quantitative trait loci, QTL) that are associated (some "suggestive," some "significant") with specific sleep/wake traits. In only one case has a QTL linked a specific gene to a specific trait: retinoic acid receptor-β affects EEG cortical synchrony.[398] A preliminary report has been recently reported finding many QTLs ($N = 52$) correlated with many different sleep/wake traits in a large segregating cross ($N = 269$ mice) of two inbred strains.[399] Such reports suggest an expanded understanding of sleep's genetic underpinnings may be on the horizon. Rapid advances in mouse genomics suggest the possibility that a number of specific genes and molecular pathways will soon be associated with specific sleep/wake traits in mice. In addition, much more extensive analysis of sleep/wake phenotypes on a large battery of inbred mouse strains whose genomes are being fully sequenced should also lead to new discoveries on the genes and genetic networks underlying sleep/wake traits.[400]

Transgenic animal models focused on sleep and circadian rhythms offer the potential to identify novel genes and genetic pathways underlying sleep disorders. Translatability of mouse mutants appears to be robust as many of mutants expected to have circadian effects or sleep alterations, based on established human pharmacology, do in fact show effects that are consistent with pharmacology in man and animal models (see Table 12.2 for examples). Many of the sleep and circadian mutants described to date are part of established pathways identified as important for sleep/wake regulation. Examples include knockout animals in the GABAergic, histaminergic, serotonergic, dopaminergic, and adrenergic transmitter pathways. Mutant mice such as the glycine receptor knockout have revealed genes that have unexpectedly played a role in sleep.[417] These have added additional information about the role of novel genes in modulation of sleep/wake behavior.

Table 12.2 Genetically manipulated mice with reported sleep or circadian effects

Name of gene	Sleep effect	Reference
ALDH1	Abnormal sleep pattern	401
BMAL1/ARNTL/MOP3	Circadian rhythm	402 403
Brn-3.1 [Pou4f3]	Circadian rhythm	404
Cadps 2	Circadian rhythm	405
CaV 3.1	Abnormal sleep pattern	406
CB1 receptor	Circadian rhythm	407
Clock	Circadian rhythm	408
CREM	Circadian rhythm	409
Cry1/2	Circadian rhythm	410
DBP	Sleep consolidation and EEG activity	411
Dec1 and Dec2	Circadian rhythm	412
DRD3	Abnormal sleep pattern Circadian rhythm	413 414
GABRb2, GABRb1	Abnormal sleep pattern	415
Ghrelin	Abnormal sleep pattern, homeostasis	416
Glra1 (glycine receptor)	Long sleep times, anesthetic sensitivity	417
Histamine 1 receptor	Abnormal NREM sleep	418

Table 12.2 (Continued)

Name of gene	Sleep effect	Reference
Kcnma1	Circadian rhythm	419
Kv 3.1 and 3.3	Fragmented NREM, long duration REM	420
Kv 1.2	Decreased NREM sleep	421
Leptin	Altered sleep regulation	368
M3/M2 receptors	Decreased REM/altered theta activity	422
MAOA	Decreased ethanol-induced sleep	423
Mat2a	Circadian rhythm	424
Math5	Circadian entrainment defects	425
MOP3	Circadian rhythm	403
Mtap6	Circadian rhythm	426
NPAS 2	Abnormal sleep and circadian patterns	427
NPY 1/2 receptors	Abnormal sleep pattern/REM	428
Rev-erbα	Circadian rhythms	429
Opn4	Circadian rhythm (entrainment)	430
Per1, 2, 3	Circadian rhythm	431 432
PGD2	Rebound sleep effects	433
PKR2	Circadian rhythm (output)	434
PRF1	Circadian rhythm	435
Rab3a	Circadian activity/sleep homeostasis	436
Slc6a4 (SERT)	Abnormal sleep pattern	437
SXR	Abnormal sleep pattern	438
Glra1 (glycine receptor)	Long sleep times, anesthetic sensitivity	417
TNF R	Decreased REM, increased NREM	439
TSHR	Abnormal sleep pattern	440
VPAC2	Circadian disruption	441
Wocko	Circadian activity	442

Human Studies

Potential genetic determinants of human sleep began with descriptive studies in monozygotic and dizygotic twins when Webb and Campbell[443] recorded 14 identical and 14 fraternal young adult twin pairs during one night of sleep. Sleep onset latencies, awakenings during sleep, sleep stage changes, and REM amounts were significantly correlated in identical twins but not between fraternal twins. Linkowski, Mendlewicz and their colleagues provided the most comprehensive studies of sleep in monozygotic and dizygotic twins by recording full polysomnography over repeated nights to find strong genetic influence on Stages III and IV sleep.[444,445] Genetic effects on REM sleep were inconclusive, and no genetic effects were found for total sleep, period of sleep, sleep onset, or REM latency. Unfortunately, the relatively small sample size of the studies precludes any firm conclusions about the genetic control of other sleep/wake traits. Indeed, the entire field suffers a lack of genetic human association studies on sufficiently large populations ($\approx$1000 individuals) to foster meaningful discussion regarding whether or not specific genomic regions are associated with specific sleep/wake traits. However, a recent association study involving a self-completion sleep questionnaire[446] indicates that such information may be available in the near future.

In support of the twin data for the genetic control of human sleep are studies that have quantified inter-individual variability on standard polysomnogram (PSG)-assessed variables of sleep structure in a controlled laboratory environment. For these studies, inter-individual variability is compared across sleep nights either under-baseline or under-sleep deprivation conditions to evaluate the stability, robustness, or magnitude of the sleep/wake trait. One recent study[447] revealed considerable trait inter-individual variability for almost all of the 18 PSG-assessed sleep variables, which confirmed earlier work indicating individual variability using fewer traits or less comprehensive methods of analysis. Individual sleep trait studies are often criticized as influenced by environmental factors, habit formations, traits acquired in development, or developed over the course of a lifetime. However, trait variability between individuals in the context of similar trait variability between strains of inbred mice suggests at least partial genetic control of human individual differences for sleep/wake traits.

CANDIDATE GENES FOR SLEEP/WAKE TRAITS

As noted earlier in this review, a number of neurochemicals (e.g., cytokines), neuropeptides (e.g., hypocretin), neurotransmitter (e.g., GABA), and other molecules (e.g., adenosine) have been implicated in either the regulation of sleep or wake and/or the response to sleep deprivation. Thus, many genes can be expected to ultimately be involved in the regulation of the sleep/wake cycle. However, the fact that there are multiple neurotransmitters, receptors, molecules, etc. involved in regulating sleep/wake states does not mean there is not a "core" molecular-genetic control network acting at the cellular level, which regulates fundamental sleep/wake traits. By analogy, the circadian clock system in the SCN contains a vast array of neurochemicals, neurotransmitters and neuropeptides,[448] and an alteration in any one of these may influence overall circadian timing. However, these molecules do not represent the molecular circadian clock itself; instead, the core molecular circadian clock consists of an intracellular transcriptional-translational feedback loop(s) that can generate 24 h signals at the intracellular level.[449] Are there similar core molecular networks that underlie genetically controlled sleep/wake traits such as total wake time, duration of REM bouts, SWA, etc.? Indeed, the analogy with the circadian clock system is particularly appropriate for sleep/wake traits as a number of circadian clock genes themselves have emerged as important genetic components for multiple aspects of sleep and wake regulation.[450]

The first mammalian circadian clock gene was discovered in a forward mutagenesis program in which the heterozygous mutant animal had a circadian period 1 h longer than wild-type mice while homozygous animals had a circadian period in constant darkness of about 27–28 h, and the activity rhythm of these animals often deteriorated into arrhythmicity.[449] While the mutant gene, *Clock*, was expected to alter the period of the sleep/wake cycle since it altered the period of the rest-activity cycle based on locomotor activity,[449] unexpectedly, when sleep/wake patterns were examined, we (FT) found that *Clock/Clock* mice exhibit a high amount of wake time (+1–2 h/day versus wild-type mice) with a reciprocal decrease in NREM sleep time under both 12:12 L:D and constant dark conditions.[451] Furthermore, following short-term sleep deprivation, the homozygous Clock mutant recover less REM sleep time compared to wild-type mice. These data represented the first demonstration that an alteration in the function of a core circadian clock gene could have a direct impact on the amount of sleep produced and on the recovery response to sleep loss, and opened the door to further inquiries into how circadian clock genes might influence the sleep/wake cycle at many levels.[450]

Subsequent studies of sleep in mice deficient in one or more core circadian clock genes showed an altered response to sleep deprivation including diminished duration, consolidation, or EEG delta power.[452,453] The relatively recent finding that transcriptional-translational feedback loop(s) of known circadian clock genes exist in many areas of brain and peripheral tissues[454] raises the possibility that circadian clock genes are influencing sleep/wake traits independently of any alterations at the level of the SCN. Furthermore, there is now extensive evidence linking circadian clock genes with metabolic molecular network providing another avenue for how alterations in clock genes could modulate sleep/wake behavior (e.g., by altering energy metabolism, activity levels, endocrine function).[58] For example, we have demonstrated that *Clock* mutant mice develop increased adiposity and symptoms of the metabolic syndrome.[58] Similarly *Bmal1*$^{-/-}$ mice may have altered glucose homeostasis and develop joint disease, which leads to abnormalities in locomotor activity, and the *Bmal1* gene even plays a role in molecular pathways related to adipogenesis.[450] It will be important to gain a better understanding of the multiple molecular pathways in which *Clock*, *Bmal1*, and other circadian genes are involved in sleep and metabolic regulation independent of their core circadian function. Because clock genes have been identified in a variety of central and peripheral tissues, there is likely to be anatomical specificity of function at the physiological and molecular levels for both metabolism and sleep and wakefulness. Indeed, had sleep/wake traits rather than circadian properties (e.g., period of rhythms) first been characterized in mice carrying mutations or deletions in what are now seen as "canonical circadian clock genes," these genes might have been called "canonical sleep genes." Indeed, it may well be that many "core" circadian and sleep genes may turn out to be one and the same genes.

DRUG DISCOVERY AND PHARMACOLOGIC TARGETS FOR THE TREATMENT OF SLEEP DISORDERS

Currently no cures exist for insomnia, sleep apnea, narcolepsy or EDS, so pharmacological treatment for these disorders are symptomatically driven. Insomnia is a worldwide disease of widely varying presentation so the diagnosis rates are low, at perhaps less than 20%, partly because patients are not sufficiently motivated to go their physicians or do so only after failed attempts to self-medicate with alcohol, over-the-counter (OTC), or herbal treatments. Popular self-treatment options include antihistamines, valerian root and other herbs and teas, and OTC melatonin. Recently, there has been increased availability of OTC pain medications combining OTC pain relievers with "sleep aids" – typically antihistamine compounds. The ease and availability of these options make them popular, but their use may mask accurate diagnosis and availability to well-studied scientifically proven treatments.

According to the National Disease and Therapeutic Index for 1987–1996 (recapitulated in Table 12.3), the 10 drugs most often prescribed for insomnia in the United States were (in alphabetical order by generic name): alprazolam, amitriptyline, clonazepam, doxepin, flurazepam, lorazepam, temazepam, trazodone, triazolam, and zolpidem. Of note, only flurazepam, temazepam, triazolam, and zolpidem are approved hypnotics. The remaining listed agents are antidepressants (amitriptiline, doxepin, and trazodone) or anxiolytics (alprazolam, clonazepam, and lorazepam) with sleep-induction side effects. Actions of these compounds are mechanistically similar, but regulatory labeling factors drive the prescribing habits of physicians away from hypnotics toward approved anxiolytic and antidepressant compounds.[301] Approved hypnotic use in the United States is generally limited to nightly administration for 1–2 weeks duration for hypnotics, while compounds with the same mechanism of action that are approved as antidepressants or anxiolytics are not as dose period-limited. Thus, physicians can prescribe more doses of anxiolytics for longer periods of time to benefit a patient suffering chronic insomnia. Dose titration ability for anxiolytics and antidepressants is also much greater than for hypnotics, giving physicians more dose options for treating their patients. Further, concerns around chronic anxiolytic and antidepressant use are not as great as the perceived potential for abuse with chronic hypnotic use – even though the compounds have the same basic activities. When combined with behavioral modifications (e.g., weight loss, sleep hygiene, scheduled naps) sleep pharmacological treatment is more effective for not only the treatment of primary insomnia, but also when insomnia is comorbid with other behavioral disorders including depression (cf., Refs. 455, 458, 459).[ix]

The current classes of hypnotics have focused on efficacy for promoting sleep onset. An unmet medical need in the insomnia market is the absence of drugs that promote sleep maintenance without causing rebound insomnia or next-day residual effects, and improve both subjective and objective measurements of restorative sleep.

[ix]Behavioral therapies are seen as an important adjunct to pharmacological treatment of many disorders. For further discussion please refer to Millan, The discovery and development of pharmacotherapy for psychiatric disorders: a critical survey of animal and translational models, and perspectives for their improvement in this volume.

Table 12.3 Drugs currently in use for the treatment of sleep disorders

Mechanism of action	Generic name	Brand name	FDA approved?
Insomnia			
Benzodiazepines	Alprazolam	Xanax®/Niravam®	
	Clonazepam	Klonopin®	
	Estazolam	ProSom®/Eurodin®	Yes
	Flurazepam	Dalmane®/Dalmadorm®	Yes
	Quazepam	Doral®/Dormalin®	Yes
	Lorazepam	Ativan®/Temesta®	
	Temazepam	Restoril®/Euhypnos®	Yes
	Triazolam	Halcion®/Novodorm®	Yes
GABAergic Non-benzodiazepines	Zapelon	Sonata®	Yes
	Zoldipem	Ambien®	Yes
	Zoldipem CR	Ambien CR®	Yes
	Eszoplicone	Lunesta®	Yes
	Zoplicone	Imovane®	
Melatonin MT$_{1/2}$	Ramelteon	Rozerem®	Yes
Antidepressant TCA	Amitriptiline	Elavil®/Endep®	
	Doxepin	Aponal®/Sinipin®	
Antidepressant SSRI	Trazodone	Desyrel®	
Sleep apnea			
	Modafinil[a]	Provigil®	Yes
Excessive daytime sleepiness/narcolepsy			
	D-amphetamine	Dexedrine®	Yes
	Methylphenidate	Ritalin®	Yes
	Modafinil	Provigil®	Yes
	Sodium oxybate	Xyrem®	Yes

Sources: National Disease and Therapeutic Index for 1987–1996, Atalay[455] and Roth.[456]
[a]*Adjunct therapy for daytime sleepiness associated with sleep apnea.[457]*

By changing the formulation of short-acting non-benzodiazepines to controlled-release forms, some compounds are starting to address the middle/late night insomnia that can occur following the elimination of the compound during the sleep phase (cf., Ambien CR®). While such reformulations address the duration of effect, they do not address problems associated with mechanism of action of these compounds.

Stimulants (modafinil, amphetamines, and methylphenidate) are approved and effective therapy for EDS according to the latest practice parameters issued by the American Academy of Sleep Medicine.[460] Stimulants work by increasing activating neurotransmitter levels across the neuroaxis and with minimal pharmacologic selectivity. Amphetamines and their derivatives increase CNS monoamines by a variety of mechanisms, mainly increased transmitter release and specific uptake inhibition.[461] Global CNS monoamine release increases always promote wakefulness, metabolism, and muscle activity – a necessary set of pharmacologic effects for patients with EDS.

An exception to stimulant treatment for EDS is sodium oxybate (Xyrem®; gamma-hydroxybutyrate). Approved in 2005 for nighttime dosing to increase delta sleep, it has shown some benefit on next-day alertness.[462,463] Sodium oxybate increases SWS and reduces arousals from sleep, suggesting that Xyrem's next-day benefits result from improved post-dosing sleep rather than disease modification. Unfortunately, the half-life of this compound requires twice nightly dosing to assure consistent nocturnal sleep. Both improving nocturnal sleep and promoting daytime wakefulness appear to meet the palliative need to reduce EDS in patients with sleep disorders.

Currently, no pharmacological treatment exists for sleep apnea,[464] although treatment with modafinil appears to be effective in treating the daytime sleepiness associated with sleep apnea.[457]

As discussed above, there is a significant unmet medical need in the sleep disorders therapeutic area due to generally low diagnoses rates, low presentation rates of patients, under-appreciation of the seriousness of the consequences of sleep disorders, fear of withdrawal/tolerance effects and other cultural beliefs about sleep loss and sleep therapeutics. A strong and specific demand exists for drugs with new mechanisms that are non-scheduled, have very clean safety/tolerability profiles, and are approved for long-term use.[x]

Several new mechanisms of action to affect changes in sleep appear to be in clinical development currently that may represent alternative future options for treating insomnia. Anticipated to be available soon are compounds that act as antagonists at the serotonin 2 receptor ($5-HT_{2A}$). These compounds act to suppress stimulatory effects of serotonin at these G-protein-coupled receptors. The compounds ketanserin and ritanserin are $5-HT_{2A}$ preferring compounds that are reported to increase SWS.[465] The benefit of such compounds could be increasing "deep" sleep or SWS that may be associated with both cognitive improvement and subjective feelings of restorative sleep. Uncertain effects on sleep onset are a potential weakness with this mechanism of action, and it will be of interest to see whether these compounds can enhance sleep onset as well as increase sleep maintenance through enhancement of SWS. A combination approach including both a short half-life non-benzodiazepine and $5-HT_{2A}$ compound may provide a better alternative therapeutic approach with both sleep onset and potential for enhancement of SWS.

---

[x] For a further discussion on the regulatory aspects and scheduling of new drugs, please refer to Rocha *et al.*, Development of medications for heroin and cocaine addiction and regulatory aspects of abuse liability testing

Another mechanism of action of compounds entering later phase clinical trials are antagonists of Hypocretin 1 and 2 receptors. Recent data demonstrates the efficacy of these compounds in sleep onset and increased amounts of REM and NREM sleep.[466] Whether Hcrt antagonism can provide long-term unscheduled use along with subjective and objective benefits remains to be seen in longer term studies. Ongoing questions regarding the role of this therapeutic approach (dual orexin receptor antagonism) and the risk of cataplexy/narcolepsy will need to be addressed as these compounds move through larger clinical trials in later stages of development.

HOW TO CHANGE SLEEP PHARMACEUTICAL DISCOVERY

Future sleep and wake-promoting compounds will succeed only by exceeding efficacy of current compounds. The past 100 years of neurophysiology research has only recently focused on small cell groups, like the hypocretin-producing cells, and described their role in modulation of natural sleep. The discovery that genetic alteration of these specific cell groups also caused narcolepsy strongly implicates genetics as the approach most likely to identify underlying mechanisms for other sleep disorders. Even if genetic modifications alone are not sufficient to produce complex sleep disorders like insomnia, single nucleotide polymorphism (SNP)-related propensities towards sleep problems are likely to guide our selection for the next generation of sleep compounds.

Sleep pharmaceutical discovery needs to exceed current efficiencies by going beyond arousal state quantification to include sleep disruption, effects of chronic versus acute responses, and more precise localization of sleep behavior. Locomotion and EEG carried our research for the first 80 years, but today more complex quantification of these signals are being used to detect more precise biologic responses to good or poor quality sleep. For example, discoveries linking slow wave EEG activities to learning[467-469] have provided neurophysiologic support for sleep as a synapse-modifying process in the cortex.[470,471] Sleep processes are likely being recorded at some distance from the sites of sleep's critical action – we just do not know how far.

The consequences of sleep disorders are typically quantified using sleep itself as the critical outcome measure – or worse – subjective reports of sleep. New methods for measurement coupled with advanced algorithmic analysis are launching sleep discovery forward. While we long knew that people could learn without sleep, only recently have we discovered what they cannot learn without sleep[331,472,473] and what compensations are made to mask our behavioral deficiencies during sleep deprivation.[474] Brain imaging to uncover lost or re-directed brain processes during acute and chronic sleep loss informs our need to learn which physiologic measures best index sleep-repairing pharmaceuticals.

Translational sleep measures abound when comparing animal models to human clinical conditions. While the models are not perfect simulations of the sleep disorders, they do capture the EEG and behavioral changes related to natural and experimentally induced poor sleep. But, as described above, today we use a circular logic based on viewing sleep as a homeostatic process to claim that sleep is repaired when sleep is returned to near-baseline levels. Viewing sleep as a physiologic process susceptible to long-term plasticity will force us to both improve our sleep-sensing measures and require us to include chronic monitoring of sleep and wake sequelae before we declare pharmacologic success for modifying sleep patterns. Chronic monitoring using measures and experimental designs amenable to detecting subtle chronic effects are now common in many animal models, but are still very costly to be considered in many clinical studies. The value of long-term epidemiologic studies like the Framingham heart health study will be seen in more accurate measures of efficacy and in providing reverse translational guidance such as human genetics.

CONCLUSIONS

Animal models of normal and disordered sleep necessarily contain the primary endpoints of clinical interest – sleep onset, sleep architecture, and the ability to measure next-day effects (sleepiness, cognition, metabolism, etc.). While comparative studies have quantified which sleep variables are more or less similar between species, these studies tend to be summaries of all day sleeping patterns or the propensity for specific sleep states during specific portions of the circadian cycle. Quantitative polysomnographic assessment of normal sleep and pharmacologic effects of novel compounds on different species find validity for rodents and primates as useful models to predict PK/PD relationships for potential pharmaceuticals in humans (cf., Ref. 475). Respecting cross-species differences does not invalidate animal models for testing sleep pharmaceuticals, but rather points out how evolutionary differences have modified the neural physiology of sleep. Strain differences for sleep responses to stress provide an even better example of how acknowledging, and working with, evoked sleep differences between species as a genetic guide in our selection of animal sleep models and new sleep mechanisms.

Potentially every animal model of a CNS disorder offers an opportunity to examine how sleep pattern modification might alter the pathology of that disorder. For example, both the rat and monkey model for Parkinson's Disease (ICV injection of 6-OHDA and systemic MPTP administration respectively) produces a decrease in wake-period wakefulness and an increase in sleep-period wakefulness as compared with sham-control animals (Doran, unpublished observations[476]).[xi] Like Parkinson's patients, these animals have disrupted sleep, EDS, and evidence for excessive motor activity during sleep. Additionally, animal models of PD appear to produce state dissociations between the neurophysiologic systems monitored using EEG, EOG, and EMG sensors of polysomnography. Improving animal models for any CNS disorder known to disrupt human sleep is a strong candidate for evaluating sleep's translational effects in those animal models.

Mathematical reductions of EEG activity across days of normal or disrupted sleep are the cornerstone of our knowledge that sleep is a homeostatic process in humans.

[xi] Please refer to Merchant *et al.*, Animal models of Parkinson's disease to aid drug discovery and development, in Volume 2, *Neurologic Disorders* for a detailed discussion of animal models of Parkinson's disease.

EEG SWA in human sleep recordings decreases exponentially during normal sleep but starts at higher levels and then decreases more slowly during sleep that follows prolong sleep deprivation (see Ref. 477 for a review). Similarly, numerous species, including rodents (reviewed in Ref. 478) and monkeys[479] show an increase in SWA after short periods of sleep deprivation or sleep disruption. However, both rats[480,481] and monkeys[482] show limited EEG SWA responses to chronic sleep loss. By expecting allostatic changes in sleep processes after chronic experimental or pharmacologic manipulation, we may improve our animal and human models and gather the most accurate information about pathologic arousal state control. Fortunately, technology developments, and the ubiquity of the EEG, allow sleep research to test and treat sleep, and sleep-related disorders like obesity, as chronic problems for which we can monitor the effects of long-term treatments. Ambulatory polysomnography in patient's homes is an .example of how human clinical studies are ready to mirror the long-term telemetry recordings already common in many animal sleep laboratories.

Animal models of sleep, including changes in sleep due to age and disease, are a versatile set of laboratory tools to help uncover both the neurophysiology of arousal state control and the daytime complaints arising from a variety of medical disorders. Sleep measurements are fully translatable across multiple phyla. Pharmacologic changes in sleep and EEG patterns are variable between species but the abundance of species available allows species-specific pharmacologic differences to be isolated for discovery rather than viewed as an impediment to translation. Sleep naturally crosses all disciplines of physiology and neuroscience. Such ubiquity makes animal models of sleep easily accessible and discernible scientific methods for improving human health.

WHERE ARE THE NOVEL MEDICINES?

There are many issues to be considered and hurdles to overcome in the development of novel sleep therapeutics. Not least among these is the importance of establishing alternative measures to traditional efficacy measurements that more adequately capture the benefits that novel agents might uniquely provide to sleep and wakefulness. Current expectations of efficacy for novel insomnia treatments are improved subjective and objective measures of sleep onset. These expectations are based on comparing sedation induced by novel mechanisms to standard non-benzodiazepine effects of traditional compounds. Non-benzodiazepines have been engineered to minimize impact on next-day cognitive functioning by designing compounds with short half-lives and rapid onset to produce fast sleep onset but clearance before awakening. Although these compounds provide objective and subjective data for rapid sleep onset (and increased maintenance when formulated appropriately), it is unclear whether they are returning normal sleep to insomniac patients.

Understanding and capitalizing on the functional benefits of improved sleep architecture should be the driving force for novel sleep drug discovery. Unfortunately, based on expense and time required to screen multiple mechanisms for effects on sleep and our lack of understanding of specific health consequences of insomnia versus other sleep disorders, it is difficult to ascertain which clinical measures should be the focus of insomnia drug development. Clearly, effects on mood and cognition are linked to poor sleep (see above), but the physiologic systems that impact these outcome measures are unclear so we are left with crude animal measures of sleep to predict the vagaries of the human mood and subjective experience. A better understanding of specific correlations between sleep architecture and functional outcomes should drive drug discovery. Future drug discovery still needs to account for aging and disease processes because functional benefits of improved sleep architecture may be age-limited by residual "plasticity" of the CNS. For neurodegenerative diseases where sleep effects are abundant, even the best sleep compounds might not be able to generate benefit because sleep or wake-promoting networks might be damaged or permanently compromised in these patients.

New efforts to bring novelty to pharmacological sleep disorder treatment will require: (1) novel measures for objectively diagnosing sleep disorders, (2) quantifying the restorative efficacy of sleep, (3) easily obtained measures to demonstrate that ideal sleep "quality" has been attained, and (4) showing functional "life" changes of the resultant sleep changes benefiting patients. Until we understand the functional links between sleep architecture and effects on immune, CNS, mood, and metabolic function, we cannot adequately construct experiments able to measure progress towards these goals. It is likely that we will uncover the physiology/functional links through novel genetic approaches by revealing genetic networks and regulatory systems controlling sleep and wake. With this knowledge, we may be able to determine the "best" translational measures of sleep.

ACKNOWLEDGMENTS

The authors would like to thank all respective laboratory personnel and colleagues (too numerous to mention) who contributed to the original work described in this chapter. We also thank Anthony Gotter and Chris Winrow for help with Table 12.2, and Susan Garson for help with references. Preparation of this chapter supported in part by NIH RO1 HL/MH59658, RO1MH61755, and RO1AG020584.

REFERENCES

1. American Academy of Sleep Medicine. (2001). *International Classification of Sleep Disorders, Revised: Diagnostic and Coding Manual*. American Academy of Sleep Medicine, Rochester, MN.
2. Partinen, M. and Hublin, C. (2000). Epidemiology of sleep disorders. In Kryger, M.H., Roth, T., and Dement, W.C. (eds.), *Principles and Practice of Sleep Medicine*. W.B. Saunders, Philadelphia, pp. 558–579.
3. Hossain, J.L. and Shapiro, C.M. (2002). The prevalence, cost implications, and management of sleep disorders: An overview. *Sleep Breath*, 6(2):85–102.
4. Walsh, J.K. (2004). Clinical and socioeconomic correlates of insomnia. *J Clin Psychiatry*, 65(Suppl 8):13–19.
5. Buysse, D.J. (2005). Insomnia state of the science: An evolutionary, evidence-based assessment. *Sleep*, 28(9):1045–1046.

6. Ford, D.E. and Kamerow, D.B. (1989). Epidemiologic study of sleep disturbances and psychiatric disorders. An opportunity for prevention?. *JAMA*, 262(11):1479-1484.

7. Hajak, G. (2000). Insomnia in primary care. *Sleep*, 23(Suppl 3):S54-sS63.

8. Hohagen, F. *et al.* (1993). Prevalence and treatment of insomnia in general practice. A longitudinal study. *Eur Arch Psychiatry Clin Neurosci*, 242(6):329-336.

9. Leger, D. *et al.* (2000). Prevalence of insomnia in a survey of 12,778 adults in France. *J Sleep Res*, 9(1):35-42.

10. Chilcott, L.A. and Shapiro, C.M. (1996). The socioeconomic impact of insomnia. An overview. *Pharmacoeconomics*, 10(Suppl 1):1-14.

11. Leger, D. (1994). The cost of sleep-related accidents: A report for the National Commission on Sleep Disorders Research. *Sleep*, 17(1):84-93.

12. Leger, D., Levy, E., and Paillard, M. (1999). The direct costs of insomnia in France. *Sleep*, 22(Suppl 2):S394-S401.

13. Stoller, M.K. (1994). Economic effects of insomnia. *Clin Ther*, 16(5):873-897. discussion 854

14. Walsh, J.K. and Engelhardt, C.L. (1999). The direct economic costs of insomnia in the United States for 1995. *Sleep*, 22(Suppl 2):S386-S393.

15. Hajak, G. (2001). Epidemiology of severe insomnia and its consequences in Germany. *Eur Arch Psychiatry Clin Neurosci*, 251(2):49-56.

16. Novak, M. *et al.* (2004). Increased utilization of health services by insomniacs – an epidemiological perspective. *J Psychosom Res*, 56(5):527-536.

17. Simon, G.E. and VonKorff, M. (1997). Prevalence, burden, and treatment of insomnia in primary care. *Am J Psychiatry*, 154(10):1417-1423.

18. Roth, T. (2005). Prevalence, associated risks, and treatment patterns of insomnia. *J Clin Psychiatry*, 66(Suppl 9):10-13.

19. Roth, T. (2001). The relationship between psychiatric diseases and insomnia. *Int J Clin Pract Suppl*(116):3-8.

20. Culpepper, L. (2005). Insomnia: A primary care perspective. *J Clin Psychiatry*, 66(Suppl 9):14-17.

21. Schramm, E. *et al.* (1995). Mental comorbidity of chronic insomnia in general practice attenders using DSM-III-R. *Acta Psychiatr Scand*, 91(1):10-17.

22. Stores, G. and Crawford, C. (1998). Medical student education in sleep and its disorders. *J R Coll Physicians Lond*, 32(2):149-153.

23. American Psychiatric Association. (1994). *Diagnostic and Statistical Manual of Mental Disorders*, 4th edition. American Psychiatric Association, Washington, DC.

24. World Health Organization. (1992). *The ICD-10 classification of mental and behavioral disorder: Diagnostic criteria for research*. World Health Organization, Geneva.

25. Kupfer, D.J. *et al.* (1984). Application of automated REM and slow wave sleep analysis: I. Normal and depressed subjects. *Psychiatry Res*, 13(4):325-334.

26. Kupfer, D.J. *et al.* (1985). Electroencephalographic sleep of younger depressives. Comparison with normals. *Arch Gen Psychiatry*, 42(8):806-810.

27. Roth, T. and Ancoli-Israel, S. (1999). Daytime consequences and correlates of insomnia in the United States: Results of the 1991 National Sleep Foundation Survey. II. *Sleep*, 22(Suppl 2):S354-S358.

28. Mellinger, G.D., Balter, M.B., and Uhlenhuth, E.H. (1985). Insomnia and its treatment. Prevalence and correlates. *Arch Gen Psychiatry*, 42(3):225-232.

29. Terzano, M.G. *et al.* (2004). Studio Morfeo: Insomnia in primary care, a survey conducted on the Italian population. *Sleep Med*, 5(1):67-75.

30. Wilson, K.G. *et al.* (2002). Major depression and insomnia in chronic pain. *Clin J Pain*, 18(2):77-83.

31. Mallon, L., Broman, J.E., and Hetta, J. (2002). Sleep complaints predict coronary artery disease mortality in males: A 12-year follow-up study of a middle-aged Swedish population. *J Intern Med*, 251(3):207–216.

32. Leppavuori, A. *et al.* (2002). Insomnia in ischemic stroke patients. *Cerebrovasc Dis*, 14(2):90–97.

33. Thase, M.E. (2005). Correlates and consequences of chronic insomnia. *Gen Hosp Psychiatry*, 27(2):100–112.

34. Sateia, M.J. and Nowell, P.D. (2004). Insomnia. *Lancet*, 364(9449):1959–1973.

35. Buysse, D.J. *et al.* (1994). Clinical diagnoses in 216 insomnia patients using the International Classification of Sleep Disorders (ICSD), DSM-IV and ICD-10 categories: A report from the APA/NIMH DSM-IV Field Trial. *Sleep*, 17(7):630–637.

36. Weyerer, S. and Dilling, H. (1991). Prevalence and treatment of insomnia in the community: Results from the Upper Bavarian Field Study. *Sleep*, 14(5):392–398.

37. Katz, D.A. and McHorney, C.A. (2002). The relationship between insomnia and health-related quality of life in patients with chronic illness. *J Fam Pract*, 51(3):229–235.

38. Guilleminault, C. and Bassiri, A. (2005). Clinical features and evaluation of obstructive sleep apnea-hypopnea syndrome and the upper airway resistance syndrome. In Kryger, M.H., Roth, T., and Dement, W.C. (eds.), *Principles and Practices of Sleep Medicine*. Elsevier Saunders, Philadelphia, pp. 1043–1052.

39. Pack, A.I. (2006). Advances in sleep-disordered breathing. *Am J Respir Crit Care Med*, 173(1):7–15.

40. Gozal, D., Daniel, J.M., and Dohanich, G.P. (2001). Behavioral and anatomical correlates of chronic episodic hypoxia during sleep in the rat. *J Neurosci*, 21(7):2442–2450.

41. Peppard, P.E. *et al.* (2000). Prospective study of the association between sleep-disordered breathing and hypertension. *N Engl J Med*, 342(19):1378–1384.

42. Young, T. *et al.* (1997). Population-based study of sleep-disordered breathing as a risk factor for hypertension. *Arch Intern Med*, 157(15):1746–1752.

43. Punjabi, N.M. *et al.* (2003). Sleep-disordered breathing, glucose intolerance, and insulin resistance. *Respir. Physiol Neurobiol*, 136(2–3):167–178.

44. Punjabi, N.M. and Polotsky, V.Y. (2005). Disorders of glucose metabolism in sleep apnea. *J Appl Physiol*, 99(5):1998–2007.

45. Punjabi, N.M. *et al.* (2004). Sleep-disordered breathing, glucose intolerance, and insulin resistance: The Sleep Heart Health Study. *Am J Epidemiol*, 160(6):521–530.

46. Benca, R.M. (2007). Narcolepsy and excessive daytime sleepiness: Diagnostic considerations, epidemiology, and comorbidities. *J Clin Psychiatry*, 68(Suppl 13):5–8.

47. Zeman, A. *et al.* (2004). Narcolepsy and excessive daytime sleepiness. *BMJ*, 329(7468): 724–728.

48. Silber, M.H. *et al.* (2002). The epidemiology of narcolepsy in Olmsted County, Minnesota: A population-based study. *Sleep*, 25(2):197–202.

49. Ohayon, M.M. *et al.* (2002). Prevalence of narcolepsy symptomatology and diagnosis in the European general population. *Neurology*, 58(12):1826–1833.

50. Longstreth, W.T., Jr *et al.* (2007). The epidemiology of narcolepsy. *Sleep*, 30(1):13–26.

51. Nishino, S. *et al.* (2000). Hypocretin (orexin) deficiency in human narcolepsy. *Lancet*, 355(9197):39–40.

52. Peyron, C. *et al.* (2000). A mutation in a case of early onset narcolepsy and a generalized absence of hypocretin peptides in human narcoleptic brains. *Nat Med*, 6(9):991–997.

53. Nishino, S. (2007). Narcolepsy: Pathophysiology and pharmacology. *J Clin Psychiatry*, 68(Suppl 13):9–15.

54. Baumann, C.R. *et al.* (2006). Hypocretin (orexin) deficiency predicts severe objective excessive daytime sleepiness in narcolepsy with cataplexy. *J Neurol Neurosurg Psychiatry*, 77(3):402–404.

55. Mignot, E. *et al.* (2002). The role of cerebrospinal fluid hypocretin measurement in the diagnosis of narcolepsy and other hypersomnias. *Arch Neurol*, 59(10):1553–1562.

56. Scammell, T.E. *et al.* (2001). Narcolepsy and low CSF orexin (hypocretin) concentration after a diencephalic stroke. *Neurology*, 56(12):1751–1753.

57. Mignot, E. (1998). Genetic and familial aspects of narcolepsy. *Neurology*, 50(2 Suppl 1):S16–S22.

58. Turek, F.W. *et al.* (2005). Obesity and metabolic syndrome in circadian clock mutant mice. *Science*, 308(5724):1043–1045.

59. Ganjavi, H. and Shapiro, C.M. (2007). Hypocretin/Orexin: A molecular link between sleep, energy regulation, and pleasure. *J Neuropsychiatry Clin Neurosci*, 19(4):413–419.

60. Siegel, J.M. (2004). Hypocretin (orexin): Role in normal behavior and neuropathology. *Annu Rev Psychol*, 55:125–148.

61. Scammell, T.E. (2001). Wakefulness: An eye-opening perspective on orexin neurons. *Curr Biol*, 11(19):R769–R771.

62. Bloch, G. and Robinson, G.E. (2001). Chronobiology. Reversal of honeybee behavioural rhythms. *Nature*, 410(6832):1048.

63. Kaiser, W. and Steiner-Kaiser, J. (1983). Neuronal correlates of sleep, wakefulness and arousal in a diurnal insect. *Nature*, 301(5902):707–709.

64. Siegel, J.M. (1995). Phylogeny and the function of REM sleep. *Behav Brain Res*, 69(1–2):29–34.

65. Zhdanova, I.V. *et al.* (2001). Melatonin promotes sleep-like state in zebrafish. *Brain Res*, 903(1–2):263–268.

66. Max, L.W. (1935). Action current responses in deaf-mutes during sleep, sensory stimulation and dreams. *J Comp Physiol [A]*, 19(469):486.

67. Loomis, A.L., Harvey, E.N., and Hobart, G. (1935). Further observations on the potential rhythms of the cerebral cortex during sleep. *Science*, 82(2122):198–200.

68. Loomis, A.L., Harvey, E.N., and Hobart, G. (1935). Potential rhythms of the cerebral cortex during sleep. *Science*, 81(2111):597–598.

69. Kleitman, N. (1963). *Sleep and Wakefulness*. University of Chicago Press, Chicago.

70. Caton, R. (1875). The electric currents of the brain. *British Medical Journal*, 2:278.

71. Berger, H. (1929). šber das Elektroenkephalogramm des Menschen. *Arch Psychiatr Nervenkr*, 87:527–570.

72. Dement, W. (1958). The occurrence of low voltage, fast, electroencephalogram patterns during behavioral sleep in the cat. *Electroencephalogr Clin Neurophysiol*, 10(2):291–296.

73. Aserinsky, E. and Kleitman, N. (1953). Regularly occurring periods of eye motility, and concomitant phenomena, during sleep. *Science*, 118(3062):273–274.

74. Parmeggiani, P.L. (2005). Physiologic regulation in sleep. In Kryger, M.H., Roth, T., and Dement, W.C. (eds.), *Principles and Practices of Sleep Medicine*. Elsevier Saunders, Philadelphia, pp. 185–191.

75. Schenck, C.H. *et al.* (1986). Chronic behavioral-disorders of human REM sleep-a new category of parasomnia. *Sleep*, 9(2):293–308.

76. Schenck, C.H. *et al.* (1987). Rapid eye movement sleep behavior disorder. A treatable parasomnia affecting older adults. *JAMA*, 257(13):1786–1789.

77. Cooley, J.W. and Tukey, J.W. (1965). An algorithm for the machine calculation of complex Fourier series. *Math Comput*, 19:297–301.

78. Borbely, A.A. (1982). A two process model of sleep regulation. *Hum Neurobiol*, 1(3):195–204.

79. Bremer, F. (1935). Cerveau "isole" et physiologie du sommeil. *Comptes Rendus de la Societe de Biologie (Paris)*, 118:1235–1241.

80. Moruzzi, G. and Magoun, H.W. (1949). Brain stem reticular formation and activation of the EEG. *Electroencephalography and Clinical Neurophysiology*, 1:455–473.

81. Batini, C. *et al.* (1958). Presistent patterns of wakefulness in the pretrigeminal midpontine preparation. *Science*, 128(3314):30–32.

82. Hess, W.R. (1925). Über die Wechselbeziehungen zwischen psychischen und vegetativen Funktionen. *Schweiz Arch Neurol Psychiat*, 16:36–55.

83. Eguchi, K. and Satoh, T. (1980). Characterization of the neurons in the region of solitary tract nucleus during sleep. *Physiol Behav*, 24(1):99–102.

84. von Economo, C. (1930). Sleep as a problem of localization. *J Nerv Ment Dis*, 71(3):249–259.

85. Nauta, W.J.H. (1946). Hypothalamic regulation of sleep in rats. An experimental study. *J Neurophysiol*, 9:285–316.

86. McGinty, D.J. and Sterman, M.B. (1968). Sleep suppression after basal forebrain lesions in the cat. *Science*, 160(833):1253–1255.

87. Sterman, M.B. and Clemente, C.D. (1962). Forebrain inhibitory mechanisms: Sleep patterns induced by basal forebrain stimulation in the behaving cat. *Exp Neurol*, 6:103–117.

88. Swett, C.P. and Hobson, J.A. (1968). The effects of posterior hypothalamic lesions on behavioral and electrographic manifestations of sleep and waking in cats. *Arch Ital Biol*, 106(3):283–293.

89. Ranson, S.W. (1939). Somnolence caused by hypothalamic lesions in the monkey. *Arch Neurol Psychiat*, 41(1):1–23.

90. Watanabe, T. *et al.* (1984). Distribution of the histaminergic neuron system in the central nervous system of rats: A fluorescent immunohistochemical analysis with histidine decarboxylase as a marker. *Brain Res*, 295(1):13–25.

91. Lin, J.S. *et al.* (1989). A critical role of the posterior hypothalamus in the mechanisms of wakefulness determined by microinjection of muscimol in freely moving cats. *Brain Res*, 479(2):225–240.

92. Stephan, F.K. and Zucker, I. (1972). Circadian rhythms in drinking behavior and locomotor activity of rats are eliminated by hypothalamic lesions. *Proc Natl Acad Sci USA*, 69(6):1583–1586.

93. Moore, R.Y. and Eichler, V.B. (1972). Loss of a circadian adrenal corticosterone rhythm following suprachiasmatic lesions in the rat. *Brain Res*, 42(1):201–206.

94. Mouret, J. *et al.* (1978). Suprachiasmatic nuclei lesions in the rat: Alterations in sleep circadian rhythms. *Electroencephalogr Clin Neurophysiol*, 45(3):402–408.

95. Ibuka, N. and Kawamura, H. (1975). Loss of circadian rhythm in sleep-wakefulness cycle in the rat by suprachiasmatic nucleus lesions. *Brain Res*, 96(1):76–81.

96. Ibuka, N., Inouye, S.I., and Kawamura, H. (1977). Analysis of sleep-wakefulness rhythms in male rats after suprachiasmatic nucleus lesions and ocular enucleation. *Brain Res*, 122(1):33–47.

97. de Lecea, L. *et al.* (1998). The hypocretins: Hypothalamus-specific peptides with neuroexcitatory activity. *Proc Natl Acad Sci USA*, 95(1):322–327.

98. Sakurai, T. *et al.* (1998). Orexins and orexin receptors: A family of hypothalamic neuropeptides and G protein-coupled receptors that regulate feeding behavior [see comments]. *Cell*, 92(4):573–585.

99. Peyron, C. *et al.* (1997). Distribution of immunoreactive neurons and fibers for a hypothalamic neuropeptide precursor related to secretin. *Soc Neurosci Abs*, 23:2032.

100. Sutcliffe, J.G. *et al.* (1997). Two novel hypothalamic peptides related to secretin derived from a single neuropeptide precursor. *Soc Neurosci Abs*, 23:2032.

101. Peyron, C. *et al.* (1998). Neurons containing hypocretin (orexin) project to multiple neuronal systems. *J Neurosci*, 18(23):9996–10015.

102. Nambu, T. *et al.* (1999). Distribution of orexin neurons in the adult rat brain. *Brain Res*, 827(1–2):243–260.

103. Chen, C.T. *et al.* (1999). Orexin A-like immunoreactivity in the rat brain. *Neurosci Lett*, 260(3):161-164.

104. Harrison, T.A. *et al.* (1999). Hypothalamic orexin A-immunoreactive neurons project to the rat dorsal medulla. *Neurosci Lett*, 273(1):17-20.

105. Date, Y. *et al.* (1999). Orexins, orexigenic hypothalamic peptides, interact with autonomic, neuroendocrine and neuroregulatory systems. *Proc Natl Acad Sci USA*, 96(2): 748-753.

106. van den Pol, A.N. (1999). Hypothalamic hypocretin (orexin): Robust innervation of the spinal cord. *J Neurosci*, 19(8):3171-3182.

107. Horvath, T.L. *et al.* (1999). Hypocretin (orexin) activation and synaptic innervation of the locus coeruleus noradrenergic system. *J Comp Neurol*, 415:145-159.

108. Hagan, J.J. *et al.* (1999). Orexin A activates locus coeruleus cell firing and increases arousal in the rat. *Proc Natl Acad Sci USA*, 96(19):10911-10916.

109. Sakurai, T. *et al.* (2005). Input of orexin/hypocretin neurons revealed by a genetically encoded tracer in mice. *Neuron*, 46(2):297-308.

110. Yoshida, K. *et al.* (2005). Afferents to the orexin neurons of the rat brain. *J Comp Neurol*, 494(5):845-861.

111. Soffin, E.M. *et al.* (2002). SB-334867-A antagonises orexin mediated excitation in the locus coeruleus. *Neuropharmacology*, 42(1):127-133.

112. Liu, R.J., van den Pol, A.N., and Aghajanian, G.K. (2002). Hypocretins (orexins) regulate serotonin neurons in the dorsal raphe nucleus by excitatory direct and inhibitory indirect actions. *J Neurosci*, 22(21):9453-9464.

113. Brown, R.E. *et al.* (2001). Orexin A excites serotonergic neurons in the dorsal raphe nucleus of the rat. *Neuropharmacology*, 40(3):457-459.

114. Yamanaka, A. *et al.* (2002). Orexins activate histaminergic neurons via the orexin 2 receptor. *Biochem Biophys Res Commun*, 290(4):1237-1245.

115. Eriksson, K.S. *et al.* (2001). Orexin/hypocretin excites the histaminergic neurons of the tuberomammillary nucleus. *J Neurosci*, 21(23):9273-9279.

116. Bayer, L. *et al.* (2001). Orexins (hypocretins) directly excite tuberomammillary neurons. *Eur J Neurosci*, 14(9):1571-1575.

117. Takahashi, K. *et al.* (2002). Effects of orexin on the laterodorsal tegmental neurons. *Psychiatry Clin Neurosci*, 56(3):335-336.

118. Burlet, S., Tyler, C.J., and Leonard, C.S. (2002). Direct and indirect excitation of laterodorsal tegmental neurons by hypocretin/orexin peptides: Implications for wakefulness and narcolepsy. *J Neurosci*, 22(7):2862-2872.

119. Eggermann, E. *et al.* (2001). Orexins/hypocretins excite basal forebrain cholinergic neurons. *Neuroscience*, 108(2):177-181.

120. Korotkova, T.M. *et al.* (2003). Excitation of ventral tegmental area dopaminergic and nondopaminergic neurons by orexins/hypocretins. *J Neurosci*, 23(1):7-11.

121. Borgland, S.L. *et al.* (2006). Orexin A in the VTA is critical for the induction of synaptic plasticity and behavioral sensitization to cocaine. *Neuron*, 49(4):589-601.

122. van den Pol, A.N. *et al.* (1998). Presynaptic and postsynaptic actions and modulation of neuroendocrine neurons by a new hypothalamic peptide, hypocretin/orexin. *J Neurosci*, 18(19):7962-7971.

123. Tamura, T. *et al.* (1999). Orexins, orexigenic hypothalamic neuropeptides, suppress the pulsatile secretion of luteinizing hormone in ovariectomized female rats. *Biochem Biophys Res Commun*, 264(3):759-762.

124. Pu, S. *et al.* (1998). Orexins, a novel family of hypothalamic neuropeptides, modulate pituitary luteinizing hormone secretion in an ovarian steroid-dependent manner. *Regul Pept*, 78(1-3):133-136.

125. Mitsuma, T. *et al.* (1999). Effects of orexin A on thyrotropin-releasing hormone and thyrotropin secretion in rats. *Horm Metab Res*, 31(11):606–609.

126. Lopez, M. *et al.* (1999). Orexin receptors are expressed in the adrenal medulla of the rat. *Endocrinology*, 140(12):5991–5994.

127. Shirasaka, T. *et al.* (1999). Sympathetic and cardiovascular actions of orexins in conscious rats. *Am J Physiol*, 277(6 Pt 2):R1780–R1785.

128. Samson, W.K. *et al.* (1999). Cardiovascular regulatory actions of the hypocretins in brain. *Brain Res*, 831(1–2):248–253.

129. Kunii, K. *et al.* (1999). Orexins/hypocretins regulate drinking behaviour. *Brain Res*, 842(1):256–261.

130. Takahashi, N. *et al.* (1999). Stimulation of gastric acid secretion by centrally administered orexin-A in conscious rats. *Biochem Biophys Res Commun*, 254(3):623–627.

131. Chemelli, R.M. *et al.* (1999). Narcolepsy in orexin knockout mice: Molecular genetics of sleep regulation. *Cell*, 98(4):437–451.

132. Lin, L. *et al.* (1999). The sleep disorder canine narcolepsy is caused by a mutation in the hypocretin (orexin) receptor 2 gene. *Cell*, 98(3):365–376.

133. Hara, J. *et al.* (2001). Genetic ablation of orexin neurons in mice results in narcolepsy, hypophagia, and obesity. *Neuron*, 30(2):345–354.

134. Gerashchenko, D. *et al.* (2001). Hypocretin-2-saporin lesions of the lateral hypothalamus produce narcoleptic-like sleep behavior in the rat. *J Neurosci*, 21(18):7273–7283.

135. Gerashchenko, D. *et al.* (2003). Effects of lateral hypothalamic lesion with the neurotoxin hypocretin-2-saporin on sleep in Long-Evans rats. *Neuroscience*, 116(1):223–235.

136. Willie, J.T. *et al.* (2003). Distinct narcolepsy syndromes in Orexin receptor-2 and Orexin null mice: Molecular genetic dissection of Non-REM and REM sleep regulatory processes. *Neuron*, 38(5):715–730.

137. Kilduff, T.S. and Peyron, C. (2000). The hypocretin/orexin ligand-receptor system: Implications for sleep and sleep disorders. *Trends Neurosci*, 23(8):359–365.

138. Nitz, D. and Siegel, J. (1997). GABA release in the dorsal raphe nucleus: Role in the control of REM sleep. *Am J Physiol*, 273(1 Pt 2):R451–R455.

139. Gritti, I., Mainville, L., and Jones, B.E. (1994). Projections of GABAergic and cholinergic basal forebrain and GABAergic preoptic-anterior hypothalamic neurons to the posterior lateral hypothalamus of the rat. *J Comp Neurol*, 339(2):251–268.

140. Gervasoni, D. *et al.* (1998). Electrophysiological evidence that noradrenergic neurons of the rat locus coeruleus are tonically inhibited by GABA during sleep. *Eur J Neurosci*, 10(3):964–970.

141. Nitz, D. and Siegel, J.M. (1997). GABA release in the locus coeruleus as a function of sleep/wake state. *Neuroscience*, 78(3):795–801.

142. Kiyashchenko, L.I. *et al.* (2002). Release of hypocretin (orexin) during waking and sleep states. *J Neurosci*, 22(13):5282–5286.

143. Torterolo, P. *et al.* (2003). Hypocretinergic neurons are primarily involved in activation of the somatomotor system. *Sleep*, 26(1):25–28.

144. Mileykovskiy, B.Y., Kiyashchenko, L.I., and Siegel, J.M. (2005). Behavioral correlates of activity in identified hypocretin/orexin neurons. *Neuron*, 46(5):787–798.

145. Lee, M.G., Hassani, O.K., and Jones, B.E. (2005). Discharge of identified orexin/hypocretin neurons across the sleep-waking cycle. *J Neurosci*, 25(28):6716–6720.

146. Majde, J.A. and Krueger, J.M. (2005). Links between the innate immune system and sleep. *J Allergy Clin Immunol*, 116(6):1188–1198.

147. Krueger, J.M. *et al.* (2001). The role of cytokines in physiological sleep regulation. *Ann N Y Acad Sci*, 933:211–221.

148. Opp, M., Obal, F., Jr, and Krueger, J.M. (1989). Corticotropin-releasing factor attenuates interleukin 1-induced sleep and fever in rabbits. *Am J Physiol*, 257(3 Pt 2):R528–R535.

149. Ehlers, C.L., Reed, T.K., and Henriksen, S.J. (1986). Effects of corticotropin-releasing factor and growth hormone-releasing factor on sleep and activity in rats. *Neuroendocrinology*, 42(6):467–474.

150. Chastrette, N. *et al.* (1990). Proopiomelanocortin (POMC)-derived peptides and sleep in the rat. Part 2 – Aminergic regulatory processes. *Neuropeptides*, 15(2):75–88.

151. Piper, D.C. *et al.* (2000). The novel brain neuropeptide, orexin-A, modulates the sleep-wake cycle of rats. *Eur J Neurosci*, 12(2):726–730.

152. Winsky-Sommerer, R. *et al.* (2004). Interaction between the corticotropin-releasing factor system and hypocretins (orexins): A novel circuit mediating stress response. *J Neurosci*, 24(50):11439–11448.

153. Chastrette, N., Cespuglio, R., and Jouvet, M. (1990). Proopiomelanocortin (POMC)-derived peptides and sleep in the rat. Part 1 – Hypnogenic properties of ACTH derivatives. *Neuropeptides*, 15(2):61–74.

154. Riehl, J. *et al.* (2000). Chronic oral administration of CG-3703, a thyrotropin releasing hormone analog, increases wake and decreases cataplexy in canine narcolepsy. *Neuropsychopharmacology*, 23(1):34–45.

155. Nishino, S. *et al.* (1997). Effects of thyrotropin-releasing hormone and its analogs on daytime sleepiness and cataplexy in canine narcolepsy. *J Neurosci*, 17(16):6401–6408.

156. Broberger, C. and McCormick, D.A. (2005). Excitatory effects of thyrotropin-releasing hormone in the thalamus. *J Neurosci*, 25(7):1664–1673.

157. Hemmeter, U. *et al.* (1998). Effects of thyrotropin-releasing hormone on the sleep EEG and nocturnal hormone secretion in male volunteers. *Neuropsychobiology*, 38(1):25–31.

158. Zini, I. *et al.* (1984). Actions of centrally administered neuropeptide Y on EEG activity in different rat strains and in different phases of their circadian cycle. *Acta Physiol Scand*, 122(1):71–77.

159. Ehlers, C.L. *et al.* (1997). Electrophysiological actions of neuropeptide Y and its analogs: New measures for anxiolytic therapy?. *Neuropsychopharmacology*, 17(1):34–43.

160. Szentirmai, E. and Krueger, J.M. (2006). Central administration of neuropeptide Y induces wakefulness in rats. *Am J Physiol Regul Integr Comp Physiol*, 291(2):R473–R480.

161. Antonijevic, I.A. *et al.* (2000). Neuropeptide Y promotes sleep and inhibits ACTH and cortisol release in young men. *Neuropharmacology*, 39(8):1474–1481.

162. Held, K. *et al.* (2006). Neuropeptide Y (NPY) shortens sleep latency but does not suppress ACTH and cortisol in depressed patients and normal controls. *Psychoneuroendocrinology*, 31(1):100–107.

163. Revell, V.L. and Eastman, C.I. (2005). How to trick mother nature into letting you fly around or stay up all night. *J Biol Rhythms*, 20(4):353–365.

164. Krauchi, K. *et al.* (1997). Early evening melatonin and S-20098 advance circadian phase and nocturnal regulation of core body temperature. *Am J Physiol*, 272(4 Pt 2):R1178–R1188.

165. Wirz-Justice, A. *et al.* (2004). Evening melatonin and bright light administration induce additive phase shifts in dim light melatonin onset. *J Pineal Res*, 36(3):192–194.

166. Revell, V.L. *et al.* (2006). Advancing human circadian rhythms with afternoon melatonin and morning intermittent bright light. *J Clin Endocrinol Metab*, 91(1):54–59.

167. Lewy, A.J. *et al.* (2005). Melatonin entrains free-running blind people according to a physiological dose-response curve. *Chronobiol Int*, 22(6):1093–1106.

168. Verret, L. *et al.* (2003). A role of melanin-concentrating hormone producing neurons in the central regulation of paradoxical sleep. *BMC Neurosci*, 4:19.

169. Hanriot, L. *et al.* (2007). Characterization of the melanin-concentrating hormone neurons activated during paradoxical sleep hypersomnia in rats. *J Comp Neurol*, 505(2):147–157.

170. Roky, R., Valatx, J.L., and Jouvet, M. (1993). Effect of prolactin on the sleep-wake cycle in the rat. *Neurosci Lett*, 156(1–2):117–120.

171. Obal, F., Jr *et al.* (1989). Prolactin, vasoactive intestinal peptide, and peptide histidine methionine elicit selective increases in REM sleep in rabbits. *Brain Res*, 490(2):292–300.

172. Riou, F., Cespuglio, R., and Jouvet, M. (1981). Hypnogenic properties of the vasoactive intestinal polypeptide in rats. *C R Seances Acad Sci III*, 293(12):679–682.

173. Fang, J., Payne, L., and Krueger, J.M. (1995). Pituitary adenylate cyclase activating polypeptide enhances rapid eye movement sleep in rats. *Brain Res*, 686(1):23–28.

174. Ahnaou, A. *et al.* (1999). Long-term enhancement of REM sleep by the pituitary adenylyl cyclase-activating polypeptide (PACAP) in the pontine reticular formation of the rat. *Eur J Neurosci*, 11(11):4051–4058.

175. Ahnaou, A. *et al.* (2000). Muscarinic and PACAP receptor interactions at pontine level in the rat: Significance for REM sleep regulation. *Eur J Neurosci*, 12(12):4496–4504.

176. Sangiah, S. *et al.* (1982). Sleep: Sequential reduction of paradoxical (REM) and elevation of slow-wave (NREM) sleep by a non-convulsive dose of insulin in rats. *Life Sci*, 31(8):763–769.

177. Danguir, J. and Nicolaidis, S. (1984). Chronic intracerebroventricular infusion of insulin causes selective increase of slow wave sleep in rats. *Brain Res*, 306(1–2):97–103.

178. Obal, F., Jr *et al.* (1998). Changes in sleep in response to intracerebral injection of insulin-like growth factor-1 (IFG-1) in the rat. *Sleep Res Online*, 1(2):87–91.

179. Lu, J. *et al.* (2006). A putative flip-flop switch for control of REM sleep. *Nature*, 441(7093):589–594.

180. Daan, S., Beersma, D.G.M., and Borbely, A.A. (1984). Timing of human sleep-recovery process gated by a circadian pacemaker. *American Journal of Physiology*, 246(2):R161–R178.

181. Sterling, P. and Eyer, J. (1988). Allostasis: A new paradigm to explain arousal pathology. In Fisher, S. and Reason, J. (eds.), *Handbook of Life Stress, Cognition and Health*. John Wiley & Sons, New York, pp. 629–649.

182. Van Dongen, H. *et al.* (2003). Trait-like inter-individual differences in the expression of REM sleep. *Sleep*, 26:A51–A51.

183. Price, N.J. *et al.* (2002). Sleep physiology following 88h total sleep deprivation: Effects of recovery sleep duration. *Sleep*, 25:A92–A93.

184. Kim, Y. *et al.* (2007). Sleep response to chronic partial sleep restriction in old rats. *Sleep*, 30:A32–A33.

185. Finelli, L.A. *et al.* (2000). Dual electroencephalogram markers of human sleep homeostasis: Correlation between theta activity in waking and slow-wave activity in sleep. *Neuroscience*, 101(3):523–529.

186. Dinges, D.F., Maislin, G., and Van Dongen, H. (2001). Chronic sleep restriction: Relation of sleep structure to daytime sleepiness and performance. *Sleep*, 24:A28–A29.

187. Dinges, D.F. (2006). The state of sleep deprivation: From functional biology to functional consequences. *Sleep Med Rev*, 10(5):303–305.

188. Carskadon, M.A. and Dement, W.C. (1981). Cumulative effects of sleep restriction on daytime sleepiness. *Psychophysiology*, 18(2):107–113.

189. Carskadon, M.A. and Dement, W.C. (1985). Sleep loss in elderly volunteers. *Sleep*, 8(3):207–221.

190. McEwen, B.S. (2006). Sleep deprivation as a neurobiologic and physiologic stressor: Allostasis and allostatic load. *Metabolism*, 55(10 Suppl 2):S20–S23.

191. Edgar, D.M., Dement, W.C., and Fuller, C.A. (1993). Effect of SCN lesions on sleep in squirrel monkeys: Evidence for opponent processes in sleep-wake regulation. *J Neurosci*, 13(3):1065–1079.

192. Chou, T.C. *et al.* (2002). Afferents to the ventrolateral preoptic nucleus. *J Neurosci*, 22(3):977–990.

193. Abrahamson, E.E., Leak, R.K., and Moore, R.Y. (2001). The suprachiasmatic nucleus projects to posterior hypothalamic arousal systems. *Neuroreport*, 12(2):435–440.

194. Aston-Jones, G. *et al.* (2001). A neural circuit for circadian regulation of arousal. *Nat Neurosci*, 4(7):732–738.
195. Fujiki, N. *et al.* (2001). Changes in CSF hypocretin-1 (orexin A) levels in rats across 24 hours and in response to food deprivation. *Neuroreport*, 12(5):993–997.
196. Zeitzer, J.M. *et al.* (2003). Circadian and homeostatic regulation of hypocretin in a primate model: Implications for the consolidation of wakefulness. *J Neurosci*, 23(8):3555.
197. Geyer, M.A. and Markou, A. (1995). Animal models of psychiatric disorders. In Bloom, F.E. and Kupfer, D.J. (eds.), *Psychopharmacology. The Fourth Generation of Progress*. Raven Press, New York, pp. 787–798.
198. Jouvet, M. (1967). The states of sleep. *Sci Am*, 216(2):62–68.
199. Jouvet, M. (1969). Biogenic amines and the states of sleep. *Science*, 163(862):32–41.
200. Jouvet, M., Michel, F., and Mounier, D. (1960). Comparative electroencephalographic analysis of physiological sleep in the cat and in man. *Rev Neurol (Paris)*, 103:189–205.
201. Steriade, M. (1992). Basic mechanisms of sleep generation. *Neurology*, 42(7 Suppl 6):9–17.
202. Steriade, M., McCormick, D.A., and Sejnowski, T.J. (1993). Thalamocortical oscillations in the sleeping and aroused brain. *Science*, 262(5134):679–685.
203. Morrison, A.R. (1988). Paradoxical sleep without atonia. *Arch Ital Biol*, 126(4):275–289.
204. Morrison, A.R., Sanford, L.D., and Ross, R.J. (2000). The amygdala: A critical modulator of sensory influence on sleep. *Biol Signals Recept*, 9(6):283–296.
205. Lydic, R., McCarley, R.W., and Hobson, J.A. (1983). The time-course of dorsal raphe discharge, PGO waves, and muscle tone averaged across multiple sleep cycles. *Brain Res*, 274(2):365–370.
206. Lydic, R., McCarley, R.W., and Hobson, J.A. (1983). Enhancement of dorsal raphe discharge by medial pontine reticular formation stimulation depends on behavioral state. *Neurosci Lett*, 38(1):35–40.
207. Jouvet, M., Michel, F., and Courjon, J. (1960). EEG study of physiological sleep in the intact, decorticated and chronic mesencephalic cat. *Rev Neurol (Paris)*, 102:309–310.
208. Jouvet, M. and Mounier, D. (1961). Demonstration of nervous structures responsible for rapid cortical activity, in the course of physiological sleep. *J Physiol (Paris)*, 53:379–380.
209. Chase, M.H., McGinty, D.J., and Sterman, M.B. (1968). Cyclic variation in the amplitude of a brain stem reflex during sleep and wakefulness. *Experientia*, 24(1):47–48.
210. Steriade, M., Domich, L., and Oakson, G. (1986). Reticularis thalami neurons revisited: Activity changes during shifts in states of vigilance. *J Neurosci*, 6(1):68–81.
211. Steriade, M., Kitsikis, A., and Oakson, G. (1979). Excitatory-inhibitory processes in parietal association neurons during reticular activation and sleep-waking cycle. *Sleep*, 1(4):339–355.
212. Sterman, M.B. and Clemente, C.D. (1968). Basal forebrain structures and sleep. *Acta Neurol Latinoam*, 14(1):228–244.
213. Sterman, M.B. and Wyrwicka, W. (1967). EEG correlates of sleep: Evidence for separate forebrain substrates. *Brain Res*, 6(1):143–163.
214. Swisher, J.E. (1962). Manifestations of "activated" sleep in the rat. *Science*, 138:1110.
215. Tang, X. *et al.* (2005). Rat strain differences in sleep after acute mild stressors and short-term sleep loss. *Behav Brain Res*, 160(1):60–71.
216. Tang, X., Yang, L., and Sanford, L.D. (2005). Rat strain differences in freezing and sleep alterations associated with contextual fear. *Sleep*, 28(10):1235–1244.
217. Tang, X. and Sanford, L.D. (2005). Home cage activity and activity-based measures of anxiety in 129P3/J, 129 × 1/SvJ and C57BL/6J mice. *Physiol Behav*, 84(1):105–115.
218. Rabat, A. *et al.* (2004). Deleterious effects of an environmental noise on sleep and contribution of its physical components in a rat model. *Brain Res*, 1009(1–2):88–97.
219. Rabat, A. *et al.* (2005). Chronic exposure to an environmental noise permanently disturbs sleep in rats: Inter-individual vulnerability. *Brain Res*, 1059(1):72–82.

220. Murillo-Rodriguez, E. *et al.* (2004). The diurnal rhythm of adenosine levels in the basal forebrain of young and old rats. *Neuroscience*, 123(2):361-370.

221. Carskadon, M.A. and Dement, W.C. (2005). Normal human sleep: An overview. In Kryger, M.H., Roth, T., and Dement, W.C. (eds.), *Principles and Practices of Sleep Medicine*. Elsevier Saunders, Philadelphia, pp. 13-23.

222. Tang, X., Yang, L., and Sanford, L.D. (2007). Individual variation in sleep and motor activity in rats. *Behav Brain Res*, 180(1):62-68.

223. Renger, J.J. *et al.* (2004). Sub-chronic administration of zolpidem affects modifications to rat sleep architecture. *Brain Res*, 1010(1-2):45-54.

224. van Lier, H. *et al.* (2004). Effects of diazepam and zolpidem on EEG beta frequencies are behavior-specific in rats. *Neuropharmacology*, 47(2):163-174.

225. Feinberg, I., Maloney, T., and Campbell, I.G. (2000). Effects of hypnotics on the sleep EEG of healthy young adults: New data and psychopharmacologic implications. *J Psychiatr Res*, 34(6):423-438.

226. Visser, S.A. *et al.* (2003). Dose-dependent EEG effects of zolpidem provide evidence for GABA(A) receptor subtype selectivity in vivo. *J Pharmacol Exp Ther*, 304(3):1251-1257.

227. Patat, A. *et al.* (1994). EEG profile of intravenous zolpidem in healthy volunteers. *Psychopharmacology (Berl)*, 114(1):138-146.

228. Balzamo, E. *et al.* (1977). Nonhuman primates: Laboratory animals of choice for neurophysiologic studies of sleep. *Lab Anim Sci*, 27(5 Pt 2):879-886.

229. Porrino, L.J. *et al.* (2005). Facilitation of task performance and removal of the effects of sleep deprivation by an ampakine (CX717) in nonhuman primates. *PLoS Biol*, 3(9):e299.

230. Adey, W.R., Kado, R.T., and Rhodes, J.M. (1963). Sleep: Cortical and subcortical recordings in the chimpanzee. *Science*, 141:932-933.

231. Freemon, F.R., McNew, J.J., and Adey, W.R. (1969). Sleep of unrestrained chimpanzee: Cortical and subcortical recordings. *Exp Neurol*, 25(1):129-137.

232. Freemon, F.R., McNew, J.J., and Adey, W.R. (1971). Chimpanzee sleep stages. *Electroencephalogr Clin Neurophysiol*, 31(5):485-489.

233. Hanley, J. *et al.* (1968). Chimpanzee performance: Computer analysis of electroencephalograms. *Nature*, 220(5170):879-881.

234. Hanley, J. *et al.* (1969). Combined telephone and radiotelemetry of the EEG. *Electroencephalogr Clin Neurophysiol*, 26(3):323-324.

235. Bert, J. and Pegram, V. (1969). The sleep electroencephalogram in Cercopithecinae: Erythrocerbus patas and Cercopithecus aethiops sabaeus. *Folia Primatol (Basel)*, 11(1):151-159.

236. Adams, P.M. and Barratt, E.S. (1974). Nocturnal sleep in squirrel monkeys. *Electroencephalogr Clin Neurophysiol*, 36(2):201-204.

237. Wexler, D.B. and Moore-Ede, M.C. (1985). Circadian sleep-wake cycle organization in squirrel monkeys. *Am J Physiol*, 248(3 Pt 2):R353-R362.

238. Abelson, J.F. *et al.* (2005). Sequence variants in SLITRK1 are associated with Tourette's Syndrome. *Science*, 310(5746):317-320.

239. Bert, J. (1973). Similarities and differences in the sleep of 2 baboons, Papio hamadryas and Papio papio. *Electroencephalogr Clin Neurophysiol*, 35(2):209-211.

240. Bert, J. *et al.* (1975). The sleep of the baboon, Papio papio, under natural conditions and in the laboratory. *Electroencephalogr Clin Neurophysiol*, 39(6):657-662.

241. Bert, J. *et al.* (1975). Influence of the environment on the regulation of diurnal vigilance in the baboon. *Rev Electroencephalogr Neurophysiol Clin*, 5(4):331-334.

242. Bert, J. *et al.* (1978). Experimental kuru in the rhesus monkey: A study of EEG modifications in the waking state and during sleep. *Electroencephalogr Clin Neurophysiol*, 45(5):611-620.

243. Kripke, D.F. *et al.* (1968). Clinical and laboratory notes. Nocturnal sleep in rhesus monkeys. *Electroencephalogr Clin Neurophysiol*, 24(6):582-586.

244. Lagarde, D. and Milhaud, C. (1990). Electroencephalographic effects of modafinil, an alpha-1-adrenergic psychostimulant, on the sleep of rhesus monkeys. *Sleep*, 13(5):441-448.

245. Crofts, H.S. *et al.* (2001). Investigation of the sleep electrocorticogram of the common marmoset (Callithrix jacchus) using radiotelemetry. *Clin Neurophysiol*, 112(12): 2265-2273.

246. Zweizig, J.R. *et al.* (1967). The design and use of an FM-AM radiotelemetry system for multi-channel recording of biological data. *IEEE Trans Biomed Eng*, 14(4):230-238.

247. Breton, P., Gourmelon, P., and Court, L. (1986). New findings on sleep stage organization in squirrel monkeys. *Electroencephalogr Clin Neurophysiol*, 64(6):563-567.

248. Campbell, S.S. and Tobler, I. (1984). Animal sleep: A review of sleep duration across phylogeny. *Neurosci Biobehav Rev*, 8(3):269-300.

249. Hermant, J.F., Rambert, F.A., and Duteil, J. (1991). Awakening properties of modafinil: Effect on nocturnal activity in monkeys (*Macaca mulatta*) after acute and repeated administration. *Psychopharmacology (Berl)*, 103(1):28-32.

250. Lagarde, D. *et al.* (1995). Interest of modafinil, a new psychostimulant, during a sixty-hour sleep deprivation experiment. *Fundam Clin Pharmacol*, 9(3):271-279.

251. Zhdanova, I.V. *et al.* (2002). Melatonin promotes sleep in three species of diurnal nonhuman primates. *Physiol Behav*, 75(4):523-529.

252. Zhdanova, I.V. *et al.* (1995). Sleep-inducing effects of low doses of melatonin ingested in the evening. *Clin Pharmacol Ther*, 57(5):552-558.

253. Middleton, B., Arendt, J., and Stone, B.M. (1997). Complex effects of melatonin on human circadian rhythms in constant dim light. *J Biol Rhythms*, 12(5):467-477.

254. Yukuhiro, N. *et al.* (2004). Effects of ramelteon (TAK-375) on nocturnal sleep in freely moving monkeys. *Brain Res*, 1027(1-2):59-66.

255. Borja, N.L. and Daniel, K.L. (2006). Ramelteon for the treatment of insomnia. *Clin Ther*, 28(10):1540-1555.

256. Paul, M.A. *et al.* (2004). Sleep-inducing pharmaceuticals: A comparison of melatonin, zaleplon, zopiclone, and temazepam. *Aviat Space Environ Med*, 75(6):512-519.

257. Bliwise, D.L. (1993). Sleep in normal aging and dementia. *Sleep*, 16(1):40-81.

258. Bowersox, S.S., Floyd, T., and Dement, W.C. (1984). Electroencephalogram during sleep in the cat: Age effects on slow-wave activity. *Sleep*, 7(4):380-384.

259. Ho, K.S. and Sehgal, A. (2005). Drosophila melanogaster: An insect model for fundamental studies of sleep. *Methods Enzymol*, 393:772-793.

260. Mendelson, W.B. and Bergmann, B.M. (1999). EEG delta power during sleep in young and old rats. *Neurobiol Aging*, 20(6):669-673.

261. Stone, W.S. (1989). Sleep and aging in animals. Relationships with circadian rhythms and memory. *Clin Geriatr Med*, 5(2):363-379.

262. Takeuchi, T. and Harada, E. (2002). Age-related changes in sleep-wake rhythm in dog. *Behav Brain Res*, 136(1):193-199.

263. Welsh, D.K., Richardson, G.S., and Dement, W.C. (1986). Effect of age on the circadian pattern of sleep and wakefulness in the mouse. *J Gerontol*, 41(5):579-586.

264. Mendelson, W.B. and Bergmann, B.M. (2000). Age-dependent changes in recovery sleep after 48 hours of sleep deprivation in rats. *Neurobiol Aging*, 21(5):689-693.

265. Adam, M. *et al.* (2006). Age-related changes in the time course of vigilant attention during 40 hours without sleep in men. *Sleep*, 29(1):55-57.

266. Blatter, K. *et al.* (2006). Gender and age differences in psychomotor vigilance performance under differential sleep pressure conditions. *Behav Brain Res*, 168(2):312-317.

267. Philip, P. *et al.* (2004). Age, performance and sleep deprivation. *J Sleep Res*, 13(2):105–110.

268. Carrier, J. *et al.* (2001). The effects of age and gender on sleep EEG power spectral density in the middle years of life (ages 20-60 years old). *Psychophysiology*, 38(2):232–242.

269. Cajochen, C. *et al.* (2006). Age-related changes in the circadian and homeostatic regulation of human sleep. *Chronobiol Int*, 23(1–2):461–474.

270. Munch, M. *et al.* (2004). The frontal predominance in human EEG delta activity after sleep loss decreases with age. *Eur J Neurosci*, 20(5):1402–1410.

271. Munch, M. *et al.* (2007). Is homeostatic sleep regulation under low sleep pressure modified by age?. *Sleep*, 30(6):781–792.

272. Ancoli-Israel, S. (2005). Sleep and aging: Prevalence of disturbed sleep and treatment considerations in older adults. *J Clin Psychiatry*, 66(Suppl 9):24–30. quiz 42-3

273. Desarnaud, F. *et al.* (2004). The diurnal rhythm of hypocretin in young and old F344 rats. *Sleep*, 27(5):851–856.

274. Downs, J.L. *et al.* (2007). Orexin neuronal changes in the locus coeruleus of the aging rhesus macaque. *Neurobiol Aging*, 28(8):1286–1295.

275. Manaceine, M. (1897). *Sleep: Its Physiology, Pathology, Hygiene, and Psychology, Contemporary Science Series.* Walter Scott, London.

276. Kleitman, N. (1927). Studies on the physiology of sleep. V. Some experiments on puppies. *Am J Physiol*, 84:386–395.

277. Balzano, S. *et al.* (1990). Effect of total sleep deprivation on 5′-deiodinase activity of rat brown adipose tissue. *Endocrinology*, 127(2):882–890.

278. Rechtschaffen, A. and Bergmann, B.M. (1995). Sleep deprivation in the rat by the disk-over-water method. *Behav Brain Res*, 69(1–2):55–63.

279. Rechtschaffen, A. and Bergmann, B.M. (2002). Sleep deprivation in the rat: An update of the 1989 paper. *Sleep*, 25(1):18–24.

280. Rechtschaffen, A. *et al.* (1989). Sleep deprivation in the rat: X. Integration and discussion of the findings. *Sleep*, 12(1):68–87.

281. Rechtschaffen, A. *et al.* (1983). Physiological correlates of prolonged sleep deprivation in rats. *Science*, 221(4606):182–184.

282. Bast, T.H. and Loevenhart, A.S. (1927). Studies in experimental exhaustion due to lack of sleeo. I. Introduction and methods. *Am J Physiol*, 82:121–126.

283. Cordova, C.A. *et al.* (2006). Sleep deprivation in rats produces attentional impairments on a 5-choice serial reaction time task. *Sleep*, 29(1):69–76.

284. McCoy, J.G. *et al.* (2007). Experimental sleep fragmentation impairs attentional set-shifting in rats. *Sleep*, 30(1):52–60.

285. Zager, A. *et al.* (2007). Effects of acute and chronic sleep loss on immune modulation of rats. *Am J Physiol Regul Integr Comp Physiol*, 293(1):R504–R509.

286. Meerlo, P. *et al.* (2002). Sleep restriction alters the hypothalamic-pituitary-adrenal response to stress. *J Neuroendocrinol*, 14(5):397–402.

287. Dinges, D.F. (2004). Sleep debt and scientific evidence. *Sleep*, 27(6):1050–1052.

288. Allison, K.C. *et al.* (2005). Neuroendocrine profiles associated with energy intake, sleep, and stress in the night eating syndrome. *J Clin Endocrinol Metab*, 90(11):6214–6217.

289. Dinges, D.F. *et al.* (1995). Sleep deprivation and human immune function. *Adv Neuroimmunol*, 5(2):97–110.

290. Dinges, D.F. *et al.* (1994). Leukocytosis and natural killer cell function parallel neurobehavioral fatigue induced by 64 hours of sleep deprivation. *J Clin Invest*, 93(5): 1930–1939.

291. Dickstein, J.B. and Moldofsky, H. (1999). Sleep, cytokines and immune function. *Sleep Med Rev*, 3(3):219–228.

292. Borbely, A.A. *et al.* (1989). Sleep initiation and initial sleep intensity: Interactions of homeostatic and circadian mechanisms. *J Biol Rhythms*, 4(2):149–160.

293. Banks, S. and Dinges, D.F. (2007). Behavioral and physiological consequences of sleep restriction. *J Clin Sleep Med*, 3(5):519-528.

294. Everson, C.A. and Toth, L.A. (2000). Systemic bacterial invasion induced by sleep deprivation. *Am J Physiol Regul Integr Comp Physiol*, 278(4):R905-R916.

295. McKenna, J.T. *et al.* (2007). Sleep fragmentation elevates behavioral, electrographic and neurochemical measures of sleepiness. *Neuroscience*, 146(4):1462-1473.

296. Toth, L.A. and Rehg, J.E. (1998). Effects of sleep deprivation and other stressors on the immune and inflammatory responses of influenza-infected mice. *Life Sci*, 63(8):701-709.

297. Toth, L.A. and Verhulst, S.J. (2003). Strain differences in sleep patterns of healthy and influenza-infected inbred mice. *Behav Genet*, 33(3):325-336.

298. Van Dongen, H.P.A. and Dinges, D.F. (2003). Investigating the interaction between the homeostatic and circadian processes of sleep-wake regulation for the prediction of waking neurobehavioural performance. *J Sleep Res*, 12(3):181-187.

299. Van Dongen, H.P.A. and Dinges, D.F. (2003). Sleep debt and cumulative excess wakefulness. *Sleep*, 26(3):249.

300. Andersen, M.L. *et al.* (2005). Endocrinological and catecholaminergic alterations during sleep deprivation and recovery in male rats. *J Sleep Res*, 14(1):83-90.

301. Roehrs, T. and Roth, T. (2004). Sleep disorders: An overview. *Clin Cornerstone*, 6(Suppl 1C):S6-s16.

302. Nicholson, A.N. *et al.* (1986). Sleep after transmeridian flights. *Lancet*, 2(8517):1205-1208.

303. Michaud, J.C. *et al.* (1982). Mild insomnia induced by environmental perturbations in the rat: A study of this new model and of its possible applications in pharmacological research. *Arch Int Pharmacodyn Ther*, 259(1):93-105.

304. Paterson, L.M. *et al.* (2007). A translational, caffeine-induced model of onset insomnia in rats and healthy volunteers. *Psychopharmacology (Berl)*, 191(4):943-950.

305. Shigemoto, Y. *et al.* (2004). Participation of histaminergic H1 and noradrenergic alpha 1 receptors in orexin A-induced wakefulness in rats. *Brain Res*, 1023(1):121-125.

306. Shinomiya, K. *et al.* (2003). Effects of short-acting hypnotics on sleep latency in rats placed on grid suspended over water. *Eur J Pharmacol*, 460(2-3):139-144.

307. Shinomiya, K. *et al.* (2004). Effects of three hypnotics on the sleep-wakefulness cycle in sleep-disturbed rats. *Psychopharmacology (Berl)*, 173(1-2):203-209.

308. Bonnet, M.H. and Arand, D.L. (1992). Caffeine use as a model of acute and chronic insomnia. *Sleep*, 15(6):526-536.

309. Bonnet, M.H. (1993). Cognitive effects of sleep and sleep fragmentation. *Sleep*, 16(8 Suppl):S65-S67.

310. Hindmarch, I. *et al.* (2000). A naturalistic investigation of the effects of day-long consumption of tea, coffee and water on alertness, sleep onset and sleep quality. *Psychopharmacology (Berl)*, 149(3):203-216.

311. Horne, J.A. and Reyner, L.A. (1996). Counteracting driver sleepiness: Effects of napping, caffeine, and placebo. *Psychophysiology*, 33(3):306-309.

312. Schwierin, B., Borbely, A.A., and Tobler, I. (1996). Effects of N6-cyclopentyladenosine and caffeine on sleep regulation in the rat. *Eur J Pharmacol*, 300(3):163-171.

313. Ising, H. and Kruppa, B. (2004). Health effects caused by noise: Evidence in the literature from the past 25 years. *Noise Health*, 6(22):5-13.

314. Wilkinson, R.T. and Campbell, K.B. (1984). Effects of traffic noise on quality of sleep: Assessment by EEG, subjective report, or performance the next day. *J Acoust Soc Am*, 75(2):468-475.

315. Horne, J.A. *et al.* (1994). A field study of sleep disturbance: Effects of aircraft noise and other factors on 5,742 nights of actimetrically monitored sleep in a large subject sample. *Sleep*, 17(2):146-159.

316. Thiessen, G.J. and Lapointe, A.C. (1983). Effect of continuous traffic noise on percentage of deep sleep, waking, and sleep latency. *J Acoust. Soc Am*, 73(1):225–229.

317. Basner, M., *et al*. (2007). Aircraft noise: Effects on macro- and microstructure of sleep, *Sleep Med*. DOI:10.1016/j.sleep.2007.07.002.

318. Bonnet, M.H. (1986). Performance and sleepiness as a function of frequency and placement of sleep disruption. *Psychophysiology*, 23(3):263–271.

319. Bonnet, M.H. and Arand, D.L. (2003). Clinical effects of sleep fragmentation versus sleep deprivation. *Sleep Med Rev*, 7(4):297–310.

320. Rabat, A. *et al*. (2006). Chronic exposure of rats to noise: Relationship between long-term memory deficits and slow wave sleep disturbances. *Behav Brain Res*, 171(2):303–312.

321. Okuma, T. and Honda, H. (1978). Model insomnia, noise, and methylphenidate, used for the evaluation of hypnotic drugs. *Psychopharmacology (Berl)*, 57(2):127–132.

322. Saletu, B., Grunberger, J., and Sieghart, W. (1985). Nocturnal traffic noise, sleep, and quality of awakening: Neurophysiologic, psychometric, and receptor activity changes after quazepam. *Clin Neuropharmacol*, 8(Suppl 1):S74–S90.

323. Saletu, B. *et al*. (1987). Therapy of multi-infarct dementia with nicergoline: Double-blind, clinical, psychometric and EEG imaging studies with 2 dosage schedules. *Wien Med Wochenschr*, 137(22):513–524.

324. Stone, B.M. *et al*. (2002). Noise-induced sleep maintenance insomnia: Hypnotic and residual effects of zaleplon. *Br J Clin Pharmacol*, 53(2):196–202.

325. Cluydts, R. *et al*. (1995). Antagonizing the effects of experimentally induced sleep disturbance in healthy volunteers by lormetazepam and zolpidem. *J Clin Psychopharmacol*, 15(2):132–137.

326. Pawlyk, A.C. *et al*. (2008). Stress-induced changes in sleep in rodents: Models and mechanisms. *Neurosci Biobehav Rev*, 32(1):99–117.

327. Smith, C. (1985). Sleep states and learning: A review of the animal literature. *Neurosci Biobehav Rev*, 9(2):157–168.

328. Smith, C. (1995). Sleep states and memory processes. *Behav Brain Res*, 69(1–2):137–145.

329. Stickgold, R. (2006). Neuroscience: A memory boost while you sleep. *Nature*, 444(7119):559–560.

330. Stickgold, R. and Walker, M.P. (2005). Sleep and memory: The ongoing debate. *Sleep*, 28(10):1225–1227.

331. Stickgold, R. and Walker, M.P. (2007). Sleep-dependent memory consolidation and reconsolidation. *Sleep Med*, 8(4):331–343.

332. Liu, X., Tang, X., and Sanford, L.D. (2003). Fear-conditioned suppression of REM sleep: Relationship to Fos expression patterns in limbic and brainstem regions in BALB/cJ mice. *Brain Res*, 991(1–2):1–17.

333. Sanford, L.D. *et al*. (2003). Influence of shock training and explicit fear-conditioned cues on sleep architecture in mice: Strain comparison. *Behav Genet*, 33(1):43–58.

334. Sanford, L.D., Yang, L., and Tang, X. (2003). Influence of contextual fear on sleep in mice: A strain comparison. *Sleep*, 26(5):527–540.

335. Sanford, L.D., Fang, J., and Tang, X. (2003). Sleep after differing amounts of conditioned fear training in BALB/cJ mice. *Behav Brain Res*, 147(1–2):193–202.

336. Hendricks, J.C. *et al*. (1987). The English bulldog: A natural model of sleep-disordered breathing. *J Appl Physiol*, 63(4):1344–1350.

337. Schotland, H.M. *et al*. (1996). Quantitative magnetic resonance imaging of upper airways musculature in an animal model of sleep apnea. *J Appl Physiol*, 81(3):1339–1346.

338. Veasey, S.C. *et al*. (2001). The effects of ondansetron on sleep-disordered breathing in the English bulldog. *Sleep*, 24(2):155–160.

339. Ramadan, W. *et al*. (2007). Sleep apnea is induced by a high-fat diet and reversed and prevented by metformin in non-obese rats. *Obesity (Silver Spring)*, 15(6):1409–1418.

340. Brennick, M.J. *et al.* (2006). Phasic respiratory pharyngeal mechanics by magnetic resonance imaging in lean and obese zucker rats. *Am J Respir Crit Care Med*, 173(9):1031–1037.
341. Radulovacki, M., Trbovic, S., and Carley, D.W. (1996). Hypotension reduces sleep apneas in Zucker lean and Zucker obese rats. *Sleep*, 19(10):767–773.
342. Philip, P. *et al.* (2005). An animal model of a spontaneously reversible obstructive sleep apnea syndrome in the monkey. *Neurobiol Dis*, 20(2):428–431.
343. Strollo, P.J., Jr, Atwood, C.W., Jr, and Sanders, M.H. (2005). Medical therapy for obstructive sleep apnea-hypopnea syndrome. In Kryger, M.H., Roth, T., and Dement, W.C. (eds.), *Principles and Practices of Sleep Medicine*. Elsevier Saunders, Philadelphia, pp. 1053–1065.
344. Decker, M.J. *et al.* (2003). Episodic neonatal hypoxia evokes executive dysfunction and regionally specific alterations in markers of dopamine signaling. *Neuroscience*, 117(2):417–425.
345. Gozal, E. *et al.* (2001). Developmental differences in cortical and hippocampal vulnerability to intermittent hypoxia in the rat. *Neurosci Lett*, 305(3):197–201.
346. Row, B.W. *et al.* (2007). Impaired spatial working memory and altered choline acetyltransferase (CHAT) immunoreactivity and nicotinic receptor binding in rats exposed to intermittent hypoxia during sleep. *Behav Brain Res*, 177(2):308–314.
347. Meyers, L. (2005). Sleep apnea and diabetes. *Diabetes Forecast*, 58(7):32.
348. Vgontzas, A.N., Bixler, E.O., and Chrousos, G.P. (2003). Metabolic disturbances in obesity versus sleep apnoea: The importance of visceral obesity and insulin resistance. *J Intern Med*, 254(1):32–44.
349. Iturriaga, R. *et al.* (2006). Chronic intermittent hypoxia enhances carotid body chemosensory responses to acute hypoxia. *Adv Exp Med Biol*, 580:227–232.
350. Gozal, E. *et al.* (2005). Tyrosine hydroxylase expression and activity in the rat brain: Differential regulation after long-term intermittent or sustained hypoxia. *J Appl Physiol*, 99(2):642–649.
351. Veasey, S.C. *et al.* (2004). Long-term intermittent hypoxia in mice: Protracted hypersomnolence with oxidative injury to sleep-wake brain regions. *Sleep*, 27(2):194–201.
352. Gozal, D. and Kheirandish-Gozal, L. (2007). Neurocognitive and behavioral morbidity in children with sleep disorders. *Curr Opin Pulm Med*, 13(6):505–509.
353. Dematteis, M. *et al.* (2007). Intermittent hypoxia induces early functional cardiovascular remodeling in mice. *Am J Respir Crit Care Med*, 177(2):227–235.
354. Tartar, J.L. *et al.* (2006). Hippocampal synaptic plasticity and spatial learning are impaired in a rat model of sleep fragmentation. *Eur J Neurosci*, 23(10):2739–2748.
355. Sforza, E. and Haba-Rubio, J. (2005). Night-to-night variability in periodic leg movements in patients with restless legs syndrome. *Sleep Med*, 6(3):259–267.
356. Sforza, E. *et al.* (1999). EEG and cardiac activation during periodic leg movements in sleep: Support for a hierarchy of arousal responses. *Neurology*, 52(4):786–791.
357. Gozal, D. and Kheirandish-Gozal, L. (2007). Cardiovascular morbidity in obstructive sleep apnea: Oxidative stress, inflammation, and much more. *Am J Respir Crit Care Med*.
358. Everson, C.A. and Crowley, W.R. (2004). Reductions in circulating anabolic hormones induced by sustained sleep deprivation in rats. *Am J Physiol Endocrinol Metab*, 286(6):E1060–E1070.
359. Koban, M. and Swinson, K.L. (2005). Chronic REM-sleep deprivation of rats elevates metabolic rate and increases UCP1 gene expression in brown adipose tissue. *Am J Physiol Endocrinol Metab*, 289(1):E68–E74.
360. Koban, M., Le, W.W., and Hoffman, G.E. (2006). Changes in hypothalamic corticotropin-releasing hormone, neuropeptide Y, and proopiomelanocortin gene expression during chronic rapid eye movement sleep deprivation of rats. *Endocrinology*, 147(1):421–431.
361. Bodosi, B. *et al.* (2004). Rhythms of ghrelin, leptin, and sleep in rats: Effects of the normal diurnal cycle, restricted feeding, and sleep deprivation. *Am J Physiol Regul Integr Comp Physiol*, 287(5):R1071–R1079.

362. Kok, S.W. *et al*. (2003). Hypocretin deficiency in narcoleptic humans is associated with abdominal obesity. *Obes Res*, 11(9):1147–1154.

363. Zhang, S. *et al*. (2007). Sleep/wake fragmentation disrupts metabolism in a mouse model of narcolepsy. *J Physiol*, 581(Pt 2):649–663.

364. Knutson, K.L. *et al*. (2007). The metabolic consequences of sleep deprivation. *Sleep Med Rev*, 11(3):163–178.

365. Spiegel, K. *et al*. (2004). Brief communication: Sleep curtailment in healthy young men is associated with decreased leptin levels, elevated ghrelin levels, and increased hunger and appetite. *Ann Intern Med*, 141(11):846–850.

366. Jenkins, J.B. *et al*. (2006). Sleep is increased in mice with obesity induced by high-fat food. *Physiol Behav*, 87(2):255–262.

367. Minet-Ringuet, J. *et al*. (2004). A tryptophan-rich protein diet efficiently restores sleep after food deprivation in the rat. *Behav Brain Res*, 152(2):335–340.

368. Laposky, A.D. *et al*. (2006). Altered sleep regulation in leptin-deficient mice. *Am J Physiol Regul Integr Comp Physiol*, 290(4):R894–R903.

369. Laposky, A.D., *et al*. (2007). Sleep and circadian rhythms: Key components in the regulation of energy metabolism. *FEBS Lett*.

370. Williams, K.E. *et al*. (2006). Multiple vaccine and pyridostigmine interactions: Effects on EEG and sleep in the common marmoset. *Pharmacol Biochem Behav*, 84(2):282–293.

371. De Saint, H.Z. *et al*. (1997). Active immunization of rats against insulin beta subunits: Effects on sleep and feeding. *Physiol Behav*, 61(5):649–651.

372. Lange, T. *et al*. (2003). Sleep enhances the human antibody response to hepatitis A vaccination. *Psychosom Med*, 65(5):831–835.

373. Spiegel, K., Sheridan, J.F., and Van Cauter, E. (2002). Effect of sleep deprivation on response to immunization. *JAMA*, 288(12):1471–1472.

374. Krueger, J.M., Majde, J.A., and Obal, F. (2003). Sleep in host defense. *Brain Behav Immun*, 17(Suppl 1):S41–S47.

375. Krueger, J.M. and Obal, F., Jr (2003). Sleep function. *Front Biosci*, 8:d511–d519.

376. Medori, R. *et al*. (1992). Fatal familial insomnia, a prion disease with a mutation at codon 178 of the prion protein gene. *N Engl J Med*, 326(7):444–449.

377. Gambetti, P., Parchi, P., and Chen, S.G. (2003). Hereditary Creutzfeldt-Jakob disease and fatal familial insomnia. *Clin Lab Med*, 23(1):43–64.

378. Lugaresi, E. *et al*. (1986). Fatal familial insomnia and dysautonomia with selective degeneration of thalamic nuclei. *N Engl J Med*, 315(16):997–1003.

379. Montagna, P. (2005). Fatal familial insomnia: A model disease in sleep physiopathology. *Sleep Med Rev*, 9(5):339–353.

380. Thannickal, T.C. *et al*. (2000). Reduced number of hypocretin neurons in human narcolepsy. *Neuron*, 27(3):469–474.

381. Maret, S. and Tafti, M. (2005). Genetics of narcolepsy and other major sleep disorders. *Swiss Med Wkly*, 135(45–46):662–665.

382. Cirelli, C., Gutierrez, C.M., and Tononi, G. (2004). Extensive and divergent effects of sleep and wakefulness on brain gene expression. *Neuron*, 41(1):35–43.

383. Cirelli, C. (2002). How sleep deprivation affects gene expression in the brain: A review of recent findings. *J Appl Physiol*, 92(1):394–400.

384. Terao, A. *et al*. (2003). Region-specific changes in immediate early gene expression in response to sleep deprivation and recovery sleep in the mouse brain. *Neuroscience*, 120(4):1115–1124.

385. Terao, A. *et al*. (2003). Differential increase in the expression of heat shock protein family members during sleep deprivation and during sleep. *Neuroscience*, 116(1):187–200.

386. Terao, A. *et al.* (2006). Gene expression in the rat brain during sleep deprivation and recovery sleep: An Affymetrix GeneChip study. *Neuroscience*, 137(2):593–605.

387. Mackiewicz, M. *et al.* (2007). Macromolecule biosynthesis: A key function of sleep. *Physiol Genomics*, 31(3):441–457.

388. Konopka, R.J. and Benzer, S. (1971). Clock mutants of Drosophila melanogaster. *Proc Natl Acad Sci USA*, 68(9):2112–2116.

389. Pittendrigh, C.S. (1960). Circadian rhythms and the circadian organization of living systems. *Cold Spring Harb Symp Quant Biol*, 25:159–184.

390. Hendricks, J.C. *et al.* (2003). Modafinil maintains waking in the fruit fly Drosophila melanogaster. *Sleep*, 26(2):139–146.

391. Pitman, J.L. *et al.* (2006). A dynamic role for the mushroom bodies in promoting sleep in Drosophila. *Nature*, 441(7094):753–756.

392. Shaw, P. (2003). Awakening to the behavioral analysis of sleep in Drosophila. *J Biol Rhythms*, 18(1):4–11.

393. Cirelli, C. (2003). Searching for sleep mutants of Drosophila melanogaster. *Bioessays*, 25(10):940–949.

394. Cirelli, C. *et al.* (2005). Reduced sleep in Drosophila Shaker mutants. *Nature*, 434(7037):1087–1092.

395. Dugovic, C., *et al.* (2004). A heritable mutation, "Sleepless", promotes active sleep in neonatal mice and wake in adults.

396. O'Hara, B.F. *et al.* (2007). Genomic and proteomic approaches towards an understanding of sleep. *CNS Neurol Disord Drug Targets*, 6(1):71–81.

397. Valatx, J.L., Bugat, R., and Jouvet, M. (1972). Genetic studies of sleep in mice. *Nature*, 238(5361):226–227.

398. Maret, S. *et al.* (2005). Retinoic acid signaling affects cortical synchrony during sleep. *Science*, 310(5745):111–113.

399. Yang, H.S., *et al.* (2007). A genome-wide quantitative trait loci analysis of multiple sleep-wake traits in [C57BL/6J x BALB/cByJ x C57LB/6J F1] N2 mice in 37th Annual Meeting Society for Neuroscience. San Diego, CA, USA.

400. Owens-Ream, J. *et al.* (2007). Systematic study of 20 sleep-wake phenotypes in 15 inbred mouse strains.

401. Deltour, L., Foglio, M.H., and Duester, G. (1999). Metabolic deficiencies in alcohol dehydrogenase Adh1, Adh3, and Adh4 null mutant mice. Overlapping roles of Adh1 and Adh4 in ethanol clearance and metabolism of retinol to retinoic acid. *J Biol Chem*, 274(24):16796–16801.

402. Kondratov, R.V. *et al.* (2003). BMAL1-dependent circadian oscillation of nuclear CLOCK: Posttranslational events induced by dimerization of transcriptional activators of the mammalian clock system. *Genes Dev*, 17(15):1921–1932.

403. Bunger, M.K. *et al.* (2000). Mop3 is an essential component of the master circadian pacemaker in mammals. *Cell*, 103(7):1009–1017.

404. Murakami, D.M. *et al.* (2002). Evidence for vestibular regulation of autonomic functions in a mouse genetic model. *Proc Natl Acad Sci USA*, 99(26):17078–17082.

405. Sadakata, T. *et al.* (2007). Impaired cerebellar development and function in mice lacking CAPS2, a protein involved in neurotrophin release. *J Neurosci*, 27(10):2472–2482.

406. Anderson, M.P. *et al.* (2005). Thalamic Cav3.1 T-type Ca_2^+ channel plays a crucial role in stabilizing sleep. *Proc Natl Acad Sci USA*, 102(5):1743–1748.

407. Cota, D. (2007). CB1 receptors: Emerging evidence for central and peripheral mechanisms that regulate energy balance, metabolism, and cardiovascular health. *Diabetes Metab Res Rev*, 23(7):507–517.

408. Vitaterna, M.H. *et al.* (1994). Mutagenesis and mapping of a mouse gene, Clock, essential for circadian behavior. *Science*, 264(5159):719–725.

409. Maldonado, R. *et al.* (1999). Altered emotional and locomotor responses in mice deficient in the transcription factor CREM. *Proc Natl Acad Sci USA*, 96(24):14094–14099.
410. van der Horst, G.T. *et al.* (1999). Mammalian Cry1 and Cry2 are essential for maintenance of circadian rhythms. *Nature*, 398(6728):627–630.
411. Franken, P. *et al.* (2000). The transcription factor DBP affects circadian sleep consolidation and rhythmic EEG activity. *J Neurosci*, 20(2):617–625.
412. Honma, S. *et al.* (2002). Dec1 and Dec2 are regulators of the mammalian molecular clock. *Nature*, 419(6909):841–844.
413. Narita, M. *et al.* (2002). Intensification of the development of ethanol dependence in mice lacking dopamine D(3) receptor. *Neurosci Lett*, 324(2):129–132.
414. Yujnovsky, I. *et al.* (2006). Signaling mediated by the dopamine D2 receptor potentiates circadian regulation by CLOCK:BMAL1. *Proc Natl Acad Sci USA*, 103(16):6386–6391.
415. Blednov, Y.A. *et al.* (2003). Deletion of the alpha1 or beta2 subunit of GABAA receptors reduces actions of alcohol and other drugs. *J Pharmacol Exp Ther*, 304(1):30–36.
416. Szentirmai, E. *et al.* (2007). Spontaneous sleep and homeostatic sleep regulation in ghrelin knockout mice. *Am J Physiol Regul Integr Comp Physiol*, 293(1):R510–R517.
417. Quinlan, J.J. *et al.* (2002). Mice with glycine receptor subunit mutations are both sensitive and resistant to volatile anesthetics. *Anesth Analg*, 95(3):578–582.
418. Huang, Z.L. *et al.* (2006). Altered sleep-wake characteristics and lack of arousal response to H3 receptor antagonist in histamine H1 receptor knockout mice. *Proc Natl Acad Sci USA*, 103(12):4687–4692.
419. Meredith, A.L. *et al.* (2006). BK calcium-activated potassium channels regulate circadian behavioral rhythms and pacemaker output. *Nat Neurosci*, 9(8):1041–1049.
420. Joho, R.H., Marks, G.A., and Espinosa, F. (2006). Kv3 potassium channels control the duration of different arousal states by distinct stochastic and clock-like mechanisms. *Eur J Neurosci*, 23(6):1567–1574.
421. Douglas, C.L. *et al.* (2007). Sleep in Kcna2 knockout mice. *BMC Biol*, 5(1):42.
422. Goutagny, R. *et al.* (2005). Paradoxical sleep in mice lacking M3 and M2/M4 muscarinic receptors. *Neuropsychobiology*, 52(3):140–146.
423. Popova, N.K. *et al.* (2000). Altered behavior and alcohol tolerance in transgenic mice lacking MAO A: A comparison with effects of MAO A inhibitor clorgyline. *Pharmacol Biochem Behav*, 67(4):719–727.
424. Kim, J.S. *et al.* (2005). Methionine adenosyltransferase:adrenergic-cAMP mechanism regulates a daily rhythm in pineal expression. *J Biol Chem*, 280(1):677–684.
425. Wee, R. *et al.* (2002). Loss of photic entrainment and altered free-running circadian rhythms in math5-/- mice. *J Neurosci*, 22(23):10427–10433.
426. Brun, P. *et al.* (2005). Dopaminergic transmission in STOP null mice. *J Neurochem*, 94(1):63–73.
427. Dudley, C.A. *et al.* (2003). Altered patterns of sleep and behavioral adaptability in NPAS2-deficient mice. *Science*, 301(5631):379–383.
428. Naveilhan, P. *et al.* (2001). Distinct roles of the Y1 and Y2 receptors on neuropeptide Y-induced sensitization to sedation. *J Neurochem*, 78(6):1201–1207.
429. Sato, T.K. *et al.* (2004). A functional genomics strategy reveals Rora as a component of the mammalian circadian clock. *Neuron*, 43(4):527–537.
430. Panda, S. *et al.* (2002). Melanopsin (Opn4) requirement for normal light-induced circadian phase shifting. *Science*, 298(5601):2213–2216.
431. Zheng, B. *et al.* (2001). Nonredundant roles of the mPer1 and mPer2 genes in the mammalian circadian clock. *Cell*, 105(5):683–694.
432. Bae, K. *et al.* (2001). Differential functions of mPer1, mPer2, and mPer3 in the SCN circadian clock. *Neuron*, 30(2):525–536.
433. Qu, W.M. *et al.* (2006). Lipocalin-type prostaglandin D synthase produces prostaglandin D2 involved in regulation of physiological sleep. *Proc Natl Acad Sci USA*, 103(47):17949–17954.

434. Cheng, M.Y. *et al.* (2002). Prokineticin 2 transmits the behavioural circadian rhythm of the suprachiasmatic nucleus. *Nature*, 417(6887):405–410.

435. Arjona, A. and Sarkar, D.K. (2006). The circadian gene mPer2 regulates the daily rhythm of IFN-gamma. *J Interferon Cytokine Res*, 26(9):645–649.

436. Kapfhamer, D. *et al.* (2002). Mutations in Rab3a alter circadian period and homeostatic response to sleep loss in the mouse. *Nat Genet*, 32(2):290–295.

437. Wisor, J.P. *et al.* (2003). Altered rapid eye movement sleep timing in serotonin transporter knockout mice. *Neuroreport*, 14(2):233–238.

438. Xie, W. *et al.* (2000). Humanized xenobiotic response in mice expressing nuclear receptor SXR. *Nature*, 406(6794):435–439.

439. Deboer, T., Fontana, A., and Tobler, I. (2002). Tumor necrosis factor (TNF) ligand and TNF receptor deficiency affects sleep and the sleep EEG. *J Neurophysiol*, 88(2):839–846.

440. Segall, M.A., French, T.A., and Weiner, N. (1996). Effect of neonatal thyroid hormone alterations in CNS ethanol sensitivity in adult LS and SS mice. *Alcohol*, 13(6):559–567.

441. Harmar, A.J. *et al.* (2002). The VPAC(2) receptor is essential for circadian function in the mouse suprachiasmatic nuclei. *Cell*, 109(4):497–508.

442. Sollars, P.J. *et al.* (1996). Altered circadian rhythmicity in the Wocko mouse, a hyperactive transgenic mutant. *Neuroreport*, 7(7):1245–1248.

443. Webb, W.B. and Campbell, S.S. (1983). Relationships in sleep characteristics of identical and fraternal twins. *Arch Gen Psychiatry*, 40(10):1093–1095.

444. Linkowski, P. (1999). EEG sleep patterns in twins. *J Sleep Res*, 8(Suppl 1):11–13.

445. Linkowski, P. *et al.* (1991). Genetic determinants of EEG sleep: A study in twins living apart. *Electroencephalogr Clin Neurophysiol*, 79(2):114–118.

446. Gottlieb, D.J., O'Connor, G.T., and Wilk, J.B. (2007). Genome-wide association of sleep and circadian phenotypes. *BMC Med Genet*, 8(Suppl 1):S9.

447. Tucker, A.M., Dinges, D.F., and Van Dongen, H.P. (2007). Trait interindividual differences in the sleep physiology of healthy young adults. *J Sleep Res*, 16(2):170–180.

448. Rosenwasser, A.M. and Turek, F.W. (2005). Chronobiology: Sleep and the circadian clock. In Kryger, M.H., Roth, T., and Dement, W.C. (eds.), *Principles and Practice of Sleep Medicine*. Elsevier, Philadelphia, pp. 351–362.

449. Vitaterna, M.H., Pinto, L.H., and Turek, F.W. (2005). Molecular genetic basis for mammalian circadian rhythms. In Kryger, M.H., Roth, T., and Dement, W.C. (eds.), *Principles and Practice of Sleep Medicinem*. Elsevier, Philadelphia, pp. 363–374.

450. Laposky, A.D., Turek, F.W. (2008). Animal circadian rhythms vertebrate: Circadian genes and the sleep-wake cycle. In: L.R. Squire (ed.), *New Encyclopedia of Neuroscience*, Elsevier, New York, 2008, pp. in press.

451. Naylor, E. *et al.* (2000). The circadian clock mutation alters sleep homeostasis in the mouse. *J Neurosci*, 20(21):8138–8143.

452. Laposky, A. *et al.* (2005). Deletion of the mammalian circadian clock gene BMAL1/Mop3 alters baseline sleep architecture and the response to sleep deprivation. *Sleep*, 28(4):395–409.

453. Wisor, J.P. *et al.* (2002). A role for cryptochromes in sleep regulation. *BMC Neurosci*, 3:20.

454. Panda, S. *et al.* (2002). Coordinated transcription of key pathways in the mouse by the circadian clock. *Cell*, 109(3):307–320.

455. Atalay, H. (2006). Insomnia: Recent developments in definition and treatment. *Prim Care Community Psychiatry*, 11(2):81–91.

456. Roth, T. (2007). Narcolepsy: Treatment issues. *J Clin Psychiatry*, 68(Suppl 13):16–19.

457. Schwartz, J.R. *et al.* (2003). Modafinil as adjunct therapy for daytime sleepiness in obstructive sleep apnea: A 12-week, open-label study. *Chest*, 124(6):2192–2199.

458. Kupfer, D.J. (1999). Pathophysiology and management of insomnia during depression. *Ann Clin Psychiatry*, 11(4):267–276.

459. Thase, M.E. (2006). Depression and sleep: Pathophysiology and treatment. *Dialogues Clin Neurosci*, 8(2):217–226.

460. Morgenthaler, T.I. *et al.* (2007). Practice parameters for the treatment of narcolepsy and other hypersomnias of central origin. *Sleep*, 30(12):1705–1711.

461. Fleckenstein, A.E. *et al.* (2007). New insights into the mechanism of action of amphetamines. *Annu Rev Pharmacol Toxicol*, 47:681–698.

462. Robinson, D.M. and Keating, G.M. (2007). Sodium oxybate: A review of its use in the management of narcolepsy. *CNS Drugs*, 21(4):337–354.

463. Black, J. and Houghton, W.C. (2006). Sodium oxybate improves excessive daytime sleepiness in narcolepsy. *Sleep*, 29(7):939–946.

464. Erman, M.K. (2006). Selected sleep disorders: Restless legs syndrome and periodic limb movement disorder, sleep apnea syndrome, and narcolepsy. *Psychiatr Clin North Am*, 29(4):947–967. Abstract viii–ix

465. Sharpley, A.L. *et al.* (1994). Slow wave sleep in humans: Role of 5-HT2A and 5-HT2C receptors. *Neuropharmacology*, 33(3–4):467–471.

466. Brisbare-Roch, C. *et al.* (2007). Promotion of sleep by targeting the orexin system in rats, dogs and humans. *Nat Med*, 13(2):150–155.

467. Axmacher, N. *et al.* (2007). The role of sleep in declarative memory consolidation – direct evidence by intracranial EEG. *Cereb Cortex*, 18(3):500–507.

468. Fogel, S.M. *et al.* (2007). Sleep spindles and learning potential. *Behav Neurosci*, 121(1):1–10.

469. Ji, D. and Wilson, M.A. (2007). Coordinated memory replay in the visual cortex and hippocampus during sleep. *Nat Neurosci*, 10(1):100–107.

470. Tononi, G., Massimini, M., and Riedner, B.A. (2006). Sleepy dialogues between cortex and hippocampus: Who talks to whom?. *Neuron*, 52(5):748–749.

471. Walker, M.P. and Stickgold, R. (2006). Sleep, memory, and plasticity. *Annu Rev Psychol*, 57:139–166.

472. Karni, A. *et al.* (1994). Dependence on REM sleep of overnight improvement of a perceptual skill. *Science*, 265(5172):679–682.

473. Stickgold, R. *et al.* (2001). Sleep, learning, and dreams: Off-line memory reprocessing. *Science*, 294(5544):1052.

474. Drummond, S.P., Gillin, J.C., and Brown, G.G. (2001). Increased cerebral response during a divided attention task following sleep deprivation. *J Sleep Res*, 10(2):85–92.

475. Madsen, S.M. *et al.* (1983). Pharmacokinetics of the gamma-aminobutyric acid agonist THIP (Gaboxadol) following intramuscular administration to man, with observations in dog. *Acta Pharmacol Toxicol (Copenh)*, 53(5):353–357.

476. Almirall, H. *et al.* (1999). Nocturnal sleep structure and temperature slope in MPTP treated monkeys. *J Neural Transm*, 106(11–12):1125–1134.

477. Achermann, P. and Borbely, A.A. (2003). Mathematical models of sleep regulation. *Front Biosci*, 8:s683–s693.

478. Tobler, I. and Borbely, A.A. (1986). Sleep EEG in the rat as a function of prior waking. *Electroencephalogr Clin Neurophysiol*, 64(1):74–76.

479. David, J., Grewal, R.S., and Wagle, G.P. (1975). Restricted sleep regime in rhesus monkeys: Differential effect of one night's sleep loss and selective REM deprivation. *Life Sci*, 16(9):1375–1385.

480. Kim, Y. *et al.* (2007). Repeated sleep restriction in rats leads to homeostatic and allostatic responses during recovery sleep. *Proc Natl Acad Sci USA*, 104(25):10697–10702.

481. Rechtschaffen, A. *et al.* (1999). Effects of method, duration, and sleep stage on rebounds from sleep deprivation in the rat. *Sleep*, 22(1):11–31.

482. Klerman, E.B. *et al.* (1999). Circadian and homeostatic influences on sleep in the squirrel monkey: Sleep after sleep deprivation. *Sleep*, 22(1):45–59.

Translational Models for the 21st Century: Reminiscence, Reflections, and Some Recommendations

Paul Willner[1], Franco Borsini[2] and Robert A. McArthur[3]

[1]Department of Psychology, Swansea University, Swansea, Wales, UK
[2]sigma-tau S.p.A., Pomezia, Roma, Italy
[3]McArthur and Associates GmbH, Ramsteinerstrasse, Basel, Switzerland

INTRODUCTION

This series has provided a systematic overview of translational research in psychopharmacology that integrates the perspectives of academics, industrial pharmacologists, and clinicians, in therapeutic areas representing three broad therapeutic domains, neurological disorders, psychiatric disorders, and reward/impulse control disorders. An earlier attempt to systematize translational research in psychopharmacology summarized the scope of the endeavor as follows:

> The problem of using animal behavior to model human mental disorders is, explicitly or implicitly, the central preoccupation of psychopharmacology. The idea that psychiatric disorders might be modeled in animals provides the basis for a substantial proportion of current research; and research that does not employ behavioral models directly is usually justified by reference to its eventual benefits, in terms of an understanding of the human brain and the development of more effective and safer therapies.[1]

In effect, the principle that translation from animals to humans is both possible and necessary underpins and justifies the whole field of preclinical psychopharmacology.

The forerunner to the present series, *Behavioural Models in Psychopharmacology: Academic, Theoretical and Industrial Perspectives*[2] was intended to generalize an approach first outlined in a more focused earlier review of animal models of depression.[3] These publications introduced four significant ideas: that drug screening tests should not be thought of as models and differ in their practical and evidential requirements; that academics, industrial pharmacologists, and clinicians view preclinical behavioral models from different perspectives, based on their different professional aspirations; that it is important to establish, or at least, estimate, the validity of animal models of psychiatric disorders; and that this is best achieved by considering validity from different aspects that reflect different bodies of evidence.

In the 20 or so years since these ideas were first introduced, they have achieved a wide degree of acceptance, and the first two are very apparent in the structure and content

Animal and Translational Models for CNS Drug Discovery,
Vol. 1 of 3: Psychiatric Disorders
Robert McArthur and Franco Borsini (eds), Academic Press, 2008

457

of the present series. The three approaches to the validation of animal models that were outlined in these publications, using terms borrowed from the realm of psychometric testing, were predictive validity ("performance in the test predicts performance in the condition being modeled"), face validity ("there are phenomenological similarities between the two"), and construct validity ("the model has a sound theoretical rationale").[2] This analysis has since become standard, as seen, for example, in recent reviews of animal models of anxiety[4] and schizophrenia.[5] Indeed, these principles are now so well established that many contributors to the present series begin their discussions by considering the face, predictive, and construct validity of the models used and being developed in their therapeutic areas.[i] The extent to which these concepts have become absorbed into the language of psychopharmacology is demonstrated by the fact that they are now almost always used without attribution to the original publications.

Much has changed in terms of model development in the last 20 years; particularly in neurology. As has been discussed in the neurological therapeutic areas surveyed in this series, much of the work has been developed more recently, and it is noticeable that these chapters tend to have a different flavor to those chapters surveying psychiatric and reward deficit disorders, being heavily dominated by genetic and genomic models. In psychiatry, on the other hand, while these areas have also been heavily influenced by the genomic revolution, in behavioral terms, models of depression, anxiety, schizophrenia, or substance abuse have seen relatively little development. That is not to say that there have not been developments in the procedures by which models of depressed-like, anxious-like, schizophrenic-like or substance-abuse-like behaviors can be assessed. Indeed, there is now a significantly greater choice of procedures. However, the newer developments are largely more sophisticated variants on procedures that were well established prior to 1990.

Schizophrenia represents perhaps the one major therapeutic area where a significant shift in emphasis has been evident over the past 20 years. From the discovery of neuroleptics in the early 1950s[6,7] and the establishment of the dopamine hypothesis of schizophrenia,[8] drug discovery and development of pharmaceuticals used to treat the positive, that is, psychotic, symptoms of schizophrenia have centered around impairment of excessive dopaminergic function. Effects of mesolimbic dopaminergic imbalance have been relatively straightforward to model, mainly using changes in locomotion.[ii] Notwithstanding the importance of dopamine in schizophrenia,

---

[i]For further and detailed discussions regarding criteria of validity, the reader is invited to refer to discussions, for example, by Steckler *et al.*, Developing novel anxiolytics: Improving preclinical detection and clinical assessment; Large *et al.*, Developing therapeutics for bipolar disorder: From animal models to the clinic; Joel *et al.*, Animal models of obsessive–compulsive disorder: From bench to bedside via endophenotypes and biomarkers, in Volume 1, *Psychiatric Disorders*; Lindner *et al.*, Development, optimization and use of preclinical behavioral models to maximize the productivity of drug discovery for Alzheimer's Disease; Merchant *et al.*, Animal models of Parkinson's Disease to aid drug discovery and development, in Volume 2, *Neurologic Disorders*; Koob, The role of animal models in reward deficit disorders: Views from academia; Markou *et al.*, Contribution of animal models and preclinical human studies to medication development for nicotine dependence, in Volume 3, *Reward Deficit Disorders*.

[ii]Please refer to Jones *et al.*, Developing new drugs for schizophrenia: From animals to the clinic, in Volume 1, *Psychiatric Disorders*. For further discussion regarding models and procedures in schizophrenia research.

awareness of the influence of other neurotransmitters such as serotonin, glutamate and GABA has led to considerable research into the role of these and their interactions with dopamine.[9,10] Pharmaceutical interest in glutamate in schizophrenia has been particularly fruitful with the development of the metabotropic glutamate$_{2/3}$ (mGlu$_{2/3}$) receptor agonist LY2140023, which appears to be as effective as olanzapine (Zyprexa®) as an antipsychotic in a Phase II trial.[11,12] mGlu$_{2/3}$ receptor agonists have been discovered and characterized using classical locomotor activity procedures or pharmacological interaction studies,[13-15] but it is interesting to note that they also show positive effects on newer procedures that have been developed to assess drug effects on models of negative (i.e., social withdrawal, lack of affect and drive, poverty of speech) and cognitive symptoms of schizophrenia.[15,16] Such procedures include sensory gating and pre-pulse inhibition,[17] sustained or focused attention,[18,19] and impaired social interaction.[20] Furthermore, greater awareness of neurodevelopmental and environmental factors of schizophrenia has led to the establishment of models such as neo-natal hippocampal lesions,[21] and to attempts to model effects of peripartum complications as risk factors of schizophrenia.[22]

Stress as a predisposing factor, the role of the hypothalamo-pituitary-adrenal (HPA) axis and reactions to stress influenced by the environment and development, are themes discussed not only in the chapters of the Psychiatry volume, such as depression,[23] anxiety,[24] bipolar disorders,[25] and attention deficit hyperactivity disorder (ADHD),[26] but also the chapters representing the reward and impulse deficit disorders; disorders that share a high psychiatric component.[27-29] Consequently, major efforts have been made to model the effects of chronic stress and influences of development on psychiatric, reward deficit, and impulse control disorders. Behavioral developments in these areas are concerned almost exclusively with the ways in which stressors are applied and their effects evaluated. The procedures used to evaluate these changes have not changed markedly in the past 20 years. However, the way in which these procedures are used has been greatly influenced by the "endophenotypic" approach to considering psychiatric disorders and how to model aspects of these disorders.[23,24,iii] Similarly, models of reward and impulse disorders continue to be dominated by self-administration and place conditioning procedures. There is certainly a greater use of more sophisticated procedures, such as second order or progressive ratio reinforcement schedules[30,iv] but the procedures themselves have been well established for decades.[31]

Nevertheless, despite the relatively minor changes in the behavioral methodologies, research in these "traditional" areas of translational modeling is markedly different from 20 years, ago, since they too have been transformed by the genomic revolution, which now dominates and largely determines directions of change, dwarfing developments in behavioral technologies. Almost every chapter in this series bears witness to the fact

---

iii Please refer to McArthur and Borsini, preface to this volume, "What do *you* mean by translational research? An enquiry through animal and translational models for CNS drug discovery," and references within for further discussion on endophenotypes and deconstructing behavioral syndromes.

iv See also Koob, The role of animal models in reward deficit disorders: Views from academia; and Rochas *et al.*, Development of medications for heroin and cocaine addiction and regulatory aspects of abuse liability testing in Volume 3, *Reward Deficits Disorders*.

that current research is highly productive in proposing new models of aspects of psychiatric and impulse control disorders that, like the new neurological models, are based almost exclusively on the use of genetically modified animals.[32,33] Molecular biology has also had a huge impact on the understanding of intracellular processes, particularly in relation to those intracellular sequelae of transmitter–receptor interactions that result in changes in gene expression. These developments were driven in part by the recognition that successful pharmacotherapy for psychiatric disorders – depression in particular – often requires chronic drug treatment. Consequently, there is an increasing use in preclinical studies of chronic dosing strategies modeled on the time course of clinical action, leading to a search for the biochemical mechanisms that underlie slowly developing neuroadaptive changes and the identification of a plethora of novel intracellular targets.[34-38]

A similar dynamic is apparent in relation to the understanding of brain structure and function, which serves as the context for translational research. Twenty years ago, psychopharmacology was preoccupied almost exclusively with neurotransmitters; specifically the monoamines dopamine, norepinephrine and serotonin, acetylcholine and GABA, and their receptors. There had been a shift away from the original paradigm that saw the brain as a "biochemical soup," with a recognition that the anatomical site of action was also a crucial consideration, but little attention was paid to the underlying neural circuitry. Over the past 20 years, progress in understanding neurotransmitters and their receptors has been slowly incremental, particularly in relation to glutamatergic and peptidergic systems, as well as the cannabinoid systems, which represent the only major truly novel development. On the other hand, the understanding of brain circuitry has increased exponentially. The importance of dopamine and the mesolimbic and nigrostriatal systems in terms of movement (Parkinson's) and mood (schizophrenia), helped focus research on a more "neural systems" approach. Subsequently, examination of the relationships and interactions between neurotransmitter and neuromodulators within discrete neural circuits has helped to clarify neural substrates of behavioral processes, with the result that the basic operating principles of the brain are being increasingly well understood.[39-41] The parallel development of cognitive neuroscience has been accompanied by technological innovations, most notably, brain scanning methodologies, which have promoted a substantial growth of studies in human participants that complement the traditional work in animal models.

Over the past two decades, then, it is the dramatic developments in molecular biology and in behavioral and cognitive neuroscience, rather than developments in psychopharmacology itself, that have had the major impact on both the theory and practice of translational research, as exemplified by the contributions that comprise the present series. And the fundamental dilemma of psychopharmacology was already apparent 20 years ago, and remains so today: that following an early "golden age" all of the investment in academic and industrial research has produced tiny returns by way of novel pharmacotherapies. For 30, perhaps 40, years now, psychopharmacological research has not substantially changed the pharmacological armamentarium with which to treat devastating and life-threatening behavioral disorders. It has often been pointed out, but bears repeating, that it was 1958, now half a century ago, when the first publication appeared on the clinical efficacy of tricyclic[42] and monoamine oxidase inhibiting[43] antidepressants which, together with neuroleptics a few years earlier[6,7] and benzodiazepines a few years later,[44,45] completed the triad of innovations that have dominated clinical psychopharmacology ever since. Shortly afterwards, basic pharmacotherapy for neurologic disorders was revolutionized by the elucidation of the role of dopamine in Parkinson's disease[46,47] followed by the use of *L*-dopa in its treatment.[48] The concept of neurologic disorders related to neurotransmitter deficiency and its treatment by replacement of the neurotransmitter was one of the driving forces behind the research into acetylcholine potentiation by cholinesterase inhibitors in Alzheimer's disease,[49] which culminated with the registration of tacrine (Cognex®), a pro-cholinergic drug for dementia, in 1993.

Subsequent clinical developments following all of these innovations have been disappointingly unimpressive. For example, second or third generation antidepressants cannot be claimed as pharmacological innovations, since they target known properties of tricyclics, that is, serotonin and/or noradrenergic inhibition; furthermore, the efficacy of these drugs as antidepressants is increasingly questioned.[50] Atypical neuroleptics retain as an essential feature the major property of typical neuroleptics, dopamine receptor antagonism, tempered by additional properties, typically, serotonin receptor antagonism; they offer no new mechanism and very limited clinical advantage, and the prototype of this class of drug, clozapine (Clozaril®), was introduced as long ago as 1989. As indicated above, the early signs of efficacy of the mGlu$_{2/3}$ receptor agonist LY404039,[11] offers some hope of moving beyond dopaminergic compounds in the treatment of schizophrenia,[12] but this development is still at a very early stage. Acetylcholinesterase inhibition has been the standard treatment for dementia since the introduction of tacrine in 1993. Tacrine is hardly ever prescribed now: donepezil (Aricept®) is one of the drugs of choice, but even this "gold standard" is of limited effectiveness and duration.[51,52] Glutamatergic drugs offer some hope of a genuinely novel approach but the clinical efficacy of, in particular, memantine (Ebixa®/Namenda®) is extremely modest.[53,54] In Parkinson's disease, there has been no improvement, as monotherapy at least, on *L*-dopa. In contrast, new drugs have been approved for the treatment of reward deficit disorders such as alcoholism [naltrexone (Vivitrol®/Revia®) and acamprosate (Campral®)], nicotine abuse [varenicline (Chantix®/Champix®), bupropion (Zyban®)], and heroin abuse [methadone (Dolophine®), buprenorphine (Subutex®), and buprenorphine/naloxone (Suboxone®)]. These drugs, however, treat the symptoms of these disorders, and in the case of heroin abuse, the treatment is limited to replacement of heroin. We are still waiting for more effective drugs to be developed for all therapeutic indications surveyed in this book series.

And the certainties of 20–30 years ago have been questioned. Two major issues have emerged in the development and use of psychotherapeutics for the treatment of behavioral disorders: the placebo response, or the ability of certain patients to recover without medication,[50,55,56] and treatment-resistance,[57-59] which has led to initiatives such as the STAR*D trial.[60] For psychiatric indications the traditional triad of anxiety, depression, and schizophrenia are no longer viewed as self-contained entities: comorbidity is recognized as a major factor in the phenomenology of these disorders.[61] Traditional medications for one indication have now become drugs of choice for another. For example, selective serotonin reuptake inhibitor (SSRI) antidepressants such as fluoxetine (Prozac®), paroxetine (Paxil®), sertraline (Zoloft®), fluvoxamine (Luvox®), or escitalopram (Lexapro®) are all approved by the US Food and Drug Administration (FDA) for the treatment of various anxiety disorders. SSRIs as well as tricyclic antidepressants such as imipramine (Tofranil®) and desipramine (Norpramin®) indeed are now considered first-line treatment for general anxiety disorder.[62] Anti-epileptics such as lamotrigine (Lamictal®) are being used to treat depression, while antipsychotics such as olanzapine, as well as lamotrigine, are treatments of choice for bipolar disorder.[v] Research into previously under-treated disorders such as obsessive–compulsive disorder (OCD), ADHD, or autistic spectrum disorders has also contributed to a blurring of the boundaries of traditional psychiatry.[vi] The gradual realization that psychiatric disorders are etiologically complex,[63] and that it is unrealistic to take a simple view that one pill might "cure" depression, or anxiety, or schizophrenia, has important implications for the modeling of these disorders.

What has gone wrong? Perhaps the most frustrating thing of all is that there is no clear answer to this question. One potential explanation lies in the wide anatomical distribution of most drug receptors, and the likelihood that systemically administered drugs have multiple effects that may in some cases be mutually antagonistic. Studies in genomic models employing regionally specific conditional knockouts and other genetic techniques[64-71] may go some way to addressing this issue. However, another, more disturbing, potential explanation arises from a consideration of the validity of psychiatric diagnoses. The predominant contemporary approach to diagnosis, based on the use of diagnostic criteria, defines disorders in terms of lists of symptoms, with patients typically required to display one or more items from each of a list of core and subsidiary symptoms.[72,73] It has frequently been pointed out that this can lead to a situation in which two patients who share the same diagnosis may not share any symptoms in common.[74] There have been attempts to introduce a different approach based around a systematic focus on specific symptoms,[75-77] but the failure of this eminently sensible alternative testifies to the hegemony of diagnostic criteria in determining what constitutes permissible clinical research design.[vii]

There have, of course, been numerous instances where compounds are identified in animal models as having clinical potential. However, it is now almost routine for novel pharmacotherapies, identified in models that are assessed as having a high degree of validity, to fail in the clinic. Just as examples, ondansetron, a 5-HT$_3$ receptor antagonist, was reported to antagonize scopolamine-induced effects in marmosets[78] but not in humans;[79] talsaclidine, a muscarinic receptor agonist, did not exert the same effects on muscarinic M$_2$ and M$_3$ receptors in animals and humans,[80] while repinotan, a 5-HT$_{1A}$ receptor agonist, reduced the neurological deficit in animal models of stroke

---

[v] Please refer to Large *et al.*, Developing therapeutics for bipolar disorder: From animal models to the clinic, in Volume 1, *Psychiatric Disorders*, for further discussion of psychotherapeutics for bipolar disorder.

[vi] Please refer to Joel *et al.*, Animal models of obsessive–compulsive disorder: From bench to bedside via endophenotypes and biomarkers; and Tannock *et al.*, An integrative assessment of attention deficit hyperactivity disorder: From biological comprehension to the discovery of novel therapeutic agents for a neurodevelopmental disorder, in Volume 1, *Psychiatric Disorders*.

[vii] Please refer to McEvoy and Freudenreich, Issues in the design and conductance of clinical trials, in Volume 1, *Psychiatric Disorders*; and Schneider, Issues in design and conduct of clinical trials for cognitive-enhancing drugs, in Volume 2, *Neurologic Disorders*, for further discussion regarding changes to standard clinical trial design.

but not in humans.[81] Other 5-HT$_{1A}$ receptor agonists, flibanserin, and gepirone[23,82,83] were found to be active in the majority of animal models sensitive to antidepressants but failed in clinical trials. TCH346 and CEP1347 seemed very promising as antiparkinsonian agents in preclinical experiments but failed in clinical trials.[84] Tramiprosate (Alzhemed) was found to reduce β-amyloid brain and plasma levels in animals[85] and cerebrospinal levels in humans,[86] but failed to meet its primary endpoint in a Phase III clinical study,[87,viii] although there are claims that significant reductions in hippocampal atrophy were observed with Alzhemed and that the drug itself will be distributed as a food supplement. [88]

How are we to understand these predictive failures? They might represent a failure of the model to predict clinical efficacy, but there are several other potential explanations. One, suggested above, is that a clinical trial could fail to recognize a successful compound because the population of participants identified by the use of diagnostic criteria is clinically heterogeneous. Another explanation, given that drugs are usually administered to animals at much higher doses than they are to people, even after taking into account inter-species scaling factors, is that a clinical failure could reflect the use of an inefficient clinical dose.[23,25,28,84,89-93] Or there could be pharmacokinetic/metabolism issues; in particular, problems with bioavailability, which account for a high proportion of failures at an early stage of clinical testing.[89,91,93] Also, other considerations that go beyond scientific matters, involving corporate policies and politics, may contribute to these predictive failures.[94,95] On the other side of the coin, it is also important to recognize that successful clinical trials may not always be all they seem. In particular, recent meta-analyses of antidepressant efficacy have drawn attention to the fact that, for a variety of reasons, positive outcomes are much more likely to be published than negative outcomes, and that when all of the data are taken into account, antidepressants appear significantly less efficacious than has been generally assumed.[55,96,97] There is no reason to suppose that this is a problem peculiar to antidepressants.

In the search for alternative ways forward, two new concepts have been embraced within translational research: endophenotypes and biomarkers.[ix] Biomarkers are essential to follow the progress of a disorder and the effects of therapeutic intervention. In terms of translational research, the same biomarker of the disorder should be mirrored in the animal model. However, so far very few biomarkers have been validated and this remains a focus of intensive research and of great concern (cf., [50,84,91,93,98-100]). As discussed in the preface to this volume, there is a notable proposal that the concept of validity for biomarkers should be deconstructed into face, predictive and construct dimensions, as used routinely to evaluate the validity of translational models.[101]

As discussed in many chapters of this book series, endophenotypes refer to the heritable, state-independent and family-associated characteristics of a disorder that can be linked to a candidate gene or gene region, which can help in the genetic analysis

---

[viii] See Schneider, Issues in design and conduct of clinical trials for cognitive-enhancing drugs, in Volume 2, *Neurologic Disorders*, for further discussion on primary and secondary endpoints in Alzheimer clinical trials.

[ix] Please refer to McArthur and Borsini, preface to this volume, "What do *you* mean by translational research? An enquiry through animal and translational models for CNS drug discovery," and references within for further discussion on endophenotypes and biomarkers.

of the disorder.[102-104] An endophenotypic approach to modeling requires as a first step the identification of "… critical components of behavior (or other neurobiological traits) that are more representative of more complex phenomena" ([102] p. 641). To date, there are very few putative behavioral endophenotypes that actually meet the five criteria proposed by Gottesman and Gould[102] of: (1) a specific association with the illness of interest; (2) heritability; (3) state-independence; (4) greater prevalence among ill relatives than in the general population (familial association) and (5) than in well relatives (co-segregation). For example, Hasler and colleagues[105] reviewed eight putative behavioral endophenotypes of depression, and concluded that only one of them, anhedonia, met all five of these criteria, as well as a sixth criterion, plausibility. (A second candidate, increased stress sensitivity, also scored highly in Hasler's analysis, but does not show a specific association with depression.) Two putative biological endophenotypes (REM sleep abnormalities and a depressive response to tryptophan depletion) also appeared to meet all six criteria.

For the purposes of the present book series, it is important to distinguish between clinical endophenotypes and translational models of clinical endophenotypes. Taking anhedonia as a putative endophenotype for depression, two distinct considerations clearly apply to a putative model of this putative endophenotype. Consider first Hasler's plausibility criterion. The question of plausibility is reflected in Miczek's 1st principle for translational models, *The translation of preclinical data to clinical concerns is more successful when the development of experimental models is restricted in their scope to a cardinal or core symptom of a psychiatric disorder.*[120] Plausibility is intimately related to construct validity, so it is also essential to verify the construct. The anhedonia endophenotype (an internal construct) is inferred in a translational model from the presence of a variety of different exophenotypes (observable behaviors) such as decreased sucrose intake, increased brain stimulation reward threshold, or impaired place conditioning;[106,107] therefore it is important to evaluate a range of appropriate behavioral endpoints rather than relying on a single procedure.[x] The second, and perhaps more obvious, but also more demanding, consideration is that the Gottesman and Gould criteria imply a change in the focus of model building, moving away from the traditional preoccupation with environmental precipitants of behavioral change to encompass a search for susceptible individuals. Strategies to achieve this objective include inbreeding[108,109] or genetic modification[110,111] to produce putatively anhedonic strains, and the identification of susceptible and resilient individuals within strains.[112,113] What needs to be recognized is that having identified susceptible individuals, a rigorous program of further research is needed to demonstrate face validity, which in this context means that the model conforms to the range of criteria that apply to a clinical endophenotype. For example, a genetically produced trait is by definition heritable, but may not show individual differences in response to stress; conversely, traits identified as individual differences may not be heritable; and both of these approaches raise questions of specificity and state-independence.

---

[x] See also Miczek's 3rd principle, *Preclinical data are more readily translated to the clinical situation when they are based on converging evidence from at least two, and preferably more, experimental procedures, each capturing cardinal features of the modeled disorder.*

While recognizing that the nature of translational modeling is changing, it remains important to retain the strengths of the traditional approach, such as the emphasis on validation of models. Indeed, as discussed in the preface to this volume, concepts of validity are also intimately involved in the establishment of human models of behavioral disorders in experimental medicine, as well as the establishment of biomarkers and endophenotypes.[101,114] There are several reasons to maintain this focus. Firstly, the use of a taxonomy of predictive, face and construct validity,[3,115] or similar alternative taxonomies,[116,117] ensures that when the merits of different models are compared, like is compared with like. Secondly, the practice of assessing validity along several dimensions challenges the predominant view within the pharmaceutical industry that pharmacological isomorphism is the paramount consideration, which incorporates the potentially unhelpful implication that novel agents must resemble known drugs in their spectrum of action. Thirdly, attention to validity forces the proponents of a particular procedure (perhaps one developed in their own laboratory) to engage a self-critical awareness of the model's weaknesses in addition to its strengths, and discourages the publication of over-zealous or biased claims that could be misleading to others. And fourthly, an overt discussion of validity will serve as a context for the selection and adoption of models by the increasing population of workers entering the field of translational modeling from molecular biology rather than from behavioral sciences.

In addition to the translational initiatives of training non-behavioral scientists in behavioral methods and analyses,[xi] a further issue that merits some reflection is the – largely unrecognized – increase in the volume of translational research emanating from the world's developing economies. This can be illustrated by the pattern of submissions to one of the major journals in the field, *Behavioral Pharmacology*, with similar trends in submissions to at least one other major journal (Personal Communication from the editor). In 2007, 20% of submissions to *Behavioral Pharmacology* were from four non-traditional sources: China, India, Brazil, and Iran, the majority of these papers reporting translational research. To take India as an example, submissions during the 1990s were only 0.2% of the total, rising to 2% in the 5 years from 2000 to 2004, and almost 4% in 2005–2007. The most dramatic change has been in submissions from China, mirroring the emergence of the Chinese economy, with submissions languishing at well below 0.5% for the 15 years to 2004 (and these largely from one laboratory), rising suddenly to well over 5% in 2005–2007. However, the growth of research in developing economies is not well integrated into the wider scientific community. With rare exceptions[118] scientists in developing countries have little direct contact with the mainstream scientific community, and therefore miss out on both the apprenticeship model of scientific training and the background of informal discourse, particularly the conversations that take place outside the formal sessions at scientific meetings. One important consequence of this dislocation is that claims made in the literature may be accepted more readily by scientists outside the mainstream, where investigators with access to the oral tradition and the informal chatter might be more skeptical. Behavioral pharmacology in

---

[xi] Please refer to http://www.ncrr.nih.gov/clinical_research_resources/clinical_and_translational_science_awards/index.asp, http://www.mrc.ac.uk/ApplyingforaGrant/InternationalOpportunites/fp7/index.htm for government-sponsored translational research training initiatives.

developing countries also is typically home grown, lacking the scientific cultural roots that come from a tradition of research and development in the area. There is a clear need for positive steps to enable engagement and integration between scientists in developing and developed economies. The European Behavioral Pharmacology Society has for many years achieved some success in meeting these objectives by offering financial support for attendance at scientific meetings to scientists in the developing economies of Eastern Europe. Models of outreach are now needed that can be applied globally, to support the development of behavioral pharmacology in general and translational research in particular, in emerging scientific communities. Academic institutions, scientific journals, learned societies, and the pharmaceutical industry will all have a role to play in shaping the new landscape.

Some considerations on the future DSM-V are also appropriate. Limitations to the current diagnostic paradigms described in the DSM-IV indicate that description of syndromes may never successfully uncover their underlying etiologies. Thus, in the agenda for preparing DSM-V (http://www.dsm5.org), a series of events is planned to try to overcome this limitation. First, a series of "white papers" is contemplated, with the aim of encouraging a research agenda that goes beyond our current thinking to integrate pieces of information from a wide variety of sources and technology. Neuroscience is the subject of one of these "white papers," aimed at developing a basic, clinical neuroscience, and genetics research agenda to guide the development of a future pathophysiological-based diagnostic classification. The working group focused on four main domains: (1) better animal models for the major psychiatric disorders; (2) genes that help determine abnormal behavior in animal models; (3) imaging studies in animals to understand better the nature of imaged signals in humans; and (4) functional genomics and proteomics involved in psychiatric disorders. Second, research conferences are planned to discuss several topics, among which is "stress-induced and fear circuitry disorders." A special session will also be dedicated to gender effects. Thus, we hope that the present series of books may also serve as another basis for discussion of how neuroscience can improve the diagnostic criteria of mental and nervous illnesses.

We end with some reflections on the scope of this project. Its predecessor[2] aimed to integrate academic, industrial, and clinical perspectives through a sequential construction process. Each section of the book had three chapters. The introductory chapter, which set out the concept of the project[1] was written first and forwarded to the academic authors in each therapeutic area, whose chapters were provided to the industrial authors, and finally, the academic and industrial chapters were forwarded to the clinical authors. The present project has taken a more adventurous approach, in which groups of academic, industrial, and clinical authors were established by the editors and were asked to write collaboratively. The introductory chapters to each volume, "What do *you* mean by translational research?" explain that this was done in order "to simulate the conditions of the creation of an industrial Project team" in which the combined talents and expertise of the project members are called together for a clearly defined goal. We can apply the, by now conventional, methodology to assess the validity of this attempt at simulation. There is certainly some face validity: in both the literary and industrial settings, the members of project teams "are all committed to achieving the goals set out by consensus" but "need not know each other. . .". Also, in some therapeutic areas "the authors were not able to establish an effective team", which reflects the reality that not all project teams are successful. In common with the majority of newly introduced models, predictive validity is less compelling, and only time will tell whether "what appears to be a novel and unusual way of working will become the norm." And as is so often the case, construct validity is elusive. The observation that "for many, this has been a challenging and exhilarating experience, forcing a paradigm shift from how they have normally worked" implies a theory of the role of paradigm shift in drug discovery. New paradigms are the bedrock of scientific revolutions[119] and the current explosion of knowledge that results from the transformations of psychopharmacology by systems neuroscience and behavioral genomics, as discussed earlier in this chapter, can certainly be understood in this light. We nurture the hope that adoption of the project-team approach might inject a comparable creative impetus into drug discovery!

REFERENCES

1. Willner, P. (1991). Behavioural models in psychopharmacology. In Willner, P. (ed.), *Behavioural Models in Psychopharmacology: Theoretical, Industrial and Clinical Perspectives*. Cambridge University Press, Cambridge, pp. 3–18.

2. Willner, P. (ed.) (1991). *Behavioural Models in Psychopharmacology: Theoretical, Industrial and Clinical Perspectives*. Cambridge University Press, Cambridge.

3. Willner, P. (1984). The validity of animal models of depression. *Psychopharmacology (Berl)*, 83(1):1–16.

4. Fendt, M. (2005). Animal models of fear and anxiety. In Koch, M. (ed.), *Animal Models of Neuropsychiatric Diseases*. Imperial College Press, London, pp. 293–336.

5. Koch, M. (2005). Animal models of schizophrenia. In Koch, M. (ed.), *Animal Models of Neuropsychiatric Diseases*. Imperial College Press, London, pp. 337–402.

6. Delay, J. and Deniker, P. (1955). Neuroleptic effects of chlorpromazine in therapeutics of neuropsychiatry. *J Clin Exp Psychopathol*, 16(2):104–112.

7. Delay, J., Deniker, P., and Harl, J.M. (1952). Therapeutic use in psychiatry of phenothiazine of central elective action (4560 RP). *Ann Med Psychol (Paris)*, 110(2:1):112–117.

8. Carlsson, A. (1977). Does dopamine play a role in schizophrenia? *Psychol Med*, 7(4):583–597.

9. Carlsson, M. and Carlsson, A. (1990). Schizophrenia: A subcortical neurotransmitter imbalance syndrome?. *Schizophr Bull*, 16(3):425–432.

10. Carlsson, A. (1995). Neurocircuitries and neurotransmitter interactions in schizophrenia. *Int Clin Psychopharmacol*, 10(Suppl 3):21–28.

11. Patil, S.T., Zhang, L., Martenyi, F., Lowe, S.L., Jackson, K.A., Andreev, B.V. *et al.* (2007). Activation of mGlu2/3 receptors as a new approach to treat schizophrenia: A randomized Phase 2 clinical trial. *Nat Med*, 13(9):1102–1107.

12. Conn, P.J., Tamminga, C., Schoepp, D.D., and Lindsley, C. (2008). Schizophrenia: Moving beyond monoamine antagonists. *Mol Interv*, 8(2):99–107.

13. Rorick-Kehn, L.M., Perkins, E.J., Knitowski, K.M., Hart, J.C., Johnson, B.G., Schoepp, D.D. *et al.* (2006). Improved bioavailability of the mGlu2/3 receptor agonist LY354740 using a prodrug strategy: *In vivo* pharmacology of LY544344. *J Pharmacol Exp Ther*, 316(2):905–913.

14. Woolley, M.L., Pemberton, D.J., Bate, S., Corti, C., and Jones, D.N. (2008). The mGlu2 but not the mGlu3 receptor mediates the actions of the mGluR2/3 agonist, LY379268, in mouse models predictive of antipsychotic activity. *Psychopharmacology (Berl)*, 196(3):431–440.

15. Harich, S., Gross, G., and Bespalov, A. (2007). Stimulation of the metabotropic glutamate 2/3 receptor attenuates social novelty discrimination deficits induced by neonatal phencyclidine treatment. *Psychopharmacology (Berl)*, 192(4):511–519.

16. Greco, B., Invernizzi, R.W., and Carli, M. (2005). Phencyclidine-induced impairment in attention and response control depends on the background genotype of mice: Reversal by the mGLU(2/3) receptor agonist LY379268. *Psychopharmacology (Berl)*, 179(1):68–76.

17. Geyer, M.A. and Braff, D.L. (1987). Startle habituation and sensorimotor gating in schizophrenia and related animal models. *Schizophr Bull*, 13(4):643–668.

18. Robbins, T.W. (2002). The 5-choice serial reaction time task: Behavioural pharmacology and functional neurochemistry. *Psychopharmacology (Berl)*, 163(3–4):362–380.

19. Robbins, T.W. (2000). Animal models of set-formation and set-shifting deficits in schizophrenia. In Myslobodsky, M. and Weiner, I. (eds.), *Contemporary Issues in Modeling Psychopathology*. Kluwer Academic, Boston, MA, pp. 247–258.

20. Sams-Dodd, F. (1996). Phencyclidine-induced stereotyped behaviour and social isolation in rats: A possible animal model of schizophrenia. *Behav Pharmacol*, 7(1):3–23.

21. Lipska, B.K., Swerdlow, N.R., Geyer, M.A., Jaskiw, G.E., Braff, D.L., and Weinberger, D.R. (1995). Neonatal excitotoxic hippocampal damage in rats causes post-pubertal changes in prepulse inhibition of startle and its disruption by apomorphine. *Psychopharmacology (Berl)*, 122(1):35–43.

22. Jones, D.N.C., Gartlon, J.E., Minassian, A., Perry, W., and Geyer, M.A. (2008). Developing new drugs for schizophrenia: From animals to the clinic. In McArthur, R.A. and Borsini, F. (eds.), *Animal and Translational Models for CNS Drug Discovery: Psychiatric Disorders*. Academic Press, Elsevier, New York.

23. Cryan, J.F., Sánchez, C., Dinan, T.G., and Borsini, F. (2008). Developing more efficacious antidepressant medications: Improving and aligning preclinical and clinical assessment tools. In McArthur, R.A. and Borsini, F. (eds.), *Animal and Translational Models for CNS Drug Discovery: Psychiatric Disorders*. Academic Press, Elsevier, New York.

24. Steckler, T., Stein, M.B., and Holmes, A. (2008). Developing novel anxiolytics: Improving preclinical detection and clinical assessment. In McArthur, R.A. and Borsini, F. (eds.), *Animal and Translational Models for CNS Drug Discovery: Psychiatric Disorders*. Academic Press, Elsevier, New York.

25. Large, C.H., Einat, H., and Mahableshshwarkar, A.R. (2008). Developing new drugs for bipolar disorder (BPD): From animal models to the clinic. In McArthur, R.A. and Borsini, F. (eds.), *Animal and Translational Models for CNS Drug Discovery: Psychiatric Disorders*. Academic Press, Elsevier, New York.

26. Tannock, R., Campbell, B., Seymour, P., Ouellet, D., Soares, H., Wang, P. *et al.* (2008). Towards a biological understanding of ADHD and the discovery of novel therapeutic approaches. In McArthur, R.A. and Borsini, F. (eds.), *Animal and Translational Models for CNS Drug Discovery: Psychiatric Disorders*. Academic Press, Elsevier, New York.

27. Little, H.J., McKinzie, D.L., Setnik, B., Shram, M.J., and Sellers, E.M. (2008). Pharmacotherapy of alcohol dependence: Improving translation from the bench to the clinic. In McArthur, R.A. and Borsini, F. (eds.), *Animal and Translational Models for CNS Drug Discovery: Reward Deficit Disorders*. Academic Press, Elsevier, New York.

28. Markou, A., Chiamulera, C., and West, R.J. (2008). Contribution of animal models and preclinical human studies to medication development for nicotine dependence. In McArthur, R.A. and Borsini, F. (eds.), *Animal and Translational Models for CNS Drug Discovery: Reward Deficit Disorders*. Academic Press, Elsevier, New York.

29. Williams, W.A., Grant, J.E., Winstanley, C.A., and Potenza, M.N. (2008). Current concepts in the classification, treatment and modelling of pathological gambling and other impulse control disorders. In McArthur, R.A. and Borsini, F. (eds.), *Animal and Translational Models for CNS Drug Discovery: Reward Deficit Disorders*. Academic Press, Elsevier, New York.

30. Czachowski, C.L. and Samson, H.H. (1999). Breakpoint determination and ethanol self-administration using an across-session progressive ratio procedure in the rat. *Alcohol Clin Exp Res*, 23(10):1580–1586.

31. Goudie, A.J. (1991). Animal models of drug abuse and dependence. In Willner, P. (ed.), *Behavioural Models in Psychopharmacology: Theoretical, Industrial and Clinical Perspectives*. Cambridge University Press, Cambridge, pp. 453–484.

32. Cryan, J.F. and Holmes, A. (2005). Model organisms: The ascent of mouse: advances in modelling human depression and anxiety. *Nat Rev Drug Discov*, 4(9):775–790.

33. Holmes, A., le Guisquet, A.M., Vogel, E., Millstein, R.A., Leman, S., and Belzung, C. (2005). Early life genetic, epigenetic and environmental factors shaping emotionality in rodents. *Neurosci Biobehav Rev*, 29(8):1335–1346.

34. Nibuya, M., Nestler, E.J., and Duman, R.S. (1996). Chronic antidepressant administration increases the expression of cAMP response element binding protein (CREB) in rat hippocampus. *J Neurosci*, 16(7):2365–2372.

35. Blom, J.M., Tascedda, F., Carra, S., Ferraguti, C., Barden, N., and Brunello, N. (2002). Altered regulation of CREB by chronic antidepressant administration in the brain of transgenic mice with impaired glucocorticoid receptor function. *Neuropsychopharmacology*, 26(5):605–614.

36. Fujimaki, K., Morinobu, S., and Duman, R.S. (2000). Administration of a cAMP phosphodiesterase 4 inhibitor enhances antidepressant-induction of BDNF mRNA in rat hippocampus. *Neuropsychopharmacology*, 22(1):42–51.

37. Warner-Schmidt, J.L. and Duman, R.S. (2007). VEGF is an essential mediator of the neurogenic and behavioral actions of antidepressants. *Proc Natl Acad Sci USA*, 104(11):4647–4652.

38. Nestler, E.J., Gould, E., Manji, H., Buncan, M., Duman, R.S., Greshenfeld, H.K. *et al.* (2002). Preclinical models: Status of basic research in depression. *Biol Psychiatr*, 52(6):503–528.

39. Goldman-Rakic, P.S. (1987). Development of cortical circuitry and cognitive function. *Child Dev*, 58(3):601–622.

40. LeDoux, J. (2003). The emotional brain, fear, and the amygdala. *Cell Mol Neurobiol*, 23(4–5):727–738.

41. Clark, A.S., Schwartz, M.L., and Goldman-Rakic, P.S. (1989). GABA-immunoreactive neurons in the mediodorsal nucleus of the monkey thalamus. *J Chem Neuroanat*, 2(5):259–267.

42. Kuhn, R. (1958). The treatment of depressive states with G 22355 (imipramine hydrochloride). *Am J Psychiatr*, 115(5):459–464.

43. Kline, N.S. (1958). Clinical experience with iproniazid (marsilid). *J Clin Exp Psychopathol*, 19(2, Suppl 1):72–78. discussion 8–9.

44. Tobin, J.M., Bird, I.F., and Boyle, D.E. (1960). Preliminary evaluation of librium (Ro 5-0690) in the treatment of anxiety reactions. *Dis Nerv Syst*, 21(Suppl 3):11–19.

45. Kerry, R.J. and Jenner, F.A. (1962). A double blind crossover comparison of diazepam (Valium, Ro5-2807) with chlordiazepoxide (Librium) in the treatment of neurotic anxiety. *Psychopharmacologia*, 3:302–306.

46. Birkmayer, W. and Hornykiewicz, O. (1962). The *L*-dihydroxyphenylalanine (*L*-DOPA) effect in Parkinson's syndrome in man: On the pathogenesis and treatment of Parkinson akinesis. *Arch Psychiatr Nervenkr Z Gesamte Neurol Psychiatr*, 203:560–574.

47. Hornykiewicz, O. (1966). Dopamine (3-hydroxytyramine) and brain function. *Pharmacol Rev*, 18(2):925–964.

48. Hornykiewicz, O.D. (1970). Physiologic, biochemical, and pathological backgrounds of levodopa and possibilities for the future. *Neurology*, 20(12):1–5.

49. Bartus, R.T., Dean, R.L., Beer, B., and Lippa, A.S. (1982). The cholinergic hypothesis of geriatric memory dysfunction. *Science*, 217(4558):408–414.

50. Kirsch, I., Deacon, B.J., Huedo-Medina, T.B., Scoboria, A., Moore, T.J., and Johnson, B.T. (2008). Initial severity and antidepressant benefits: A meta-analysis of data submitted to the Food and Drug Administration. *PLoS Med*, 5(2(e45)):260–268.

51. Lindner, M.D., McArthur, R.A., Deadwyler, S.A., Hampson, R.E., and Tariot, P.N. (2008). Development, optimization and use of preclinical behavioral models to maximise the

productivity of drug discovery for Alzheimer's disease. In McArthur, R.A. and Borsini, F. (eds.), *Animal and Translational Models for CNS Drug Discovery: Neurologic Disorders*. Academic Press, Elsevier, New York.

52. Schneider, L.S. (2008). Issues in design and conduct of clinical trials for cognitive-enhancing drugs. In McArthur, R.A. and Borsini, F. (eds.), *Animal and Translational Models for CNS Drug Discovery: Neurologic Disorders*. Academic Press, Elsevier, New York.

53. McShane, R., Areosa Sastre, A., and Minakaran, N. (2006). Memantine for dementia. *Cochrane Database Syst Rev*, 2006(2). CD003154.

54. National Institute for Health and Clinical Excellence. (2006). NICE technology appraisal guidance 111. *Donepezil, Galantamine, Rivastigmine (Review) and Memantine for the Treatment of Alzheimer's Disease*. National Institute for Health and Clinical Excellence, London.

55. Kirsch, I. and Sapirstein, G. (1998). Listening to Prozac but hearing placebo: A meta-analysis of antidepressant medication. *Prev Treat*, 1(Article 0002a):1-13.

56. Khan, A., Kolts, R.L., Rapaport, M.H., Krishnan, K.R., Brodhead, A.E., and Browns, W.A. (2005). Magnitude of placebo response and drug-placebo differences across psychiatric disorders. *Psychol Med*, 35(5):743-749.

57. Peuskens, J. (1999). The evolving definition of treatment resistance. *J Clin Psychiatr*, 60(Suppl 12):4-8.

58. Souery, D., Oswald, P., Massat, I., Bailer, U., Bollen, J., Demyttenaere, K. *et al.* (2007). Clinical factors associated with treatment resistance in major depressive disorder: Results from a European Multicenter Study. *J Clin Psychiatr*, 68(7):1062-1070.

59. Fava, G.A., Ruini, C., and Rafanelli, C. (2005). Sequential treatment of mood and anxiety disorders. *J Clin Psychiatr*, 66(11):1392-1400.

60. Rush, A.J., Trivedi, M.H., Wisniewski, S.R., Nierenberg, A.A., Stewart, J.W., Warden, D. *et al.* (2006). Acute and longer-term outcomes in depressed outpatients requiring one or several treatment steps: A STAR*D report. *Am J Psychiatr*, 163(11):1905-1917.

61. Kessler, R.C., McGonagle, K.A., Zhao, S., Nelson, C.B., Hughes, M., Eshleman, S. *et al.* (1994). Lifetime and 12-month prevalence of DSM-III-R psychiatric disorders in the United States. Results from the National Comorbidity Survey. *Arch Gen Psychiatr*, 51(1):8-19.

62. Davidson, J.R. (2001). Pharmacotherapy of generalized anxiety disorder. *J Clin Psychiatr*, 62(Suppl 11):46-50. discussion 1-2.

63. Tsuang, M.T., Glatt, S.J., and Faraone, S.V. (2006). The complex genetics of psychiatric disorders. In Runge, M.S. and Patterson, C. (eds.), *Principles of Molecular Medicine*, Humana Press, Totowa, NJ, pp.1184-1190.

64. Zeller, A., Crestani, F., Camenisch, I., Iwasato, T., Itohara, S., Fritschy, J.M. *et al.* (2008). Cortical glutamatergic neurons mediate the motor sedative action of diazepam. *Mol Pharmacol*, 73(2):282-291.

65. Gaveriaux-Ruff, C. and Kieffer, B.L. (2007). Conditional gene targeting in the mouse nervous system: Insights into brain function and diseases. *Pharmacol Ther*, 113(3): 619-634.

66. Monteggia, L.M., Luikart, B., Barrot, M., Theobold, D., Malkovska, I., Nef, S. *et al.* (2007). Brain-derived neurotrophic factor conditional knockouts show gender differences in depression-related behaviors. *Biol Psychiatr*, 61(2):187-197.

67. Chen, A.P., Ohno, M., Giese, K.P., Kuhn, R., Chen, R.L., and Silva, A.J. (2006). Forebrain-specific knockout of B-raf kinase leads to deficits in hippocampal long-term potentiation, learning, and memory. *J Neurosci Res*, 83(1):28-38.

68. Xiao, D., Bastia, E., Xu, Y.H., Benn, C.L., Cha, J.H., Peterson, T.S. *et al.* (2006). Forebrain adenosine A2A receptors contribute to *L*-3,4-dihydroxyphenylalanine-induced dyskinesia in hemiparkinsonian mice. *J Neurosci*, 26(52):13548-13555.

69. Nguyen, N.K., Keck, M.E., Hetzenauer, A., Thoeringer, C.K., Wurst, W., Deussing, J.M. *et al.* (2006). Conditional CRF receptor 1 knockout mice show altered neuronal activation pattern to mild anxiogenic challenge. *Psychopharmacology (Berl)*, 188(3):374–385.

70. Valverde, O., Mantamadiotis, T., Torrecilla, M., Ugedo, L., Pineda, J., Bleckmann, S. *et al.* (2004). Modulation of anxiety-like behavior and morphine dependence in CREB-deficient mice. *Neuropsychopharmacology*, 29(6):1122–1133.

71. Bingham, N.C., Anderson, K.K., Reuter, A.L., Stallings, N.R., and Parker, K.L. (2008). Selective loss of leptin receptors in the ventromedial hypothalamic nucleus results in increased adiposity and a metabolic syndrome. *Endocrinology*, 149(5):2138–2148.

72. American Psychiatric Association (ed.). (1994). *Diagnostic and Statistical Manual of Mental Disorders.* 4th edition. American Psychiatric Association, Washington, DC.

73. World Health Organization (2007). *International Statistical Classification of Diseases*, 10th revision, 2nd edition. World Health Organization, Geneva.

74. Fibiger, H.C. (1991). The dopamine hypotheses of schizophrenia and mood disorders: Contradictions and speculations. In Willner, P. and Scheel-Kruger, J. (eds.), *The Mesolimbic Dopamine System: From Motivation to Action.* John Wiley, Chichester, UK, pp. 615–638.

75. Costello, C.G. (ed.) (1993). *Symptoms of Depression.* John Wiley, New York.

76. Parker, G., Roy, K., Wilhelm, K., Mitchell, P., and Hadzi-Pavlovic, D. (2000). The nature of bipolar depression: Implications for the definition of melancholia. *J Affect Disord*, 59(3):217–224.

77. Parker, G., Hadzi-Pavlovic, D., Wilhelm, K., Hickie, I., Brodaty, H., Boyce, P. *et al.* (1994). Defining melancholia: Properties of a refined sign-based measure. *Br J Psychiatr*, 164(3):316–326.

78. Carey, G.J., Costall, B., Domeney, A.M., Gerrard, P.A., Jones, D.N., Naylor, R.J. *et al.* (1992). Ondansetron and arecoline prevent scopolamine-induced cognitive deficits in the marmoset. *Pharmacol Biochem Behav*, 42(1):75–83.

79. Broocks, A., Little, J.T., Martin, A., Minichiello, M.D., Dubbert, B., Mack, C. *et al.* (1998). The influence of ondansetron and m-chlorophenylpiperazine on scopolamine-induced cognitive, behavioral, and physiological responses in young healthy controls. *Biol Psychiatr*, 43(6):408–416.

80. Wienrich, M., Meier, D., Ensinger, H.A., Gaida, W., Raschig, A., Walland, A. *et al.* (2001). Pharmacodynamic profile of the M1 agonist talsaclidine in animals and man. *Life Sci*, 68(22–23):2593–2600.

81. Lutsep, H.L. (2002). Repinotan bayer. *Curr Opin Investig Drugs*, 3(6):924–927.

82. Blier, P. and Ward, N.M. (2003). Is there a role for 5-HT1A agonists in the treatment of depression?. *Biol Psychiatr*, 53(3):193–203.

83. Scrip. (2007). *FDA Rejects Fabre Kramer Antidepressant Gepirone ER.* Scrip. 3310:24.

84. Merchant, K.M., Chesselet, M.-F., Hu, S.-C., and Fahn, S. (2008). Animal models of Parkinson's disease to aid drug discovery and development. In McArthur, R.A. and Borsini, F. (eds.), *Animal and Translational Models for CNS Drug Discovery: Neurologic Disorders.* Academic Press, Elsevier, New York.

85. Wright, T.M. (2006). Tramiprosate. *Drugs Today (Barc)*, 42(5):291–298.

86. Aisen, P.S., Gauthier, S., Vellas, B., Briand, R., Saumier, D., Laurin, J. *et al.* (2007). Alzhemed: A potential treatment for Alzheimer's disease. *Curr Alzheimer Res*, 4(4):473–478.

87. Scrip. (2007). *Neurochem Shares Fall after Alzheimer Disappointment.* Scrip. 3289/90:24.

88. Neurochem Inc. (2007). We are Neurochem Quarterly Report. Third Quarter ended September 30, 2007. Laval, Quebec, Canada.

89. Winsky, L. and Brady, L. (2005). Perspective on the status of preclinical models for psychiatric disorders. *Drug Discovery Today: Disease Models*, 2(4):279–283.

90. Dourish, C.T., Wilding, J.P.H., and Halford, J.C.G. (2008). Anti-obesity drugs: From animal models to clinical efficacy. In McArthur, R.A. and Borsini, F. (eds.), *Animal and Translational Models for CNS Drug Discovery: Reward Deficit Disorders.* Academic Press, Elsevier, New York.

91. Hunter, A.J. (2008). Animal and translational models of neurological disorders: An industrial perspective. In McArthur, R.A. and Borsini, F. (eds.), *Animal and Translational Models for CNS Drug Discovery: Neurologic Disorders*. Academic Press, Elsevier, New York.

92. McEvoy, J.P. and Freudenreich, O. (2008). Issues in the design and conductance of clinical trials. In McArthur, R.A. and Borsini, F. (eds.), *Animal and Translational Models for CNS Drug Discovery: Psychiatric Disorders*. Academic Press, Elsevier, New York.

93. Millan, M.J. (2008). The discovery and development of pharmacotherapy for psychiatric disorders: A critical survey of animal and translational models, and perspectives for their improvement. In McArthur, R.A. and Borsini, F. (eds.), *Animal and Translational Models for CNS Drug Discovery: Psychiatric Disorders*. Academic Press, Elsevier, New York.

94. Cuatrecasas, P. (2006). Drug discovery in jeopardy. *J Clin Invest*, 116(11):2837–2842.

95. McArthur, R. and Borsini, F. (2006). Animal models of depression in drug discovery: A historical perspective. *Pharmacol Biochem Behav*, 84(3):436–452.

96. Kirsch, I., Moore, T.J., Scoboria, A., and Nicholls, S.S. (2002). The emperor's new drugs: An analysis of antidepressant medication data submitted to the US Food and Drug Administration. *Prev Treat*, 5(1):1–23.

97. Turner, E.H., Matthews, A.M., Linardatos, E., Tell, R.A., and Rosenthal, R. (2008). Selective publication of antidepressant trials and its influence on apparent efficacy. *N Engl J Med*, 358(3):252–260.

98. Bartz, J., Young, L.J., Hollander, E., Buxbaum, J.D., and Ring, R.H. (2008). Preclinical animal models of autistic spectrum disorders (ASD). In McArthur, R.A. and Borsini, F. (eds.), *Animal and Translational Models for CNS Drug Discovery: Psychiatric Disorders*. Academic Press, Elsevier, New York.

99. Montes, J., Bendotti, C., Tortarolo, M., Cheroni, C., Hallak, H., Speiser, Z. *et al.* (2008). Translational research in ALS. In McArthur, R.A. and Borsini, F. (eds.), *Animal and Translational Models for CNS Drug Discovery: Neurologic Disorders*. Academic Press, Elsevier, New York.

100. Wagner, L.A., Menalled, L., Goumeniouk, A.D., Brunner, D.P., and Leavitt, B.R. (2008). Huntington disease. In McArthur, R.A. and Borsini, F. (eds.), *Animal and Translational Models for CNS Drug Discovery: Neurologic Disorders*. Academic Press, Elsevier, New York.

101. Lesko, L.J. and Atkinson, A.J.J. (2001). Use of biomarkers and surrogate endpoints in drug development and regulatory decision making: Criteria, validation, strategies. *Annu Rev Pharmacol Toxicol*, 41:347–366.

102. Gottesman, I.I. and Gould, T.D. (2003/4/1). The endophenotype concept in psychiatry: Etymology and strategic intentions. *Am J Psychiatr*, 160(4):636–645.

103. Bearden, C.E. and Freimer, N.B. (2006). Endophenotypes for psychiatric disorders: Ready for primetime?. *Trends Genet*, 22(6):306–313.

104. Cannon, T.D. and Keller, M.C. (2006). Endophenotypes in the genetic analyses of mental disorders. *Annu Rev Clin Psychol*, 2(1):267–290.

105. Hasler, G., Drevets, W.C., Manji, H.K., and Charney, D.S. (2004). Discovering endophenotypes for major depression. *Neuropsychopharmacology*, 29(10):1765–1781.

106. Willner, P. (1997). Validity, reliability and utility of the chronic mild stress model of depression: A 10-year review and evaluation. *Psychopharmacology (Berl)*, 134(4):319–329.

107. Willner, P., Muscat, R., and Papp, M. (1992). Chronic mild stress-induced anhedonia: A realistic animal model of depression. *Neurosci Biobehav Rev*, 16(4):525–534.

108. Bekris, S., Antoniou, K., Daskas, S., and Papadopoulou-Daifoti, Z. (2005). Behavioural and neurochemical effects induced by chronic mild stress applied to two different rat strains. *Behav Brain Res*, 161(1):45–59.

109. Pucilowski, O., Overstreet, D.H., Rezvani, A.H., and Janowsky, D.S. (1993). Chronic mild stress-induced anhedonia: Greater effect in a genetic rat model of depression. *Physiol Behav*, 54(6):1215–1220.

110. Martin, M., Ledent, C., Parmentier, M., Maldonado, R., and Valverde, O. (2002). Involvement of CB1 cannabinoid receptors in emotional behaviour. *Psychopharmacology (Berl)*, 159(4):379–387.

111. Mormede, C., Castanon, N., Medina, C., Moze, E., Lestage, J., Neveu, P.J. *et al.* (2002). Chronic mild stress in mice decreases peripheral cytokine and increases central cytokine expression independently of IL-10 regulation of the cytokine network. *Neuroimmunomodulation*, 10(6):359–366.

112. Bergstrom, A., Jayatissa, M.N., Mork, A., and Wiborg, O. (2008). Stress sensitivity and resilience in the chronic mild stress rat model of depression; an *in situ* hybridization study. *Brain Res*, 1196:41–52.

113. Strekalova, T., Gorenkova, N., Schunk, E., Dolgov, O., and Bartsch, D. (2006). Selective effects of citalopram in a mouse model of stress-induced anhedonia with a control for chronic stress. *Behav Pharmacol*, 17(3):271–287.

114. Littman, B.H. and Williams, S.A. (2005). The ultimate model organism: Progress in experimental medicine. *Nat Rev Drug Discov*, 4(8):631–638.

115. Willner, P. (1991). Methods for assessing the validity of animal models of human psychopathology. In Boulton, A., Baker, G., and Martin-Iverson, M. (eds.), *Neuromethods: Animal Models in Psychiatry I*, Vol. 18. Humana Press, Inc, pp. 1–23.

116. Geyer, M.A. and Markou, A. (1995). Animal models of psychiatric disorders. In Bloom, F.E. and Kupfer, D.J. (eds.), *Psychopharmacology, The Fourth Generation of Progress*. Raven Press, New York, pp. 787–798.

117. Geyer, M.A. and Markou, A. (2002). *The role of preclinical models in the development of psychotropic drugs*. American College of Neuropsychopharmacology, New York. pp. 445–455.

118. Li, Q., Zhao, D., and Bezard, E. (2006). Traditional Chinese medicine for Parkinson's disease: A review of Chinese literature. *Behav Pharmacol*, 17(5–6):403–410.

119. Kuhn, T.S. (1996). *The Structure of Scientific Revolutions*, 3rd edition. The University of Chicago Press, Chicago, IL.

120. Miczek, K.A. (2008). Challenges for translational psychopharmacology research – the need for conceptual principles. In McArthur, R.A. and Borsini, F. (eds.), *Animal and Translational Models for CNS Drug Discovery: Psychiatric Disorders*. Academic Press: Elsevier, New York.

Index

Printed and bound by CPI Group (UK) Ltd, Croydon, CR0 4YY

03/10/2024

01040301-0017